D1760374

Joost J. L. M. Bierens (Ed.)

Handbook on Drowning

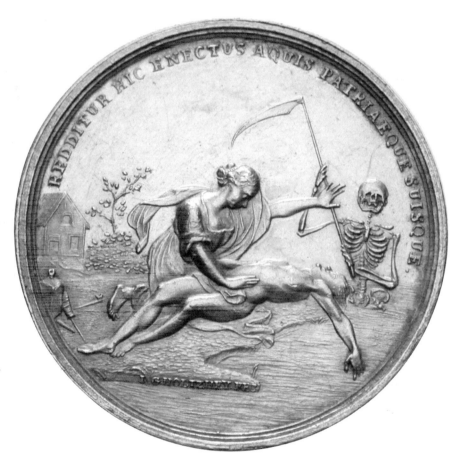

Since 1767, the Maatschappij tot Redding van Drenkelingen in Amsterdam, rewards succesful rescuers with this medal in bronze, silver or gold. The medal represents Charity leaning over a drowning victim and warding off Death as he wields his scythe.

Joost J. L. M. Bierens (Ed.)

Handbook on Drowning

Prevention, Rescue, Treatment

With 87 Figures, 9 in Colour and 52 Tables

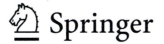 Springer

Joost J. L. M. Bierens MD PhD MCDM
Professor in Emergency Medicine
Department of Anesthesiology
VU University Medical Center
PO Box 7057
1007 MB Amsterdam
The Netherlands

ISBN-10   3-540-43973-0   Springer-Verlag Berlin Heidelberg New York
ISBN-13   978-3-540-43973-8   Springer-Verlag Berlin Heidelberg New York

Libary of Congress Control Number: 2005932048

This work is subjekt to copyright. All rights are reserved, whether the whole or part of the material is concerned, specifically the rights of translation, reprinting, reuse of illustrations, recitation, broadcasting, reproduction on microfilms or in any other way, and storage in data banks. Duplication of this publication or parts thereof is permitted only under the provisions of the German Copyright Law of September 9, 1965, in its current
version, and permission for use must be obtained from Springer-Verlag. Violations are liable to prosecution
under the German Copyright Law.

Springer is a part of Springer Science+Business Media
springeronline.com

© Springer-Verlag Berlin Heidelberg 2006

Printed in Germany

The use of general descriptive names, registered names, trademarks, etc. in this publications does not imply,
even in the absence of a specific statement, that such names are exempt from the relevant protective laws
and regulations and therefore free for general use.

Product liability: The publishers cannot guarantee the accuracy of any information about dosage and application contained in this book. In every individual case the user must check such information by consulting
the relevant literature.

Editor: Dr. Ute Heilmann, Heidelberg
Desk Editor: Hiltrud Wilbertz, Heidelberg
Typesetting: Satz-Druck-Service, Leimen
Production: Pro Edit GmbH, Heidelberg
Cover-Design: Friedo Steinen-Broo, EStudio Calamar, Spain
Printed on acid-free paper   21/3151Re   5 4 3 2 1 0

Foreword

by Jan-Carel van Dorp

The board of Governors of the *Maatschappij tot Redding van Drenkelingen* is happy to introduce this congress book, the fruit of much effort in recent years of many devoted researchers in the fields of prevention, rescue and treatment of drowned people. It is a compilation of the results of their successful studies, as laid down during the World Congress on Drowning held in Amsterdam on 26–28 June 2002.

Background

Through the ages death by drowning, like so many other causes, was accepted as a part of life. Water brings life, water takes life; burial follows. It was not until the 17th or even as late as the 18th century that it became apparent that people could be effectively rescued by bystanders, that many seemingly dead drowning victims only died after burial and that some of them could have been saved from this fate had they received medical attention.

In Europe it was the so-called Age of Enlightenment, with changing attitudes towards fellow man and social initiatives underway, including the founding of charitable societies. At that time three noblemen in Amsterdam realised that too many victims who had fallen in the waters of Amsterdam were left to their fate and died. Hence, in 1767, they founded a society for the rescue of drowning victims, *de Maatschappij tot Redding van Drenkelingen*. Their initiative was widely applauded.

In the years that followed other cities in Holland started their own initiatives. Great interest was shown by France, Russia, Austria, England, Switzerland and Denmark, as well as the cities of Venice, Hamburg and New York and similar foundations were created in some of these places.

Since its foundation the *Maatschappij tot Redding van Drenkelingen* has devoted itself to promoting everything that would lead to or improve the prevention, rescue and treatment of drowning victims. The means by which it has done this are discussed in the following sections.

Proclamations

Both the public and the authorities needed to be made aware of the duty to rescue drowning victims and resuscitate them. Therefore, a publicity campaign was started proclaiming that a drownee should be removed from the water, taken indoors, rubbed and warmed. To this end, posters were hung around the city in churches, coffee shops, beer shops and pubs.

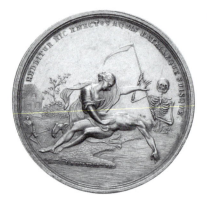

Fig. 1 Medal offered to rescuers of a drowning victim

Promotion of the Development of Resuscitation Methods

The methods of the time were crude, ranging from rolling the body over a barrel to inserting smoke in the intestines via the anus. Some people, however, realised at that time that more victims may have survived if these treatments had not been applied. Even worse was the fact that not much was known about the state of 'apparent death'. This ignorance persisted right up until the beginning of the 20th century, and it would last until the middle of that century before the effectiveness of mouth-to-mouth resuscitation was recognized.

So for more than one and a half centuries victims were subjected to the old methods of being hung from their feet, tickled with a feather under the nose and in the throat or inflated with smoke before slowly more effective methods became known.

Rewarding Successful Rescuers

In order to encourage bystanders to intervene and help drowning victims, rewards were offered to successful rescuers in the form of either a sum of money or a medal. The sum of money was much coveted as a possible reward and many cases of gallant rescues were reported, although on closer scrutiny some appeared to be forged cases.

The medal was designed in 1767, the year of the foundation of the *Maatschappij tot Redding van Drenkelingen* (**Fig. 1**). It shows a woman representing Charity leaning over a drowning victim and warding off Death as he wields his scythe. The reverse side of the medal has room for a personalised inscription.

Present Activities

The *Maatschappij tot Redding van Drenkelingen* continued these activities till far into the 20th century, first confined to the city of Amsterdam and later on expanding to the rest of the Netherlands.

It concentrates on the same three fields: publicity, research and awarding medals. Publicity comprises a variety of activities such as television adverts that are shown on prime time television, instruction stickers with pictures of the mouth-to-mouth resuscitation method that are widely distributed and the yearly report containing a survey of the activities of the *Maatschappij tot Redding van Drenkelingen*. It is distributed to specific groups in the Netherlands such as watersports organisations, schools, municipalities, and swimming pool organisations.

The *Maatschappij tot Redding van Drenkelingen* supports students and researchers in their research activities on all matters within its scope. An example of a research project – in this case of significant size – supported by the *Maatschappij tot Redding van Drenkelingen* is the World Congress on Drowning.

Awarding medals is another important activity. Rescuers greatly appreciate being rewarded for their deeds. At the request of the *Maatschappij tot Redding van Drenkelingen* mayors confer the medals on recipients. The local press is usually present, which is a good way to spread the message. In its 235 years of existence the *Maatschappij tot Redding van Drenkelingen* has awarded medals in some 6770 cases of successful rescue.

In 1995, the anaesthesiologist Joost Bierens drew the attention of the *Maatschappij tot Redding van Drenkelingen* to the world-wide dimension of drowning, the need to further develop rescue methods, co-ordinate research and to aim for consensus in these fields. The need for this was indeed confirmed in a quick survey that year, undertaken by the *Maatschappij tot Redding van Drenkelingen* with experts in different disciplines in many countries. They almost unanimously applauded the idea of a World Congress on Drowning.

Thus in 1997, 230 years after its founding, the *Maatschappij tot Redding van Drenkelingen* undertook to organise the World Congress on Drowning 2002, the first of its kind. The reasons were clear: the immense number of drowning victims world-wide, the lack of research co-ordination in the different parts of the world and the need for a consensus on treatment.

The content of the congress was new with a multitude of disciplines, and therefore unlike the many existing congresses. It required an individual and innovative approach and constant designing, rethinking and adjusting.

Professionals in roughly ten different fields related to prevention, rescue and treatment were asked to organise task forces and to lead their task force members in assessing the situation in their fields. The members of the task forces were spread all over the world. For them e-mail proved the ideal mode of communication. In Holland a steering group was set up, each member being an expert and counterpart for a task force leader.

In 1999, 2000 and 2001 the task force leaders convened with the steering group in Amsterdam. Goals were set, mutual adjustments made, progress monitored and the modes and forms of presentation at the congress were discussed.

A website was opened: www.drowning.nl on which all results of the research were amassed and which has remained operational since the congress.

The PR advisors Hill and Knowlton set up a PR campaign in a score of international magazines, as well as in the Dutch newspapers and on TV, which promoted the congress very successfully.

Finally, on 26–28 June 2002 the World Congress took place in The RAI convention centre in Amsterdam, followed the day after by "Dutch Day". Some 500 people from around the world learned about the latest developments in their field, as well as in adjoining fields.

There were posters, plenary sessions and parallel sessions, an exhibition and a specialised bookshop. Many contacts were made and the congress book (which you now hold in your hand) was announced.

The Royal Netherlands Sea Rescue Institution (KNRM) organised workshops and a splendid demonstration on the North Sea coast. There were social events such as the reception held by the Mayor and Elders of the City of Amsterdam, a lively dinner event put on for congress visitors in the old West-Indisch House in the heart of the city.

Constant assessment of the results of the congress meetings resulted in provisional recommendations that were presented in the closing session on Friday afternoon 28 June 2002.

The results of the international congress were conveyed to the some 350 visitors of "Dutch Day" on Saturday 29 June 2002; and there too satisfaction was expressed.

After reviewing the results of the congress the Board of Governors of the *Maatschappij tot Redding van Drenkelingen*, together with the steering group and the task force leaders, has come to the conclusion that a significant deepening of knowledge has been achieved in the fields of prevention, rescue and treatment. Many institutions, as well as individuals, have each in their way contributed to the success of the congress and deserve a word of gratitude.

How to Proceed?

Although there is great satisfaction at what has already been achieved, it is now clear that we have only just started on the long path towards the necessary research and development.

We hope to receive suggestions on how to proceed and invite comments and ideas to be sent to the address of the *Maatschappij tot Redding der Drenkelingen*.

It is with gratitude to all those who contributed to it that we recommend this Handbook on Drowning.

The Board of Governors
Jan-Carel van Dorp
Chairman *Maatschappij tot Redding van Drenkelingen*

Foreword

by Prof. Dr. Johannes Knape MD PhD

Death by drowning is unexpected and unwanted in most cases and is as old as the world. Nevertheless death by drowning was considered by many to be inevitable, the consequences of drowning to be irreversible and drowning itself in some cultures to be an act of a Higher Power. This attitude has discouraged people and even put them off taking initiatives to explore potential alternative approaches to drowning, as has been the case with sudden cardiac death for a long time.

But times have changed. The first society in the world active in the field of trying to improve the outcome of drowning victims, *de Maatschappij tot Redding van Drenkelingen* (The Society to Rescue People from Drowning), was established in Amsterdam in 1767. Other societies, such as the Royal Humane Society in London, England, soon followed this example. The growing realisation that human initiatives and activities of various kinds could result in a reduction in the number of drowning victims caused rescue societies to be set up and scientific attention on the problem of drowning from various sources to increase.

The (re-)invention of effective resuscitation techniques by the late Peter Safar (1924–2003) in 1960 meant a revolution in the prospects of victims of sudden cardiac arrest. The scientific activities which Safar and his group developed has also caused an upturn in interest in drowning victims. It seems that the same may hold true for drowning as for cardiac arrest victims and that better prospects are on the horizon. To quote Safar: "it is great when we can arrange death to come back later".

Thus many disciplines felt that a lot of progress had been made for drowning victims in the last decades of the 20th century. On the other hand it was surprising that research papers on the subject of drowning were scarce and that research meetings in this field were few. It was not surprising then that, in 1995, the oldest society in the field of drowning in the world, the *Maatschappij tot Redding van Drenkelingen*, took the initiative to organise a meeting where experts on all aspects of drowning (epidemiology, prevention and innovation in technology, rescue, resuscitation, medical aspects, hypothermia, water-related disasters and diving) could meet and discuss these issues.

The World Congress on Drowning, which was held in Amsterdam in 2002 for the first time, gathered hundreds of world experts from various fields of expertise to speak, listen, discuss and learn from one another.

This Handbook on Drowning is the first ever compilation of knowledge on drowning. It has been written by a great number of the experts at the World Congress, by the various task forces, as well as other individuals.

It is unique in that it also contains the documents which were the result of the various consensus meetings during the World Congress and the final recommendations of the World Congress on Drowning. It has become a unique state of the art document on drowning today.

The authors, section editors and the editor, Professor Joost Bierens, sincerely hope that the contents of this book will inspire the reader to be increasingly creative in preventing drowning and in improving the chances for drowning victims in the future. If this handbook manages to prevent one case of death due to drowning, then its making was worthwhile. It is the conviction of the authors of this book that far greater progress in the improvement of the fate of drowning victims is possible due to the efforts of many.

Prof. Dr. Johannes Knape MD PhD
Chairman of the Foundation Drowning 2002 and of the scientific steering group World Congress on Drowning

Foreword

by MARGIE PEDEN PHD

It is estimated that nearly 400,000 people drowned worldwide in 2002, making it the second leading cause of unintentional death globally after road traffic crashes. The overwhelming majority of these drowning deaths occurred in low- and middle-income countries. In fact, China and India alone accounted for just over 40% of all the drowning deaths. Data on non-fatal drowning morbidity is hard to estimate since these data are not available in many low- and middle-income countries.

Among the various age groups, children under 5 years of age have the highest drowning mortality rates worldwide. Some other major risk factors include alcohol consumption while swimming, boating, fishing, floods, uncovered water wells, transportation in unsafe or overcrowded vessels and epilepsy. Access to water is obviously the most important risk factor for drowning.

Drowning, however, can be prevented. There are many interventions which have been evaluated in high income countries but few have been tested in the developing world. Nevertheless, the four main principles for drowning prevention remain the same: remove the hazard, create barriers, protect those at risk and counter the damage. Further research on interventions in developing countries is urgently required and public health professionals have a major role to play in most of these prevention activities. The WHO constitutional mandate, as the leading co-ordinating agency for international public health, places it in a unique position to guide a science-based programme of activities in drowning prevention.

WHO has been concerned with the health aspects of water and water supply for many years through its department of Sustainable Development and Healthy Environments. Of particular concern has been the management of recreational waters which is one aspect of drowning prevention. To this end the WHO issued Guidelines for Safe Recreational Waters in 2003 which includes a chapter on drowning prevention. Furthermore, the Department of Injuries and Violence Prevention at WHO has recently begun to look at the issue of drowning prevention, particularly in low- and middle-income countries, and raising general awareness about the problem. WHO Injury Surveillance and Survey Guidelines will guide less-resourced countries to assess the magnitude of their injury problem, including that of drowning.

Human resources in the area of drowning prevention are few and far between, particularly in developing countries. The time to act is now. We all need to work together to prevent drowning worldwide. WHO therefore compliments the organisers of the First World Congress on Drowning, held in the Netherlands in June 2002, for bringing together experts in the field, developing a standardised definition for drowning and for subsequently developing this Handbook on Drowning which gathers together all that we know about the epidemiology, prevention and advocacy of this neglected epidemic.

Margie Peden PhD
Coordinator Unintentional Injuries Prevention
Department of Injuries and Violence Prevention World Health Organization

Foreword

by B. Chris Brewster

The International Life Saving Federation (ILS) is driven by a mission to enhance the safety and preservation of human life in the aquatic environment. We were extremely pleased to collaborate with the *Maatschappij tot Redding van Drenkelingen* in the tremendously successful effort to convene the historic World Congress on Drowning 2002. This was a seminal event that established critical benchmarks in drowning prevention procedures, as well as setting a course for future improvements to further our trademark goal: *World Water Safety*. This confluence of purpose of so many scholarly people, like the joining of streams into a mighty river, will unquestionably benefit all the people of the world.

ILS endeavours to lead the worldwide effort to reduce injury and death in, on, and around the water. Through ILS and our member federations, lifesaving research, development, education, and rescue information is generated and disseminated globally. We continually work to advocate with national governments and non-governmental organisations to establish drowning as a public safety issue. We advance lifesaving and drowning prevention by co-ordinating and facilitating the work of national lifesaving organisation, facilitating information exchange through research and dissemination of best practice, working with member organisations to establish and support lifesaving organisations in geographic areas where they do not exist, developing lifesaving by acting as the international federation for lifesaving sport, and by co-operating with other international bodies with shared goals.

The greatest value of the World Congress on Drowning 2002 is leadership toward identifying obstacles to water safety and proposing steps to remove them. The International Life Saving Federation will continue our ongoing leadership in this area, including taking action to implement recommendations made at the congress. We have now established a Lifesaving Commission composed of a rescue committee, education committee, medical committee, development committee, and drowning report committee. This commission is well prepared to address major recommendations of the World Congress on Drowning.

Since the congress, ILS has adopted the new definition of drowning and has fulfilled another of the congress recommendations by publishing international beach safety warning flag standards. The ILS rescue committee already serves as a forum for investigating and validating the efficacy of rescue techniques. This committee is now working on development of international beach safety sign standards. The rescue committee will also further congress recommendations on use of personal watercraft in rescue, optimal visual scanning techniques, and use of the incident command system in aquatic rescue.

Through our education committee, ILS intends to serve as the world body for teachers of water safety and swimming, emphasizing the value of these skills to all the people of the world. The education committee will evaluate the use of ILS training guidelines to promote the wearing of lifejackets to prevent drowning.

ILS embraces the congress recommendation of teaching basic resuscitation skills to rescuers and lay persons. Through the co-ordination of our development committee, ILS is continually helping increase the number of lifesaving organisations throughout the world, while our education committee identifies best practice training standards for new and existing lifesaving organisations. As recommended at the congress, our standards call for all lifesaving organisations to include basic resuscitation skills for all participants. ILS member lifesaving federations can also help further the congress recommendations of helping encourage a balance between safety and profitability of recreational diving, as well as promoting the safety of diving fishers.

The World Congress on Drowning was the most impressive gathering of medical personnel focussed on drowning and water related injury in the history of lifesaving. Through the ILS medical committee, medical system organization which was recommended to improve drowning process outcomes will be encouraged and the results will be critically appraised for educational purposes. New medical terminology recommendations will also be encouraged through ILS medical committee leadership and within our member organizations. Several ILS medical position statements will be forthcoming to further the recommendations of the congress, including those related to spinal immobilisation techniques.

As suggested by the World Congress on Drowning, ILS intends to develop the *World Drowning Report* to facilitate uniform reporting of drowning cases through a single international source of data registration, both from developing and developed nations. The ILS *World Drowning Report* will also encourage adoption of standardised definitions, as suggested at the Congress.

In summary, the International Life Saving Federation embraces the opportunity to utilise the progress made at the World Congress on Drowning 2002 to advance the cause of drowning prevention throughout the world. We commend the organisers and commit ourselves to fulfilling the ultimate goal of the congress: worldwide drowning prevention.

B. Chris Brewster
Chairman of the ILS Lifesaving Commission

Foreword

by Peter B. Bennett PhD DSc

A few years ago I was invited to speak at a meeting in Florida on scuba diving safety and accidents. It was concentrated around a pressure chamber for recompression of divers stricken with decompression sickness, or the "bends". Conjointly there was a display with brochures and coloring books for small children organized by local volunteers on drowning. It concentrated on trying to make the general public, and especially those with swimming pools, aware of the dangers of drowning and, as far as possible, how to avoid this risk and what to do in a drowning emergency.

With some 9000 drownings in the US per year, it became very clear to me that there was simply insufficient awareness of this problem among the public. This was compounded for me by the fact that the 100 deaths in the US per year from scuba diving are usually primarily listed as 'drowning' by coroners in conjunction with other diving hazards.

The Divers Alert Network (DAN), a non-profit diving safety association, provides a great deal of education on what to do in scuba diving emergencies and first aid. This includes giving 100% oxygen and possibly the use of automated external defibrillators (AED). DAN has extensive international training schemes in this area.

Very often, in swimming pool drownings, among others, it may take over 30 minutes for an emergency team to arrive. During that time, if the individual is not breathing, it will be too late. After a period of some 4 minutes it becomes progressively more difficult to achieve a recovery unless the victim has been in very cold water.

Clearly, to my thinking, it would be a good idea for individuals with swimming pools, or owners of boats to have a course on emergency oxygen and AED use so that they can provide vital emergency first aid before the professional teams arrives.

It was these thoughts that drove me to stimulate the interest of the International Divers Alert Network to support this Congress on Drowning.

Although I have since retired, I hope that others will take up the concept and concentrate on a broad program of education to help prevent drowning and, if it does happen, how to provide emergency care.

Peter B. Bennett PhD DSc
Founder, Former President DAN America
Emeritus Chairman International DAN
Professor of Anesthesiology
Duke University Medical Center

Introduction

This is a unique book for those involved in aquatic incidents and, more specifically, for those involved in one way or another with drowning incidents. Although some books on drowning have been published, this book serves a well-defined cause: to reduce the number of drownings and to improve outcome in drowning victims.

The book is the culmination of a process that started in Amsterdam in 1996 on the initiative of the *Maatschappij tot Redding van Drenkelingen* (Society to Rescue People from Drowning, established in 1767) and has involved several hundred experts who came together at the World Congress on Drowning held in May 2002. During that congress these experts, from a wide variety of different backgrounds and specialties, held interactive sessions. It is this active participation and multidisciplinary co-operation that makes this book unique.

For example, some authors have practical lifelong experience with aquatic emergencies, but have never written about their expertise before. Others are experts in a particular field of research related to the issue of drowning, but have hardly ever enjoyed (or have even feared) one of the many activities associated with water. Thus, practical down-to-earth information is combined with latest scientific data.

Because of this level of collaboration there may be some overlap or contradiction of information in some of the chapters, and not all sections will be of practical use for all readers. However, all readers will undoubtedly find a lot of information that is relevant for them within the 12 sections. Even though some sections may be less applicable to their field of involvement, this information may serve to emphasise that their involvement in the prevention, rescue or treatment of drowning is only one part of a worldwide process and that collaboration with other partners on a local, national and international level is worthwhile and often even essential.

Although the authors come from all over the world it is unfortunate that the low-income areas, where most drownings occur, are underrepresented. This fact confronts us with the greatest challenge at the moment: how can we involve the low-income countries in the struggle against drowning, not instead of grappling with other major political, social and economic problems, but in addition to these struggles? International organisations such as the World Health Organisation (WHO), the International Maritime Organisation (IMO), the International Life Saving Federation (ILS), the International Life Boat Federation (ILF), the International Red Cross and Red Crescent Societies (IRCRCF) and the Divers Alert Network (DAN) will hopefully find ways to work together to combat drownings in low-income countries.

The 2004 tsunami in Asia with tens of thousands of deaths, most of them by drowning, has resulted in an increased global awareness of the unpredictable and devastating power of water. All those who are familiar with the aquatic environment already knew this and may even have experienced this themselves. Although the tragedy in Asia was on an unprecedented scale and caused immeasurable sadness, the total number of drowning victims each year worldwide is about three times that of the 2004 tsunami disaster. This immense number refers to individual drowning, without public media coverage, but resulting in the same intensity of grief and pain for those who remain behind. If the information in this book stimulates actions that would reduce even 1% of all drownings each year, and help to prepare for future aquatic catastrophes, this means that our joint efforts would already save thousands of lives each year.

Summarised below are the main items to be found in this book.

Section 1 covers some historical elements: the history of the initiating body (the *Maatschappij tot Redding van Drenkelingen*), the development of faster and safer lifeboats, the role that drownings have played in the very first developments of resuscitation, and an overview of the projects related to the World Congress on Drowning. The final chapter in Section 1 will bring back good memories to those involved, and gives others a realistic impression of the work being done.

Section 2 presents extensive epidemiological data from around the world. At the time these data were collected for the World Congress on Drowning, this was the first attempt to gain a global overview of the problem and since then, also stimulated by the World Congress on Drowning, several other new initiatives have taken place to improve data collection. The new, more practical, definition of drowning will be of great importance in the endeavour to generate more complete and reliable worldwide data.

In Section 3 several options for drowning prevention strategies are summarized. It became clear to all participants that the drowning process evolves very quickly and that death can occur in just a few minutes. Therefore, prevention will be the most effective approach to reduce the number of drownings. To achieve this, a permanent multi-focus approach of combined organisations is needed.

The organisational aspects of rescue are addressed in Section 4, while the practical aspects of rescue are covered in Section 5. Both sections give an extensive overview of what is happening in the area of water rescue. Although these rescues may differ greatly depending on the location (for example swimming pool, river, ocean), the developments occurring at one place may still be of practical use in other areas. It is noteworthy that as a result of the congress the international exchange of information, experiences, projects and research increasingly takes place in the pragmatic and practical arena.

The following five sections deal with medical aspects. Initially, it was assumed that the medical aspects would be the main focus of this project. However, soon after the project started, it became clear that prevention and rescue are more important in reducing the number of drownings than the medical care given after the victim is taken out of the water. Nevertheless, having medical aspects as the initial focus for the project meant that many medical experts were prepared to contribute their expertise and a wide variety of medical issues could be described from different viewpoints. The medical aspects therefore still represent the majority of themes in the book. Section 6 addresses several resuscitation topics, and highlights the fact that drowning can only be survived when the immediate bystander starts with resuscitation. This section also includes a chapter on the Utstein-style guidelines for the registration of drowning which, when used in future studies, will help to better understand the resuscitation of drowning.

Section 7 deals with several aspects of the treatment of drowning victims in the hospital setting. Experts in emergency and intensive care treatment, as well as specialists in circulatory and respiratory problems, indicate which therapies are preferred.

The extrapolation of current knowledge on hypoxic brain damage to the specific situation of the drowning victim is the focus of Section 8. The information provided offers a unique scholarly background in the understanding and treatment of the often severe neurological complications after drowning.

Section 9 offers a combination of scientific and practical information on immersion hypothermia. Drowning by immersion occurs by means of a mechanism other than submersion. This section reviews the pathophysiological and practical consequences.

Section 10 addresses water-related disasters. The impact of such disasters is now painfully evident, but at the time this project started, few were so acutely aware of the extent of the potential disaster of water and the related risks of drowning. In view of the very latest knowledge concerning the 2004 tsunami, and the 2005 floods in Louisiana caused by hurricane Katrina, some chapters may have been written with a different perspective. Nevertheless, this section still provides an important theoretical basis for the actions that need to be taken to reduce the risk of drowning as a result of water-related disasters.

In Section 11 the results of a joint effort by the world's leading medical divers are summarized. The section covers prevention, rescue and treatment of the drowned diver and includes some important recommendations for future initiatives.

Several aspects of the drowning victim who has not survived are dealt with in Section 12. Although this particular area was not originally considered when preparing the project, it became clear that a lot of expertise is available on the search procedures, forensic aspects and jurisdiction related to persons who died by drowning.

For me, as project co-ordinator of the project World Congress on Drowning and co-ordinating editor of this *Handbook on Drowning Rescue, Prevention and Treatment*, it was a challenge to keep track of the continuous developments related to the dynamics of the project, and a great privilege to work with such an outstanding and dedicated group over several years. I consider their commitment, support and comradeship to be the most important reasons why the initiative, taken by a small national organisation, has become a worldwide success. The members of the steering group in the Netherlands, the international group of task force leaders, as well as each individual task force member were particularly important in the steps toward the World Congress on Drowning held in Amsterdam in 2002, and in the publication of this book in 2005.

This book marks the end of a period spanning three decades between my first day as a lifeguard on one of the most remote beaches in the Netherlands, and the worldwide upgrading of all available knowledge in the field of drowning prevention, rescue and treatment as a professor in Emergency Medicine. As such, this book is for me an acknowledgement of my emotional links with the sea and the resulting intellectual challenges to find a way to tackle the problem of drowning. Most of the work towards achieving this has been done by the hundreds of volunteers who, one way or another, have contributed to the process. I will be grateful to each of them for the rest of my life. This book is a tribute to them, their families, their loved ones, and to those they sadly lost by drowning. My special thanks go to the three board members of the Foundation Drowning 2002, Hans Knape, chairman of the scientific steering committee, Rutger Count Schimmelpenninck, chairman of the *Maatschappij tot Redding van Drenkelingen* during the course of the project, and vice-admiral retired of the Royal Netherlands Navy, former Commander-in-Chief, Herpert van Foreest esq. Their continuing support and input kept the process going.

The book is published as a tool that will further reduce the number of drownings and improve the outcome. This means that the readers are challenged not only to read this book and put the information into practice, but also to co-ordinate local, regional, national or international initiatives in their own fields of expertise, competencies and jurisdiction. In this way the snowball will continue to roll and become even larger.

The future activities observed throughout the world may well be a reason for the *Maatschappij tot Redding van Drenkelingen* to start a second initiative under their patronage.

Joost J. L. M. Bierens MD PhD MCDM

Contents

Section 11
Breath-Hold, SCUBA and Hose Diving   **587**

Section editors: DAVID ELLIOTT and ROB VAN HULST
Authors: ALFRED BOVE, JIM CARUSO, GLEN EGSTROM,
DAVID ELLIOTT, DES GORMAN, ROB VAN HULST,
MAIDA TAYLOR and JÜRG WENDLING

Section 12
Investigation of Drowning Accidents   **617**

Section editor: JEROME MODELL

List of Contributors

Stathis Avramidis, MSc
European Lifeguard Academy Greece,
El. Venizelou 12A,
18533 Kastella-Pireas, Greece

Wolfgang Baumeier, Dipl. Ing, MD
Department of Anaesthesiology,
University Hospital Schleswig-
Holstein, Campus Lübeck,
Ratzeburger Allee 160, 23538 Lübeck,
Germany

Peter Barss, MD, ScD, MPH, DTMH, FACEPM, FRCPC
United Arab Emirates University
Faculty of Medicine and Health
Sciences,
PO Box 17666, Al Ain,
United Arab Emirates

Steve Beerman, MD, BSc, BSR, CCFP, FCFP
Lifesaving Society Canada,
287 McArthur Avenue,
Ottawa Ontario, K1L 6P3, Canada

Elizabeth Bennett, MPH, CHES
Children's Hospital and Regional
Medical Center, Health Eduction,
PO Box 50020/S-217, Seattle,
WA 98145-5020, USA

Robert A. Berg, Professor, MD
The University of Arizona
College of Medicine,
1501 N Campbell Avenue, Tucson,
AZ 85724-5073, USA

Roger E. Bibbings, MBE, BA, FIOSH, RSP
Royal Society for the Prevention of
Accidents, RoSPA House,
Edgbaston Park, 353, Bristol Road,
Birmingham B5 7ST, UK

Joost J. L.M. Bierens, Professor, MD, PhD, MCDM
Department of Anesthesiology,
VU University Medical Center,
De Boelelaan 1117,
1081 HV Amsterdam,
The Netherlands

Jenny Blitvich, PhD
School of Human Movement
and Sport Sciences,
University of Ballarat, Victoria 3353,
Australia

Eke Boesten, LLM, PhD
Celebesstraat 86,
2585 TP The Hague,
The Netherlands

Leo L. Bossaert, Professor, MD, PhD
University Hospital Antwerp,
Department of Intensive Care,
Wilrijkstraat 10, 2610 Antwerp,
Belgium

Alfred A. Bove, Professor, MD
Cardiology Section,
Temple University Medical School,
3401 N. Broad Street, Philadelphia,
PA 19140, USA

Christine M. Branche, PhD
National Center for Injury
Prevention and Control,
Centers for Disease Control
and Prevention,
4770 Buford Highway NE,
Mailstop K-63,
Atlanta GA 30431-3724, USA

Helge Brandstrom, MD
Department of University Hospital,
Anaesthesiology and Intensive Care,
Umea, Sweden

Ruth A. Brenner, MD, MPH
National Institute of Child Health
and Human Development,
National Institutes of Health,
Department of Health and Human
Services, Room 7B03-7510,
6100 Executive Blvd, Bethesda,
MD 20892-7510, USA

B. Chris Brewster
United States Lifesaving Association,
3850 Sequoia Street,
San Diego, CA 92109, USA

Rob K. Brons, LLM
Chief Fire Officer,
Fire and Rescue The Hague Region,
PO Box 52158, 2505 CD The Hague,
The Netherlands

**Christopher J. Brooks, OMM, CD,
MBChB, DAvMed, FFOM**
Research & Development,
Survival Systems Limited,
Dartmouth, Nova Scotia, Canada

David Calabria
D&D Technologies (USA), Inc.,
7731 Woodwind Drive,
Huntington Beach, CA 92647, USA

Ian M. Calder, MD
University of Cambridge, Thorpe,
Huntingdon Road,
Cambridge CB3 0LG, UK

Jim Caruso, MD
1413 Research Blvd,
Rockville, MD 20850, USA

Davide Chiumello, MD
Istituto di Anestesia e Rianimazione,
Universita' degli Studi di Milano,
Ospedale Maggiore Policlinico-
IRCCS, Via Francesco Sforza 35,
20122 Milano, Italy

**Veronique G.J.M. Colman,
Professor, PhD**
Faculty of Movement and
Rehabilitation Sciences,
Catholic University Leuven,
Tervuursevest 101, 3001 Leuven,
Belgium

Peter N. Cornall
Water and Leisure Safety,
Royal Society for the Prevention of
Accidents, RoSPA house,
Edgbaston Park, 353 Bristol Road,
Birmingham B5 7ST, UK

**Günter Cornelissen, Dipl.Pol,
Dipl.Ing**
DIN Deutsches Institut für Normung
eV, Verbraucherrat,
Postfach 301107, 10772 Berlin,
Germany

Hein A. M. Daanen, Professor, PhD
Department of
Performance & Comfort,
TNO Human Factors, PO Box 23,
3769 ZG Soesterberg,
The Netherlands

Peter Dawes
Surf Life Saving Queensland,
PO Box 3747,
South Brisbane QLD 4101, Australia

Michel B. Ducharme, PhD
Human Protection
and Performance Group,
Operational Medicine Section,
Defence Research and Development,
1133 Sheppard Avenue West, Toronto,
Ontario, M3M 3B9, Canada

Glen Egstrom, PhD
University of California Los Angeles,
Department of Physiological Sciences,
3440 Centinela Avenue, Box 951606,
Los Angeles, CA 90095-1606, USA

**David H. Elliott OBE, Professor, MD,
DPhil, FRCP, FFOM**
40, Petworth Road, Rockdale,
Haslemere, Surrey GU27 2HX, UK

Mike Espino
American Red Cross National
Headquarters,
8111 Gatehouse Road, 6th floor,
Falls Church, Virginia 22042, USA

Marit Farstad, MD
Department of Anesthesia
and Intensive Care,
Institute for Surgical Sciences,
Haukeland University Hospital,
5021 Bergen, Norway

**Peter J Fenner AM, MD, DRCOG,
FACTM, FRCGP**
School of Medicine, James Cook
University, Townsville, Queensland,
PO Box 3080, North Mackay,
Qld 4740, Australia

Adam P. Fischer, MD
Department of Cardiovascular
Surgery, Centre Hospitalier
Universitaire Vaudois,
Rue du Bugnon 46, 1011 Lausanne,
Switzerland

Andrea Gabrielli, MD
Division of Critical Care Medicine
University of Florida, 1600 Sw Archer
Road, Gainesville, FL 32610-0254,
USA

**Luciano Gattinoni, Professor, MD,
PhD**
Maggiore Hospital, Department of
Anesthesia and Intensive Care,
Via F. Sforza 35, 20122 Milan, Italia

Harry P.M.M. Gelissen, MD
Radboud University Medical Centre,
Department of Intensive Care,
PO Box 9101,
6500 HB Nijmegen, The Netherlands

**Gordon G. Giesbrecht, Professor,
MD, PhD**
211 Max Bell Centre,
University of Manitoba,
Winnipeg, MB, R3T 2N2, Canada

Julie Gilchrist, MD
National Center for Injury
Prevention and Control, Centers for
Disease Control and Prevention,
Division of Unintentional Injury
Prevention, 4770 Buford Highway NE,
Mailstop K-63, Atlanta, GA 30341,
USA

**Frank St. C. Golden, MB, MD, BCh,
PhD**
15 Beech Grove, Gosport,
Hants PO12 2EJ, UK

Des Gorman, Professor, MD
Occupational Medicine Unit,
University of Auckland,
Private Bag 92019, Auckland,
New Zealand

Ralph S. Goto
Ocean Safety and Lifeguard Services
Division, City and County of
Honolulu, 3823 Leahi Avenue,
Honolulu, HI 96815, Hawaii

Shirley A. Graves, MD
University of Florida,
College of Medicine, PO Box 100254,
Gainesville, FL 32610, USA

Tom Griffiths, EdD
Aquatics and Safety Office,
Penn State University, Department
of Intercollegiate Athletics,
University Park, PA 16802, USA

Ivar Grøneng
Norwegian Maritime Directorate,
PO Box 8123, 0032 Oslo,
Norway

Ton Haasnoot
KNRM (Royal Netherlands Sea
Rescue Institution),
PO Box 434, 1970 AK IJmuiden,
The Netherlands

Katrina Haddrill
New South Wales Department of
Tourism, Sport and Recreation,
PO Box 1422, Silverwater NWS 2128,
Australia

Jack J. Haitsma, MD, PhD
Department of Anesthesiology,
Erasmus University Medical Centre,
PO Box 1738, 3000 DR Rotterdam,
The Netherlands

Anthony J. Handley, MD, FRCP
40 Queens Road, Colchester,
Essex CO3 3PB, UK

W. Andrew Harrell, Professor, PhD
Centre for Experimental Sociology,
University of Alberta, 5-21 Tory,
Edmonton, Alberta T6G 2H4, Canada

Walter Hasibeder, MD
Department of Anesthesiology
and Intensive Care Medicine,
Krankenhaus der Barmherzigen
Schwestern, Schlossberg 1,
4910 Ried im Innkreis, Österreich

Balt Heldring, LLM
PC Hooftstraat 204,
1071 CH Amsterdam,
The Netherlands

Walter Hendrick
PO Box 548, Hurley, NY 12443,
USA

Robyn M. Hoelle, MD
Emergency Medicine,
University of Florida,
PO Box 14347,
Gainesville, FL 32604, USA

James D. Howe Jr
Honolulu Emergency Services
Department, Ocean Safety and
Lifeguard Services Division,
3823 Leahi Avenue,
Honolulu Hawaii 96815

Paul Husby, Professor, MD, PhD
Department of Anesthesia
and Intensive Care, Institute for
Surgical Sciences,
Haukeland University Hospital,
5021 Bergen, Norway

Ahamed H. Idris, Professor, MD
Surgery and Emergency Medicine,
University of Texas Southwestern
Medical Center,
5323 Harry Hines Blvd, Dallas,
TX 75390-8579, USA

Udo M. Illievich, Professor, MD
Neuroanesthesiology and Critical
Care, Clinic of Anesthesia and
General Intensive Care,
Medical University of Vienna,
1090 Vienna, Austria

Nicolaas J.G. Jansen, MD, PhD
Pediatric Intensive Care Unit,
Wilhelmina Children's Hospital,
University Medical Center Utrecht,
PO Box 85090, 3508 AB Utrecht,
The Netherlands

Bas N. Jonkman, MsC
Delft University of Technology,
Faculty of Civil Engineering,
PO Box 5044, 2628 CS Delft,
The Netherlands

Cor J. Kalkman, Professor, MD, PhD
Division of Perioperative Care,
Anesthesia, Emergency Medicine
and Pain Management,
University Medical Center Utrecht,
PO Box 85500, 3508 GA Utrecht,
The Netherlands

Laurence M. Katz, MD
University of North Carolina
at Chapel Hill,
Department of Emergency Medicine,
Neurosciences,
101 Manning Dr,
Chapel Hill, NC 27599, USA

Gabriel Kinney
Business Development,
Martime Systems and Sensors,
Lockheed Martin, Syracuse,
New York NY 13221 4840, USA

Alexandra Klimentopoulou, MD
1st Department of Pediatrics,
Athens University Medical School,
Aghia Sophia Children's Hospital,
Thivon & Levadias str,
11527 Athens, Greece

**Johannes T.A. Knape, Professor,
MD, PhD**
Division of Perioperative Care,
Anesthesiology, Emergency Medicine
and Pain Management,
University Medical Center Utrecht,
PO Box 85500, 3508 GA Utrecht,
The Netherlands

**Olive C. Kobusingye, MD, MBChB,
M.Med (Surg), MPH**
WHO Regional Office for Africa,
PO Box 6, Brazzaville,
Republic of Congo

Patrick M. Kochanek, MD
Safar Center for Resuscitation
Research, Department of Critical
Care Medicine,
University of Pittsburgh School of
Medicine,
3434 Fifth Ave,
Pittsburgh, PA 15260, USA

Amanda Kost, LLD
Fire Department of The Hague,
PO Box 52155,
2505 CD The Hague,
The Netherlands

Gerard D. Laanen, MSc
Ministry of Transport,
Public Work and Water Management,
PO Box 20906, 2500 EX The Hague,
The Netherlands

Burhard Lachmann, MD, PhD
Department of Anaesthesiology,
Erasmus Medical Center,
PO Box 1738, 3000 DR Rotterdam,
The Netherlands

John Langley, PhD
Injury Prevention Research Unit,
Department of Preventive and Social
Medicine, Dunedin School of
Medicine, University of Otago,
PO Box 913, Dunedin,
New Zealand

**Laurie J. Lawrence, Dip Phys Ed,
Dip Ed, BA**
D&D Technologies Inc, PO Box 379,
Sydney, Brookvale, NSW 2100,
Australia

John Leech, Lt Cdr, MNI, MIIMS
Irish Water Safety Association,
The Long Walk, Galway, Ireland

Jennifer M. Lincoln, MS
4230 University Drive, Suite 310,
Anchorage Alaska 99508, USA

Bo Løfgren, MD
Department of Cardiology,
Research Unit, Aarhus University
Hospital, Skejby Sygehus,
Brendstrupgaardsvej 100,
8200 Aarhus N, Denmark

John B. Long
Royal Life Saving Society,
Commonwealth Headquarters,
River House, High Street, Broom,
Warks, England B50 4HN, UK

Marilyn Lyford, BHsc
The Royal Life Saving Society
Australia (NSW Branch), PO Box 753,
Gladesville NSW 1675, Australia

**Peter MacGregor, RSP MIFire DMS,
FIM MIOSH**
Royal Society for the Prevention of
Accidents, RoSPA House,
Edgbaston Park, 353 Bristol Road,
Birmingham B5 7ST, UK

Ian Mackie, AM, FRACP †

Martin H.E. Madern
Fire Department of The Hague,
PO Box 52155,
2505 CD The Hague,
The Netherlands

Denise M. Mann, BS, EMT-P
12006 Glenway, Houston,
TX 77070, USA

Ruy Marra
Superfly, Estrada das Canoas,
1476 casa 2 Sao Conrado,
22610-210 Rio de Janeiro,
Brasilia

**Fernando Neves Rodrigues
Martinho, PhD**
Casa Patrão de Salva Vidas Ezequiel
Seabra, Praia de Angeiras 4455 –
204 – Lavra, Matosinhos,
Portugal

Germ Martini
KNRM (Royal Netherlands Sea
Rescue Institution),
PO Box 434, 1970 AK IJmuiden,
The Netherlands

John T. McVan, MEd
United States Military Academy,
Aquatic Instruction,
735 Brewerton Road,
West Point, NY 10966, USA

Bart-Jan T.J. Meursing, MD
Canisius-Wilhelmina Hospital,
Weg door Jonkerbos 100,
6532 SZ Nijmegen,
The Netherlands

Robyn J. Meyer, MD, MS
Department of Pediatrics,
The University of Arizona College
of Medicine,
1501 N Campbell Avenue, Tucson,
AZ 85724-5073, USA

Andrej Michalsen, MD, MPH
University Medical Center Utrecht,
Division of Perioperative Care,
Anesthesia, Emergency Medicine
and Pain Management,
PO Box 85500, 3508 GA Utrecht,
The Netherlands

Rebecca Mitchell, MA, MOHS
Injury Prevention and Policy Branch,
New South Wales Health,
North Sydney, Australia

Jerome H. Modell, MD, DSc (Hon)
Department of Anesthesiology,
University of Florida,
College of Medicine,
PO Box 100254,
Gainesville, FL 32610, USA

Jaap Molenaar
NIBRA (Netherland Institute for Fire
Service and Disaster Management),
PO Box 7010, 6801 HA Arnhem,
The Netherlands

Kevin Moran, MEd
Centre for Health and Physical
Education,
Symonds Street, 74 Epsom Av.,
Private Bag 92601, Epsom, Auckland,
New Zealand

Luiz Morizot-Leite, MS
Beach and Marine Safety,
Miami Dade County Fire Rescue,
10800 Collings Avenue,
North Miami Beach, FL 33154, USA

Peter Morley, MD
Intensive Care Unit,
Royal Melbourne Hospital,
Parkville, Grattan Street,
Melbourne Victoria 3050,
Australia

Bengt Nellgård MD, PhD
Neuro Intensive Care Unit,
Sahlgrenska University Hospital,
413 45 Gothenburg, Sweden

Martin J. Nemiroff, MD
US Public Health Service/
US Coast Guard,
20829 Via Colombard,
Sonoma California CA 95476 – 8059,
USA

Michael A. Oostman
1912 Dimmitt Court,
Bloomington, IL 61704, USA

**Linda Papa, MD, CM, MSc, CCFP,
FRCP(C), FACEP**
Department of Emergency Medicine,
University of Florida College of
Medicine, PO Box 100186,
Gainesville FL 32610-0186, USA

Luis-Miguel Pascual-Gómez
Buena Vista 4, Esc-3, 2-b,
40006 Segovia, Spain

John Pearn, Professor, MD, AM, RFD
Department of Paediatrics and Child Health, University of Queensland, Royal Children's Hospital, Herston, Brisbane, Queensland 4029, Australia

Margie M. Peden, PhD
Department of Injuries and Violence Prevention,
World Health Organization,
Appia Avenue 20, 1211 Geneva 27, Switzerland

Tommaso Pellis, MD
Cardiac Mechano-Electric Feedback Lab, The University Laboratory of Physiology, Oxford, OX1 3PT, UK

Paul E. Pepe, MD, MPH, FACP, FCCM, FACEP, FCCP
Emergency Medicine Administration, 5323 Harry Hines Blvd, MC 8579, Dallas, TX 75390-8579, USA

David E. Persse, MD
The City of Houston Emergency Medical Services, USA

Ulrik Persyn, Professor, PhD
Faculty of Movement and Rehabilitation Sciences,
Catholic University Leuven,
Tervuursevest 101, 3001 Leuven, België

Eleni Petridou, MD, MPH
Department of Hygiene and Epidemiology,
Athens University Medical School, 75 Mikras Asias Street, Goudi, 115 27 Athens, Greece

Francesco A. Pia, PhD
Pia Consulting Services,
3 Boulder Brae Lane, Larchmont, NY 10538-1105, USA

Sjaak Poortvliet
Association of Water Boards,
PO Box 80200, 2508 GE The Hague, The Netherlands

Rolf Popp, Dipl.-Ing
Binnenschiffahrts-
Berufsgenossenschaft,
Präventionsbezirk West D IV-1, Frankenweg 2, 56337 Eitelborn, Germany

Linda Quan, Professor, MD, MPH
Department of Pediatrics,
Children's Hospital and Regional Medical Center,
4800 Sand Point Way NE cm-09, Seattle, WA 98105, USA

Slim Ray, PhD
CFS Press, 68 Finalee Avenue, Asheville NC 28803, USA

Monique Ridder, MSc, PhD
Christelijke Hogeschool Windesheim, PO Box 10090, 8000 GB Zwolle, The Netherlands

Rienk Rienks, MD, PhD
Heart Lung Center,
Central Military Hospital,
Heidelberglaan 100, 3584 CX Utrecht, The Netherlands

Wim H.J. Rogmans, PhD
Consumer Safety Institute,
PO Box 75169, 1070 AD Amsterdam, The Netherlands

Marcia L. Rom, JD
Alaska Injury Prevention Center,
3701 East Tudor, Suite 105,
Anchorage, AK 99508, USA

**Peter Safar, Professor, MD,
DSc (hon) †**

Takefumi Sakabe, professor, MD
Department of Anesthesiology and
Resuscitology, Yamaguchi University
School of Medicine,
1-1-1 Minami-Kogushi, Ube,
Yamaguchi, 755-8505, Japan

Paloma Sanz
Morillo n° 11,, 1° D, 40002 Segovia,
Spain

Justin P. Scarr, BEd, MBA (MGSM)
The Royal Life Saving Society
Australia, Suite 201,
3 Smail Street, Broadway, NSW 2007,
Australia

**Gert-Jan Scheffer, Professor, MD
PhD**
Radboud University Medical Centre,
Department of Anesthesiology,
UMC St. Radboud Nijmegen,
PO Box 9101, 6500 HB Nijmegen,
The Netherlands

Rutger J. Schimmelpenninck, LLM
Keizersgracht 814,
1017 EE Amsterdam,
The Netherlands

Adee Schoon, PhD
Leiden University,
Institute of Biology,
Animal Behaviour Group,
PO Box 9516, 2300 RA Leiden,
The Netherlands

**Michael Schwindt, Professor, Dipl.-
Pädagoge**
Rolandstraße 35, 31137 Hildesheim,
Germany

Ian Scott, PhD
PO Box 302, Abbotsford,
Victoria 3067, Australia

Jim Segerstrom, MICP
Special Rescue Services Group,
World Rescue Service, PO Box 4686,
Sonora CA 95370, USA

Andrew D. Short, Professor, PhD
Coastal Studies Unit,
School of Geosciences,
University of Sydney, Sydney,
NSW 2006, Australia

Antony Simcock, MD, MB BS, FRCA
Royal Cornwall Hospital, Truro,
Cornwall TR1 3LJ, UK

Brian V. Sims
Royal Life Saving Society – United
Kingdom, River House, High Street,
Broom, Warwickshire B50 4HN, UK

Paul E. Sirbaugh, DO, FAAP, FACEP
Texas Children's Hospital,
6621 Fannin Ste A210,
MC 1-1481, Houston, TX 77030, USA

Robert M. Slomp, Msc
Works and Water Management
Department Water Systems,
Safety Against Flooding,
Ministry of Transport, Public,
Postbus 17, 8200 AA Lelystad,
The Netherlands

Gordon S. Smith, MD, MPH
Liberty Mutual Research Institute
for Safety, 71 Frankland Road,
Hopkinton, Massachusetts 01748,
USA

Luiz Smoris

Robert K. Stallman, PhD
Sandvollvn. 80, 1400 Ski,
Norway

Alan M. Steinman, MD, MPH
1135 Harrington Place,
DuPont, WA 98327, USA

Carla St-Germain, BA, BEd
Education, Lifesaving Society,
287 McArthur Avenue,
Ottawa, Ontario K1L 6P3, Canada

John A. Stoop, PhD
Faculteit TBM,
Technical University,
PO Box 5015, 2600 GA Delft,
The Netherlands

Martin Stotz, MD
Bloomsburry Institute of Intensive
Care, The Middlesex Hospital,
Mortimer Street, London, W1T 3AA,
UK

David Szpilman, MD
Socieda Brasiliera de Salvamento
Aquatico, Av. das Américas 3555,
bloco 2, sala 302, Barra da Tijuca,
Rio de Janeiro, Brasil 22631-004

Richard Ming Kirk Tan
73 Farrer Drive,
#02-01 Sommerville Park,
Singapore 259280, Singapore

Greg Tate
Royal Life Saving Society Australia,
Floreat Forum, Perth WA 6014,
Australia

Maida Taylor, MD
785 Foerster Street,
San Francisco, CA 94127, USA

Andreas Theodorou, MD
Pediatric Critical Care Medicine,
Department of Pediatrics,
The University of Arizona Health
Sciences Center, PO Box 245073,
Tucson, AZ 85724-5073, USA

Lambert Thijs, Professor, MD, PhD
Department of Intensive Care,
VU University Medical Centre,
PO Box 7057, 1007 MB Amsterdam,
The Netherlands

Peter Tikuisis, PhD
Human Modelling Group,
Simulation, Modelling,
Acquisition, Rehersal,
and Training Section, Defence
Research and Development Canada,
1133 Sheppard Avenue West, Toronto,
Ontario, M3M 3B9, Canada

Michael Tipton, Professor, MD
Institute of Biomedical &
Biomolecular Sciences,
Department of Sport & Exercise
Science, University of Portsmouth,
Portsmouth PO1 2DT, UK

**Nigel M. Turner, MB, ChB, FRCA,
EDICM**
Pediatric Intensive Care Unit ,
Wilhelmina Children's Hospital,
University Medical Center Utrecht,
PO Box 85090, 3508 AB Utrecht,
The Netherlands

Wolfgang Ummenhofer, MD, PhD
Department of Anesthesia,
University Hospital, Basel,
Switzerland

Ed van Beeck, MD, PhD
Institute Public Health Care,
Erasmus University Rotterdam,
PO Box 1738, 3000 DR Rotterdam,
The Netherlands

Giel van Berkel, MD
Beatrixziekenhuis, PO Box 90,
4200 AB Gorinchem,
The Netherlands

Pieter van der Torn, MD, DEnv
Foundation for Cooperation of
Technique & Care,
Blankenburgerpark 154,
3042 HA Rotterdam,
The Netherlands

Josephus P.J. van Gestel, MD, PhD
Pediatric Intensive Care Unit,
Wilhelmina Children's Hospital,
University Medical Center Utrecht,
PO Box 85090, 3508 AB Utrecht,
The Netherlands

Robert A. van Hulst, MD, PhD
Diving Medical Center,
Royal Netherlands Navy,
PO Box 10.000, 1780 CA Den Helder,
The Netherlands

Joost van Nueten
Belgium Medical Crash Team
– Sea Eagles vzw,
Vloeiende 26, 2950 Kapellen,
Belgium

**Adrianus J. van Vught, Professor,
MD, PhD**
Pediatric Intensive Care Unit,
Wilhelmina Children's Hospital,
University Medical Center Utrecht,
PO Box 85090, 3508 AB Utrecht,
The Netherlands

Hans Vandersmissen
KNRM (Royal Netherlands Sea
Rescue Institution),
PO Box 434, 1970 AK IJmuiden,
The Netherlands

Karel R.R. Vandevelde, MD
Emergency Department,
AZ Sint-Jan,
Ruddershove 10, 8000 Brugge,
Belgium

Harald Vervaecke, PhD
International Life Saving Federation,
Gemeenteplein 26, 3010 Leuven,
Belgium

**Jean-Louis Vincent, Professor, MD,
PhD**
Department of Intensive Care,
Erasme University Hospital,
Route de Lennik 808, 1070 Brussels,
Belgium

Michael Vlasto, FRIN, FNI
The Royal National Lifeboat
Institution (RNLI), West Quay Road,
Poole, Dorset BH15 1HZ, UK

Wiebe de Vries, MSc
Royal Foundation of National
Organisation Providing Accident
Rescue Services and First Aid
"The Orange Cross",
Scheveningseweg 44,
2517 KV Den Haag,
The Netherlands

Beat H. Walpoth, MD, FAHA
Cardiovascular Research,
Service for Cardiovascular Surgery,
Department of Surgery, HUG,
University Hospital, 1211 Geneva 14,
Switzerland

David S. Warner, Professor, MD
Department of Anesthesiology,
Box 3094, Duke University Medical
Center, Durham, NC 27710, USA

Joop B.A. Weijers
Institute for Civil Engineering,
PO Box 17, 2628 CS Delft,
The Netherlands

**Max Harry Weil, MD, PhD, ScD
(Hon), Distinguished University
Professor**
35100 Bob Hope Drive,
Rancho Mirage, CA 92270, USA

Jürg Wendling, MD
Fbg du Lac 67, 2505 Biel-Bienne,
Switzerland

Volker Wenzel, Professor, MD, PhD
Department of Anesthesiology and
Critical Care Medicine, Innsbruck
Medical University, Anichstrasse 35,
6020 Innsbruck, Austria

Peter G. Wernicki, MD
Pro sports, 1355 37th Street,
Vero Beach, FL 32960, USA

Andrew G. Whittaker, BHMS
Victorian Aquatic Industry
Council, 44–46 Birdwood Street,
Box Hill South, Victoria 3128,
Australia

Sip E. Wiebenga
KNRM (Royal Netherlands Sea
Rescue Organisation), PO Box 434,
1970 AK IJmuiden,
The Netherlands

Jane Wigginton, Professor, MD
University of Texas Southwestern
Medical Center,
5323 Harry Hines Blvd.,
Dallas, TX 75390-8579, USA

Klaus Wilkens, PhD
Holunderweg 5, 21365 Adendorf,
Germany

Ann M. Williamson
NSW Injury Risk Management
Research Centre,
University of New South Wales,
Sydney NSW 2052, Australia

Robert L. Williamson, BS, MS
Marine Sonic Technology, Ltd.,
5508 George Washington Memorial
Highway, PO Box 730,
White Marsh, VA 23183-0730, USA

John R. Wilson, Professor, MSc, PhD
Institute for Occupational
Ergonomics,
University of Nottingham,
Nottingham NG7 2RD, UK

Michael Woodroffe
International Lifeboat Federation c/o
The Royal National Lifeboat
Institution, West Quay Road,
Poole, Dorset, BH15 1HZ, UK

Rick Wright
Rescue and Education Commission,
International Life Saving Federation,
PO Box 451, Swansea NSW 2281,
Australia

Andrea Zaferes
Lifeguard Systems/RIPTIDE,
PO Box 548, Hurley, NY 12443, USA

Durk F. Zandstra, MD, PhD
Intensive Care,
Onze Lieve Vrouwe Gasthuis,
PO Box 95500, 1090 HM Amsterdam,
The Netherlands

Edward Zwitser
KNRM (Royal Netherlands Sea
Rescue Institution), PO Box 434,
1970 AK IJmuiden, The Netherlands

Other Contributors:
Blanca Barrio, Spain
Santiago Pinto, Spain

History

Section editor: JOOST BIERENS

1.1
Brief History of *Maatschappij tot Redding van Drenkelingen* (The Society to Rescue People from Drowning)

BALT HELDRING

From June 26 until 29, 2002, the World Congress on Drowning was held in Amsterdam. More than 500 participants from over 40 countries joined in an intensive program. The congress was initiated by the *Maatschappij tot Redding van Drenkelingen*, the Dutch Society to Rescue People from Drowning. The Society was founded in 1767 and is the first organisation to have been involved in the resuscitation of drowning people. The publication of the *Handbook on Drowning* provides a good opportunity for a brief history of the Society.

A drowning victim is often referred to as 'near-dead'. Although it is only relatively recently that we have learned resuscitation measures, attempts to help drowning victims have a long history. An illustration dating back to 1237 BC shows the king of Aleppo being held upside down by two helpers after being rescued from the river Orontes. Apparently, even 3000 years ago, people had some idea that doing something is important to save a life: hold the victim upside down, pump his belly. Although the treatment seems inappropriate today, the principle of taking some initiative to save a life is still the current slogan of the Society: Do something!

In the centuries that followed, however, this attitude changed. In a law dating from 1476, Mary of Burgundy ruled:

You may pull the body out of the water, but if he appears dead, then leave his feet in the water.

A penalty of more than 30 florins was imposed if a body was removed from the water before the coroner had had the opportunity to inspect it. The problem in those days was that people did not know how to tell whether a person was dead, or nearly dead, with the result they did not consider the possibility of resuscitating the 'near-dead'.

On October 7, 1766, Abraham Calcoen, bailiff (*baljuw*) of Amstelland (Amsterdam and the surrounding region), published an article on drowning and mentioned the need to lend a helping hand. His advice was to assist the drowning victim by:
- Warming him up in front of a big fire
- Opening his intestines through the rear with a pair of bellows or a tobacco pipe or a sharp knife
- Rubbing him warm with a woollen cloth or a brush
- Letting his blood
- Rubbing his head with alcohol

The Amsterdam merchant Jacob de Clerq sympathized with the victims whose fate it was to be taken out of the water without verifying whether they were actually dead and who were then buried. De Clerq discussed this issue with the Baptist vicar Cornelis van Engelen, who was also a journalist with the magazine *The Philosopher*. On August 24, 1767, Van Engelen wrote an article in the same magazine in which he provided detailed information on how best to help a drowning person. Van Engelen propagated that rescuers should be given a financial reward and that the costs of housing of a drowning victim should be paid as well as his medical care costs.

This issue of the magazine was distributed in a number of towns and provinces throughout the Netherlands and resulted in many reactions.

On October 26, 1767, at the request of De Clerq and Van Engelen, a number of Amsterdam dignitaries gathered at the house of De Clerq to further develop the ideas set out in Van Engelen's article in *The Philosopher*. On that same day, the Society was founded and held its first board meeting. The aims of the Society were to:

- Encourage resuscitation of drowning victims
- Promote knowledge on resuscitation methods.

It was decided that bronze, silver or gold medals, as well as certificates of appreciation, were to be awarded and that compensation would be paid in some cases.

The article by Van Engelen was summarized in a *Proclamation*, of which 10,000 copies were distributed throughout the country. One negative result of this wide-scale initiative was that many false reports were received from people who were only interested in receiving a monetary reward. A positive result was that within a few years 28 local and provincial governments issued decrees.

Another positive result was that the idea spread to other countries. In 1768, a decree was issued in Venice, Italy. Also in 1768, the *Gesellschaft zur Rettung Ertrunkener* was founded in Hamburg, Germany. In around 1772, a society with similar aims was founded in France. In 1774, the 'Humane Society for the Recovery of Persons Apparently Dead by Drowning' was founded in England. Switzerland followed in 1775 and Denmark in 1797.

Initially, the board of the Society held meetings every 3 weeks. As of 1861, board meetings were held four or five times a year. This reduced frequency was possible, as it still is today, without endangering the affairs of the Society since the board is assisted by a secretarial department.

For the first 75 years, the board meetings were held at various locations, usually in Amsterdam guesthouses or inns. In 1846, the Society acquired the stately building at Rokin 114, at one of the canals in the centre of Amsterdam. Ever since, board meetings have been held there. At the end of the 20th century, this building was sold, but the Society maintained the permanent right to use the meeting room. Effectively, nothing has changed in the meeting room since the 19th century.

This is also true for the structure of the Board of the Society. Fairly soon after their appointment, new members of the board become chairman. They remain so for 2 years. Tradition has it that after his resignation, the former chairman remains an ordinary and thereafter an honorary member of the board. On average, members have remained on the board for 20 years. Seven members were 'on board', so to speak, for more than 40 years!

The Society would not be able to do its work without the help of its advisory board members. These are medical doctors who advise the board on rescue cases at every meeting .

On June 14, 2004, the Society held its 2,596th board meeting. In the course of the past 237 years, more than 6800 awards have been granted. That is an average of about 30 a year.

The annual report of the Society in 2003 mentions 26 successful rescue attempts and awards.

Nowadays, in addition to its initial aims, the Society focuses on:

- Instruction in schools
- Video material
- Television advertising
- Articles in magazines

Also, the Society awards grants and subsidies to scientists and researchers. Naturally, the Society was a major initiator and financial supporter of the World Congress on Drowning held in 2002.

The Society was founded 237 years ago, but is nevertheless still young at heart and intends to continue its work to prevent drowning, as well as to rescue and treat drowning victims.

It all started locally in Amsterdam in 1767, back in the 18th century. Today the organization is active throughout the Netherlands. During the 237 years of its existence, the Society has made an important contribution to the development of methods and treatments that help to prevent drowning. Now, at the beginning of the 21st century, this contribution is still needed, even after 237 years.

Acknowledgements. With special thanks to the authors of the commemorative book *Ideals on life and death* [1], published in 1992 for the occasion of the 225th anniversary of the Society.

References

1. Brokken HM, Frijhoff WTM (1992) Idealen op leven en dood. Gedenkboek van de Maatschappij tot Redding van Drenkelingen 1767–1992. Hollandse Historische Reeks, Den Haag

1.2
Two Centuries of Searching for Safe Lifeboats

HANS VANDERSMISSEN, TON HAASNOOT

In the Spring of 1824, Sir William Hillary initiated the launching of Britain's *Society for the Preservation of Life from Shipwreck*, today's Royal National Lifeboat Institution (RNLI). This precedent, combined with a disaster in the autumn of the same year in which six lifeboat men and three other victims drowned off Huisduinen (□ **Fig. 1.1**), near Den Helder, triggered the founding

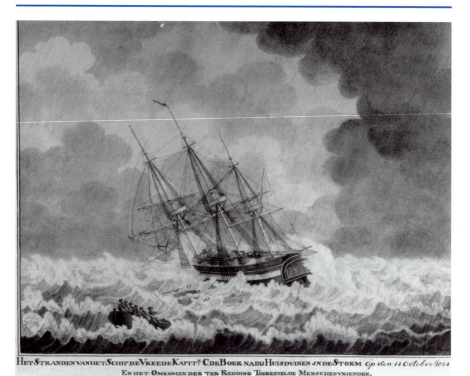

HET STRANDEN VAN HET SCHIP DE VREEDE KAPIT. C DE BOER NABIJ HUISDUINEN IN DE STORM *op den 14 October 1824*
EN HET OMKOMEN DER TER REDDING TOEGESNELDE MENSCHENVRIENDEN,

◘ **Fig. 1.1.** The shipwreck of *'De Vreede'* in 1824 in which six lifeboat men and three casualties drowned triggered the founding of two Dutch lifeboat societies

of two Dutch lifeboat societies: one in Rotterdam, covering the coast between France and The Hague (Belgium was still part of the Netherlands at that time) and one in Amsterdam to cover the coast north of The Hague.

1.2.1
Staying Afloat

The founding father of the northern society, whaler and merchant Barend van Spreekens, introduced 28-ft *Groenlandse sloepen* (a type of Dutch whaleboat) as lifeboats: light, narrow (5.5-ft beam) and made unsinkable with rush. The founder of the society to the south, merchant, ship owner and avid researcher of lifeboat safety, Willem van Houten Jr, designed a self-draining 25-ft clinker double ender, made unsinkable with copper air boxes in the sides and bottom, and with a bulky cork fender all round. In these clinker or 'lapstrake' built boats, the planks overlap each other, affording watertight, light and strong boats. Though rather similar to the crafts used in the north, Van Houten's boats, at over 7 ft, were beamier and stiffer, allowing six double thwarts for 12 rowers, instead of the whaleboat's six single thwarts and an extra seventh. This was a left over from whaling times, when the harpooner would row on the leeside, which also proved useful in lifesaving. In 1852, the design of Van Houten came eighth in the Duke of Northumberland Award for lifeboat innovation.

For the crews, the young societies bought 'lifesaving harnesses': coats of cork that severely hampered movement but probably offered some insulation. In general, safety was sought in making craft unsinkable, either by rush or by airtight metal tanks. The problem with cockpits was (and is) that either they are shallow and self-draining, or deep and protective but prone to swamping. With a high watertight cockpit sole ('foot waling') the centre of gravity of a swamped boat is high, and stability consequently low before it has shed the water. Also, with the high weight of the rowers, stability would be bad even without water sloshing around and their stroke would be too vertical and rather ineffective, with a greater risk of the oar flying from the rowlock. Designers consequently tried to keep thwarts low and the cockpit sole as near to the waterline as possible – 10 cm (4") turned out to be the optimum – with one-way valves in the relieving pipes. The Van Houten design was probably the world's first genuinely self-draining lifeboat.

Another interesting design submitted for the Duke of Northumberland Award was that of James and Edward Pellew-Plenty, a 24-ft lifeboat, at 8-ft rather beamy, and pulled with eight oars (paddles). Its sections showed triangular air cases inside the boat, with rounded slopes, leaving only a narrow foot waling, shaped to shed incoming water easily. The water that remained was concentrated amidships, where it least disturbed stability and could rapidly be sent through the relieving pipes.

1.2.2
Self-Righting Lifeboats

Though self-draining was considered crucial, self-righting was seen as desirable by a number of entries for the Duke of Northumberland Award. In these designs, big airtight end-boxes and heavy ballast keels rendered the craft quite unstable when inverted, so that they would roll the right way up again. The extra windage and weight, however, did nothing for the lightness and low profile that rowers need. Since none of the entries was exactly what the committee had hoped for, they set to work themselves, starting with the most promising design by James Beeching.

Beeching's clinker built boat was pulled by 12 rowers on six double thwarts. It had internal water ballast tanks and an iron exterior keel. The boat hoisted foresail, lug and mizzen (a lug is a fore-and-aft sail hoisted on a yard alongside the mast; a mizzen is a sail hoisted on a small mast aft in any vessel), but had only the long, shallow iron keel and a deep, narrow, coble-like rudder for lateral resistance. Eight 6" and four 4" relieving pipes ensured the rapid discharge of water. Like most contemporary lifeboats, the craft had a bulky cork rubbing strake all round, which also gave 'end'-stability and reserve buoyancy. The committee also borrowed ideas from the interesting design of James Peake, which featured large scuppers as well as relieving pipes, and sloping air cases like the Pellew-Plenty boat. The fore and aft air cases left a narrow passageway free in the middle, for access to stem and sternpost.

By incorporating these early innovations in their own design, the RNLI developed what came to be known as the *Beeching-Peake SR (Self Righting) lifeboat,* designed in fact mainly by Beeching. From 1866 the northern Dutch lifeboat society bought three of these, one 28 ft, the later two 36 ft with 7'10" beams. Two were stationed in succession at Den Helder, where, between 1876 and 1911, the legendary coxswain, Dorus Rijkers, launched 38 times and saved 497 lives. The southern Dutch lifeboat society ordered nine 31-ft Beeching Peakes from the shipyard Rotterdamsch Welvaren with 8-ft 4-in beams. Their weight and windage made the self-righters impractical for beach launching, however, and too heavy for rowing against anything over a fresh breeze, with the 2 hp 'elbow steam' that a well-trained crew could wrench out of their muscles. The Dutch only used these boats from ports where steam tugs were also stationed, such as Den Helder, IJmuiden and Hook of Holland. Normal practice was to tow the lifeboat to windward of a casualty, from where it rowed and sailed towards the wreck.

1.2.3
Light and Steady

Crews had a big say in the type of boat they volunteered to risk their lives in and most preferred light, manoeuvrable, stiff boats over self-righting craft. Self-draining, however, was considered essential. One problem with self-righting boats was that they still shed their crews when they capsized. After the boat had righted itself, getting on board again was often impossible, with the heavy woollen clothes and leather sea boots of the day, not to mention the cork cuirasses. Unfortunately, no boat could be made so stable as to rule out capsizing entirely.

In 1850, the Terschelling boatbuilder, Rotgans, built a 28-ft carvel elmwood-on-oak self-draining pulling boat, with fine ends and an 8-ft beam. Its limited weight, guaranteeing stability and good handling in rough seas, made this particular design suitable for beach launching and coastal operations. The Rotgans lifeboat rowed easily and had a strong influence on the standard type of lifeboat distributed by the north Dutch lifeboat society after 1858. The standard type had a straight stem and stern post for maximum waterline length and was normally steered by a rudder, but the coxswain could ship a sweep (an extra long oar used for steering). Many had centreboards and (two-mast) ketch rigs with foresail and standing lugsails. Some stations preferred more reserve buoyancy in the ends and a lighter boat. As a result De Krim, on the isle of Texel, and the fishing village of Katwijk had eight-oar clinker double enders with overhanging spoon bow and stern post. The relatively short keel made the sweep steered boats highly manoeuvrable (**Fig. 1.2**).

Both societies deployed clinker built *vlet*-type inshore lifeboats: a kind of Norsk pram, with peculiar rounded, stemless spoon bow and transom stern. They varied in size from 18 ft to 30 ft. All *vlets* had sailing rigs and were unsinkable with copper air cases. Their round sections with stout bilge side keels made these

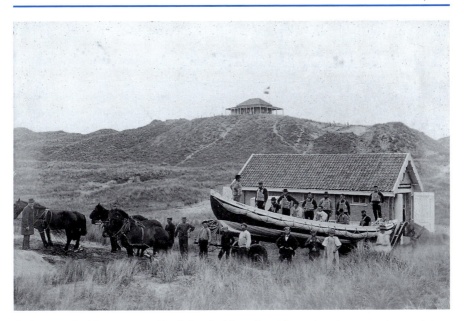

■ Fig. 1.2. A highly manoeuvrable clinker double ender with overhanging spoon bow and stern post. These boats were located in the village behind the dunes. When put into action, the local horses were gathered to bring the boat into the water. The seven rescuers then had to row to the endangered ship. This often took several hours

craft light to row and buoyant, and perfect for hauling out on the Den Helder sea dike. Watermen like Dorus Rijkers worked with such *vlet* boats on the open Texel Roads.

1.2.4
Steam and Tunnels

In 1850, the southern Dutch lifeboat society, with a constant selection of pioneering Rotterdam shipbuilders on the board, had probably the world's first iron lifeboats. They were conceived and built by famous clipper and iron pioneer Fop Smit, founding father of the IHC Holland shipyard and Smit International towage and salvage, who built six of these excellent, though short lived, craft. A friend and client of Fop, the equally famous ship-owner Willem Ruys – founding father of today's Nedlloyd – meanwhile promoted galvanised corrugated steel lifeboats made by the American C. Francis. They were 30% lighter and 65% cheaper than wooden boats, but the crews disagreed with the distribution of buoyancy and did not trust them. Practical tests revealed that stability was indeed less than desirable.

In 1893, the southern Dutch society was also the first to go for mechanical power, with a hydraulic steam lifeboat from John Thornycroft and in 1909 a similar vessel from Feyenoord shipyard of Rotterdam. These hydraulic lifeboats

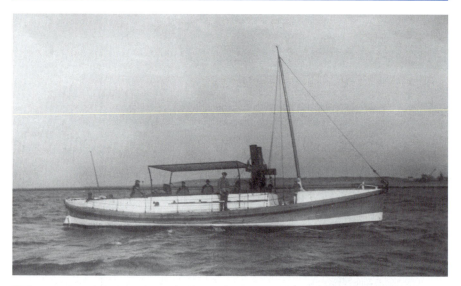

◘ Fig. 1.3. Toward the end of the eighteenth century, when steam ships replaced sailing boats, steam rescue boats were also developed. This figure shows a rescue boat assisting a sailing boat in serious conditions

were ideal for the Dutch coast and its many shallows: with nozzles rather than propellers for propulsion, no vulnerable spinning components that would hit the sand. Thanks to Thornycroft's clever positioning of the nozzles, the boats were extremely manoeuvrable, moving sideways with the same ease as forward and astern and ideal for coming alongside wrecks on lee shores. Although the positioning of the steam engine and boiler produced a high centre of gravity and was therefore bad for stability, the water intakes for the hydraulic system in the bottom of the boat partly compensated for this: the crafts were sucked into the water. Both steamers served successfully, also in very heavy weather, in which a pulling lifeboat would not have achieved anything (◘ Fig. 1.3). Sadly, the Thornycroft steamer capsized in 1921, the annus horribilis of the Dutch lifeboat service, drowning six of its seven crew. In 1929, the Feyenoord boat was lost with all hands. The Dutch had had it with steam, although their hydraulic British sisters had fared much better.

The secretary of the North Dutch society, H. de Booy, had never contemplated steam because of the danger of the fires being extinguished if the boat were swamped. The loss of propulsion and of the steadying intake of water through the bottom would then no longer compensate for the lack of initial stability. De Booy preferred petrol engines in purpose-designed motor lifeboats and ordered one in 1907 from Daan Goedkoop's Amsterdam Kromhout shipyard – still active today as a shipbuilding museum. The unsinkable motor lifeboat *Jhr Mr J.W.H. Rutgers van Rozenburg*, with a 45-hp Brooke's engine in a dedicated engine room, was arguably the first in history with a tunnel-protected propeller for safe operations in shallow seas. The next step in lifeboat evolution was in 1910 with the 38-ton, 58-ft motor lifeboat *Brandaris I* with a 76-hp Kromhout paraffin engine, giving

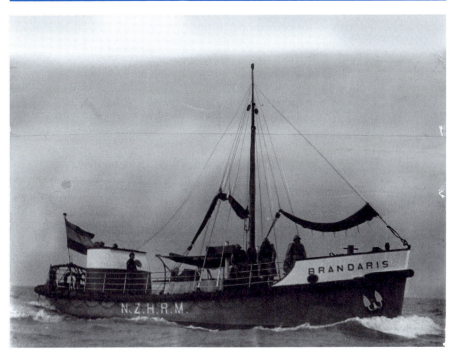

◻ Fig. 1.4. In the beginning of the twentieth century, the first models of motorised rescue boats had a watertight engine room, a heavy bronze crew shelter aft and a jumping net

nearly 9 knots and 40 h endurance. It boasted the first jumping net above deck, to break a survivor's fall when jumping from higher decks. The vessel rescued 231 people before being lost with all hands in 1921.

1.2.5
Surface Submarine

Motorisation went ahead, with both northern and southern societies ordering motor lifeboats. Special orders included the 24 hp *C.A. den Tex*, built in galvanised steel, with controllable pitch propeller in 1917, and in 1923, the 60-ft *Brandaris II*, the northern society's first twin screw boat with two 45-hp single-cylinder Kromhout engines. Construction in mild steel, with watertight engine room, twin screws working in tunnels, stout rubber fender all around, heavy bronze crew shelter aft, a jumping net and efficiently limited equipment, were now the standard for the safe and economical Dutch lifeboats (◻ Fig. 1.4).

From 1922, the northern society gradually replaced its beach-launched pulling boats with the 4.5-ton, 34-ft *Eierland* clinker built motor lifeboats. These wooden Danish double enders were originally powered by 11-hp Ferri petrol engines for 5 knots service speed. As a precaution, they also shipped ten oars and emergency sails. These fine sea boats, with an excellent safety record, were later fitted with 30-hp Fordson petrol engines and then with 65-hp Perkins diesels after the Second World War, which produced speeds of up to 7.5 knots. However, the 24-m^2 emergency rig was retained. While the prototype had been imported from Denmark, the other 12 boats were built by the Taat Brothers of Katwijk.

After several lifeboat disasters in 1921, a famous lifeboat coxswain, Mees Toxopeus, suggested a new type of self-righting lifeboat *like a submarine on the surface*, completely watertight and with fully enclosed conning position. Ernst Vossnack, a professor of naval architecture at Delft University and adviser to both lifeboat societies, as well as Jan Niestern, a Delfzijl shipbuilder, translated the idea into a design. Heavy keel plating and a righting tank under one side deck, which filled with water after capsizing, provided the self-righting momentum from inverted imbalance. Torpedo boat hatches, ventilators with snorkel balls to stop water entering the inverted boat, each engine in its own watertight engine room and mercury switches to stop the engines beyond an inclination of 100°, were some of the revolutionary features. In 1927, the 62-ft, 50-ton *Insulinde* was launched, soon followed by its sister ship *Neeltje Jacoba*. Their length-to-beam ratio of 4:64 (usual was 3:86) and boiler-type hulls made these ballasted bottles not exactly comfortable at sea but extremely seaworthy and efficient as lifeboats.

All post-WWII big self-righters from *Prins Hendrik* (1951) onwards were further developments of the *Insulinde* design. In the 1960s, the northern Dutch lifeboat society built five *Carlot*-class self-righters and the southern society three *Javazee*-class self-righters. The *Carlot*-class was low in the water, a helpful feature when working among casualties, and had double screws with a single rudder. The *Javazee*-type, operating in the busy approaches to the ports of Rotterdam and Flushing, was designed for accommodating large numbers of survivors and had double screws as well as double rudders, which made them more manoeuvrable. Two 140-hp Kromhout diesels gave the *Carlot*-class a service speed of 10.6 knots; the *Javazee*'s two 200-hp GM diesels produced 10.75 knots.

1.2.6
The Advent of Rigid Inflatable Boats

The big Dutch motor self-righters have an excellent safety record: since entering service in 1927, they have never suffered a fatal accident, despite having frequently been out at sea in the worst of weather. By the time the last of the *Carlot*- and *Javazee*-class boats entered service, however, a change of 'client' was already unmistakable, with yachting casualties and medical services increasing while merchant ships became safer. This coincided with the development of high-speed rigid inflatable boats (RIBs) in Britain. Both northern and southern Dutch lifeboat societies embraced the concept and, in particular following their merger in 1991 to become the *Koninklijke Nederlandse Redding Maatschappij* (KNRM) (the Royal Netherlands Sea Rescue Institute), embarked on an ambitious new building program. All conventional craft have since been replaced with fast RIBs.

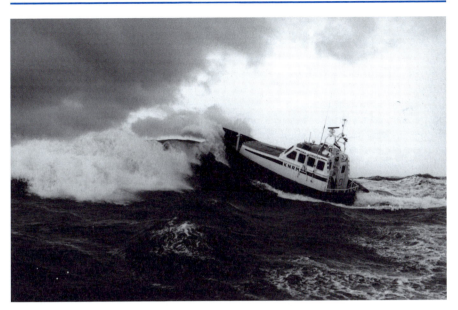

Fig. 1.5. Fast and manoeuvrable rigid inflatable boats (RIBs) were developed in the last decades of the twentieth century. Each RIB can float on its hulls without the tubes, but they can also float on the tubes alone

RIBs completely changed the lifeboat men's seamanship 'battle-drill', not to say that instincts were turned upside down. Beaching a conventional boat, or running it before breaking seas, the coxswain would use a drogue to keep the sternpost of the boat to the waves. A drogue is a cone-shaped and very strong canvas bag with the towline attached to the open base and a small opening in the top. It is also called a 'sea anchor'. A small craft may ride out a gale behind such a drogue. North Sea waves, charging at speeds of up to 25 knots in extreme weather conditions, would otherwise overtake – or even overwhelm – a boat in such conditions.

RIB crews will more often choose an active approach. In order to be able to stay ahead of North Sea waves, all KNRM RIBs have top speeds of 34 knots or more. Because the boats are so fast and manoeuvrable, the helmsman has the means to outwit sudden groundswells or freak waves, which was impossible in conventional boats. Add to this active seaworthiness a high degree of redundancy. For instance, each engine has its own fuel and electrical system, so that having two engines does not double the chance of engine failure. The KNRM's RIBs can float on their hulls without the tubes, but they can also float on the tubes alone if, for instance, a suspended container would be hit at full speed, ripping the hull open. Despite the high level of redundancy in crucial systems, however, the bosun's locker of the lifeboats is kept as empty as possible, only storing tools of proven usefulness on rescue missions (**Fig. 1.5**).

1.2.7
A Small Step for Mankind, But a Giant Leap for the Sailor

The remarkable thing is that many aspects of early pulling lifeboats are still found but perfected in modern RIBs. The big cork fender around Henry Greathead's *Original* of 1790 vintage, added reserve buoyancy, stability and shock absorbing properties, just as the tubes of a modern RIB do. Modern RIBs can do heroic things in weather that would have kept rowing lifeboat crews ashore. What would only half a century ago have been a day-long struggle, may now take an hour. However, there is one aspect which, over two centuries of progress, has barely improved for the lifeboat man: his creature comforts. On board an RIB, while being tossed from wave crest to wave crest in a freezing winter gale, crews may be forgiven for idealising the beauty, leisurely pace and warming-up sports of a pulling lifeboat.

Lifeboats have become safer and more powerful, but they are also called out under far worse conditions. Life on a lifeboat is still not for the meek or the weak-hearted. Modern lifeboats today are crammed with the latest technology in navigation, communication, boat handling and propulsion, and it requires courage as well as thorough knowledge and hard training to be a lifeboat man or woman.

As with the old pulling boats, RIB crews may end up in the water, especially crews of smaller RIBs. Contrary to their forebears, however, they are perfectly prepared for this eventuality. With modern fabric technology, heavy weather garments and survival suits can be made to keep you warm, even in icy cold water; modern life jackets provide buoyancy without hampering movement. Thanks to these attributes, sending a swimmer from a lifeboat or a rescue helicopter is often the most efficient way of getting a line across to a casualty. But this requires intensive survival training and physical strength and modern lifeboat men and women spend more time training than actually saving lives.

In the old days you needed brawn and bravery, today brains, bravery and training, to handle the dream of all lifeboat men since Sir William Hillary: a well-equipped RIB. The RIB may be a small step for mankind, but it is a giant leap for the sailor.

1.3
The History of Resuscitation

BART JAN MEURSING

Probably since prehistory, human beings have been helping and rescuing each other in times of danger and threat. The earliest recorded resuscitations can be found, according to most authors, in the Bible. The text in Genesis 2:7, Kings 17:17–22 and 4:32–35 suggests that people at that time were at least familiar with a technique that resembles our current artificial exhaled air ventilation. However, those paragraphs could also only tell us about a 'miracle'.

In ancient times death was considered as a special form of sleep. No wonder the early rescuers used painful stimuli to waken the victim. Some methods were even brutal: hitting the victim hard in the face, touching him with glowing coal or iron, even sticking needles into the victim.

1.3.1
Resuscitation in Ancient Times

Resuscitation in ancient times was focussed in particular on restoring ventilation. The treatment of the King of Chyryba (Aleppo) is probably one of the oldest preserved recorded stories of a resuscitation. The King was thrown into the Orontes river by the furious Egyptian pharaoh Ramses II and almost drowned. One can still admire in the Rameseum at Thebe the gravures of the rescue treatment given to the King by his soldiers. Soldiers lift their King by his feet probably with the idea of draining water from his lungs. So it may be that the history of resuscitation started with the history of resuscitation in drowning.

In ancient China one used a method in which the victim was positioned on his stomach on the back of an ox with both arms hanging on one side, both legs on the other. The rescuer held the victim in place while he brought the ox into gallop.

With the barrel-roll method, in use in Europe in the Middle Ages, the victim was put on his stomach on the barrel. The rescuer grabbed both feet and rolled the victim to and fro using the barrel. With our current knowledge, it is likely that the changes in intrathoracic and intra-abdominal pressures that occurred during each of these methods caused some circulation.

In the seventh century before Christ the *Pneuma* theory was postulated by Greek philosophers. If the *Pneuma* could leave the body of the victim with his last breath, it meant that immortality was achieved. Based on this theory, punishments like hanging and strangulating were horrible ways of dying and only preserved for criminals. A nobleman was allowed to die, if his sentence required it, by poison or the sword. Drowning was considered to be particularly bad since Galen postulated that the weight of water on the epiglottis during submersion obstructed the airway, thereby hindering the *Pneuma* to leave the body. Efforts were frequently undertaken to free the *Pneuma* after the victim was salvaged. Hippocrates (460–370 BC) suggested in his work *Prognosticon* that a priest could blow the *Pneuma* back into the body by inserting a tube into the trachea. The importance of an unobstructed airway was clearly recognised but based on a different theoretical concept. The tracheotomy was invented, probably for this reason, only a 100 years later by Asclepiades (128–56 BC).

In addition to the Bible there are also two papers dating back to ancient times in which rescue breathing was described as a known technique. The Midrash Rabbah (a bible commentary written by a rabbi in the period 1900–1100 BC) explained the name of Puah, a midwife, from the book Exodus: "Puah was her name because she used to revive the newly born with her own breath".

Also the Babylonian Talmud (written between 200 and 500 AC) accurately describes the mouth-to-mouth rescue breathing method: "One should hold the newly born in a way that it can not fall and one blows one's own exhaled air in the nose of the child."

With the downfall of the Roman empire the development of new medical ideas and theories ceased. Not until the 16th century did a new era in resuscitation begin.

1.3.2
The "Dark Ages" for the Drowned

Between the 11th and the 16th centuries, a ship's cargo was considered more important than its sailors in the event of a shipwreck. Often sailors were watched as they drowned with no attempts being made at rescue.

Moreover, both the legal system and the authorities were opposed to rescue efforts insofar as it was obligatory to leave the victim "with its feet hanging in the water". The victim was not to be transported until a representative of the Law had judged the situation and classified the cause of death as accidental, criminal assault or suicide. An example is the Great Privilege issued by Maria van Bourgondie in 1476. Other laws and orders with similar messages followed up until the beginning of the 18th century.

1.3.3
The Experiments of Vesalius

Scientific interest in resuscitation slowly developed from the mid 16th century beginning with Vesalius (born as Andre van Wezel in Brussels, 1514–1564). Andreas Vesalius (◘ **Fig. 1.6**) worked as a professor in Padua, Bologna and Pisa. He performed animal experiments in which he showed that, for an adequate function of the heart, ventilation was necessary. After opening the chest, bilateral pneumothorax resulted in collapse of the lungs and quick deterioration of the circulation. Positive pressure ventilation via the trachea did expand the lungs again, thereby improving the function of the heart and circulation. The experiments were described in his book *De Fabrica Humana Corporis* (Basel 1555) and repeated over and over by several scientists and proved to be correct. With the exception of midwifes, nobody actually put the knowledge into practice. Only some 200 years later William Tossach (1744) published the first article on mouth-to-mouth ventilation in an adult victim. In 1732, Tossach, a Scottish surgeon, came to the rescue of James Blair, a miner rescued from the pit: "There was not the least pulse in either heart or arteries, and not the least breathing could be observed: so that he was in all appearance dead. I applied my mouth close to his, and exhaled as strong as I could: but having neglected to close his nostrils all the air came out of them. Wherefore taking hold of them with one hand, and holding my other on his breast, I blew again my breath as strong as I could, raising his chest fully with it; and immediately I felt six or seven quick beats of the heart."

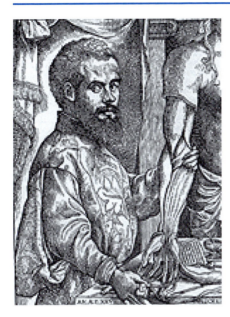

Fig. 1.6. Andreas Vesalius who demonstrated the effectiveness of exhaled air resuscitation

Slowly, scientists were realising that signs of death were not always irreversible. William Cullen (1712–1790, professor at Edinburgh and Glasgow) described "the vital principle" in 1774 in which he states: "death is only irreversible after the neurons have died".

1.3.4
The First Pioneers in Resuscitation of the Drowned

The Swiss priest Sebastian Albinus is probably the first who actively promoted resuscitative efforts in drowning victims. He published a booklet in 1670 in which he described several techniques to resuscitate the drowned victim. Some of these techniques were taught to him by his parents who owned a watermill.

King Louis XV of France was the first who recognised the importance of the government and law in the rescue process and the treatment of drowned persons. A publication of Reaumor (1683–1767) on how to save a drowning victim was circulated through France in 1740 by order of King Louis. The law was also changed. Rescuing a drowning victim was no longer punishable. In the Netherlands the law was changed by the mayor and aldermen of Amstelland in 1767.

1.3.5
Maatschappij tot Behoudenis van de Drenkeling

In 1767, the *Maatschappij tot Redding van Drenkelingen* (Society to Rescue People from Drowning, initially named in Dutch *Maatschappij tot Behoudenis van Drenkelingen*) was established in Amsterdam. This society had three objectives: The first was to reduce the fear and bias associated with touching a drowned victim, the second was to stimulate scientific research and the third was to educate the public in the best way to rescue and preserve the lives of a drowning victims. Billboards were put up in the harbour cities of the Netherlands announcing the most helpful methods. Some treatments, viewed through the prism of present day understanding, may appear trivial: "At first, one should blow tobacco smoke into the anus of the victim by means of a pipe or a pair of bellows. The quicker and the more forceful this blowing will be done, the better it will be". Tobacco smoke insufflation was probably brought to Europe from the New World where Indians had practised the technique on their sudden dead. Despite the fact that in 1811 Sir Benjamin Brodie (1783–1862) already demonstrated in experiments that the technique could be lethal due to nicotine poisoning, it was still used up until 1860.

Other techniques advertised on the billboards, however, were very appropriate: "... but it is also very important and useful when one of the witnesses presses his mouth against the victims mouth and while he with one hand closes the nostrils, tries immediately to inflate the lungs of the victim. Yes, we judge this action as of equal importance as the blowing into the anus".

Other cities and countries followed the example of Amsterdam society, for instance Venice and Milan in 1768, Paris in 1771 and London (called the Royal Humane Society) in 1774. Methods to restore ventilation were considered important because: "What makes that restoration of breathing is very likely the most important step, is what happens during the birth of a baby. When there is too much time lost between the ending of this, for the foetus typical, lifestyle and the start of respirations then the foetus will lose all possibilities for this new life form and all signs of life will disappear. The child seems to be dead and will die for sure if there is no air forced into the lungs thereby taking away the cause of death".

A discussion started about which technique was better, mouth-to-mouth or bellows ventilation, and arose many issues. Fothergill wrote on the subject: "It was suggested to me that one should prefer bellows ventilation in these cases in stead of mouth-to-mouth technique. However, some one who has experience with the mouth-to-mouth technique will prefer this because: 1. a bellows is not always at hand; 2. the strength of the breath from a rescuer can normally be tolerated by the victim. This limit of tolerance can not be determined using bellows; 3. the warm and humid breath of a rescuer could have a better influence on circulation instead the cold air coming from a bellows".

Research was also stimulated by the various societies. Charles Kite (1768–1811) developed an apparatus which had many similarities with the modern defibrillator. He used a so-called bottle of Leiden (the earliest type of capacitor) which he charged with a electrification machine. Using two cables he connected the capacitor to two copper poles. These poles were placed across the thorax of the patient using wooden handles. By placing the two poles on the thorax the capacitor gave off its electrical charge.

The annals of the Royal Humane Society has the records of the first use of this machine during the resuscitation of Sophia Greenhill in 1775. Mr Squires, a surgeon at the Middlesex Hospital, treated her successfully with several shocks. In the Netherlands the method was successfully deployed and recorded for the first time in 1861.

The first endotracheal intubation was published in 1780 and both oral and nasotracheal routes were described. Bellows were used to ventilate the patient via the endotracheal route. After the role of oxygen in human metabolism was clarified by the work of Priestly, Scheele and Lavoisier, purified oxygen stored in pigs bladder was added to the ventilation gas to create a higher oxygen content. All these advanced ventilation techniques, however, were lost and forgotten for a century because of the complications that occurred during positive pressure ventilation.

1.3.6
The Rise of the Push-and-Pull Techniques

In 1829 the French physician Jean Jacques Leroy d'Etioles (1798–1860) published an article in which the potential hazards of positive pressure ventilation were demonstrated. He showed that forceful ventilation with bellows could lead to pneumothorax and, with continued ventilation, could lead to death. This publication was interpreted in such a way that physicians believed that the lungs of a victim of sudden death could not bear positive pressure ventilation. In 1837 the Royal Human Society removed bellows – and mouth-to-mouth ventilation – from the list of advised treatments. A variety of techniques for artificial ventilation were suggested and developed. They all had the physiology of normal ventilation as a basis. During inspiration the techniques created a larger volume of the thorax (pull) thereby creating a negative intrathoracic pressure and imitating normal ventilation. By pushing on the chest the thorax volume was reduced and expiration induced. The different push-and-pull techniques were so numerous that the Royal Human Society had to appoint a study group which would evaluate the existing scientific material and make an official recommendation as to which technique should be used by rescuers. Among the more than 100 techniques, some were positively tested. The best remembered include: the Hall, the Silvester, the Schäfer and the Holger Nielson technique.

The push-and-pull technique also had an influence on medicine. Patients with respiratory insufficiency due to respiratory muscle paralysis caused by the poliomyelitis virus infection were stabilised and ventilated by using a so-called iron lung (☐ Fig. 1.7). Only the head of the patient was sticking out of this iron lung. Around the neck of the patient a rubber seal guaranteed air-tight closure of the iron lung. Air was squeezed out or sucked into the patient by varying air pressure inside the 'lung'. This mechanical lung was the catalyst in the rediscovery of the mouth-to-mouth ventilation technique. During the polio epidemic of 1949 many

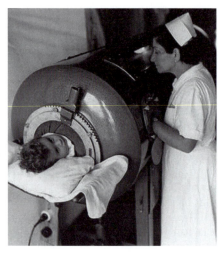

Fig. 1.7. The iron lung in use in a child paralysed in the course of a poliomyelitis infection

iron lungs were used. However, they were not fail-proof. If a lung broke down, physicians and nurses had no other alternative than to practice mouth-to-mouth ventilation (or bag-mask ventilation) because the head was the only accessible part of the body. In 1952 J.O. Elam, an anaesthesiologist, showed by measuring carbon dioxide and oxygen content of the blood of patients that the technique was effective in maintaining adequate blood gases. This was only published in 1958. In that year the American National Red Cross, the National Academy of Sciences and the National Research Council, brought together in an Ad Hoc Panel on Manual Methods of Artificial Respiration, advised that the mouth-to-mouth technique should replace the push-and-pull techniques. Vesalius, who was sentenced by the Inquisition to make a pilgrimage, eventually got science on his side.

1.3.7
The Rediscovery of External Cardiac Massage

The introduction of chloroform as an anaesthetic increased the incidence of sudden death during surgery. By looking directly at the heart, it was shown that these deaths were caused by the occurrence of ventricular fibrillation (VF). The electrocardiogram was not yet discovered and direct vision was the only method of distinguishing this from an asystole. VF was treated by injecting potassium into the heart. This caused asystole which in its turn was treated by injecting epinephrine. In 1947 the first defibrillator for internal use was used successfully by Claude Beck. It took another 12 years before the external defibrillator was developed and used successful. Kouwenhoven, Jude and Knickerbocker discovered by coincidence that thorax compression prior to defibrillation could increase the defibrillation success rate. Mouth-to-mouth ventilation, chest compression and shocks were once again reunited for the first time since 1829.

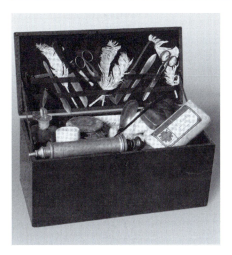

Fig. 1.8. The first aid box for drowning victims. Some of its contents are visible: tobacco clysters apparatus, feathers to tickle the nostrils, a rectal fumigator. These and other articles of historical resuscitation equipment are displayed in the entrance to the boardroom of the governors of the *Maatschappij tot Redding van Drenkelingen* in Amsterdam

After thorough instruction, preserving and sometimes restoring vital functions became possible for laymen.

1.3.8
Recognising, Helping and Saving Drowning Victims

This is a completely different story. It starts perhaps (at least as far as Amsterdam is concerned) in 1796. Night guards were given lanterns and ropes and drags were positioned near bridges and locks.

In October 1824 a desperate rescue effort to save the sailors of the stranded vessel "*De Vreede*" resulted in tragedy: all rescuers were drowned. This was the cue for the founding of the coastal rescue societies (northern and southern Dutch rescue societies). Slowly these organisations grew and were able to position more vessels along the coast. They eventually fused in 1991 to the Royal Netherlands Sea Rescue Institute.

In the year 1866 the Vondel park in Amsterdam was opened to the public. With its many ponds the incidence of drowning created the need for a first aid shelter for drowning victims. This wooden building was made possible with the support of the *Maatschappij*. They also created a first aid box (**Fig. 1.8**) containing a variety of tools and instruments for use in the revival of drowning victims. These boxes were in place and maintained between 1866 and 1913.

In 1909 the Royal Society for Rescue and First Aid in Accidents (the Orange Cross) was established in the Netherlands. Slowly, by streamlining and fusion, the many organisations, some professional but most voluntarily, made it possible for large numbers of drowning victims to be rescued, treated and finally to recover to complete health.

1.4
The World Congress on Drowning:
A Move Towards the Future

JOOST BIERENS and HANS KNAPE

Although much progress has been made in the diagnosis and treatment of patients who have suffered an acute myocardial event and require resuscitation, many people became aware that little progress had been made in the resuscitation of drowning victims. It was felt by many that the pathophysiological processes in drowning, which led the patient to a resuscitation situation, were fundamentally different from the cardiac patient and therefore needed a different approach in terms of diagnosis and treatment. Other observations were that therapeutic innovations were limited, outcome had not improved and reliable international data on the incidence of drowning were lacking.

The board of governors of the *Maatschappij tot Redding van Drenkelingen* (founded in Amsterdam, the Netherlands, in 1767), being the oldest society to promote the rescue of drowning victims in the world, realized the importance of collecting information about this problem from around the world, and of trying to bring various experts together to discuss these matters. The objective was to improve outcome for drowning victims and, even more importantly, to reduce the number of drowning victims.

During the 1990s, the idea to organise a World Congress on Drowning gradually evolved in the wake of a medical PhD thesis on drowning [1]. This PhD thesis was partly sponsored by the *Maatschappij tot Redding van Drenkelingen* (*De Maatschappij*).

Apart from the conclusions based on the epidemiological and clinical studies presented in the thesis, this thesis clearly showed that very limited scientific development in the field of drowning had occurred during the last 30 years.

This interesting but also disturbing and worrying observation motivated *De Maatschappij* to request the supervisor of that PhD thesis, Dr. Hans Knape (also in his role as medical adviser to the board of governors of *De Maatschappij*), together with the PhD candidate to investigate how to bring the apparently neglected tragedy of drowning to the attention of researchers, relevant organisations and institutions, policymakers and politicians (see **Table 1.1**).

This chapter describes the evolution of this initiative, the results attained and the lessons learned.

1.4.1
From Process to Project

A conceptual framework was developed. First, an international network of experts had to be established to make an inventory of existing knowledge and experience and to disseminate this information to all those experts. In this way, the body of knowledge would be upgraded at the highest possible level on a world-wide scale. The ultimate objective of the inventory was to use the accumulated

■ **Table. 1.1.** Observations, motivations and expectations to start in 1996 the World congress on Drowning [3]

- Each year an estimated number of 150,000 people die from drowning. At least the same number of victims (but probably 2–20 times that number) are admitted to hospital for observation and treatment
- Hardly any data are available about drowning in third world countries, except that water-related disasters frequently result in large numbers of victims
- Initiatives to improve prevention, rescue and treatment of drowning are often on a once-only basis and have therefore been unable to achieve durable impact
- Many organisations and institutions have ties with the prevention, rescue and treatment of drowning victims, but none of these have this as their sole mission
- Research on the prevention, rescue and treatment of drowning victims has taken place, but no researcher or research institute has selected this subject to be of highest priority
- Long-term research programs in these fields do not exist and the existing research is always a spin-off from related fields of interest
- In recent decades, several hundred individuals have shown a commitment to contribute to the improvement of prevention, rescue and treatment of drowning victims
- The total body of knowledge, experience and expertise in the several fields is large. Individual experts, however, have access only to a small part of this knowledge. An international platform does not exist
- De Maatschappij tot Redding van Drenkelingen (Society to Rescue People from Drowning) was established in Amsterdam in 1767 with the aim to reduce the number of drowning victims. The society is still active in this field

Conclusions and expectations

- Drowning is a world-wide problem that needs to be tackled
- Reduction of drowning has to be a multidisciplinary effort
- Suitable conditions are available for a goal-oriented multidisciplinary agenda-driven and world-wide project
- Identification of the drowning problem as the focus for an international project will enable progress in this field
- Establishment of an international network will facilitate the dissemination of existing knowledge
- Planning of a world-wide conference on drowning will facilitate discussion among experts
- The conclusions, recommendations, consensus statements and visions expressed during a world-wide conference will be helpful for the related experts, organisations and institutions
- The extensive preparations of a meeting between all related experts, organisations and institutions will generate more information and more results
- The activities mentioned above would lead to a more structured and constant focus on the drowning problem.

information to generate a consensus process, to establish recommendations on current policies and practices and to establish a long-term agenda for collaborative action.

These aims should be reached by means of three lines of activities:

- A formal document with preliminary draft conclusions, recommendations and consensus statements, which would serve as the basis for personal discussions during:
- A congress, where final conclusions, recommendations and consensus statements could be established, both resulting in:
- A state-of-the-art handbook on drowning prevention, rescue and treatment.

In 1996 an enquiry was sent to some 100 key persons world-wide in order to ascertain whether the concerns and ambitions of *De Maatschappij* were shared by others. Most of these experts were identified from the medical and life-saving literature. The response to the enquiry was more than 50% which was very encouraging, and all but two responders agreed that the neglected issue of drowning needed focused and agenda-driven attention. Many suggestions were made concerning topics that needed to be addressed.

Following this international enquiry, a workshop to discuss the feasibility of an international congress on drowning was held in Utrecht, the Netherlands, in 1998, which was attended by 30 representatives of relevant Dutch organisations. The basic idea received broad national interest and support. This response convinced *De Maatschappij* of the need for the initiative and it was decided to focus on the quality of the congress program and limit the audience to opinion leaders, major stakeholders and scientists.

Based on the enquiry and the subsequent meeting, ten main drowning topics were identified:

- Epidemiology
- Prevention
- Rescue
- Resuscitation
- Hospital treatment
- Brain and spinal resuscitation
- Immersion hypothermia
- Breath hold diving, hose diving and scuba diving
- Water-related disasters
- Implementation

The board of governors of *De Maatschappij*, now convinced of the wide interest and support, decided to install two agencies: a national steering group World Congress on Drowning 2002, in 1997, and, in 1999, a Foundation Drowning 2002.

The steering group, consisting of Dutch experts on the ten topics, was asked to establish an international task force for each of the topics. International key persons were approached to join the process as a task force chairperson and to select a group of maximally eight other experts with the aim to review all available information, to identify areas of controversy or non-addressed themes, and to produce consensus documents before the actual congress started.

During these activities which lasted from 1999 to 2002, many newly identified experts were found (or they introduced themselves), thereby contributing new viewpoints for the task forces or new topics to be addressed at the congress. Also, formal contact was made with leading international bodies such as the World Health Organisation (WHO), the International Maritime Organization (IMO), the International Federation of Red Cross and Red Crescent Societies (IFRCRCS), the International Life Saving Federation (ILS), the International Lifeboat Federation (ILF), the Divers Alert Network (DAN), and the European Consumer Safety Association (ECOSA). All these organisations supported the drowning project, which gave extra impetus to the steering group and the Foundation 'Drowning 2002'.

Once a summary had been made of the available knowledge and data world-wide, this resulted in a significant expansion of the body of knowledge. Surprisingly, very important expertise was found to be available on a national level, or sometimes even on a local level. Often, this knowledge and expertise remained concealed from the outside world because, for example, it had not been translated or published, or there was a lack of time, finances or some other form of support. On other issues, it became clear that large differences in opinions existed. An important finding was that many firmly established procedures and convictions were not so much based on hard evidence, but rather on tradition, expert opinion or authority.

Another unexpected finding at that time was a WHO publication in which the annual number of over 500,000 drownings each year was reported [2].

1.4.2
The Consensus Process

One of the main goals of the project was to define consensus with regard to the three major issues: prevention, rescue and treatment. Although all task forces were instructed to try and reach consensus on the conclusions and recommendations for their particular task force, in most cases this proved to be very difficult for a variety of reasons.

Quite early in the process it became clear that the task forces were very dissimilar regarding both the focus and the body of evidence available. The timing of a consensus procedure and the communication between task force members was not always easy. Moreover, there was little experience at the end of the 1990s with setting up and carrying out a consensus procedure via the world wide web. For example, the task forces *Resuscitation*, *Hospital treatment*, *Brain and spinal cord resuscitation* and *Immersion hypothermia* had planned to produce a consensus on the best treatment protocol. However, they quickly realised that hard data and evidence were lacking for most subjects. Nevertheless, each medical task force was able to produce a robust overview of the existing literature.

The main focus of the *Epidemiology* task force was to obtain a global view on the burden of drowning world-wide. However, the task force soon realised that this goal could not be achieved without a proper definition of the concept of "drowning" and spent much time and energy reaching consensus on the definition of drowning and non-fatal drowning, which was later accepted by the congress.

The chairs of the task force *Prevention* produced a manuscript which summarised the main recommendations and strategies for drowning prevention.

The task force *Resuscitation* established a uniform registration procedure for drowning victims (Utstein style) to be used for resuscitation studies of drowned victims [3].

The task forces *Hospital treatment*, *Brain and spinal resuscitation* and *Immersion hypothermia* were able to aggregate the currently available knowledge, to identify areas of interest for research but also to transfer relevant knowledge to rescue and lifesaving communities.

The task force on *Breath hold, hose diving and scuba diving* produced a number of recommendations on prevention, rescue and treatment of diving fatalities by means of a formal consensus process between experts.

Due to the large variety of subjects on rescue and to the absence of cohesion between the subjects, each member of the task force *Rescue* developed their recommendations somewhat independently and each member defined recommendations in their own particular area of expertise. Generally, the other members accepted the authority of an individual task force member on a specific subject and the results were finally approved by all other members.

The outcomes of all task forces were submitted to the steering group, discussed at three annual meetings with all task force chairs in 1999, 2000 and 2001, and were placed on the congress website.

During the 2002 congress, formal consensus meetings were organised for the task forces on *Epidemiology, Resuscitation, Brain and spinal resuscitation, Immersion hypothermia* and *Breath hold, hose and scuba diving*. At the end of each day, the task force chairpersons and the steering group members discussed the status of the consensus process. During a plenary meeting on the last day, each task force chair was able to make recommendations, compiled with or without support of the steering group, while others were able to inform the audience about consensus statements.

1.4.3
The Organisation

The organisation of the congress evolved from the combined ambitions of just three people to the participation of more than 100 (all volunteers) just before the congress started.

The *Maatschappij tot Redding van Drenkelingen* took the initiative and sponsored the congress, both intellectually and financially. In the early stages the secretary of *De Maatschappij* helped to deal with the international enquiries, the national meetings, the correspondence and also prepared the first meeting with the task force chairpersons. The governors of *De Maatschappij* were strongly committed to organising a successful congress and provided support at all times.

The *Foundation 'Drowning 2002'* was installed in 1999. The board of the Foundation consisted of the chairman of the scientific steering group (a physician), the past chairman of *De Maatschappij* (a lawyer), and a retired vice-admiral of the Royal Netherlands Navy. The Foundation held general control on the initiative and was given the final responsibility for the total organisation of the World Congress. The Foundation also enabled a faster response to and interaction with the project coordinator and congress organiser. The board of the Foundation was mainly involved with the legal and financial aspects, the committee of recommendation, financial sponsors, public relations and promotion, as well as the social program of the congress.

Eight *task forces* were installed in 1998 and 1999 to produce a series of state-of-the-art documents with recommendations. When completed, a task force publication was distributed among the task force members for comment and was available on the website www.drowning.nl for additional input from any other experts. Eventually, over 60 documents were on the website.

Most communication between the task force members went via e-mail, which was a relatively new mode of communication at that time. Several task forces also held face-to-face meetings and telephone conferences. Three meetings between the task force chairs and the steering group were held in Amsterdam in 2000, 2001 and 2002, in order to maintain coherent and consistent progress in the various activities. These meetings also included water-related social events, and meetings with members of the board of governors of *De Maatschappij* (❑ Fig. 1.9).

In 1996 *the project coordinator* started to prepare the practical organisation of the initiative. From that moment onwards, he coordinated the contacts between the board of the Foundation 'Drowning 2002', the steering group, the task force chairs and task force members, and also supervised the progress of the task forces. A major activity was the constant search for and identification of new sources of information or expertise, combined with inviting newly identified experts, organisations, institutions, commercial parties and potential sponsors to become involved in the process and to participate in the congress. The project coordinator was supported by a secretary and, later on, by a project assistant.

The Dutch Consumer Safety Institute (*Consument en Veiligheid*) was hired in July 2000 as the official congress organisation for the international and national congresses. The Institute has a long history in drowning prevention programs in the Netherlands, and is experienced in the organisation of international meetings.

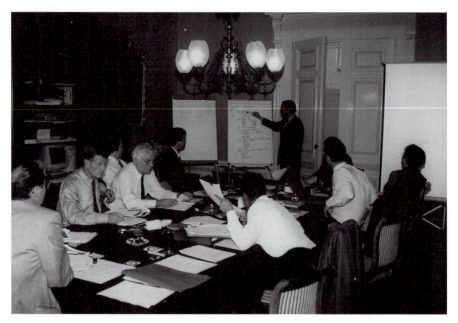

◘ Fig. 1.9. Chairpersons of the task forces and members of the steering group at the headquarters of the *Maatschappij tot Redding van Drenkelingen* during the first meeting in Amsterdam in 1999

1.4.4
Means of Communication

Flyers, brochures, newsletters, e-mail, Internet, books, personal accounts and presentations at meetings have been used to disseminate information about the congress. The logo of the congress was designed to give the project an international image.

Before the task forces started, a brochure was made available to all task force members informing them about the needs, methods and goals of the project (◘ **Fig. 1.10**) [4]. All such information, as well as papers and statements made by the task forces were available on the website www.drowning.nl from 1997 onwards.

At each phase of preparation, great care was taken to maintain a very high quality of work in order to ensure the participants that, although the subject was relatively small and *De Maatschappij* unknown, this project had a solid and reliable foundation.

Several newsletters were also produced to inform all relevant Dutch parties about the initiative.

After the congress, a booklet containing the final recommendations of the World Congress on Drowning (◘ **Fig. 1.11**) [5] was distributed, while this *Handbook on Drowning* is the final publication to emerge.

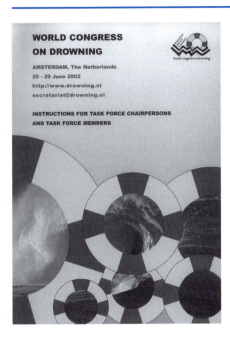

■ **Fig. 1.10.** Brochure containing the instructions for task force chairpersons and task force members [3]

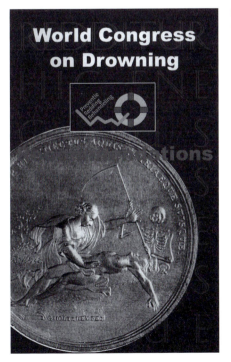

■ **Fig. 1.11.** Booklet containing the final recommendations of the World Congress on Drowning [4]

1.4.5
Financial Aspects

The evolution of the initiative is well demonstrated by the financial aspects. The initial budget for the congress was 30,000 euro but the final formal budget was almost 530,000 euro.

To obtain additional funding, a sponsoring project was set in motion. The major portion of the sponsoring of the congress was provided by *De Maatschappij*. The first external sponsoring by the *Prins Hendrik Fonds* came at a crucial point because at that moment the anticipated need to expand the project became clear. Other main sponsors included the Dutch government (the Ministry of Transport, Public Work and Water Management, the Ministry of Interior and Kingdom Relations, and the Ministry of Health, Welfare and Sports), organisations (such as the Divers Alert Network, the Royal Dutch Lifeboat Institute and *Vereniging Parkherstellingsoorden*), and industries (such as Damen Shipyard, NEDAP and ZOLL). Several other parties donated smaller funds and other forms of support.

Not included in the formal budget was the large number of supportive activities carried out by other organisations. For example, during the meetings with the task force chairpersons in 2000, the use of a private yacht was offered by a supporter of the initiative to transport the chairpersons over the Ijsselmeer from one meeting location to another. During the 2001 meeting, all participants were invited by the chairman of *De Maatschappij* to dinner at his house. The Royal Netherlands Sea Rescue Institute (KNRM) had a significant task in organising the nine pre-congress courses which took place near the harbour and on the beach at Ijmuiden. These courses had a separate budget of 25,000 euro. The Norwegian Maritime Directorate combined a study on improved personal life-saving appliances in the Netherlands with their attendance at the congress. The Smit-Tak salvage company sponsored a video wall during the congress; Vacuvin (an innovative business) invited the task force Brain and spinal resuscitation for a brainstorming session on the potential use of a newly developed device for head and body cooling; the *Reddingsbrigades Nederland* (Royal Dutch Lifesaving Association) organised the beach barbeque; PricewaterhouseCoopers gave advice on financial and fiscal aspects; Hill and Nolton produced fact sheets and supported the public relations activities; the Ministry of Defence provided logistic support for the activities outside the RAI congress centre; and the Vrije Universiteit medical centre of Amsterdam gave valuable support to the project coordinator.

1.4.6
The International World Congress on Drowning 2002

Another goal of the World Congress on Drowning was to bring together all members of the task forces who had actively participated over the years in the preparation of the statements, conclusions and consensus of a wide range of topics related to drowning.

Ample opportunity was given to all other participants of the congress to express their views on and their experience with important issues related to drowning, and to interact with the task force members during the meetings. Before the congress, 150 abstracts had been submitted for discussion.

During the congress the amount of accumulated knowledge, expertise, dedication and ambition was most impressive. Also the fact that, for the first time, over 500 people with a specific interest in drowning were gathered together was a very stimulating experience. The congress was opened with a videotaped presentation called 'To the rescue' which clearly expressed the aims of the congress. Then representatives from the World Health Organisation, the International Maritime Organisation, and the International Life Saving Federation made introductory speeches.

The task forces presented their data in the form of plenary task force sessions, discussion sessions, interdisciplinary sessions, expert meetings, research meetings, workshops, poster sessions and consensus meetings. Because the most critical issues had already been identified, these issues were high on the agenda and received extra attention during the congress. Throughout the congress, a multidisciplinary approach was used in order to learn from the various areas of interest, to connect the various disciplines involved, and to link the relevant instruments.

Other methods used to promote interactions included nine pre-congress courses (among which the first Advanced Life Support Course by the European Resuscitation Council in the Netherlands), five pre-congress meetings, 20 information booths, a permanent display of 36 video presentations on drowning-related issues from all over the world, practical demonstrations on rescue techniques, industry sponsored satellite meetings, and a bookshop with over 200 books on drowning and related issues.

The social program included receptions at the Amsterdam Town Hall and at the headquarters of *De Maatschappij*, a congress dinner, and a beach barbeque with a live rescue demonstration in the North Sea during a storm with wind force 10 on the Beaufort scale.

During the closing ceremony, the first two medals of honour of the *Maatschappij tot Redding van Drenkelingen* were offered to Jerome Modell [6] in person, and to Peter Safar [7, 8] who unfortunately could not attend the congress. Both laureates have made major contributions to our understanding of the pathophysiology, resuscitation and treatment of drowning.

In the closing remarks, three images were used to motivate participants to continue the work initiated by *De Maatschappij*:

- 'We have picked the small flowers of drowning from several branches of medicine and put them together in one vase; let's now take good care of them'
- 'We have made a small snowball which needs to keep on rolling so that it will get bigger and bigger'
- 'We built the kitchen, you brought the ingredients – now let's start cooking'

1.4.7
The National Congress (the Dutch Day on Drowning)

From the very beginning it was the intention of *De Maatschappij* to involve Dutch organisations in the various processes in order to show the importance of the congress in its entirety for the Dutch community. After the workshop held in 1998, the major Dutch stakeholders were kept updated about events. The Dutch Day on Drowning, which immediately followed the World Congress, was attended by over 300 people and was supported by many Dutch organisations. Topics and target groups included prevention, rescue, treatment and diving. This national congress was opened with the personal accounts of two rescuers and the victims that they had rescued and successfully resuscitated. The two rescuers had been honoured some time earlier by *De Maatschappij*.

Members of the steering group presented an overview of the major conclusions from the World Congress on Drowning. All invited Dutch speakers had attended the international congress and were thus able to include the most recent information in their presentations. Again, the interdisciplinary exchange of information was a major factor contributing to the success of this national meeting.

1.4.8
Results of the World Congress on Drowning

The project World Congress on Drowning 2002 has achieved a number of important aims.

A significant number of conclusions and recommendations have been agreed upon. These have been published in the booklet *Recommendations of the World Congress on Drowning* (Fig. 1.11) [5] and are published in this book.

An international and interdisciplinary network on drowning has been established. Surprisingly, during the congress people from the same country often discovered that they were investigating similar problems, without knowing about each other's involvement in their own country.

Several meetings on the prevention, rescue and treatment of drowning have and will be organised on a local, regional, national or international level. At these meetings, the major outcomes of the World Congress on Drowning were selected for key lectures. Several members of the task forces were invited to present the new information from the World Congress on Drowning at scientific meetings. Existing prevention and research initiatives received support and input, while other initiatives are being prepared.

A number of personal impressions, reports and scientific articles have been published or were included on websites of the participating organisations [9, 10]. The congress supported WHO initiatives to publish a fact sheet on drowning (◘ Fig. 1.12) [11], a book on water safety [12], and a special issue on drowning prevention in the journal *Injury Control and Safety Promotion* [13–20]. The congress venue was also used to make a television documentary on drowning to be broadcast by the National Geographic channel.

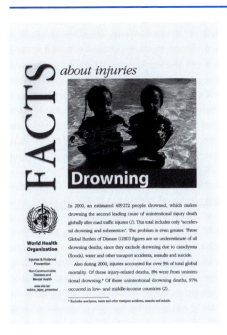

■ **Fig. 1.12.** The WHO fact sheet on drowning [10]

Many international experts on drowning, and those with special interest in the subject, were able to participate and contribute. Many friendships, informal and formal contacts have been made, resulting in inspiration, stimulation and new plans.

At a national level, the World Congress drew significant attention from the media (over 30 newspaper articles and interviews, four radio interviews and five television interviews) and resulted in several new initiatives undertaken by organisations involved in swimming instruction, fire fighting and rescue. After 2002, *De Maatschappij* received a larger number of requests to honour heroic persons who had rescued others from the water than before the congress [21].

1.4.9
Lessons Learned

Considering that the World Congress on Drowning had to start from scratch and that all the essential aspects have now been put into practice, these 'lessons learned' should not be considered as failures but rather as important items for future initiatives.

1.4.9.1
Topics

Originally, the initiative aimed to organise a medical and scientific meeting. It soon became apparent, however, that prevention and rescue were far more powerful instruments to reduce the number of drowning victims. Notably, within the rescue component, the variety of subjects addressed was far more extensive than initially estimated. Examples are the impact of different locations of possible drowning (bath tub, home, lake, swimming pool, sea), the different activities (accidental, recreation, car in water, boating), the efficacy of activities by rescuers (signals, scanning, rescue techniques), the need for and experiences with equipment (rescue tools, boats), and the consequences depending on whether the organisation was manned by professionals or volunteers. Prevention and rescue therefore received a lot of attention, not only during the planning phases but also during the congress itself.

Only a few international experts in the field of water-related disasters, flooding and boat accidents with large numbers of victims, could be invited. No international network could however be identified. This was considered to be an important item in the field of drowning. It was explained that the issue of disasters mainly involves policymakers and bureaucrats who, compared to scientists, generally have much less active international networks, tend to have a reactive attitude (as long as there are no water-related disasters, they will not include the item on the political agenda), and these people change positions often. To ensure that the issue of water-related disasters was addressed at the congress, a national task force was installed.

Unfortunately, no task force on *Implementation* could be installed even though the final success of any project will strongly depend on a successful implementation process. After the congress, the participants were motivated to take care of the implementation themselves.

In spite of careful preparations, a topic that was not identified before the congress and gradually revealed itself was the *Search for dead drowned persons*. It seems that there is a large number of international experts involved in search techniques for drowned persons, as well as in legal investigations and jurisdiction.

1.4.9.2
Interactive Expert Network

It was planned that draft versions of the work by the task forces should be available on the website for internal and external comment and discussion. However, when the drafts were available on the website, it appeared that there was no simple and cheap software to allow interactive communication so that most discussions took place between closed e-mail groups. This limited the input from other experts. When the website became managed by the congress organiser during the last 2 years, the e-mail groups worked well and it was decided that the interactive options on the website could be omitted.

Another planned activity that was confronted with technical limitations at that time, was the establishment of a database of all identified experts to facilitate communication between all those involved before and after the congress. Although data of over 2000 people were collected (including contact data, fields of expertise and interests, and the national and international organisations in which the persons were actively involved or affiliated with), the database had to be reduced to an address list because of practical problems (costs, shifts in budget, maintenance and updating).

One important lesson learned here is that for essential process tools such as an interactive website and a complete set of data for an international network of experts sufficient dedicated manpower and funds are needed.

1.4.9.3
Process Management and Project Management

An interesting observation is related to the problems that occur when the process in which the interaction between people is the central theme transfers to a project in which a certain goal has to be reached by a certain point in time.

The World Congress on Drowning started as a process which planned to involve as many experts as possible. Each new opportunity to reach the aims of the initiative needed to be explored, and active searches for experts, regular reviews of the literature, and surfing on the Internet were needed. In addition, spontaneously appearing experts, organisations and themes had to be considered within the total framework of the project. To make their involvement rewarding, all experts should have the opportunity to express their opinions and intentions, while at the same time it was necessary to ensure that progress should not be dominated by one single person or organisation. Thus, the approach was typical for such a process and required a lot of flexibility, creativity and good relationships with all involved. It was not always possible to set definite deadlines because each activity within the process also had its own time path.

When the actual organisation of the congress needed to be prepared, the congress organiser had to work according to a strict time schedule, with clear goals and arrangements: the congress had to start on 26 June 2002. For several experts, organisations and sponsors this confrontation with a more focused approach, typical for a such a project, endangered their commitment.

While it can be concluded that both the process and the project has worked very well, an important lesson is that the different roles of the process and the project – as well as the allocation of responsibilities, funds and personnel to support both aspects – need to be established in an early stage and clearly communicated throughout the initiative.

1.4.9.4
Other Aspects

A few plans that were embedded in the original concept could not be realised: for example, the plan to involve delegates from low-income countries (due to lack of sponsoring, and lack of support from appropriate organisations), and the plan to involve Spanish, Portuguese, Russian, Chinese and Japanese delegates with important expertise (due to their inability to communicate English). The construction of a swimming pool at the congress venue to demonstrate rescues and the physiological responses to immersion hypothermia was not possible due to technical and safety problems. A few other courses, as well as lunch lectures on the cultural and artistic impact of drowning, and table-top exercises on water-related disasters also had to disappear from the planning.

1.4.10
Conclusions

The initiative by the *Maatschappij tot Redding van Drenkelingen* to organise the first World Congress on Drowning has been very successful. Many results have been accomplished and these results will contribute to the reduction of drowning and the improvement in outcome; the identified goals and ambition of the initiative (◘ **Table 1.1**). The conceptual idea to organise a congress as an incentive at the end of a knowledge-exchange process was an effective method to obtain the active involvement of experts from all over the world, to structure a worldwide network of experts, and to enhance global knowledge on the prevention, rescue and treatment of drowning. Unprecedented scientific and humanitarian progress was made that will decrease the annual numbers of drowned victims, and improve the outcome after drowning.

Considering the dynamics of the initiative, it is interesting to observe that the initiative starts as an interactive, interdisciplinary and international process. Then, at a certain moment, elements of a time and target focused project interfere and eventually take over. Also, there is a transition phase between using volunteers and professionals – but both aspects are required at that time to make progress in the field of drowning prevention, rescue and treatment. Outstanding and dedicated key persons who are willing to offer their time, knowledge, experience and prestige to support a goal that reaches further than their immediate personal interest, are needed to accomplish such an endeavour.

Implementation of the recommendations of the World Congress on Drowning will be very important for the final result. For this reason, the recommendations have been distributed, or will be distributed, to all major organisations involved worldwide (among which the WHO, IMO, IFRCRCS, ILS, ILF, DAN, ECOSA) with the request to study these recommendations, to select those that are important for their organisation, and to include the implementation of relevant recommendations in their action plans. In the coming years the *Maatschappij tot Redding van Drenkelingen* will again contact experts and other organisations to establish whether the initiative has generated new activities. Based on this evaluation, a new initiative may be taken in the future.

References

1. Bierens JJLM (1996) Drowning in the Netherlands. Pathophysiology, epidemiology and clinical studies. PhD thesis, Utrecht
2. Krug R (1999) Injury. A leading cause of the global burden of disease. WHO, Geneva
3. Idris AH, Berg RA, Bierens J, et al (2003) ILCOR advisory statement. Recommended guidelines for uniform reporting of data from drowning. The "Utstein style". Circulation 108:2565–2574; Resuscitation 59:45–57

 4. Maatschappij tot Redding van Drenkelingen (1999) Instructions for task force chairpersons and task force members. World Congress on Drowning, Amsterdam
 5. Maatschappij tot Redding van Drenkelingen (2003) Recommendations of the World Congress on Drowning. Maatschappij tot Redding van Drenkelingen, Amsterdam, www.drenkeling.nl
 6. http://www.asahq.org/Newsletters/2004/07_04/rovenLecture.html
 7. Baskett PJF (2001) Peter J. Safar, the early years 1924–1961, the birth of CPR. Resuscitation 50:17–22
 8. Baskett PJF (2002) Peter J. Safar. Part two. The University of Pittsburgh to the Safar Centre for Resuscitation Research 1961–2002. Resuscitation 55:3–7
 9. Bierens JJLM, Knape JTA, Gelissen HPMM (2002) Drowning. Curr Opin Crit Care 8:578–586
10. Gilchrist J (2004) Nonfatal and fatal drownings in recreational water settings. MMWR 53:447–452
11. WHO (2003) Facts about injuries: drowning. WHO, Geneva. www.who.int/violence_injury_prevention/
12. WHO (2003) Guidelines for safe recreational water environments. Volume 1. Coastal and fresh waters. WHO, Geneva
13. Brenner RA, Saluja G, Smith GS (2003) Swimming lessons, swimming ability, and the risk of drowning. Inj Control Saf Promot 10:211-216
14. Hyder AA, Arifeen S, Begum N, et al (2003) Death from drowning: defining a new challenge for child survival in Bangladesh. Inj Control Saf Promot 10:205-210
15. Michalsen A (2003) Risk assessment and perception. Inj Control Saf Promot 10:201-204
16. Norris B, Wilson JR (2003) Preventing drowning through design–the contribution of human factors. Inj Control Saf Promot 10:217-226
17. Peden MM, McGee K (2003) The epidemiology of drowning worldwide. Inj Control Saf Promot 10:195-199
18. Rogmans W, Wilson J (2003) Editorial to the special issue on drowning prevention. Inj Control Saf Promot 10:193-194
19. Scott I (2003) Prevention of drowning in home pools–lessons from Australia. Inj Control Saf Promot 10:227-236
20. Stoop JA (2003) Maritime accident investigation methodologies. Inj Control Saf Promot 10:237–242
21. Maatschappij tot Redding van Drenkelingen (2003/2004) Jaarverslagen 2002 en 2003. Maatschappij tot Redding van Drenkelingen, Amsterdam

The Epidemiology of Drowning

TASK FORCE ON THE EPIDEMIOLOGY OF DROWNING
Section editors: CHRISTINE BRANCHE and ED VAN BEECK

Members of the Task Force on the Epidemiology of Drowning would like to celebrate the life and contributions of our colleague, Ian J. Mackie, AM FRACP, National Medical Advisor to the Royal Lifesaving Society in Australia. At the time of his death in 2002, and just before the World Congress on Drowning, he had already made important contributions to our discussions and debates based on his considerable experience in the area of drowning prevention. Dr. Mackie forced us to ask ourselves difficult questions that required us to think broadly and yet within the realm of the scientific evidence, and always with a rich sense of whit. Our chapter is better because of his meaningful contributions.

Task Force Chairs

- Christine Branche
- Ed van Beeck

Task Force Members

- Olive Kobusingye
- John Langley
- Ian Mackie[1]
- Eleni Petridou
- Linda Quan
- Gordon Smith
- David Szpilman

Other Contributors

- Joost Bierens
- Alexandra Klimentopoulou
- Jennifer Lincoln
- Jerome Modell

This section consists of portions authored by different professionals, who were responsible for the content and accuracy of their material. The merging of these contributions into a single section was reviewed and accepted by all authors. The views represented are those of members of the Task Force on the Epidemiology of Drowning, but do not necessarily represent the official views of the Centers for Disease Control and Prevention of the US Department of Health and Human Services, or any other agency of the US Federal Government. This section was authored or co-authored by an employee of the US government and is considered to be in the public domain.

2.1
Overview

Christine Branche and Ed van Beeck

Drowning is a major cause of death, disability and lost quality of life. It is a leading cause of death among children globally [5]. With 449,000 drowning deaths worldwide in 2000, it is a significant public health problem. The global

---

[1] Dr. Ian Mackie died in 2001, after he completed his portion of the section, but before the World Congress on Drowning.

mortality rate for drowning is 8.4 per 100,000 population [5]. Furthermore in 2000 1.3 million disability adjusted life years (DALYs) were lost through premature death or disability due to drowning.

The first World Congress on Drowning (WCOD) in June 2002 provided a rare opportunity for world class experts on injury and drowning to bring their expertise to bear on risk factors that place populations at highest risk for drowning. This section, prepared first as a background document for the WCOD, has been edited to include information shared during the WCOD, including a new definition of drowning. Throughout this section, experts in the science of epidemiology examine key risk factors for drowning from a worldwide perspective.

The limited international data available on drowning provides interesting contrasts. Drowning rates are higher in low-income countries and in indigenous communities [1]. The average number of unintentional drowning deaths annually in the Netherlands, for example, is 0.6 per 100,000, occurring mostly among children under 4 years of age [2, 4]. In Thailand, in 1999, more than 3000 people drowned (5.0 per 100,000). In the UK, the drowning mortality rate is 0.5 per 100,000, but in the US in 1999 it was substantially higher at 1.3 per 100,000 [3].

Research indicates that age, gender, alcohol use, socioeconomic status (as measured by income and/or education) and location are key risk factors for drowning. Young children, teenagers and older adults are at highest risk of drowning. Drowning is one of the most frequent causes of death among children ages 5 through 14 years in both genders [5]. Moreover, drowning rates can be as much as five times higher among males compared to females, and this difference is evident in every year of life from childhood through older age. Alcohol is a well-documented risk factor for drowning, and receives ample discussion in the section. As many as half of all drownings are affected by alcohol use by the victim or caregiver. Drowning occurs more frequently among persons with lower income and lower levels of education [1].

Drownings occur in the ocean, in swimming pools, in bathtubs, and in village wells. The location of a drowning or type of body of water in which it occurs also plays an important role. For example, in Japan, bathtubs are the major source of accidental drownings, especially among young children and older adults. This is probably due to a combination of sociocultural factors, including the design of the Japanese baths, which are very deep, the Japanese habit of taking frequent baths of long duration, and their habit of using very hot water. The latter can lead to a large discrepancy in temperature with the ambient air and could provoke sudden death among older adults (Y. Sorimachi, personal communication).

In this section, in an effort to advance the field, the Task Force on the Epidemiology of Drowning proposes a new definition of drowning, together with the rationale, a description of the consensus process, and suggested research directions using this new definition. This new definition is needed for consistent worldwide data collection and to better document the burden of drowning as a global public health problem. Furthermore, the Task Force appeals for better and consistent data collection on drowning worldwide so that research and prevention programs can be improved globally. Dr. Quan describes methods for estimating the burden of drowning, starting with a description of frequency and rates, classification by intent, use of E-codes, injury severity measures, various outcomes to be measured and the importance of obtaining economic cost data. Dr. Mackie describes the availability of data and data quality needed to assess the global burden of drowning. Dr. Smith describes the epidemiology and global burden of drowning, including the relevance of contributions from the International Collaborative Effort (ICE) on injury statistics. Dr. Kobusingye discusses the specific problem of drowning on the African continent. Dr. Petridou describes a comprehensive list of risk factors for drowning including sociodemographic, environmental, and behavioural factors. Dr. Langley describes a general overview of drowning prevention strategies including lifeguards, pool fencing and personal flotation devices. The reader is encouraged to examine the sections 3, 4 and 5 of this handbook which provide considerably more discussion. Finally, Ms. Lincoln describes drownings in occupational settings, specifically those in the commercial fishing industry.

References

1. Barss P, Smith GS, Baker S, Mohan D (1998) Injury prevention: an international perspective. Epidemiology, surveillance and policy. Oxford University Press, New York, NY, pp 151–165
2. Bierens JJLM (1996) Drowning in the Netherlands: pathophysiology, epidemiology and clinical studies (PhD. thesis). Utrecht, The Netherlands
3. Centers for Disease Control and Prevention. Web-based Injury Statistics Query and Reporting System (WISQARS) [Online] (2002) National Center for Injury Prevention and Control, Centers for Disease Control and Prevention (producer). Available from: http://www.cdc.gov/ncipc/wisqars [Access date: March 2003]
4. Toet H (2003) Drowning in the Netherlands: a quantitative analysis. Final paper, World Congress on Drowning, Amsterdam, The Netherlands; 26–28 June 2002. Available from: http://www.drowning.nl
5. World Health Organization (1999) Bulletin report on "Injury: a leading cause of the global burden of disease". World Health Organization, Geneva, Switzerland

2.2
Recommendations

THE TASK FORCE ON THE EPIDEMIOLOGY OF DROWNING[2]

The recommendations listed here are drawn from portions of the section as offered by the authors or from the closing session of the World Congress on Drowning.
- It is recommended that all water safety and health organizations involved (including WHO which is responsible for the International Classification of

---

[2] Christine M. Branche, Ph.D., Ed van Beeck, M.D., Ph.D. (Co-Chairs); Olive Kobusingye, M.B.Ch.B, M.Med, MPH, John Langley, Ph.D., Ian Mackie, M.D., Eleni Petridou, M.D., M.P.H., Linda Quan, M.D., Gordon Smith, M.D., M.P.H., David Szpilman, M.D.

Diseases) adopt the new definition ('drowning is the process of experiencing respiratory impairment from submersion/immersion in liquid') and include it in their glossaries.

- Researchers are invited to use the new definition and to report on the advantages and disadvantages they observe in journal articles and editorials.
- Medical research on the classification and measurement of pathophysiological changes induced by drowning should be continued.
- Researchers and practitioners involved in drowning should become aware of general recommendations on the classification and measurement of disease and injury outcomes.
- It is suggested that aquatic incidents be separated from other injuries, and responsibility for preventive strategies be handed over to existing highly competent water safety authorities (and not to those responsible for national injury surveillance activities) in countries where these organisations exist.
- Four-sided isolation swimming pool fencing is an effective protective measure. The fence should meet certain construction criteria and should separate access to the pool from access to the house (private swimming pools) or any other facility (public swimming pools).
- Because alcohol consumption in water recreation activities predisposes to drowning, vigorous action should be taken. Advertisements that encourage alcohol use during boating should be eliminated. The availability of alcohol at water recreation facilities should also be restricted.
- Pool owners are advised to learn cardio-pulmonary resuscitation and keep a telephone nearby in case of an emergency. Caregivers should never leave a child unattended in order to attend to other things, such as answering the telephone.
- Early intervention by lifeguards can improve drowning outcome.
- The World Congress on Drowning has shown that in all parts of the world many people are interested in, knowledgeable about, and need resources for both scientific and practical efforts to advance drowning prevention. Therefore, it is recommended that the drowning website (www.drowning.nl) organised by the World Congress on Drowning be continued and extended with an e-mail service. Everyone involved is encouraged to send abstracts of their published and unpublished work on drowning to this website. By sharing these findings, contributing factors and effective control measures can be identified and region-specific actions can be initiated.
- The location of drowning is recognised as a key variable in identifying measures to prevent drowning in different cultures. During the World Congress on Drowning, it was shown that in most current data systems a variable on location of drowning is missing or underreported. An improvement is highly needed. Collecting data on the location of drowning is critical to better understanding the epidemiology of drowning and for addressing prevention.

2.3
Definition of Drowning

ED VAN BEECK, CHRISTINE BRANCHE, DAVID SZPILMAN,
JEROME MODELL and JOOST BIERENS

Drowning is the process of experiencing respiratory impairment from sub-mersion/immersion in liquid

2.3.1
Rationale

Drowning is a major, but often neglected, public health problem. At the end of the 1990s, the World Bank and WHO released the *Global Burden of Disease* study. It showed that, worldwide, drowning is one of the most important causes of death [8]. For many, this was an unexpected result. *The Lancet* published an editorial on this study, stating "further down the list come the real surprises: in 1990, suicides (786,000, no. 12) far outnumbered deaths from HIV infection (312,000, no. 30); *death by drowning* (504000, no. 20) was more common than death through war (502,000, no. 21)" [1].

The unfamiliar impact of drowning on public health is partly due to an enormous lack of sound epidemiological data globally in this field. Data collection for epidemiological purposes has been hampered by the lack of a uniform and internationally accepted definition, including all relevant cases to be counted. This means the inclusion of both fatal and non-fatal cases, because the latter may have a major impact on public health as well [7]. For drowning, sound epidemiological data on non-fatal cases and their consequences are even more scarce than on fatal cases. To start solving this problem, a simple but comprehensive definition is needed. Within the framework of the first World Congress on Drowning (WCOD), such a definition was developed in order to provide a common basis for future epidemiological studies in all parts of the world. It is our hope that such a definition will lead to a better and comprehensive understanding of the burden of drowning at the population level and its main determinants globally. In addition, the definition could be of value for those involved in prevention, rescue and treatment. A global, uniform definition and its inclusion criteria will assist in clinical studies as well.

2.3.2
Consensus Procedure

When the Task Force on the Epidemiology of Drowning was established in 1998 it was well recognised that important previous work on defining drowning and related topics had started almost thirty years earlier [4]. Over the last several decades this work has been of primary importance for improving our understanding of the pathophysiology of drowning and the medical treatment of non-fatal cases [6]. By 1971, the definitions were based on a thorough understanding of the biology of drowning and helped clinicians to classify victims for purposes of their evaluation and treatment. But as explained in the rationale, we were searching for a standard definition to serve epidemiological purposes. Therefore in 1999, one Task Force member, David Szpilman, was invited to write a discussion paper on the definition of drowning, which was released on the website of WCOD (www.drowning.nl).

This paper formed the basis of a consensus procedure aimed at the development of a new definition. Over the year 2000, the paper provoked a lively electronic discussion with contributions from Task Force members and other experts (input was received from Steve Beerman, Joost Bierens, Christine Branche, Chris Brewster, Anthony Handley, Olive Kobusingye, John Langley, Stephen Leahy, Ian Mackie, Jerome Modell, James Orlowski, Eleni Petridou, Linda Quan and Gordon Smith). Based on this discussion, the Task Force on the Epidemiology of Drowning released a revised discussion paper and a set of working definitions on the website. This paper was available from the beginning of 2002, during the months preceding the conference. At the conference, two discussion sessions were held under guidance of the chairwoman of the Task Force on Epidemiology of Drowning (Christine Branche). The input for these discussions was provided by the discussion paper and working definitions of the Task Force, and by proposals of three medical experts (Joost Bierens, Jerome Modell and David Szpilman). This procedure led to consensus and the adoption of the following definition by all conference attendees in June 2002:

> *Drowning is the process of experiencing respiratory impairment from sub-mersion/immersion in liquid*

The drowning process has been well described in Chapter 6.14 on "Utstein guidelines for uniform reporting of drowning research". A short summary of this process is: "The drowning process is a continuum beginning when the patient's airway is below the surface of the liquid, usually water. This induces a cascade of reflexes and pathophysiological changes, which, if uninterrupted, may lead to death, primarily due to tissue hypoxia. A patient can be rescued at any time during the process and given appropriate resuscitative measures in which case, the process is interrupted". Impairment of the respiratory system is secondary to laryngospasm and/or aspiration of water and the consequences thereof. According to Webster's dictionary, submersion is 'to plunge under the surface of water' and immersion is described as 'to plunge or dip especially into a fluid' [3]. In any case, this definition of drowning applies when the entrance of the airway is under water, precluding the breathing of air.

In the literature, an initial lack of consensus was observed with respect to the definitions and terminology used by different water safety and health organisations, experts in the field, papers in the scientific medical literature and lay-persons. From the short description of the consensus procedure and from the new definition itself, the impression may be that this was a rather simple and straightforward process. However, it was not. This was due to the complexity of the problem. Drowning is a heterogeneous process with large variation in underlying causes, pathophysiologic changes and possible outcomes. It is characterised by a chain of events, with different experts with different perspectives involved in different parts of the chain. Therefore, reconciliation of expertise and opinions required a meticulous consensus procedure. The complexity of defining drowning is fully addressed in the final paper on this issue currently available on the drowning website [10]. This paper provides an overview of the pros and cons of inclusion and exclusion of several specific elements [10]. In this section we only provide a short summary of two main lines of the discussion: the suitability of existing definitions for epidemiological purposes and the major requirements for a new definition.

2.3.3
Suitability of Existing Definitions

Over the past decades it has been customary to use separate definitions for fatal (called *drowning*) and non-fatal cases (called *near-drowning*) respectively, and to make a further distinction between cases with or without aspiration. Modell proposed a definition in 1971 [4] and slight modifications in 1981 [5], which led to the following terminology:

- Drown(ing) without aspiration: to die from respiratory obstruction and asphyxia while submerged in a fluid medium
- Drown(ing) with aspiration: to die from the combined effects of asphyxia and changes secondary to aspiration of fluid while submerged
- Near-drown(ing) without aspiration: to survive, at least temporarily, following asphyxia due to submersion in a fluid medium
- Near-drown(ing) with aspiration: to survive, at least temporarily, following aspiration of fluid while submerged

In the past, also the terms 'dry' versus 'wet' drowning were used, but there is consensus that these terms should be abandoned.

The existing definitions were judged as difficult to use in empirical research, because they mix characteristics of the event (for example, submersion) with the pathophysiological changes (for example, asphyxia) and the outcome (for example, death). Moreover, previous attempts to describe the major characteristic of drowning by terms like 'suffocation', 'asphyxia' or 'liquid aspiration', were shown to lack both sensitivity and specificity [9]. During the consensus procedure, the pros and cons of having separate definitions for fatal and non-fatal cases were intensively debated. We concluded that an outcome classification (drowning = death, near-drowning = survival) being part of the case definition is not in accordance with the internationally accepted Utstein style, which was developed to provide a common language and terminology for investigators from different specialities [2]. Moreover, it is different from what is customary with respect to other medical conditions. It was also recognised, that the use of two separate definitions may lead to a continued underestimation of the problem. A major example is the Global Burden of Disease study [7], which completely neglected the impact of non-fatal drowning cases.

2.3.4
Major Requirements for a New Definition

A list of requirements was put forward, which formed the basis of the new definition. We agreed that the definition should be simple, inclusive (including all relevant cases) and specific (excluding irrelevant cases). Furthermore, we wanted the terminology to be in accordance with the Utstein style and other medical conditions. Therefore, the definition should not be confused with systems to describe the aetiology or to classify the outcome of the drowning process. The definition should assure that all patients have some important and preferably unique characteristic in common. We agreed that an acceptable definition meeting these requirements is: 'respiratory impairment induced by submersion/immersion in liquid'. Our intention is that the definition should include cases of drowning from all kinds of liquid aspiration, except body fluids (vomits, saliva, milk and amniotic fluid). We intend for the definition to exclude a water rescue case (these are all submersion/immersion events where no respiratory impairment is evident, whether with or without other injury, such as cervical spine injury). Furthermore, we intend for outcomes to classified as death, morbidity and no morbidity, but invite further discussion and debate in the scientific community to develop a severity classification scheme for morbidity (also, please see ▶ **Chapter 7.11** for more discussion on the topic of classifying drowning morbidity). Finally, we sought to eliminate confusing terms, like 'dry' versus 'wet' drowning. Another confusion arises from using the terms 'active' drowning and 'passive' drowning, which more than likely represent witnessed and unwitnessed drowning, respectively.

2.3.5
Use of the Definition and Research

Based on an analysis of problems with existing definitions, a list of requirements and with major input from several experts, the Task Force on the Epidemiology of Drowning has come up with a new definition. We expect this definition will support future activities in worldwide drowning research in order to gain better and comprehensive knowledge of this too often neglected public health problem. We recognise that our new definition will need to prove its value in epidemiological research and public health practice. Given that our definition accommodates both fatal and nonfatal events, we understand also that a classification scheme is needed to capture the scope of morbidity. Only from worldwide implementation can we determine whether the new definition is actually better suited for epidemiological purposes and whether the major requirements listed are met. Therefore it is recommended that all water safety and health organisations involved adopt the new definition and include it in their glossaries. WHO, which is responsible for the International Classification of Diseases, has already adopted the new definition [11]. Researchers are invited to use the new definition and to report on the advantages and disadvantages they observe in journal articles and editorials. In addition, medical research on the classification and measurement of pathophysiological changes induced by drowning should be continued. Finally, researchers and practitioners involved in drowning should become aware of general recommendations on the classification and measurement of disease and injury outcomes.

References

1. Anonymous (1997) From what will we die in 2020? Lancet 349:1263
2. Cummins RO (1993) The Utstein-style for uniform reporting of data from out of hospital cardiac arrest. Ann Emerg Med 22:37–40
3. Merriam Webster (1995) The Merriam Webster dictionary on CD ROM. Zane, Dallas, TX
4. Modell JH (1971) Pathophysiology and treatment of drowning and near-drowning. Charles C. Thomas, Springfield, IL, pp 8–9
5. Modell JH (1981) Drown versus near-drown: discussion of definitions. Crit Care Med 9:351–352
6. Modell JH (1993) Drowning: current concepts. N Engl J Med 328:253–256
7. Murray CJL (1994) Quantifying the burden of disease: the technical basis for disability-adjusted life years. Bull World Health Organ 72:429–445
8. Murray CJL, Lopez A (1997) Mortality by cause for eight regions of the world: global burden of disease study. Lancet 349:1269–1276
9. Szpilman D (1997) Near-drowning and drowning classification: A proposal to stratify mortality based on the analysis of 1831 cases. Chest 112:660–665
10 Szpilman D. Definition of drowning and water-related injuries. Final paper, World Congress on Drowning, Amsterdam, The Netherlands; June 26-28, 2002 [cited January 2003]. Available from: URL: www.drowning.nl.
11. World Health Organization (2003) Facts about injuries: drowning. World Health Organization, Geneva, Switzerland

2.4
Methods for Estimating the Burden of Drowning

Linda Quan

Drowning is a series of multifaceted and complex events that vary widely based on age and location of occurrence. Assessing the burden of drowning requires careful consideration of a number of elements [2]. As interest in and investigation of drowning injury increase, it is critical for us to count and classify them so that the magnitude of the problem can be quantified, compared over time or among regions, and tracked as interventions or emerging hazards develop. Only through use of classification systems and rigorous evaluation will we be able to identify the effects of prevention measures on the burden of drowning.

At the World Congress on Drowning, a panel agreed to define drowning as the process of experiencing respiratory impairment from submersion in a liquid medium, thereby precluding ventilation and oxygenation. Drowning victims either drown, that is die, or they survive with or without morbidity.

2.4.1
Frequency and Rates

Counting the number of drownings is the starting point for describing the burden of injury. Drowning victims usually have been ascertained as persons who seek medical care or die following their submersion. However, the lifeguarding industry measures rescues [11]. Perhaps rescues represent the real drowning population since their airway was perceived at risk. Because the number of rescues is likely to be much larger than the number of hospitalised or dead drowning victims the population of rescues might provide better statistical opportunities for testing the effectiveness of interventions. The real difficulty here is that the number of rescues is very difficult to capture.

Numbers provide more useful information when converted to a rate. The denominator for the rate can be any population or subpopulation, such as age, sex, or region, for which a number is known. Rates for survivors and deaths vary considerably amongst different age groups and by gender [12]. Drowning death rates are the most easily obtained and reported measure of drowning injury because deaths are usually reported by medical personnel and validated. Injury rates are more difficult to obtain as drowning survivors are more difficult to find. A complete assessment of drowning injury needs to include emergency department (ED) visits as well as hospitalisations.

It might be more useful to calculate drowning injury rates based on exposure to water related activities, such as number of drownings per hours of boating rather than per numbers of boaters or general population. However, these denominators are usually unavailable.

Defining and counting the numerator, such as number of drowning deaths, is not always straightforward. Counting deaths requires committing to one cause or etiologic mechanism for the death. For example, if a person drives into a river and drowns, the mechanism could be classified as either a drowning or traffic crash. One way to deal with this is to use multiple-cause of death files. The International Classification of Diseases, 10th Revision (ICD-10) helps to reconcile quality of determination of cause across countries, but variations by region or country exist [14]. With most drownings, the cause or mechanism of death is usually obvious. However, in some situations the mechanism may not be clear. Difficulty in classifying tends to occur in adults who have pre-existing medical conditions that have the potential to cause sudden death or altered mental states, and leave no obvious sign at autopsy. Some victims may have new cardiac arrhythmias from previously undetected causes. Recently described persons with prolonged QT syndrome have a congenital condition characterised by syncopal episodes caused by cardiac arrhythmias. The first evidence of their condition may be a drowning event [1]. In the future, genetic testing may help to identify this small subset of etiologic mechanisms for drowning. Ideally, a medical history of the victim, autopsy, and scene investigation are needed to make the best determination of causation and classification. Sometimes, the final determination of cause of death is subjective even when all information is available.

The following classification systems indicate ways by which to identify subgroups of drowning victims for a numerator. These classifications are described below with regard to the host (drowning victim), the agent (water), the environment and the event.

2.4.2
Classification

Drowning may be classified by intent: unintentional versus intentional (violence-related) which includes assault, homicide, child abuse or suicide. The majority of drownings are unintentional ('accidental'). Intent may be difficult to determine. The outcome of intentional drowning may be worse than that of unintentional drowning. A not infrequent dilemma occurs when an adolescent or adult swimming alone drowns: Was it unintentional or a suicide? 'Undetermined drowning' is a third category of intent used by medical examiners when it is unclear if the injury was unintentional or purposely inflicted. While medical examiners and coroners misclassify, the amount of misclassification is difficult to confirm. Emergency department and hospital personnel contribute to misclassification by failing to consider or recognise intentional injury, that is, child abuse. Yet, several studies have identified characteristics of drowning that are abuse related [6].

The ICD-9 Supplementary Classification of External Causes of Injury and Poisoning (E-Codes), in use from 1975–1998, was developed to classify intent and circumstances around injury and poisoning [13]. Thirty E-codes were developed to identify drownings involving boats and occupational injury; ten codes were developed to identify accident to watercraft causing drowning; and another ten codes for drowning involving water transport. ICD-9 codes for drowning facilitate the identification of bathtub. They do not specifically identify open water sites such as lakes, rivers, or oceans, the most common drowning site for older children adolescents and adults. While they permit identification of some recreational activities such as boating, water skiing, swimming, and diving, other sports are lumped into one code, 910.2. Swimming pool drownings are combined with 'not otherwise specified' (910.8), even though swimming pools are the most common site for drownings involving children under 5 years of age in the US. These codes specify intent and sometimes include activity with body of water; unfortunately, however, they are not complete. In 1992, the World Health Organization (WHO) revised these codes, creating ICD-10 [14] but full adoption of ICD-10 coding did not occur worldwide until later in the decade. ICD-10 does a better job of allowing identification of the type of location, the body of water involved, including open water, type of boat involved (for example, kayak, inflatable) and pre-drowning activity (for example sport, leisure, work-related). It also identifies drownings resulting from a fall into the major bodies of water as separate from drownings unrelated to falling into these bodies of water. While drowning codes for ICD-10 are an improvement over those for ICD-9, ICD-10 does not identify drownings related to motor vehicles, water skiing, diving, and swimming [8].

2.4.3
Severity of Injury

Drowning statistics usually focus on victims who use medical resources. In addition to deaths, hospitalised patients represent a severely injured group of patients. In the US, identification of patients hospitalised for drowning injury has been made easy with the development of hospital discharge registries. Upon discharge, patient records are assigned ICD-9CM codes, a system of classification of diagnoses or nature of injury or disease. The ICD-9CM code for drowning, 994.1, includes 'drowning and nonfatal drowning' [10].

In addition to ED use, many drowning victims receive initial medical care from emergency medical systems where these systems exist. Some patients never seek ED care after receiving prehospital care. As prehospital care expands its scope as an arm of hospital or a health care system, it may decrease utilisation of emergency departments. Most EMS systems maintain data sets that identify drowning and increasingly, these datasets are computerised. Thus more data will be available in the future.

2.4.4
Initial Mental Status

Severity of injury is best measured clinically. The most powerful predictor of outcome is the mental status of the drowning victim following rescue [7]. Subsequent studies show that the longer delayed the response to resuscitation or rescue, the worse the prognosis. All studies show that alertness at the scene or on arrival in the hospital predicts a good outcome [3, 7].

2.4.5
Outcome

A critical method to assess the burden of drowning injury is to determine outcome. Classification of outcome can be death, survival, and quality of survival. Most of the medical literature on paediatric drowning injury has focused on outcome and noted the extraordinary bimodal distribution: death and survival with normal function at hospital discharge.

Years of potential life lost (YPLL) is one measure that is useful in assessing the burden of mortality [5]. Drowning, like injury in general, is a major contributor to years of potential life lost because it kills young children so frequently.

There are categorisation schemes for measuring non-fatal health outcomes that are applicable to drowning [9]. These classification systems have focused on health-related quality of life, which address opportunity, health perceptions, functional states, and impairments. In 1980, the WHO developed the International Classification of Impairments, Disabilities and Handicaps, a classification system for the consequences of disease, including impairment and disability. Quality-adjusted life years (QALYS) is a measure of life and health after an injury. It measures the number of years of life remaining after the injury multiplied by a weight of the quality of life during each year of life. Specific paediatric tools exist for the evaluation of children who represent the majority of drowning survivors. Disability adjusted life years (DALY) measures were developed to assess the consequences of premature death, while also quantifying economic and social morbidity (for example, severity of disability in activities of daily living). The DALY is the sum of years of life lost and years lived with disability, adjusted for the severity of disability. The measurement is simple to calculate using a formula and life expectancy tables.

2.4.6
Costs

Economic measures of morbidity help to describe the burden of injury. Death does not measure the burden of this injury that is borne by governments and all of society. Direct costs of acute medical care costs can be estimated if they are not readily available. Charges for hospitalisation have been measured for drownings, but it generally does not include all the costs of hospitalisation, such as the fees for physicians, and is limited to acute care [4]. Direct and indirect costs incurred by the family of a drowning victim or survivor should be measured because the impact on families can be enormous with depression, divorce, job loss, all having economic effects. Direct charges for long-term care, measures of loss of productivity and other indirect costs should be included as well in order to have a full sense of the impact of drowning.

References

1. Ackerman MJ, Tester DJ, Porter CJ (1999) Swimming, a gene-specific arrhythmogenic trigger for inherited long QT syndrome. Mayo Clin Proc 74:1088–1094
2. Bonnie R, Fulco C, Liverman C (1999) Reducing the burden of injury. Institute of Medicine. National Academy Press, Washington, DC
3. Conn AW, Montes JE (1980) Cerebral salvage in near-drowning following neurological classification by triage. Can Anaesth Soc J 27:201–210
4. Ellis AA, Trent RB (1995) Hospitalizations for near drowning in California: incidence and costs. Am J Public Health 85:1115–1118
5. Gardner JW, Sanborn JS (1990) Years of potential life lost (YPLL) – what does it measure? Epidemiology 1:322–329
6. Gillenwater JM, Quan L, Feldman KW (1996) Inflicted submersion in childhood. Arch Pediatr Adolesc Med 150:298–303
7. Graf WD, Cummings P, Quan L, Brutocao D (1995) Predicting outcome of pediatric submersion victims. Ann Emerg Med 26:312–319
8. Langley JD, Chalmers DJ (1999) Coding the circumstances of injury: ICD-10 a step forward or backwards? Inj Prev 5:247–253
9. Murray C, Lopez A (1996) The Global burden of disease: a comprehensive assessment of mortality and disability from diseases, injuries and risk factors in 1990 and projected to 2020. Global Burden of Disease and Injury Series. Harvard School of Public Health, Boston, MA

10. National Center for Health Statistics (1991) International classification of diseases, clinical modi-
    fication, 9th revision. U.S. Department of Health and Human Services, Washington, DC, PHS
    91-1260
11. Priest E (1999) Drowning in a closed-water environment: lessons that can be learned. CRC Press,
    Boca Raton, FL
12. Quan L, Cummings P (2004) Characteristics of drowning according to victim's age. Injury Pre-
    vention (in press)
13. World Health Organization (1977) International statistical classification of diseases and related
    health problems – 9th revision. WHO, Geneva, Switzerland
14. World Health Organization (1992) International statistical classification of diseases and related
    health problems – 10th revision. WHO, Geneva, Switzerland

2.5
Availability and Quality of Data
to Assess the Global Burden of Drowning

IAN MACKIE[3]

Between 1921 and 1938, the League of Nations provided limited epidemiological
information. In 1955 K.W. Donald, writing for the British Medical Journal, could
find only five clinical reports of drowning in the medical literature. Today, there
are abundant sources of information on drowning. The emphasis has moved
from clinical reporting to resuscitation on to pathophysiology and clinical
management in hospitals, but since 1975 the epidemiological aspects have
dominated the literature. Data for water-related injuries are relatively sparse,
but are sorely needed.

The major purpose of collecting epidemiological data is to create and follow
the effectiveness of preventive strategies, which include education, engineering,
legislation and enforcement. There are so many varying locations and risk
factors for drowning that reporting will never be simple. Water-related injuries
similarly are extremely varied and change regularly as different types of craft
become available in different countries. ICD-9 and ICD-10 E-codes do not
identify all drowning-related deaths, and high quality collection of all water-
related incidents now requires complex and difficult examination of details from
many sources, including records from coroners and medical examiners, police,
water safety organisations and other sources, even newspapers. This must be
improved.

Several authors have expressed dissatisfaction with the present reporting
formats, which clearly require revision. These are notably Smith and Langley [3]
and Barss et al. [1]. In many less affluent countries, no details are available and
the world's most populous countries have supplied almost no information on
water-related mortality and morbidity to the World Health Organization (WHO)
or to peer-reviewed scientific journals. Most reports in the literature are regional
and not national. The most recent Australian report, however, is one of very few

---

[3] Dr. Ian Mackie died in 2001, after he completed his portion of the section, but before the World
    Congress on Drowning. His dedication to aquatic life safety was an inspiration to us all.

national reports to include all drownings, including those which are not covered by the E-codes [2].

As it concerns prevention, however, regional reports are of great value. For example, many states and counties in the US have reported their patterns of drowning, and these vary greatly from area to area. This fact reveals a further difficulty in creating a uniform coding and reporting mechanism that would be useful for national and international comparison. For example, drownings in cold climates such as Canada differ greatly from warmer countries like Australia whose data are also well documented. Much of the world literature on drowning is published from Canada, the US, and Australia. All of these countries report a decline in the incidence of unintentional drowning over the past century. Sweden and Italy have provided similar details, however, there is no indication of where or how the drownings occurred.

Toddler (ages 1 through 4 years) drowning is, undoubtedly, the best reported of all aquatic problems and dominates the literature. It is certain that toddlers die in many different locations depending on affluence, geography and other factors. In the larger cities of high income countries, the data vary from suburb to suburb. The developing countries have few if any private swimming pools, so most of their toddler drownings occur in natural waterways or in irrigation canals. This was reported from Sri Lanka in the mid 1970s.

Well-documented risk factors for drowning include age, sex, alcohol, race, epilepsy, heart and cerebral disease, type of activity, accessibility of water, climate, hypothermia, lifeguard services, types of watercraft used and degree of affluence. Some of these risk factors have been elegantly described in the scientific literature, but many, including swimming ability and availability of swimming lessons have not. Furthermore, effectiveness of legislation and enforcement require much more research. There is emerging evidence that ocean drowning is more likely in persons who live inland or who are tourists, but more details are required. Bathtub drownings have been highlighted in many reports, and some nations such as Japan have very high rates. Reasons and factors are not well reported.

In the case of suicide by drowning, most published data describe suicide alone, and usually make no comparison with other types of aquatic death in the same geographic area. Nor do they describe suicide by other methods. Most western countries report an increase in suicide rates over the past several decades, but no reports on aquatic suicides year by year are available. Clearly more research is required.

In the past decade, reports on drowning incidents in some low income countries have begun to appear in the peer-reviewed scientific journals and to come to the attention of the WHO. These drownings are universally alarming and may underestimate the real situation. The absence of agreed upon definitions of the terms 'drowning' and 'near drowning' contributes to some extent to the problem of comparing statistics as different countries use their own definitions (see ▶ Chapter 2.3). There is a strong case for those national organisations which report drownings to change their structures. Drowning and water-related injuries are incorporated into national injury surveillance departments in which the aquatic environment is usually one relatively small section. It is suggested that aquatic incidents be separated from other injuries, and responsibility for preventive strategies be handed over to existing highly competent water safety authorities in countries where these organisations exist. Many of these authorities are very strong with great expertise. Most are members of the International Lifesaving Federation (ILS).

References

1. Barss P, Smith GS, Baker S, Mohan D (1998) Injury prevention: an international perspective. Epidemiology, surveillance and policy. Oxford University Press, New York, NY
2. Mackie I (1999) Patterns of drowning in Australia, 1992 to 1997. Med J Aust 171:587–590
3. Smith GS, Langley JD (1998) Drowning surveillance: how well do E-codes identify submersion fatalities. Injury Prevention 4:135–139

2.6
The Global Burden of Drowning

2.6.1
The Global Burden of Drowning

GORDON SMITH

Drownings are an important cause of injury deaths in many countries [2, 11]. In the US, for example, drowning is the third leading cause of unintentional deaths in ages 0–4 and second for 5- to 14-year-olds. Similarly, internationally drownings are an important cause of death in many countries, although the rates vary widely from a high of 13.9 per 100,000 population in Russia, for example, to as low as 0.5 per 100,000 population in the UK (◘ Fig. 2.1). In children under age 5 years, the pattern is a little different where in addition to Russia; rates are high in Australia, US, Japan and New Zealand (◘ Fig. 2.2).

Drownings occur from a wide variety of activities depending on the country. There are two very different age groups for drowning in terms of circumstances and where they occur. Young children 0–4 years of age generally drown in bathtubs, wells, swimming pools and other bodies of water close to the home. In the age group of teenagers and adults natural bodies of water are the most common sites [2]. In general, drowning rates are higher in less developed countries and in indigenous communities such as Native Americans in the US.

In many countries, drowning ranks second to traffic injuries as a cause of unintentional injuries, especially among young and adult males. Drowning is the leading cause of unintentional injury deaths in rural areas of countries such as Sri Lanka, China and Bangladesh [2]. In some areas of Bangladesh and South China, for example, drowning is the leading cause of death among toddler-aged children. Drowning rates as high as 215 per 100,000 population have been reported in rural Bangladesh for children aged 1–4 years and 546 per 100,000 in 1-year-old males. This is due to the frequent flooding and proximity of water to the home environment. Even among adults in Bangladesh, drowning

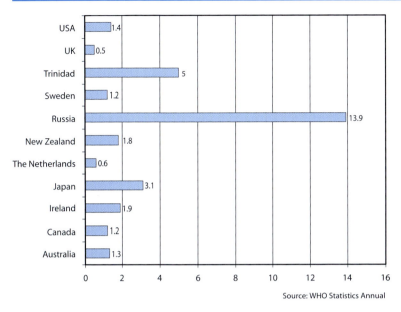

■ **Fig. 2.1.** Accidental drowning rates per 100,000 population (all ages), by country (1995)

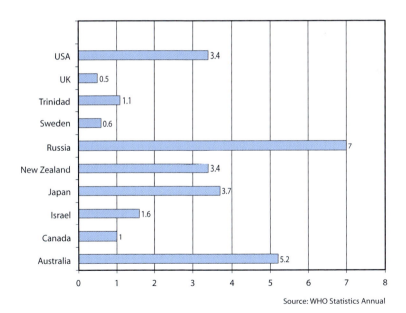

■ **Fig. 2.2.** Accidental drowning rates per 100,000 children aged 1–4 years, by country (1995)

is an important cause of death with drowning accounting for one-third of all unintentional injury deaths for women of childbearing age (15–44 years) [5]. Drowning is the third leading cause of injury death in China [7] and rates are much higher than in countries such as the US and UK. For example, rates in the US for males ages 1–4 years are seven times higher than in China and ten times higher among females. Rates are more similar in young adults but rise much more rapidly in the elderly in China, probably reflecting their high exposure to water hazards in rural areas of that country.

A study in the Highlands of Papua New Guinea, from 1971–1986 found a drowning rate of 17 per 100,000 among adult males. When overall drowning rates were age-adjusted and compared to those in Sweden, drowning rates for males were 37 times higher in Bangladesh and 20 times higher in Papua New Guinea [2]. Another study in Jalisco State, Mexico, found the highest drowning rates in ages 1–4 years (7.6/100,000) and 15–24 years of age (5.0 per 100,000) [4]. Comparable rates over a similar time period (1980–1986) for the US are 6.0 per 100,000 population for males under 5 years of age and 6.2 for males 15–24 years [1]. Russia is another country where drowning rates appear much higher. In fact as shown in ◘ Fig. 2.1, the official reported drowning rate is 13.9 per 100,000 population, almost 10 times that in the US, and 28 times that in the UK. One report in the *New York Times* [15] strongly suggests that alcohol is an important factor that contributes to the high drowning rate in Russia. From May 1 to June 21, 1999, 144 swimmers drowned in Moscow and 94% of these were recorded as 'drunk when they drowned'. Alcohol is known to greatly increase the risk of dying in aquatic environments [10]. Indepth studies of alcohol involvement in drowning are currently underway in one region of Russia. Preliminary results from a detailed review of records of medical examiners confirm that most adult drowning victims have a high blood alcohol concentration.

Much of our understanding of drowning in individual countries has come from special in-depth studies of mortality such as those discussed above. However, as discussed by Dr. Kobusingye below (► see Chapter 2.6.2), drowning data from most low-income countries are not available. In addition, because most drownings occur well before medical treatment is provided, they are much less likely to be reported by hospital-based data systems, including death registration. Most statistics underreport the true burden of drowning, especially in lowincome countries.

In comparing drowning deaths between countries, it is important to consider the definitions used. Boat-related drownings are excluded from most analyses as they are not reported separately by the World Health Organization (WHO), but listed under other transport deaths. For example, in Canada, boating deaths comprise 40% of all drownings and about 20% in the US [2]. A further reason drownings may be underestimated is that drownings resulting from floods and natural disasters are not coded as drownings, but coded as natural disasters. In some countries, tidal waves and massive floods can be a major cause of drowning mortality. Under the WHO ICD-9 rules, these would be coded as deaths due to natural and environmental causes and not be counted as drownings in official statistics. Drownings are also an important method of suicide in some countries and can also be a method of homicide [11]. In addition, some of the deaths due to undetermined intent can be due to drownings, further increasing the likelihood that the true burden of drownings will be under-represented [13]. One of the big deficiencies in current drowning data is that little information is available on the place of drowning, as ICD-9 does not identify the place except for bathtubs [9]. With the increasing implementation of ICD-10, such data should become available as it identifies bathtubs, swimming pools and natural bodies of water with specific codes.

As shown in ◘ Fig. 2.1, drowning rates vary widely by country for a sample of those countries reporting to WHO. These drownings are for accidental drownings coded as E910 only, and exclude boating, suicide, homicide, and other drownings discussed above. In an effort to better understand how important these other causes of drownings are, a series of studies were conducted under the auspices of the International Collaborative Effort (ICE) on Injury Statistics. The ICE on Injury Statistics is one of several international activities sponsored by the National Center for Health Statistics, Centers for Disease Control and Prevention, and seeks to improve the international comparability and quality of injury data. The ultimate goal is to provide the data needed to better understand the causes of injury and the most effective means of prevention. The WET ICE Collaborative Group, in an effort to better understand how drownings are coded in high-income countries, is conducting a series of studies in order to allow more valid comparisons and estimate the true burden of drowning [6, 12, 14]. More details on both ICE and the WET ICE on drowning can be found at http://www.cdc.gov/nchs/advice.htm.

While a number of studies have identified wide variations in injury rates between countries [8], it is not known if these variations are due to real differences in incidence or due, in part, to differences in coding practices for injury deaths [6, 13]. As part of the ICE on Injury Statistics, the WET ICE Collaborative Group has been using drownings as a sentinel, or tracer, condition to examine in detail the differences in injury rates in order to uncover potential problems, and differences in coding injury deaths between countries. While unintentional or 'accidental' drowning deaths were found to vary widely between countries, when drownings are examined with the matrix developed to examine injuries regardless of intent (ICD-9 Framework for Presenting Injury Mortality Data (available at http://www.cdc.gov/nchs/about/otheract/ice/matrix.htm), there was much less variation in overall drowning rates suggesting big differences in coding intent by country, rather than true differences in the drowning rates. For example, 40% of all drownings in England and Wales were coded as undetermined intent (E984), while only 5% were so coded in the US and New Zealand, and only 1% in Israel [14].

Injuries, including drownings, may also have multiple causes that are not adequately described by single underlying causes of death [14]. Multiple cause of death coding records all conditions listed on the death certificate. Many drowning deaths for example may be coded as due to other causes such as transportation, or falls. One study in New Zealand found that 17.6% of all drownings were missed as they were coded with other injuries as the underlying cause [11]. In addition, disease conditions may be coded as the underlying cause. Free text searches for the word 'drown' were used to identify multiple cause drownings in New Zealand. The traditional drowning E-codes do not identify all drownings as defined by the nature of injury codes for drowning (N991.4) or by free text search. E-codes only identified 82.4% of drownings in New Zealand and 94.0% in England. In England, 35.5% of drownings were of undetermined intent (E984) while in most other countries it was less than 5%, although in Denmark it was 12.8%. Motor vehicle traffic deaths comprise 11.4% of drownings in New Zealand but only 0.9% in Denmark. Only a small percentage of the drowning N-code deaths were coded with disease as the underlying cause. These range from 5.5% in England and Wales, to only 1.9% in the US, and 4.9% in New Zealand.

Death certificates often include medical diagnoses with the drowning deaths. For all drownings, medical conditions were the underlying cause of death for 1.9% of drownings in the US, 2.4% in Canada, 5.5% in England and Wales, and 4.9% of drownings in New Zealand. Heart disease was the underlying cause of 0.8% of drownings in the US, 0.7% in Canada, 0.4% in England and Wales and 1.1% in New Zealand. The WHO coding rules for epilepsy mentioned earlier results in considerable variation in the proportion of drownings coded with epilepsy as the underlying cause: US (0.7%), Canada (1.4%), England and Wales (4.8%) and New Zealand (1.1%).

The multiple cause of death data provide a valuable opportunity to identify all deaths due to drowning, not just those coded using standard ICD codes. The wide variation in the proportion of all drownings coded to the various underlying cause categories suggests that some of the wide variation in drowning rates between countries may, in fact, be due to differences in coding practices. Accidental drowning rates (E910) are low in England but 36% of drownings are of undetermined intent, much higher than for other countries. Even among injury deaths, the proportion of drownings classified as other causes indicate that many drowning deaths are missed by traditional E-codes. In addition, there are wide variations in selecting drowning as the underlying cause. Thus, official statistics undercount the true burden of drowning in most countries.

While differences in coding are important in understanding the burden of drowning, perhaps the most important issue in comparing drowning rates between countries is their exposure to water. This may change by area and over time [3, 8, 9]. For example, the US has experienced dramatic declines in drowning over time. While the exact causes are poorly understood, it has been suggested that this is not due necessarily to improved health care or prevention strategies, but maybe because adolescents and adults are now less active than in the past and spend less time on physical activity outdoors, thus reducing exposure to hazardous bodies of water [9].

References

1. Baker SP, O'Neill B, Ginsburg MJ, Li G (1992) The injury fact book, 2nd edn. Oxford University Press, New York
2. Barss P, Smith GS, Baker S, Mohan D (1998) Injury prevention: an international perspective. Epidemiology, surveillance and policy. Oxford University Press, New York
3. Brenner RA, Smith GS, Overpeck MD (1994) Divergent trends in childhood drowning rates, 1971 through 1988. J Am Med Assoc 271:1606–1608
4. Celis A (1991) Asfixia por inmersion en Jalisco: 1983–89. Salud Pub Mex 33:585–589

5. Fauveau U, Blanchet T (1989) Deaths from injuries and induced abortion among rural Bangla-deshi women. Soc Sci Med 29:1121–1127
6. Langlois JA, Smith GS, Baker SP, Langley J (1995) International comparisons of injury mortality in the elderly: issues and differences between New Zealand and the United States. Int J Epidemiol 24:136–143
7. Li GH, Baker SP (1991) A comparison of injury death rates in China and the United States, 1986. Am J Public Health 81:605–609
8. Smith GS, Brenner RA (1995) The changing risks of drowning for adolescents in the U.S. and effective control strategies. Adolesc Med 6:153–170
9. Smith GS, Howland JH (1999) Declines in drowning: exploring the epidemiology of favorable trends. JAMA 281:2245–2247
10. Smith GS, Keyl PM, Hadley JA, et al. (2001) Drinking and recreational boating fatalities: a population-based case-control study. JAMA 286:2974–2980
11. Smith GS, Langley JD (1998) Drowning surveillance: how well do E-codes identify submersion fatalities. Injury Prevention 4:135–139
12. Smith GS, Langlois JA, Rockett IRH (1995) International comparisons of injury mortality: hypothesis generation, ecological studies, and some data problems. In: Proceedings of the International Collaborative Effort on Injury Statistics, vol 1. National Center for Health Statistics, Hyattsville, Maryland. DHHS Publication No. (PHS) 95-1252:13:1-15. Available from: URL: http://www.cdc.gov/nchs/data/ice/ice95v1/ice_i.pdf
13. Smith GS and the WET ICE Collaborative Group (1996) International comparisons of injury mortality databases: evaluation of their usefulness for drowning prevention and surveillance. In: Proceedings of the International Collaborative Effort on Injury Statistics, vol II. Melbourne Meeting: Working Papers, Melbourne, Australia. Hyattsville, Maryland: Public Health Service, Centers for Disease Control and Prevention, National Center for Health Statistics; 1996. DHHS Publication No. (PHS) 96-1252:6:1-29. Available from: URL: http://www.cdc.gov/nchs/data/ice/ice95v2/c06.pdf
14. Smith GS (2000) International comparisons of drowning mortality: the value of multiple cause data, Chap. 20. In: Proceedings of the International Collaborative Effort on Injury Statistics, vol III, 1999. Washington DC (2nd Symposium), 2000. Available from: URL: http://www.cdc.gov/nchs/about/otheract/ice/pro-iii.htm
15. Wines M (1999) Vodka and water, a deadly mix. New York Times 4 July 1999

2.6.2
The Global Burden of Drowning: An African Perspective

Olive Kobusingye

Africa still has a huge burden of disease from infectious diseases, and non-communicable diseases are often not included in routine disease surveillance. Most African countries also lack emergency pre-hospital services, and have poor access to quality acute care at health facilities. In these conditions, patients that might have survived following a drowning incident die due to lack of prompt and appropriate care. Health facility-based surveillance never includes these deaths, as they never made it to a health facility in the first place. Also, not all deaths are certified by medically qualified people. Depending on the country and the specific local circumstances, these fatalities might appear in police mortuaries, community and other vital statistics reports, or will not be recorded anywhere. Data on drowning in Africa is thus scant, and estimating the burden is difficult. For example, in Kenya, during 1996 through 1997, only 11 incidents of non-fatal drowning, and one of fatal drowning, were recorded from all the health units in the country [1]. A hospital survey in a large teaching hospital in Egypt reported only one case of fatal drowning during a 6-month period. These data are not credible.

In 1998, a population-based community survey was conducted in a rural Ugandan district, covering 1673 households, with 7427 people. The survey investigated morbidity and mortality from injuries of all types. Drowning was the leading cause of fatal injury in the 5 years preceding the survey, responsible for 27% of all injury deaths (32.2 drowning deaths per 100,000 person-years). No disability was attributed to drowning, implying that patients either had a fatal outcome or recovered fully [2]. Most of the drowning victims were young males (average age 23.8 years) who drowned in lakes or rivers during transportation or on fishing trips. Factors indicated in the community survey included overloading of vessels, unanticipated violent weather on the lake and alcohol intoxication. No leisure boating or swimming pool events were reported. In the same country, routine hospital registries at the five largest city hospitals had no record of either fatal or non-fatal drowning, for three consecutive years, 1997–1999 [5, 6, 7].

In this and similar communities, fishing vessels are often small boats and canoes with no communication equipment, and no floatation or other rescue devices. Furthermore, there is no coast guard or rescue service, so once the boats go out on the lake, survival depends almost entirely on the ingenuity of the boat occupants and the mercy of the waters. Often, there is no record of the numbers or demographics of the people on board, so when boats capsize there is uncertainty about those involved.

In South Africa, a cross-sectional analysis of state mortuaries, forensic and police data in Metropolitan Cape Town found that drowning was responsible for 2% of all non-natural deaths in 1994 [3]. The South African National Non-natural Surveillance System (NNSM) captures all injury fatalities from a sample of mortuaries across the country. From this system, drowning was responsible for 2.3% of all non-natural deaths in 1999. Almost three out of four (73%) of these drowning deaths were clearly unintentional, 1% were homicide, and the rest were of undetermined intent [4]. The majority of the drowning victims were children younger than 9 years of age, accounting for more than one quarter of the fatalities. The most common age was 2 years (6% of all drowning fatalities). Most drownings occurred in the sea, dams or swimming pools.

The role of alcohol in drowning is poorly understood in most of Africa. In the South African surveillance system, where blood alcohol concentration (BAC) levels are routinely checked for medical and legal purposes, almost 50% of the cases were positive for alcohol, with almost one quarter exceeding 0.20 g/dl at the time of drowning.

Drowning is a big burden to Africa in terms of mortality. This burden, however, is poorly appreciated because of under-reporting.

References

1.   Kenyan Ministry of Health (1997) National summary: morbidity and mortality report 1996 and 1997. Ministry of Health, Kenya

2. Kobusingye O, Guwatudde D, Lett R (2001) Injury patterns in rural and urban uganda. Injury Prevention 7:46–50
3. Lerer LB, Matzopoulos RG, Phillips R (1997) Violence and injury mortality in the Cape Town metropole. S Afr Med J 87:298–301
4. Peden M (2000) National injury surveillance system, a profile of fatal drownings in South Africa 1999. Final report: a DACST Innovation Fund Project
5. Uganda Injury Control Center (1997) Trauma registries annual report 1997. Makerere Medical School, Kampala, Uganda
6. Uganda Injury Control Center (1998) Trauma registries annual reports 1998. Makerere Medical School, Kampala, Uganda
7. Uganda Injury Control Center (1999) Trauma registries annual reports 1999. Makerere Medical School, Kampala, Uganda

2.7
Risk Factors for Drowning

ELENI PETRIDOU and ALEXANDRA KLIMENTOPOULOU

Identifying risk factors leading to drowning is essential for developing targeted, efficient prevention strategies [16]. Drowning mortality data are rather imperfect, and they present the highest proportion of unknown external cause codes among all types of injury. Despite these shortcomings and after searching more than 600 articles in the scientific literature, research or review articles were identified that were likely to contribute to the concise presentation of the risk factors for drowning. These can be divided into two groups, those related to human factors and those related to environmental factors. In this portion of the section, we emphasise those factors which are amenable to primary prevention interventions, instead of those which are related more to healthcare delivery, and as such are amenable to secondary prevention. More specifically, sociodemographic, environmental and behavioural factors are presented in an attempt to facilitate critical review and to enable more effective implementation.

2.7.1
Sociodemographic Risk Factors

2.7.1.1
Gender

Drowning occurs more often among males, as is the case for almost all types of unintentional injury [3]. According to national data reported to the WHO, the high ranking of drowning among the leading causes of death is mainly due to the high male drowning mortality on all continents. Overall, males experience drowning three times more frequently than females in all age groups. Among children 5 years and younger, there is a much lower male to female ratio, whereas among adolescents, the gender difference largely exceeds an overall 9:1 ratio [5], with wide variation across countries. Possible explanations for this gender difference include developmental and motor skills differences (as a result of the different evolution of the sexes) and differences in environmental conditions, including exposure to water. Sociocultural reasons may also play a role, in that in some cultures, male toddlers are allowed more time for exploration than their female counterparts [19], including in water where males typically swim and are involved in water recreation more often than females. Other explanations for this gender difference should be explored.

2.7.1.2
Age

The Bulletin Report of the World Health Organization [20] indicated that drowning was one of the most frequent causes of death among children aged 5–14 years old in both genders. In the European Union member states and the US, for example, drowning is the second most frequent cause of unintentional injury death in persons ages 0–19 years [18]. The child-to-adult ratio for drowning in the US is 3:1, a relatively high ratio. Comparative data from other countries with diverse drowning incident rates seem to lead to the same estimate [12]; however, in some countries, this ratio may be reversed, depending on time activity patterns and age group interactions with water environment activities. In Greece, a country with a lengthy 16,000-kilometre coastline, the drowning mortality rate among children in 1995 was 1 per 100,000 compared to 3 per 100,000 among adults [1]. Adolescent boys, in particular, are prone to behavioural deviations, including alcohol and drug use, which are often associated with water recreational sports and watercraft driving, all of which increase the likelihood of suffering a drowning event [6]. Among adults ages 19 years and older, the victim is typically the inexperienced recreational swimmer. In contrast, drowning among adults 65 years and older can often be attributed to underlying medical conditions, such as cardiovascular disease, depression or epilepsy, rather than delinquent behaviour or lack of swimming skills. Hence, co-morbidity of underlying medical conditions should be considered when implementing drowning prevention policies.

2.7.1.3
Socio-economic Status Indicators

Social patterning in injury risk is a complex phenomenon. More specifically, socioeconomic status is an ill-defined term, and often includes variables such as education, occupation, income and sociocultural milieu. These variables cannot be easily assessed or compared across countries. Moreover, any attempt to ecologically correlate the Gross Domestic Product with drowning risk is hindered by the confounding effect of factors, such as the differential proximity of various countries with the water environment, the variable climatic conditions and the diverse time-exposure patterns.

Given these limitations, data on socioeconomic differentials of drowning risk in different countries is either lacking or insufficient, with the exception of the US. However, it seems that the relation of socioeconomic status with drowning risk is not a unidirectional phenomenon. Indeed, among children under age

5 years, the risk of drowning increases linearly with accessibility to swimming pools and other standing water facilities (such as lakes and ponds) [9]. It would be useful, therefore, to calculate the magnitude of the risk of drowning on the basis of the density of residential swimming pools per regional population so as to help advocate for the prevention of drowning in swimming pools.

Data from the US show that the overall age-adjusted drowning rate among African Americans is almost 50% higher than that among whites. The drowning incidence among African American children ages 5–19 years is more than twice that of their white counterparts. African American children ages 1–4 years, however, have a lower drowning rate compared to white children largely because drowning in this age group more frequently occurs in residential swimming [9]. It should be noted, however, that the excess of drowning among African Americans might simply reflect their lower socioeconomic status. This observation is not unique to Americans of African descent in the US. In addition, there may be cultural issues regarding the frequency of use of water for recreational purposes. In Japan, North Africa, Turkey and among Black South Africans, there are higher drowning rates, and this may be due to less frequent recreational aquatic activity [11, 21].

In Japan, bath tubs are the major source of accidental drownings, especially among young children and the elderly [11]. This is probably due to a combination of sociocultural factors in Japan, such as the design of very deep bathtubs, the habit of taking frequent and long baths, and the use of very hot water, which leads to a large discrepancy in temperature with the ambient air and could provoke sudden death in vulnerable populations.

Level of education is often used as a proxy for social background in many studies, which assess the socioeconomic differentials in injury risk [9]. Although the existing data is occasionally controversial, there is evidence to suggest that higher parental education leads to higher levels of awareness of the existing environmental risks for their children and to the development of appropriate compensatory mechanisms [9]. Therefore, one should always consider the role that the socioeconomic triangle – education, occupation, income – exert on the quality of parental supervision and hence the drowning risk during childhood. Indeed, in Greece, there is evidence that children of high school educated, non-working, and hence less distressed, mothers seem to experience fewer injury risks.

2.7.2
Environmental Risk Factors

2.7.2.1
Place of Occurrence

Place of occurrence accounts overall for most of the variability of drowning incidence observed across different countries. One could speculate that drowning incidents occurring in salt water are more prevalent in places with easy access to seawater. This seems to be the case for some countries of the Mediterranean basin. Surprisingly, however, in the US state of Florida, which has a considerable coastline, the majority of drownings occur in standing fresh water facilities (for example, swimming pools, lakes), rather than in salt water [19]. In some countries the primary, fundamental risk factor of drowning is access to swimming pools [19]. Regardless of type (in-ground, above-ground, round or rectangular, public or private) recreational swimming pools are the primary site where childhood drowning occurs.

Data for childhood drowning in swimming pools from the US Consumer Product Safety Commission show that 60% fewer drowning occur when comparing in-ground pools without four-sided fencing to in-ground pools with four-sided isolation fencing [17]. Apart from the recreational swimming pools, for children younger than 4 years, indoor water facilities like bathtubs, jetted bathtubs and basins pose a major risk for childhood drowning. There are several scientific papers, however, suggesting that bathtub drowning should always alert the clinician for the possibility of an intentionally afflicted injury [7]. Moreover, 5-gallon buckets and other large containers represent a higher drowning risk for toddlers, a fact that seems to be strongly related to developmental and anthropometric characteristics of the toddlers. In this age group, the head is relatively the heaviest part of a small child's body, so it can easily become trapped in such containers. Also, when large containers are filled with liquid, they weigh more than the child and will not tip over to allow the child to escape [3].

The relationships among age groups, drowning location and activity are not uniform and may be confounded by gender, geographical region, community, season, race and economic status [3]. Lakes, ponds, rivers and pools are the most frequent sites where drowning of children and adolescents aged 5–19 years takes place [2]. About one out of every ten drowning events among small children occur in bathtubs, whereas 5% of them are related to recreational boating. This percentage is higher in the adult age group. Four-sided isolation swimming pool fencing is an effective protective measure. The fence should meet certain construction criteria and should separate access to the pool from access to the house (private swimming pools) or any other facility (public swimming pools) [10]. The gate in the fence is the single most important component of the fence. It should be self-latching and self-closing, and should open away from the pool and be checked frequently to ensure good working order [10]. Rigid motorised pool covers, on the other hand, are not a substitute for four-sided fencing because pool covers are not likely to be used appropriately and consistently.

2.7.2.2
Climatic Conditions

Adverse climate conditions substantially increase the risk of drowning deaths. More specifically, unfamiliarity with easily changing climatic conditions is an important determinant of the risk for drowning. Furthermore, low water temperature [4] and forced lengthy stay in the water environment appear to predict a detrimental outcome once a drowning incident has occurred.

2.7.2.3
Safety Equipment and Safety Policies

The availability and accessibility of safety equipment in water transportation vessels (watercraft) are additional potential risk factors. Massive drowning events, such as sinking ships, can be caused by climatic conditions, as well as lack of safety equipment. Flotation devices such as lifejackets are indispensable on all water transportation vessels, whether for public or private use. From 1987 to 1994 five major 'drowning tragedies' have taken place in European seas with more than 4300 fatalities [13]. However, it is strongly suggested that if safety devices were more readily available, more lives would have been saved. Lack of safety equipment standards along with poor maintenance have often been raised as important risk factors. Results from European research conducted by the National Consumers' and Quality of Life Associations has shown that it is much safer travelling on a ferryboat in the Baltic or North Sea than going on a cruise in the Mediterranean [13, 14]. For a considerable number of ferryboats, however, evacuation policies, fire protection, lifejackets and lifeboats are not adequately prepared or maintained. Therefore, more work is still needed to make them safer. Moreover, safety equipment used by children while swimming (such as supporting rings) may give a false feeling of reassurance to parents. Drowning prevention and age-appropriate swimming lessons are important prevention tools.

2.7.3
Behavioural Risk Factors

Risk-taking behaviour is an important component of unintentional injury occurrence. In this context, alcohol intake is highlighted and should be considered, especially for the adolescent ages as well as for crew members in vessels that are responsible for mass transportation. Parental supervision is also of vital importance and it appears to be considerably affected by cultural, behavioural and attitude aspects.

2.7.3.1
Use of Alcohol

Alcohol use has been estimated to be involved in about 25%–50% of adolescent and adult deaths associated with water recreation [8]. A meta-analysis of alcohol involvement in fatal injuries concluded that 49% of adult drownings involved alcohol and 34% had a blood alcohol concentration (BAC) over 100 mg/dl [14]. Another important factor to consider is the alcohol consumed by parents or guardians while supervising young in water recreation activities. While many studies have documented high alcohol involvement in drownings, little work has been done to estimate the magnitude of the risks involved in alcohol use. One study of alcohol use as a risk factor in boating fatalities (most of which are due to drowning) estimates that the risk was actually greater than that observed for most studies of motor-vehicle fatalities. The risk of death was elevated even at low BAC's (odds ratio 1.3 at BAC 10 mg/dl) and increased dramatically as BAC increased until there was a 52-fold increased odds of dying while boating if the person's BAC was above 250 mg/dl [15]. Unfamiliar settings and activities along with alcohol consumption are also strong precipitating factors, a combination that makes tourists more vulnerable, having a between three and four times higher risk as reported from some countries [1].

Because alcohol consumption in water recreation activities predisposes to drowning, vigorous action should be taken. Legal limits for blood alcohol levels during water recreation activities should be mandated and enforced [5]. Advertisements that encourage alcohol use during boating should be eliminated. The availability of alcohol at water recreation facilities should also be restricted [5].

2.7.3.2
Parental Supervision

The quality of supervision provided to children by parents and other caregivers is an important factor in drowning. A 2-year-old male child, living in a home with a swimming pool in the backyard is at great risk for drowning. His risk is compounded when he is left unsupervised, even momentarily. Pool owners are advised to learn cardio-pulmonary resuscitation and keep a telephone nearby in a case of an emergency. Furthermore, caregivers should never leave a child unattended in order to attend to other things, such as answering the telephone [19]. Parental supervision serves as a compensatory mechanism for the environmental hazards. The level and the adequacy of parental supervision, therefore, reflect to a significant extent the understanding of the parents of the dangers present.

Small children can drown in a few seconds. Among children under age 4 years, tragedy occurs when the child wanders away from the house and into the swimming pool without a parent or caregiver knowing it. Therefore, it is strongly advised that parents should not install a swimming pool in their yard until their child has reached the age of 5 years [5]. Paediatricians should properly and routinely advise parents and guardians about the dangers children face when swimming or having access to different standing water facilities and containers.

Preventing drowning is an uphill battle because a lot of effort is needed. There is a consensus, however, that these efforts are necessary because drowning frequently affects healthy people during times of pleasure and leisure. The way to move forward is by studying risk factors in such a way so that effective prevention strategies can be designed.

References

1. Alexe D, Dessypris N, Petridou E (2002) Epidemiology of unintentional drowning deaths in Greece. Book of Abstracts, World Congress on Drowning 2002 Amsterdam, The Netherlands, pp 26–28
2. The American Academy of Pediatrics (1992) Drowning in infants, children and adolescents. Pediatrics 92(2):292–294
3. Baker SP, O'Neill B, Ginsburg MJ, Li G (1992) The injury fact book, 2nd edn. Oxford University Press, New York, NY
4. Bierens JJ, Velde EA van der, Berkel M van, Zanten JJ van (1990) Submersion in the Netherlands: prognostic indicators and resuscitation. Ann Emerg Med 19:1390–1395
5. Centers for Disease Control and Prevention (1998) Drowning fact sheet [Online]. National Center for Injury Prevention and Control, Centers for Disease Control and Prevention (producer). [cited September 21, 2001]. Available from: URL: http://www.cdc.gov/ncipc/factsheets/drown.htm
6. Christensen DW (1992) Near drowning. In: Rogers MC (ed) Textbook of pediatric intensive care. Williams and Wilkins, Baltimore, MD, pp 877–880
7. Gillenwater JM, Quan L, Feldman KW (1996) Inflicted submersion in childhood. Arch Ped Adolesc Med 150:298–303
8. Howland J, Hingson R (1988) Alcohol as a risk factor for drowning: a review of the literature (1950–1985). Accid Anal Prev 20:19–25
9. Laflamme L (1998) Social inequality in injury risks. Knowledge accumulated and plans for the future. Karolinska Institute, Department of Public Health Sciences, Stockholm, Sweden
10. Milliner N, Pearn J, Guard R (1980) Will fenced pools save lives? A ten-year study from Mulgrave Shire Queensland. Med J Aust 2:510–511
11. Mizuta R, Fujita H, Osamura T, et al. (1993) Childhood drownings and near-drownings in Japan. Acta Paediatr Jpn 35:186–192
12. Morgenstern H, Bingham T, Reza A (2000) Effects of pool fencing ordinances and other factors on childhood drowning in Los Angeles county, 1990–1995. Am J Public Health 90:595–601
13. Consumers' Association of Quality of Life (1998) Safety on ferryboats. „EKPIZO" Consumers' Association of Quality of Life bulletin 1:23–26
14. Smith GS, Branas CC, Miller TR (1999) Fatal non-traffic injuries involving alcohol: a meta-analysis. Ann Emerg Med 33:659–668
15. Smith GS, Keyl PM, Hadley JA, et al. (2001) Drinking and recreational boating fatalities: a population-based case-control study. JAMA 286:2974–2980
16. Spzilman D (1997) Near-drowning and drowning classification in children: a proposal to stratify mortality based on the analysis of 1831 cases. CHEST 112:660–665
17. US Consumer Product Safety Commission (1998) Backyard pool: always supervise children [cited March 17, 2003]. Available from: URL: http://www.cpsc.gov/cpscpub/chdrown/5097html
18. Wintemute GJ (1990) Childhood drowning and near drowning in the United States. Am J Dis Child 144:663–669
19. Wintemute GJ, Drake C, Wright M (1991) Immersion events in residential swimming pools: evidence for the experience effect. Am J Dis Child 101:200–203
20. World Health Organization (1999) Injury, a leading cause of global burden of disease. Bulletin Report. Violence and Injury Prevention Team, Geneva, Switzerland
21. Wyndham CH (1986) Deaths from accidents, poisoning and violence – differences between the various population groups in the RSA. S Afr Med J 69:556–558

2.8
Review of Literature on Available Strategies
for Drowning Prevention

JOHN LANGLEY

Preventive factors are best when drawn from epidemiological research findings. The bulk of this section has captured and described the definition of drowning, the importance of consistent data collection and risk factors for drowning. This portion of the section is an overview of drowning prevention strategies. More information on efforts to prevent drowning may be found in Sections 3–5.

2.8.1
Swimming Pool Fencing

The Harborview Injury Prevention and Research Center, as part of the Cochrane collaboration [3], has reviewed the impact of a number of measures to reduce drowning. Of these the most comprehensive is pool fencing. Summarising the few case-control studies that have been conducted, they conclude that isolation fencing (enclosing swimming pool only) is superior to perimeter fencing (enclosing property and pool) because perimeter fencing allows access to the pool area through the house. They also conclude that the studies have shown that pool fencing significantly reduces the risk of drowning.

Harborview has not updated its summary since 1997. Since that time another study has shed light on the issue, looking at drownings in Los Angeles over a 5-year period [7]. A case-control approach was used in which all pools in which children had drowned were cases, and other pools chosen randomly were controls, in order to examine the effectiveness of pool fencing laws. Morgenstern et al. [7] found that the overall rate of childhood drowning was not lower in pools regulated by fencing ordinances than in pools unregulated by fencing ordinances in Los Angeles County. However, they point out that this does not necessarily imply that pool fencing does not lower the risk of childhood drowning, but only that the pool fencing laws in Los Angeles have been ineffective. One suggestion they have for why this is the case is that the effectiveness of local ordinances may have been compromised because of inadequate enforcement by local building and safety authorities. Such a suggestion seems feasible, with research in New Zealand [8] and Victoria, Australia [1] showing that enforcement of pool fencing laws has been inadequate in those places also.

2.8.2
Lifesavers

Australian research has shown that the presence of livesavers seems to increase the likelihood of positive outcome. In the first study, cases of resuscitation attempts made by livesavers on Australian beaches between 1973 and 1983 were reviewed [6]. During this time, 262 resuscitation attempts by livesavers were recorded and 162 were successful. In 16% of the cases of survival, a pulse was absent at the initial assessment. It is highly likely that many of the 162 survivors would have died without livesaver intervention.

A second Australian study considered rescues at one beach with lifesavers. The key finding of this study was that survival after rescue decreased significantly with distance from the clubhouse [2]. This suggests that early intervention by livesavers can improve outcome. The importance of livesavers is further enhanced by evidence of the importance of early resuscitation.

2.8.3
Resuscitation

A case-control study of paediatric submersion victims in the US compared children with poor outcomes following immersion (cases), and with good outcomes following immersion (controls) [4]. After controlling for age, gender, duration of submersion and hypothermia, children with good outcomes were significantly more likely to have been resuscitated immediately, prior to the arrival of paramedical personnel (odds ratio 4.75, 95% confidence interval: 3.44–6.06). There do not appear to have been any epidemiological studies conducted on the effect of resuscitation on adult submersion victims, with the exception of the lifeguard studies above, which covered all age groups.

2.8.4
Swimming Training

The important points regarding swimming training, for children in particular, have been identified by Harborview. They state: "Although a number of studies have shown that swimming lessons improve one's ability to dive, swim underwater, breathe correctly, and tread water, no study has examined the more important question of whether swimming lessons and/or drown proofing courses actually prevent drownings and near-drownings". A particular concern for swimming instruction among young children is that it may increase exposure to risk by increasing the likelihood of children entering the water or encouraging over confidence once in the water [11]. However, there do not appear to be any studies which have attempted to answer this important question.

2.8.5
Personal Flotation Devices

It is highly likely that lifejackets, also called personal flotation devices (PFDs) prevent drownings. However, the epidemiological basis for this assumption appears to be unproven. In a observational study in the states of Washington and Oregon in the US, use of PFDs among boaters were observed. These authors stated: "While PFD use has not been proven to decrease drownings, the very low use of PFDs by adolescents and adults in our study suggests that infrequent PFD use may be a factor in the higher incidence of boat related drowning in these age groups" [9]. A study of fatalities in the Alaskan (US) fishing industry concluded that PFDs should be worn on the decks of vessels at all times. In 45% of the fatal man-overboard cases from 1991 to 1996, the victim was not tangled in gear and was observed falling overboard, and should have been floatable and recoverable [5]. Moreover, they observed that where entangling occurred, the body part entangled tended to be an extremity, so wearing PFDs should not increase the likelihood of entanglement. Immersion suits are also important in cold waters. The same authors concluded that the progress made during the early 1990s in reducing drowning mortality in the fishing industry has occurred primarily by keeping fishermen who have evacuated capsized or sinking vessels afloat and warm through the use of immersion suits and life rafts.

2.8.6
Barriers on Roads

No evidence has been located that barriers on roads reduce drowning. However, in New Zealand, considerable resources have been spent on placing barriers on roads next to waterways where drownings as a result of motor vehicle crashes have occurred. Assuming barriers are located in places where cars commonly leave the road and enter the water, and that barriers are effective in stopping cars leaving the road, then this strategy must reduce drownings from this cause.

2.8.7
Small Boats: Design and Actions after Capsizing

No references to articles which specifically link boat design to drownings have been identified in the literature. However, it is very likely that improvements in boat design, especially related to stability, will decrease the likelihood of drowning. With respect to the Alaskan fishing industry, it has been recommended that periodic stability reassessment and vessel inspection of all vessels should be seriously considered [5].

Commonly accepted practice following a capsize is to remain with your boat. A recent study, however, has suggested that this is not always the best advice. From a review of coroner and police reports of water-related fatalities in Canada, the responses to immersion were compared between victims and survivors of swamping and capsizing incidents where at least one person died. The authors conclude that: "The data suggest that under adverse conditions where immediate rescue is unlikely, especially for good swimmers wearing a flotation device, it is preferable to swim immediately for shore rather than stay with the boat or swim after a delay" [10].

References

1. Ashby K, Routley V, Stathakis V (1998) Enforcing legislative and regulatory injury prevention strategies. Hazard VISS 34:1–12
2. Fenner PJ, Harrison SL, Williamson JA, Williamson BD (1995) Success of surf lifesaving resuscitations in Queensland, 1973–1992. Med J Aust 163:580–583
3. Harborview Injury Prevention and Research Center (2001) Drowning scope of the problem [cited September 15, 2001]. Available from: URL: http://depts.washington.edu/hiprc/childinjury/topic/drowning/
4. Kyriacou DN, Arcinue EL, Peek C, Kraus JF (1994) Effect of immediate resuscitation on children with submersion injury. Pediatrics 94:137–142
5. Lincoln JM, Conway GA (2001) Commercial fishing fatalities in Alaska: risk factors and prevention strategies. NIOSH; September 1997 [cited September 15, 2001]. Available from: URL: http://www.cdc.gov/niosh/97163_58.html
6. Manolios N, Mackie I (1988) Drowning and near-drowning on Australian beaches patrolled by life-savers: a 10-year study, 1973–1983. Med J Aust 148:165–171
7. Morgenstern H, Bingham T, Reza A (2000) Effects of pool-fencing ordinances and other factors on childhood drowning in Los Angeles County, 1990–1995. Am J Publ Health 90:595–601
8. Morrison L, Chalmers DJ, Langley JD, et al. (1999) Achieving compliance with pool fencing legislation in New Zealand: a survey of regulatory authorities. Injury Prevention 5:114–118
9. Quan L, Bennett E, Cummings P, et al. CD (1998) Are life vests worn? A multiregional observational study of personal flotation device use in small boats. Injury Prevention 4:203–205
10. Sawyer S, Barss P (1998) Stay with the boat or swim for shore? A comparison of drowning victim and survivor responses to immersion following a capsize or swamping [Abstract]. Proceedings of the Fourth World Conference on Injury Prevention and Control; 17–20 May 1998, Amsterdam, The Netherlands
11. Smith GS (1995) Drowning prevention in children: the need for new strategies. Injury Prevention 1:216–217

2.9
Occupational Drownings

Jennifer M. Lincoln

Drowning is an occupational safety problem around the world. Any maritime occupation, including commercial fishing, commercial diving, and water transportation workers are exposed to drowning hazards. In many cases, particularly with commercial fishermen and water transportation workers, the vessel is not only the workplace, but also often their home while they spend weeks at a time at sea. A diligent search for national and international occupational drowning data was not successful. Data are not reported internationally for overall occupational drownings. Extensive research, however, has been conducted on drowning prevention and commercial fishing safety throughout the commercial fishing industry.

In the commercial fishing industry alone it is estimated that 25–40 million people are employed worldwide [2]. Fatality rates have been reported from different countries ranging from 45.8/100,000 per year (Canada 1975–1983) to as high as 414.6/100,000 per year (Alaska, US, 1980–1988) [3]. The International Labor Organization's Occupational Safety and Health Branch estimates that 24,000 fatalities occur worldwide per year in fisheries [4]. Studies have shown that drowning, presumed drowned and hypothermia are the predominant causes of death among commercial fishermen (91% in Canada, 88% in Alaska, and 78% in Ireland) [1].

Commercial fishing fatalities can be divided into the categories vessel-related events (such as vessels sinking or fire) or non-vessel-related events (such as deck injuries or falls overboard). Unfortunately, vessels with all hands lost at sea is not an unusual scenario. Weather and fatigue are usually factors in these events. Safety during commercial fishing operations depends on several things including the design of the vessel, how it is loaded, water tight integrity, the operating conditions and the experience of the skipper and crew. In the last 15 years, the safety gear which is depended upon during emergencies at sea has greatly improved [3]. Such gear includes life rafts, electronic position-indicating radio beacons (EPIRBs) and immersion suits. Inflatable personal flotation devices (PFDs) are also now available that are comfortable to wear.

By the 1990s, many countries activated new prevention programs including educational programs and safety regulations. There have been several fora worldwide that have led to development of safety guidelines for fishing vessels, including design, construction and safety training guidelines for personnel on board. Based on these and other factors, countries have developed regulations for their respective fleets. These requirements vary greatly, however. Australia, for example, has extensive licensing requirements for all classes of vessels and qualification requirements for skippers, mates, engineers and crew. Norway's fleet is heavily regulated for operation and material conditions for vessels greater than 15 meters. Requirements for vessels and personnel in the US are not as stringent [7]. In Alaska, there has been a decline in the number of fishing fatalities since the implementation of a US law requiring emergency equipment on board fishing vessels and emergency drills performed by crews. However, there has not been any primary prevention to keep fishermen out of the water in the first place [5, 6].

While high-income countries have been moving towards implementing measures to improve the safety in their own commercial fishing fleets and preventing drownings, safety at sea continues to be a very serious problem in low-income countries. Fleets may consist mainly of small and often non-motorised vessels, with limited communications, navigation and emergency equipment onboard. There are very few technically trained personnel in these countries to serve as crew members, trainers and inspectors of vessels. Infrastructure that is necessary for enforcement of regulations is lacking. This also makes launching search and rescue operations difficult because they require high levels of organisational structure and coordination. The motivation of each society to invest in fishing vessel safety may vary. The biggest challenge in these areas is to educate the authorities on the extent of the problem, to encourage discussion and to persuade them to act [4].

Commercial fishermen around the world are faced with many hazards including the risk of drowning. Measures have been implemented in several parts of the world to mitigate this problem, but more must be done. Different aspects of drowning hazards in the industry in high-income countries as well as in low-income nations should continue to be addressed. Through successful intervention programs, the drowning rate should decrease among commercial fishermen around the world.

References

1. Abraham PP (2001) International comparison of occupational injuries among commercial fishers of selected northern countries and regions. Barents Newsl Occup Health Safety 4:24
2. Anonymous (1998) Encyclopedia of occupational health and safety, 4th edn, vol III. Fishing general profile. International Labour Office, Geneva, Switzerland, p 66.2
3. (Anonymous (1998) Encyclopedia of occupational health and safety, 4th edn, vol III. Fishing health problems and disease patterns. International Labour Office, Geneva, Switzerland, p 66.14
4. Food and Agricultural Organization of the United Nations (2001) Safety at sea as an integral part of fisheries management. FAO Fisheries Circular No. 966, FAO, Rome, Italy
5. Lincoln JM, Conway GA (1999) Preventing commercial fishing deaths in Alaska. Occup Environ Med 56:691–695
6. National Institute for Occupational Safety and Health (1997) Commercial fishing fatalities in Alaska: risk factors and prevention strategies. Current Intelligence Bulletin #58. DHHS (NIOSH), Cincinnati, OH, Pub. No. 97-163
7. National Research Council, Marine Board, Committee on Fishing Vessel Safety (1991) Fishing vessel safety: blue print for a national program. National Academy Press, Washington, DC

The Prevention of Drowning

TASK FORCE ON THE PREVENTION OF DROWNING
Section editors: JOHN WILSON, HANS KNAPE and JOOST BIERENS

Task Force Chairs

- John Wilson
- Wim Rogmans

Task Force Members

- Peter Barss
- Elizabeth Bennett
- Ruth Brenner
- Moniek Hoofwijk
- Andrej Michalson
- Beverley Norris
- John Pearn
- Ian Scott

Other Contributors

- Blance Barrio
- David Calabria
- Peter Cornall
- Julie Gilchrist
- Andrew Harrell
- Katrina Haddrill
- Laurie Lawrence
- John Leech
- Maryl Lyford
- John McVan
- Rebecca Mitchell
- Kevin Moran
- Luis-Miguel Pascual-Gómez
- Frank Pia
- Santiago Pinto
- Linda Quan
- Monique Ridder
- Marcia Rom
- Paloma Sanz
- Robert Stallman
- Greg Tate
- Andrew Whittaker

3.1
Overview

JOHN WILSON and WIM ROGMANS

It is no exaggeration to say that the prime purpose of this handbook, indeed the *raison d'être* of all research and development in the field of drowning, is prevention. This is both prevention of any incident occurring in the first place, and also prevention of a drowning death if an incident takes place (that is, both primary and secondary safety). In the end, the only purpose for all the other contributions examining drowning is to reduce the incidence of death or other harmful consequence. In this section a number of contributions examine different aspects of prevention. We have not been able to include contributions from all approaches, but have touched on most of the main ones. For further information the reader should both examine other main sections in this *Handbook* and refer also to [1–8].

Following two short opening contributions from the chairpersons of the Prevention task force (▶ **Chapter 3.2 and 3.3**), the section has a contribution from Andrej Michalsen (▶ **Chapter 3.4**) on risk assessment and perception, basically making the point that in order to have any chance of sensible preventive strategies we need to understand risk and risk perception.

The next two contributions, by John Pearn and David Calabria (see ▶ **Chapter 3.5**), examine drowning in the context of children, including infanticide by drowning, while Ian Scott examines drowning at home and in the garden (▶ **Chapter 3.6**). Both make the case for a particular technical preventative strategy, namely fencing and gates around domestic pools. The first authors stress the need for such techniques to be well designed and based on good ergonomics. Scott emphasises some of these points, and makes a strong argument that any regulation and legislation must be appropriate. He also highlights the possible opposition from the community, including parents as well as others, if they feel that they might lose something by being compelled to use some technical means of prevention. However, the authors strongly argue for such a case to be made and for opposition to be overcome.

Secondary safety requires that if people are in distress in the water, some means of rescue must be on hand, whether by means of buoyancy aids, parental supervision, or official supervision. The latter is the subject of the chapter by Andrew Harrell (▶ **Chapter 3.7**), examining in particular the vigilance required of beach patrols. He stresses the need to understand what goes on in scanning behaviour of lifeguards, and also their decision biases and team behaviour, as well as the need for better job design, training and support.

Ruth Brenner, Kevin Moran, Robert Stallman, Julie Gilchrist and John McVan, in a joint chapter, examine the different aspects of a controversial question, namely the supposition that improving swimming ability in the population will decrease the risk of drowning. They quite cogently make the point that this is not necessarily so, since increased swimming ability might lead to people taking greater risks, and also that it is very difficult to define what we mean by ability in this context. It is probably not useful to think of swimming ability in general, but rather better to do so in relation to specific risks. They also stress the importance of cognitive and social factors of individuals and also of motor development, with identification of at least eight other motor abilities which are important other than just the pure ability to produce a recognisable stroke over a set distance. The authors of this part define future research needs picking up the themes of their chapter, and also make certain recommendations for the future (▶ Chapter 3.8).

In the final chapter, ▶ Chapter 3.9, Elizabeth Bennett has brought together fourteen contributions from many authorities from around the world, to describe community and national campaigns in their own countries or regions. The lessons drawn from these contributions are interesting, not so much in differences in approach between different authorities, but more in the common lessons which have been learned, about the implementation of such programs and about their outcomes. Bennett herself sets out common themes: the need to use multiple strategies but with specific targets, the need for multi-organisational collaboration in campaigns, the need for education and training to be implemented along with other more technical and design approaches, and also the need for better evaluation of successful programs.

Whilst, as explained above, not examining all possible routes to prevent drowning, it is hoped that the contributions in this section will whet the appetite of the reader to look for other ways of reducing the incidence and consequences of the potentially tragic event of drowning.

References

1. Brenner RA, Saluja G, Smith GS (2003) Swimming lessons, swimming ability, and the risk of drowning. Inj Control Saf Promot 10:211-216
2. Hyder AA, Arifeen S, Begum N, et al. (2003) Death from drowning: defining a new challenge for child survival in Bangladesh. Inj Control Saf Promot 10:205-210
3. Michalsen A (2003) Risk assessment and perception. Inj Control Saf Promot 10:201-204
4. Norris B, Wilson JR (2003) Preventing drowning through design—the contribution of human factors. Inj Control Saf Promot 10:217-226
5. Peden MM, McGee K (2003) The epidemiology of drowning worldwide. Inj Control Saf Promot 10:195-199
6. Rogmans W, Wilson J (2003) Editorial to the special issue on drowning prevention. Inj Control Saf Promot 10:193-194
7. Scott I (2003) Prevention of drowning in home pools—lessons from Australia. Inj Control Saf Promot 10:227-236
8. Stoop JA (2003) Maritime accident investigation methodologies. Inj Control Saf Promot 10:237–242

3.2
Recommendations

WIM ROGMANS and JOHN WILSON

3.2.1
The Challenges of Prevention

Of the three leading causes of unintentional injury, deaths drowning ranks third, and among infants and toddlers first. Routine hospital and other data, as well as the scarce and somewhat fragmented studies that are available at present, identify a number of suspected risk factors. Young children have a different set of risks than older persons. Childhood drowning occurs usually in bathtubs, garden ponds and swimming pools and lapses in adult supervision are one of the major causes of these incidents. For adults drownings occur more often in recreational activities such as swimming in inland or coastal waters and boating and are often associated with unfamiliarity with the risks involved in these activities or with alcohol consumption.

Unlike other public injury areas, such as car safety, pedestrian safety and fire safety, remarkably few drowning prevention programs have been formally evaluated. Those that have been evaluated appear to provide some encouragement for prevention. Also, we are observing, in at least the high income countries, a clear downward trend in fatalities due to drowning over the past century. This is certainly owing to: increased urbanisation that did not fully eliminate the dangers of surface water but at least significantly reduced exposure rates compared to rural areas; improved quality of living environments (housing and community planning); an increase in swimming abilities among the general population; and enhanced knowledge in and availability of rescue and first aid. It is doubtful, however, whether risk factors such as adult supervision at home, in the garden and at swimming pools have improved over the years. Drowning remains an issue of importance world wide and presents, in particular, a risk for vulnerable groups such as young children and ethnic minorities.

The World Congress on Drowning gives a very welcome opportunity to identify and document the state of play in drowning prevention. It highlights the gaps in knowledge and understanding of what works in drowning prevention and identifies routes for further development and for increasing the effectiveness of drowning prevention.

3.2.2
Gaps in Knowledge

Hazard identification and risk assessment are the first steps towards understanding the problem, identifying priorities in measures to be taken and continuously monitoring risks for further improvements. It is the simple structure of the plan, do, check and act cycle, which has been implemented in various environments such as safety of open water in communities, pool safety and beach safety. This has resulted in the development of tools for risk assessment; however, their application is most fragmented. As most authorities lack the time and resources for elaborate risk assessment procedures, these tools must be kept simple in use, based on best practice and shared internationally. Much more effort should be invested in establishing world wide accepted standards for risk assessment in aquatic environments.

As regards measures to prevent drowning, much of the anecdotal evidence (and the few evaluated interventions) support the belief that the best solution remains to physically separate the person from danger or, in the case of immersion, to prevent immediate drowning. These measures include barriers around private swimming pools, creating natural barriers along surface water in communities, allowing people only to swim in sections of beaches that are professionally controlled and supervised continuously, and wearing personal floatation devices. Except for pool fencing and personal floatation devices, of which the effectiveness is well researched and proven (although only if properly installed, maintained and enforced), much less is known about the effectiveness of design changes in bathtubs, toilets, buckets and garden ponds, in pool covers and pool alarms, in water edge design and treatment, in inland and coastal beach arrangements (lay out, signs and flags). Most importantly, if better design criteria and then actual designs are to be developed, and appropriate test and evaluation programs established, we need much better understanding of the relevant human factors. Better information from structured research programs is needed on adult and child capabilities and characteristics, for example on dynamic physical characteristics of strength and movement, static and dynamic measurements related to equipment fit, perception and comprehension of information and situations and risk awareness.

There are other possible solutions that address the victim and supervisors but they are even harder to prove than the previously mentioned environmental changes. These include actions such as raising general awareness of drowning risks among the general population, educating special risk groups, ensuring adequate supervision at home, in public pools and at beaches, providing early teaching swimming skills, teaching young adults life saving techniques and implementing basic training for all in resuscitation. Most of these measures should be considered as being complementary to the primary physical prevention measures that are proven to be more effective and to provide immediate protection against danger. Nevertheless, in order to increase the complementary effectiveness of measures directed to risk groups and to get the best benefits out of limited resources, much more research is needed into the role of each of these measures in reducing drowning deaths.

A special risk that is relevant in drowning prevention is boating under the influence of alcohol. This behaviour is well researched and it becomes even more hazardous in the marine environment where elements of sun, wind and spray accelerate impairment. In spite of regulations, enforcement and communication efforts the deadly combination of alcohol and water seems to be less understood by boaters than by car drivers today: a challenge for further research.

Finally, it is not known how knowledge and experiences in successfully preventing drowning can be transferred to other settings and cultures and in particular to low income countries. In spite of all cultural and economical diversity in today's world we cannot be dismissive or withhold the wider application of the results achieved in one part of the world. Such knowledge transfer programs should be better documented and evaluated.

3.2.3
Action Needed and Major Stakeholders to Be Involved

International bodies such as the World Health Organization (WHO), the International Red Cross and Red Crescent (IRCRC), the International Life Saving Federation (ILS) and the International Lifeboat Federation (ILF) should develop guidelines and tools for risk assessment and preventive measures that can be applied in a wide range of settings. The establishment of a clearing house for collecting good practice in applying these techniques and providing the various interest groups with easy access to this information should be considered.

Intergovernmental bodies such as WHO and the International Maritime Organisation (IMO), together with their member states, should review current regulations and standards related to maritime safety and water safety. Much more effort should be invested in ensuring proper regulations for pool safety (both private and public), beach safety and safety of boating (also including compulsory use of life jackets for all passengers on vessels under 24 feet in length).

Non-governmental bodies such as IRCRC and ILS should play an important role in gearing up research and development into better understanding of the relevant psychological and physical human factors, enhanced product design and the design of physical environments in order to prevent people from drowning. This should be in partnership with the maritime industry, pool manufacturers, and building industry. Private industry should develop technologies that make better personal flotation devices available that are also more comfortable to wear and therefore better accepted by people, and pool covers and barriers more suitable for both their purpose in protection and also for child safety.

Finally, all international bodies, together with national governments, should develop a consistent program for collaboration in exchange of experience in drowning prevention through research, standards, regulation, enforcement and continuous education and training. The development of national reports on drowning prevention policies might help to make the diversity in national infrastructures, prevention efforts and their outcomes more transparent.

The following recommendation was established by the task force on the prevention of drowning.

Preventive Strategies and Collaboration Are Needed

The vast majority of drownings can be prevented and prevention (rather than rescue or resuscitation) is the most important method by which to reduce the number of drownings. The circumstances and events in drowning vary across many different situations and in different countries world wide. Considerable differences exist in the locations of drowning and among different cultures. Therefore, all agencies concerned with drowning prevention – legislative bodies, consumer groups, research institutions, local authorities, designers, manufacturers and retailers – must collaborate to set up national and local prevention initiatives. These will depend on good intelligence and insightful research, and must include environmental design and equipment designs as a first route, in conjunction with education, training programs and policies which address specific groups at risk, such as children. The programs must be evaluated and the results of the evaluations must be published.

3.3
Purposes and Scope of Prevention of Drowning

JOHN WILSON and WIM ROGMANS

3.3.1
Purpose

The purpose of this section of the book is to present some of the measures that are relevant for prevention of drownings in the broadest sense. Unfortunately, scientific evidence on the efficacy of measures is scant. Therefore, we have to limit ourselves to reporting on best practices as have been developed in the various countries that have a special concern about drowning and on particular practices that seem to have gained some justification through qualitative research and quasi-experimental studies.

3.3.2
Scope

Immersion and drowning can involve:
- People, and especially children, who fall into pools, bathtubs, ponds, wells or even buckets of water
- People swimming in pools and natural bodies of water
- Boaters, sailors, windsurfers and anyone else taking part in water sports during recreation on natural or artificial bodies of water
- Individuals standing or walking on banks of canals, lakes or rivers or who get caught in flood waters, and
- Persons with impairment (alcohol, drugs, fatigue, seizures, heart attack or other health problems) while bathing, swimming or standing near water

As part of the project World Congress on Drowning a new definition of drowning was adopted: Drowning is the process of experiencing respiratory impairment from submersion/immersion in liquid (▶ **Chapter 2.3**).

By this definition drownings can be fatal or non-fatal. We therefore refer to drownings independently of the fatal or non-fatal outcome, thus including accidental submersion and immersions, since what counts for prevention is the control of all factors that may create the hazardous situation irrespective of the outcome of the event.

The predominant mechanism of injury is asphyxia, but impact injuries such as cervical cord injuries associated with diving or trauma from blades on motor boats, surf boards and so on are relevant for drowning prevention as these injuries severely handicap the person while in water and may actually lead to drowning. Attack by sharks or contact with poisonous water animals are not considered. Decompression injuries to scuba divers is dealt with in ▶ Section 11.

3.3.3
Causes and Prevention

For much of the history of humankind, accidental injuries have been perceived as acts of God beyond the control of people. If any injury prevention efforts have been made, these focused mainly on the assumed shortcomings of the victims, with energy directed to such educational measures as the production and distribution of pamphlets and posters. Although this emphasis has changed dramatically in past decades, and in particular in the domains of occupational safety and traffic safety, this victim-centred approach is still evident in policies addressing home and leisure safety.

The modern view of injury prevention does not eliminate personal responsibility, but assigns greater weight to the multitude of factors that also play an important role and some of which are more open for control. As with the outbreak of a disease, each injury is the product of more than one cause that relates to at least three different sources: the host (for instance a swimmer), the agent itself (a tide) and the environment (unsupervised beach) in which host and agent find themselves.

In diagrammatic form this view can be detailed along two dimensions (◘ Fig. 3.1):

- Type of factors involved: on the one hand human factors, such as individual characteristics and social environment, and on the other hand the physical environment, such as products involved in human activity and the physical setting. These are represented in the diagram as the horizontal dimension.
- The time dimension involved: some factors may influence human interaction with the physical environment temporarily, such as impairment by alcohol, while others may have a more continuous influence such as group norms or level of education, skills and so on.

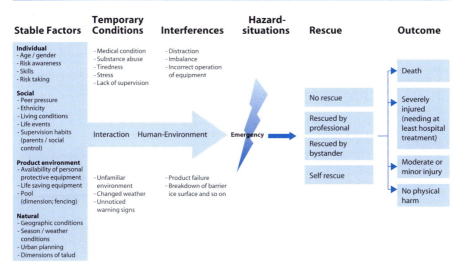

◘ Fig. 3.1. Modern concept of injury prevention, based on multiple factors. Each injury is the product of more than one cause that relates to at least three different sources: host, agent and environment

3.3.4
Routes to Prevention

In this chapter we will focus on primary and secondary prevention, efforts to control factors that may lead to a potential hazardous situation (primary prevention) or which ensure that in case of an emergency the victim can be saved from further harm effectively through proper protective equipment or skills to cope with the emergency situation (secondary prevention). Measures that improve the efficiency of rescue through bystanders is part of this consideration, while professional rescue services, first aid and emergency services are considered to be tertiary prevention measures that are dealt with in other sections of this handbook.

We can focus on three basic routes for prevention (◘ **Table 3.1**):
- Remove, reduce or change the hazard
- Change behaviour in risk taking, supervision or skills
- Prevent contact between people and the environment

However, we can go into more detail than this, and examine drowning prevention from nine inter-related standpoints. These are shown in ◘ **Table 3.2.**

□ Table 3.1. Three basic routes for prevention

Route	Means	Examples in natural water	Examples in artificial environment
1. Remove, reduce or change hazard (focus: physical environment)	Take product/service off market	Drain ponds or lakes	Lower high diving board
	Redesign system/product/environment	Clear underwater traps in fresh water recreation areas	Swimming pool covers
			Vertical distance between water surface and land surface
2. Change behaviour in risk taking/supervision/skills (focus: human being)	Raise risk awareness	Campaigning for beach safety	School swimming education programs
	Educate parents	Parent education centre programs	Safety drill in swimming pools
	Train kids	Improve training in water sports	Parent awareness of bath drownings
	Train parents and youth in rescue		
3. Prevent contact between man and environment	Guards	Separate areas for boats or surfing from bathing	Fence private swimming pools
	Barriers	Life jackets	Separate swimming training area from regular basin
	Personal protective equipment		

■ Table 3.2. Three basic routes to prevent drowning and nine interrelated standpoints

Route	Means	Examples and comments	
		Natural water	**Artificial facilities**
1. Remove hazard	Take hazard or related 'system' or product off market	Drain ponds, lakes – only in special circumstances	Close public swimming pools
2. Reduce level of hazard	Redesign of system, product or environment	Better steering and control interface for boats (power, rowing, sail)	Shallower swimming pools
		Clear underwater traps in salt or fresh water recreation areas	Lower height of diving boards
		Improved diving equipment fit	Higher lighting levels in open and public spaces
		Standards and legislation	Standards and legislation
3. Prevent access or inappropriate interaction	Guards, barriers	Fencing around open water	Swimming pool covers
	Gaps	Separate areas for power boats, swimmers and divers	Walls and fences around pools
	Place hazard out of reach	Standards and legislation	Height of bath side
			Standards and legislation
4. Barrier around individual	Personal protection equipment	Goggles, buoyancy suits, water wings, life jackets	Goggles, buoyancy suits, water wings, life jackets
5. Reduce deliberate risk taking behaviour	Education	Peer or 'hero' advice, schools, advertising	Peer or 'hero' advice, schools, advertising
	Motivation		
	Publicity		

◘ **Table 3.2.** *Cont.*

Route	Means	Examples and comments	
		Natural water	Artificial facilities
6. Increase incidence of safer behaviour	Education, training	Sailing, windsurfing, diving Safety in skill development	Swimming lessons Safety in skill development
7. Improve supervision	Technical or human observation	Closed circuit TV, parental presence, lifeguards, intelligent underwater drowning detection systems	Closed circuit TV, parental presence, lifeguards, intelligent underwater drowning detection systems
8. Recovery from hazard	Improve personal recovery	Coast guards, lifeguards, lifesaving equipment. First aid and lifesaving training for public	Coast guards, lifeguards, lifesaving equipment. First aid and lifesaving training for public
	Rescue services		
9. Remove the person from the hazardous situation	Ensure vulnerable people do not go near or in water	Legislation (probably unfeasible)	Legislation (probably unfeasible)

3.3.5
Domains of Interest

Drownings involve very different risk groups, occur in a wide variety of settings and involve a great diversity of products and physical environmental features. So the presentation of relevant measures can take different structures depending on the focus of interest one wants to underline.

For prevention measures it is relevant to take also into consideration the level of responsibility and the extent to which such responsibility is borne by public and private bodies. Following this line of reasoning there are the following domains of interest:

- The domestic area which relates to the risk of drowning in bathtubs, buckets and garden ponds, but also to the risk of privately owned swimming pools for domestic use
- Public swimming pools, educational pools, spas and other built environments for recreational swimming
- Natural bodies of water that serve as public areas for recreation and for which public authorities have made some arrangements to accommodate people for recreation such as arranged beach settings along the coast line, lakes and rivers
- Natural bodies of water which do not have a primarily recreational function, such as unsupervised coastlines, or which serve for transportation (for example canals in urban areas as well as in rural areas) or for drainage (ditches, rivers, lakes)

For each of these settings consideration should be given to risk management strategies, including risk assessment methodologies, and to the role of legislation and standardisation in ensuring the application of proper safety technologies and equipment.

3.4
Risk Assessment and Perception

ANDREJ MICHALSEN

Risk assessment helps to form the basis for prevention. The implementation and effectiveness of prevention is influenced by individual risk perception. Considering drowning, both hazard and incidence of submersion injuries are underestimated, whereas treatment options are usually overestimated. This paper aims to clarify the concepts of risk assessment and risk perception with special attention to drowning.

Life carries risks. This truism may have very distinct meanings in different parts and populations in the world of today. Whereas some check the completeness of their water skiing gear, others try to survive volcanic eruptions or floods. Air traffic controllers, for instance, need to assess the risk of alternative flight routes to certain destinations. Physicians must clarify the risks of alternative treatment options for their patients. Parents should teach the risks of certain behaviour to their children.

Before risks can be dealt with, they must be identified, characterised, and quantified. Statistically, risk denotes the probability of an untoward event, often expressed in terms of potential financial loss. As human judgement is not only based on evidence, but also on experience and anecdotal knowledge, lay assessment of risks appear to be heavily influenced by individual risk perception. Individual perception appears to be strongly influenced by personal traits and sociocultural parameters. Thus, "risk" can both relate to an objective reality and to a subjective manner of interpretation [1]. Understanding and influencing the individual perception may help to prevent the manifestation of the risk in question.

Specifically, the risk of drowning appears to be underestimated, although, according to the World Health Organization, approximately 500,000 annual deaths worldwide can be attributed to drowning in recent years. Over one-half of these deaths occur among children from 0 to 14 years of age. Still, drowning rarely catches the attention of the general public. Drowning occurs quickly and silently, it is rarely related to mass casualty scenarios, and immersion injuries are frequently linked to feelings of guilt for failed supervision, especially regarding children. Therefore, determining and communicating the risk of such injuries appear to be important components of reducing the toll of drowning.

3.4.1
Definition of Risk

Statistically, risk is the probability of an untoward event or unfavourable consequences of an event [2]. Among other things, this can refer to emotional, medical, ecological, legal, or economic consequences. In the world of insurance, for instance, risk is usually related to losses equated in financial terms. In this text, risk will specifically refer to events with medical sequelae.

3.4.2
Risk Assessment

To describe a certain risk epidemiologically, its distribution and determinants within a particular population need to be known. Based on the Framingham Heart Study, for example, the risk of developing coronary heart disease can be described using certain parameters or risk factors. Individual probabilities of developing defined outcome conditions within a certain time period can be calculated and compared with other cohort members, with a certain margin of confidence. Usually, such a risk assessment pertains to a specific population and may not necessarily be generalised to other populations without further modifications. Also, the individual risk of morbidity and mortality may differ from population-based patterns. Still, preventive efforts can be targeted within defined populations. Such efforts appear to be most successful in so-called high-risk subpopulations.

In risk assessment, risk has also been described as the product of exposure and hazard [3]. An exposure can be quantified through frequency and extent. Hazard denotes the characteristic capacity of an incident to adversely affect human health. Usually, such an incident denotes an interaction between man and his physical and biochemical environment, such as substances, structures, or organisms, with an ensuing energy transfer [4]. For instance, among US anaesthesia personnel, and given average seroprevalence rates and 0.42 percutaneous injuries with infectious material yearly, the estimated average risks of acquiring an occupational hepatitis C or human immunodeficiency

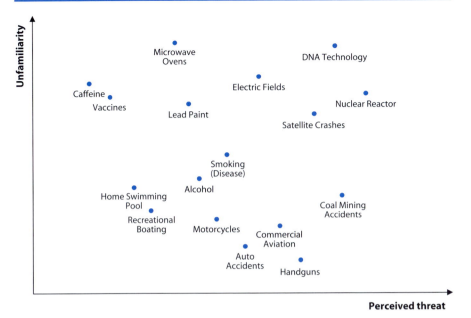

◻ Fig. 3.2. Risk perception by non-experts through positioning of a risk within a perceptual space defined by the degrees of perceived threat and unfamiliarity. (Based on [5])

virus infection within 30 work years have been calculated as approximately 0.5% and 0.05%, respectively.

Prudent risk assessment, related to the populations concerned, forms the basis for public health planning and implementation. For many of the risks of life, however, epidemiological data are difficult to ascertain. And even if objective data are available, the way in which they are interpreted may differ considerably amongst various target populations.

3.4.3
Risk Perception

Subjective perceptions reflect the interpretation of epidemiologically derived data in personal terms. The subjective assessment of the probability of an undesirable event and its seriousness can be called perceived risk. This individually perceived risk appears to rely strongly on personal traits and socio-cultural parameters, such as education, experience, habits, political orientation, beliefs, and values. Often, peer opinion, hearsay, and media coverage substitute for insufficient personal experience or knowledge [2, 5–7].

Research by Slovic and others [5, 6] has shown that the responses of non-experts to risk are closely related to the position of the risk in a perceptual space, defined by the degree of the perceived threat, the horizontal dimension, and the perceived unfamiliarity, the vertical dimension of the risk (◻ Fig. 3.2).

As to the examples in ◘ **Fig. 3.2**, nuclear reactors and DNA technology have been viewed as bearing high risks, whereas home swimming pools have been perceived as incurring small risks. The attributed positions of the risks covered do not necessarily correspond to their objective epidemiological significance. For instance, the risks of electric fields and satellite crashes appear to have been overestimated, whereas the risks of traffic accidents, handguns and swimming pools appear to have been underestimated [5].

Lay judgements of risk incorporate several aspects such as severity and controllability of the risk, willingness to be exposed and acuity of effect. Overall, such judgements have been found to be inversely related to judgements of benefit, for example the higher the perceived risk, the lower the perceived benefit, and vice versa [8]. This leads to individual acceptable risk-benefit trade-offs, where usually higher risks are accepted for voluntary activities than for involuntary hazards, and where immediate consequences are more actively avoided than late sequelae. Risks that appear obvious and controllable by the potential victims are accepted more easily than risks that appear ambiguous and uncontrollable [5, 6]. Risk perception also varies by age group, that is to say that children cannot recognise many risks in their environments, whereas adolescents often tend to seek risks, rather than to avoid them.

Individual risk-benefit trade-offs are naturally subjective and may be coloured by a number of mental biases. Recently manifested risks, such as those caused by tornadoes, are overestimated in the minds of people compared with those barely recalled, such as those caused by plague epidemics. This is called the availability or publicity bias. Also, the impact of rare risks, such as botulism or bovine spongiform encephalopathy (BSE), is often overestimated, whereas the impact of common risks, such as smoking or paediatric drowning, is underestimated. This is called compression bias. Risks leading to more fatalities per manifestation, such as ferry boat accidents, are perceived as more catastrophic than risks leading to fewer fatalities per manifestation, such as leisure boating accidents, even if the accumulated fatalities of the latter exceed those of the former [2, 6]. In fact, a considerable variation of fatality risks exists among different modes of travel. In the European Union, the fatality risks for travel with road motor vehicles, ferries, planes, or trains are 1.1, 0.33, 0.08, and 0.04 per 10^8 person-kilometres, respectively. This variation is probably not always accurately perceived by the general public.

Finally, expert risk assessment has to deal with missing evidence that may be related, among other things, to the scarcity of data, the applicability of statistical techniques or the generalisability of conclusions. Non-experts, however, may wish to be given certainty through scientific rigour and seem to be considerably troubled by the inherent and remaining uncertainty in risk assessment [6, 7]. The fact of remaining uncertainty underscores the necessity of appropriate risk communication between risk assessment experts and the populations concerned.

3.4.4
Application to Prevention

Key theories explaining health behaviour and change in health behaviour imply a central role for health education, emphasising the importance of knowledge and beliefs about health. Risk perception can be conceptualised as a set of psychosocial factors that determine whether certain situations or behaviour are viewed as risky or risk-free [9]. Efforts to modify risk perception, then, need to incorporate both the individual perceptional idiosyncrasies and the socio-economic conditions of the populations targeted. Communication and management of risk might be best structured as a process that includes conveying risk assessment data, emphasising the relevance of the risk considered to the population concerned, fostering self-responsibility, acknowledging individual concerns and personal beliefs, and striving for broad understanding through awareness and knowledge.

The majority of submersion injuries appear preventable. Yet drowning is the second leading cause of death in children aged 1–14 years in the European Union, with male toddlers being especially vulnerable. Among member states, risk fatality rates vary from 0.32 to 1.26 per 100,000 population yearly [10]. To help parents understand this rate, it can be roughly translated into "one child in a large town per year". The only strategy shown to significantly reduce drowning in private pools is continuous poolside fencing. Case control studies evaluating pool fencing interventions indicate that the odds ratio for the risk of drowning in a fenced pool compared to an unfenced pool is 0.27 [95% CI (0.16, 0.47)] [10]. Parental risk perception, however, may be different. Parents may rely on the presumed safety of the environment, the swimming skills of their children or the effectiveness of their supervision. According to a cross-sectional study on the risk perception among parents of pre-schoolers in the US, parents that have already had an experience with injury, who see their children as difficult to manage or who are experiencing stress, seem to have better awareness of potential injuries [9]. In principle, all children in or near water are at risk of drowning. How alert, then, might parents be who have not yet had an experience with childhood injuries and who perceive their children as usually calm, sensible and reasonably compliant with orders? An important preventive task will be to alert all parents and caregivers to the actual risk and the dire prognosis once a child has suffered a submersion leading to unconsciousness due to hypoxia. In fact, the single most important factor that determines outcome of submersion is the duration of the submersion and the duration and severity of the hypoxia. Therefore, the prevention of submersion injuries is of utmost importance.

Mandatory pool fencing appears to make an important contribution towards this goal. Further measures advocated to prevent drowning, although less evidence based than pool fencing, include swimming lessons for children, wearing life jackets while boating, and training in basic life support for the general public. Furthermore, personal risk communication by victims and their families, general practitioners, paediatricians, and emergency physicians, public health specialists, and teachers may modify the perception of the risk of drowning. Also, the media may play an important role, especially through educational material.

3.4.5
Conclusions

Human health behaviour is a complex and dynamic mosaic of interactions rather than a tidy set of actions and reactions. Health behaviour is influenced by the perceptions of gains and losses. The conceptualisation of risk by lay persons is more complex than conversion of human health risks to figures of morbidity and mortality by experts. Efforts to prevent diseases and injuries need to incorporate the factors that influence the risk perception of the populations targeted for interventions.

Specifically considering drowning, the populations at risk are large, because submersion is a ubiquitous risk. Both hazard and incidence of submersion injuries are widely underestimated, whereas treatment options are rather overestimated by the public. Beyond engineering and education, individual and parental alertness needs to be fostered. Submersion is a general risk in life and the principal responsibility rests with each individual or his caregivers.

Acknowledgements. Joanne Vincenten BPE, MA, Amsterdam, and Ralph Houston PhD, Manchester, have assisted in reviewing the manuscript. Their help is gratefully acknowledged. An extended article with a complete list of references can be found in [11].

References

1. Holzheu F, Wiedemann PM (1993) Perspektiven der Risikowahrnehmung. In: Bayerische Rückversicherung (ed) Risiko ist ein Konstrukt. Knesebek, München, pp 9–19
2. Kemp R (1993) Risikowahrnehmung: Die Bewertung von Risiken durch Experten und Laien – ein zweckmässiger Vergleich? In: Bayerische Rückversicherung (ed) Risiko ist ein Konstrukt. Knesebek, München, pp 109–127
3. Rider G, Milkovich S, Stool D, et al. (2000) Quantitative risk analysis. Inj Control Saf Promot 7:115–133
4. Haddon W Jr (1970) On the escape of tigers: an ecological note. Am J Public Health 60:2229–2234
5. Slovic P (1987) Perception of risk. Science 236:280–285
6. Jungermann H, Slovic P (1993) Charakteristika individueller Risikowahrnehmung. In: Bayerische Rückversicherung (Hrsg.) Risiko ist ein Konstrukt. Knesebek, München, pp 9–107
7. National Research Council (1996) Understanding risk – informing decisions in a democratic society. National Academy Press, Washington, D.C.
8. Alhakami S, Slovic P (1994) A psychological study of the inverse relationship between perceived risk and perceived benefit. Risk Anal 14:1085–1096
9. Glik D, Kronenfeld J, Jackson K (1991) Predictors of risk perceptions of childhood injury among parents of preschoolers. Health Educ Q 18:285–301
10. Vincenten J (2001) Priorities for child safety in the European Union: agenda for action. European Child Safety Alliance, Amsterdam
11. Michalsen A (2003) Risk assessment and perception. Inj Control Saf Promot 10:201–204

3.5
Prevention of Drowning in the Home and Garden

JOHN PEARN and DAVID CALABRIA

All around the world, drowning in the home, family garden or its surroundings has become a leading cause of unintentional death among children under the age of 5 years. In many tropical and sub-tropical countries, drowning has replaced motor vehicle accidents as the leading cause of all childhood deaths from injury.

Children under the age of 5 years are particularly vulnerable to home drowning accidents. The sites of such incidents include family-owned swimming pools, the family bathtub, buckets and pails, fish ponds and ornamental pools (◘ Table 3.3) [1, 2]. Child drownings at each of these sites have their individual site-specific precedents and specific approaches to prevention.

Three approaches, sequential in nature, are required if the modern epidemic of preventable child drownings is to be reduced. The first of these comprises an understanding of the site- and age-specific syndromic profiles of home drownings. The second is an analysis of preventive options; and a subsequent matching of preventative stratagems to the primary individual and specific drowning threats. Thirdly, any community in which high home-drowning rates are occurring must pursue a vigorous advocacy of prevention.

Childhood drowning fatalities do not form a spectrum of drowning incidents. They comprise a subset of quite distinct site-specific syndromes unrelated to each other except by the fact that the endpoint of drowning forms the extinction of a young life. A total of 95% of all child drownings are accidental. However, most charged with the duty of reducing child trauma eschew this adjective, and speak of unintentional child drownings. This proactive use of language is held by many to promote a non-defeatist attitude that almost all home and garden drownings involving children are completely preventable.

The primary classification of drowning trauma into unintentional child drownings and intentional child drownings, also highlights the fact that there is a subgroup, less than 2% of all infant and toddler drownings, in which drowning is the modus operandi of child homicide [5].

One generic definition of safety is that "state characterised by adequate control of physical, material or moral threats which contributes to a perception of being sheltered from danger" [6]. All approaches to the promotion of child safety are based on two underlying themes. The first of these is a fundamental philosophical and ethical stance that infants and children have a right to safety.

The second essential distinguishing feature which characterises the domain of child safety is not a philosophical one, but a pragmatic, developmental one. Young children do not have any primary or innate perception of danger. This must be taught or learned by experience.

Specifically, in the case of home drowning incidents, the peak at-risk groups, toddlers, have no perception whatsoever of the threat of water. The biggest injury killer of children, the garden in-ground swimming pool, poses no perceived threat but rather is an attractant to toddlers.

◫ **Table 3.3.** Relative rank order and percent of sites of drowning of children aged 0–5 years. Data typical of tropical and temperate developed nations. Older children (80% males) drown also in rivers, lakes and the sea. Data compiled from the Brisbane Drowning Study and other sources [1, 2]

	Percent
Private swimming pools	64
Family bathtubs	16
Creeks	11
Dams, building trenches, sewers	5
Waterholes, fish ponds	4

3.5.1
Site- and Age-Specific Home Drownings

The causes, sites, survival rates and aftermath of drowning deaths all differ when child victims are compared with adult subjects. The common pattern of adult drowning incidents involving alcohol, suicide and boating accidents are rarely encountered in the case of childhood drowning victims. In drowning incidents which occur in the home or garden, the drowning times of childhood victims are always measured in minutes rather than hours [7].

Children who drown in garden swimming pools or in the waterways of canal estates are always the victims of unintentional injury. An unknown proportion, but in the range of 10%–20%, of home bathtub drowning incidents are non-accidental. In some jurisdictions the specific crime of neonaticide applies to home drownings of newborn infants, usually in the bathroom toilet. This syndrome is very specific and has long been recognised with its sad socio-familial overtones. Such mothers are always young and often young teenagers. They are almost always single and the drowning in the bathroom toilet or bathtub occurs in the context of a concealed pregnancy followed by a solitary labour and delivery.

Infanticide is the crime of unlawful killing of a child under 1 year; and, in some jurisdictions, 1 year and 1 day. Deliberate killing of an infant, or a number of children in the family, by a mother disabled by psychosis, occurs not at birth, but in the weeks or months following a birth. Under these circumstances, drowning is in one sense a non-specific modus as the means of ending the life of a child. The perpetrator of infanticide is almost always the mother [2]. Most such perpetrators are suffering either from postnatal depression or from schizophrenia. When depressed mothers kill their infants, the site is always either the family home or in the family car. The proximity of the family bathtub, washing machine, buckets or pails means that drowning is the method of infanticide. Sometimes a mother will kill one, several or all of her children, before taking her own life. Some psychotic parents have attempted to drug their children before drowning them as the final act of killing.

At least 80% of childhood bathtub drownings are accidental. The syndrome of infant bathtub drowning is quite specific. Such fatalities and near-fatalities occur only, or virtually only, in poorer families or in those of lower socio-economic status. Such drownings afflict infants and toddlers in a very defined, age-specific window of 8–18 months of age only; with a modal age of 9–11 months. More than half such bathtub drowning incidents occur during a specific vulnerable period when family routine is suddenly or unexpectedly broken, such as occurs during acute sickness, affecting either parents or children, or in the context of marital strife. A typical scenario is that which involves a stressed mother who is attempting to cope singly with the control, bathing and feeding of several high-spirited or fractious young children. The telephone rings, or an appliance breaks, or someone calls unexpectedly at the door; and the mother leaves an infant in the care of two or three slightly older children. These latter climb out of the bath leaving the infant to drown [8].

A small proportion of children and teenagers drown, or almost drown, in the bathtub as a result of epileptic seizures. An important preventive approach here is to counsel teenagers not to take private plunge baths in a locked bathroom but rather to shower standing up.

More than 60% of drowning deaths in the home or garden occur in private swimming pools. In the US alone there are now over 12 million plastic wading pools and over 5 million surface swimming pools, of which an estimated 2 million are of the more dangerous in-ground variety. Proportionate rates are even higher in other countries such as Australia and New Zealand and in affluent communities within the larger cities in Southern Africa.

The age spectrum of home swimming pool victims is between 12 and 40 months with a modal peak between 18 and 24 months. Children in both the richest and the poorest families in society are particularly at risk. A total of 70% of toddlers who drown do so in their own garden pools. Other at risk sites are the pools of neighbours, motels, caravan or trailer park pools and the garden swimming pools of relatives whom children are visiting.

Any approach to the prevention of drowning deaths needs to be built on the understanding that these home drowning syndromes are distinct and separate. Each requires its specific focussed and targeted preventative approach.

3.5.2
Home Drownings: Preventive Options

There are three time-honoured approaches to primary prevention – education, better ergonomic design and legislation. There is a fourth, important, but still potentially unexploited, approach to the prevention of drowning. This is secondary prevention in terms of better first aid training of parents.

The educational approach to the reduction of drownings in the home is a time-honoured one [9]. In general, the belief that by raising the awareness of a threat to safety, a concerned society and parents within it would take steps to reduce the risk, has proved to be naive (◘ Table 3.4) [9].

■ **Table 3.4.** Defined child drowning syndromes in the home. Each syndrome is specific with respect to antecedent causes, immersion triggers, age vulnerability, forensic and coronial implications, post mortem investigations and ultimately, advocacy for prevention. Data from the Brisbane Drowning Study [1–6, 9–11]

Private swimming pool drownings	The commonest site of child drowning. Age range is principally from 10 months to 4 years of age with a modal peak at 18–30 months. Of those children who are pulseless and apneic whilst in the water, 50% respond to resuscitation. Toddlers who are so resuscitated are completely normal. Psychometric studies of survivors indicate that they as a group are of above average intelligence [5]
Bathtub drownings	The second most common site of fatal and near-fatal drowning in the home. Drowning in the bath comprises some eight subsets of specific and defined drowning syndromes, which include neonaticide, infanticide, crescendo child abuse, child homicide, post-epilepsy drowning and bathtub euthanasia [5]
Bucket and pail drownings	Victim ages range from 9–20 months. Contents of bucket includes water, detergent, bleach, soap, antiseptic or soiled diapers. Mortality rate exceeds 60%. Whether a subset of this immersion site-syndrome includes child homicide or child abuse has yet to be determined

Better ergonomic design is useful, but primarily as adjuncts to education and legislation.

3.5.3
Safety Legislation

As in the case of successful gun control, the reduction of poisoning fatalities and head injuries following road trauma, so too it has been found that the reduction of home drowning accidents primarily requires a legislative or regulatory approach.

The value of isolation fencing which separates the pool from the home in preventing young children from drowning death or injury has been demonstrated most effectively in Australia, where, as in other areas with warmer climates, drowning is the leading cause of accidental death among children under the age of six. Such studies have shown that the isolation fencing of swimming pools is highly effective in reducing child drownings, with the most important element being a secure, self-closing and self-latching gate [4, 10]. Legislation, therefore, is the catalyst which can reduce home pool drownings by between 40%–50%.

Safety legislation must be based upon evidence-based ergonomics data. The Australian Standard for pool fencing is one example of data which are available on which sensible legislation can be based. The alternative use of some suggested forms of protection, alarms or pool covers in lieu of fencing, are not effective in practice.

Legislation, as a stratagem for the prevention of child drownings, is never effective if used in isolation. Regular media campaigns and regular inspections with prosecutory "teeth" are needed if the continuing high rate of toddler drownings is to be further reduced.

3.5.4
Secondary Prevention: First Aid

Children who drown in the family bathtub, ornamental garden ponds or swimming pools do so with median drowning times not longer than 10 min. Under these circumstances, there is great scope for prevention – not of the drowning incident itself, but of the potential death which follows.

Many regard the approach of promoting first aid as a preventative stratagem for drowning as somewhat distasteful. Some regard it as under-emphasising the focus: the imperative of primary protection. Some feel that any compromise whatsoever of the insistence of the absolute right of young children to home safety is an abrogation of the fundamental ethical principles concerned. There is unequivocal evidence from the Brisbane Drowning Study that if the resuscitator of a child extracted from a home water hazard has received first aid training, there is potentially a 30% increased probability of achieving a save.

Bare-handed resuscitation of small children at the scene of a drowning incident is in fact easier than that performed on adult victims. The force necessary to compress the sternum, during external thoracic compression, is also much less than that required in an adult although the frequency is higher. Resuscitators thus do not become so rapidly fatigued. The flexibility of the bodies and limbs of children also makes them much less liable to injuries sustained during cardiopulmonary resuscitation. Such skills, of course, require prior training, but the rewards are very great.

3.5.5
Pursuing Prevention

The most important factor in the reduction of home drownings is neither any lack of knowledge about causes nor any short-comings concerning potentially effective stratagems. The biggest challenge is the strength of advocacy required to protect children who are at risk.

Those who work towards the reduction of childhood drownings in the home environment, embrace a task measured in decades rather than years, and years rather than months. Any review of the history of children's welfare shows that

Table 3.5. Approaches to the prevention of home drownings. Relative effectiveness of the four methods of prevention. Data from experience obtained in the Brisbane Drowning Study [9]

	Education	Ergonomic or design improvements	Legislation or regulation	Secondary prevention – first aid
Home				
Family bathtub	++	-	-	++
Spa pools	++	-	-	++
Buckets, pails	++	-	-	++
Garden				
Swimming pools (in-ground)	++	++	+++	++
Swimming pools (above ground)	++	++	++	++
Fish ponds, ornamental ponds	++	+++	+	+

whereas society will act swiftly to prevent industrial trauma and deaths sustained by adults, it will not guarantee safety of life and limb as a right to be enjoyed by children. In the UK, Lord Shaftesbury and others worked for many years to overcome that most difficult obstruction of all: the indifference or hostility of parents and indeed that of the whole community to the potential suffering of children. Many countries, regions and communities still do not have such protection. In California, for instance, somewhere between 50 and 100 toddler drownings continue to occur annually.

If legislation for child safety is successfully introduced, this requires constant monitoring to ensure that the regulations are policed. The best approach to the prevention of childhood home drownings is a combination of public education and media advocacy, combined with the underpinning of an enlightened, policed, legislative framework (Table 3.5).

Children's safety in the home, like safety elsewhere, is a relative term [3]. Not all hazards in the home can be eliminated. But hazards which can kill or leave children permanently disabled must be eliminated whenever such are identified. Safety is a dynamic state and approaches to ensure safety need to be changed, modified, implemented or abandoned, whenever the threats to children's welfare change.

The educational approach to reduce home drownings seems logical, indeed self-evident. Many types of home drownings, especially bathtub and bath-spa toddler drownings, are in reality susceptible only to this type of approach. A heightened awareness of the threat, achievable only by media campaigns, seems to be the only approach. However, much has been achieved to date in the reduction of this type of injury; and with resolute advocacy much more will be possible in the future.

References

1. Pearn J (1978) Fatal motor vehicle accidents involving Australian children. Aust Paediatr 14:74–77
2. Pearn JH (1985) Drowning. In: Dickermann JD, Lucey JF (eds) The critically ill child, 3rd edn. WB Saunders, Philadelphia, pp 129–156
3. Pearn JH (1990) The management of near drowning. In: Aochi A, Amaha A, Takeshita H (eds) Intensive critical care medicine. Excerpta Medica, Amsterdam, pp 139–146
4. Pearn JH, Nixon J (1979) An analysis of the causes of freshwater immersion accidents involving children. Accid Anal Prev 11:173–178
5. Pearn JH (2004) Drowning and near drowning. In: Busuttil A, Keeling JW (eds) Paediatric forensic medicine and pathology. Edward Arnold, London
6. Svanstrom L (2000) Evidence-based injury prevention and safety promotion. State-of-the-art. In: Moham D, Tiwari G (eds) Injury prevention and control. Taylor and Francis, London, pp 181–198
7. Pearn JH (1996) Drowning. In: The science of first aid. St John Ambulance Australia, Canberra, pp 138–147
8. Pearn JH, Brown H, Wong R, Bart R (1979) Bathtub drownings: report of seven cases. Pediatrics 64:68–70
9. Pearn JH, Nixon J (1977) Prevention of childhood drowning accidents. Med J Aust 1:616–618
10. Blum C, Shield J (2000) Toddler drowning in domestic swimming pools. Inj Prev 6:288–290

3.6
Prevention of Drowning in Home Pools

Ian Scott

Domestic swimming pools are now recognised as a substantial drowning hazard for young children. They are primarily a hazard for children under 5 years and, in particular, those aged 14 to 24 months. As an affluent and warm weather country Australia was one of the first countries to take up domestic pools in significant numbers and among the first to show what was to be a virtual epidemic of toddler drowning.

The unfortunate Australian history of domestic swimming pool drowning is of the early identification of a growing problem, the relatively early identification of means of prevention (fences and self closing gates appeared in regulation as early as 1972) and then 20 years of dithering while preventable deaths continued to occur. The resistance to action, introduction of ineffective measures, the adoption of effective regulation and then its abandonment were part of this history.

3.6.1
Development of Interventions

The basic components of the interventions to address the new epidemic of child drowning in swimming pools were identified and available relatively quickly.

By 1972 state-wide swimming pool regulation in South Australia required that pools be enclosed by a fence or permanent barrier not less than 1.1 m high and that every opening have a self closing and self latching gate or door. In fact at least one local government authority had started setting and enforcing fencing requirements for pools in 1960. By 1979 design guidelines were well enough advanced to be published as the Australian Standard on Fences and Gates for private swimming pools. Demonstrations of efficacy of the interventions were also available quickly. As early as January 1977 an analysis of a systematic sample of serious immersions reported a low and static rate of childhood swimming pool fatalities, noting the strong contrast to Brisbane, and attributed it to the presence and enforcement of a requirement that pools be enclosed.

One of the earliest safety measures developed was an Australian Standard for so-called safety covers for private swimming pools. The standard was developed at the request of the Victorian Minister for Consumer Affairs "to specify a means of protecting children 5 years of age and under against drowning in private swimming pools" and published in 1977.

3.6.2
Evaluation and Effectiveness

There are now a number of scientific studies attempting to assess the efficacy of the interventions to prevent child drowning in swimming pools.

The latest of these is a meta-analysis, undertaken as part of the Cochrane Collaboration, of the highest quality studies. Nearly 40 years after the first local ordinances required fencing of swimming pools, this meta-study reviewed the scientific evidence on the effectiveness of fencing as a means of preventing drowning. The authors concluded that, on the basis of the highest level of scientific quality, pool fencing significantly reduces the risk of drowning. The risk of drowning in a fenced pool is about one quarter of that of drowning in an unfenced pool. The risk of drowning in a pool that is fenced on all sides is 17% of that of drowning in a pool where there is access from the house to the pool.

The best evaluation of the effect of fencing pools is available from the Queensland experience. In 1991 new regulations required that all domestic swimming pools be fenced and have a child-resistant barrier, consistent with the Australian Standard, between the house and the pool. Pool owners were required to comply by a set date. There was substantial public discussion over the regulatory changes. Public awareness of the risk of domestic pools to young children could not have been higher and is likely to have influenced the fall in pool drowning from 1990.

The first point to be made in interpreting the effect of the Queensland regulation is that the pool drowning rate for children under 5 years has fallen substantially. There was a reduction in the pool drowning rate of 58% between the last year before regulation and the latest data available (1999). The fall was from 6.97 per 100,000 (15 deaths) to 2.90 per 100,000 (7 deaths). The second point to note is that the number of pools rose substantially in this period – pool ownership surveys indicating that pool numbers were 70% higher in 1997 than they had been in 1990. Allowing for this rise in the number of domestic pools the drop in drowning between 1990 and 1997 was about 72%. The third factor to take into account is that the detailed incident reports on child drowning now available show that about one-third of drownings occur in the 10% of pools that are unfenced, one-third occur when the gate is defective or propped open and 10% occur in the 50% of swimming pools with complying fences and gates.

3.6.3
Lessons

It is clear from nearly 30 years of effort to prevent child drowning in domestic swimming pools that it is difficult to set and implement performance standards in a contentious area. The lobbying of anti-fencing groups, of those affected by regulation of their existing swimming pools and by the pool construction industry proved very difficult to overcome.

Weakness of Standard-Setting Process

The organisation of the anti-fencing groups was difficult to counter because standards are developed on a consensual basis. Australia has a practical rule that revised standards will not be published if 15% of the membership of the committee disagree with its provisions. A solid majority of the committee wanted the standard to specify preferred fencing configurations or, as a compromise, to note the difference in risk associated with different configurations. The four of the 15 members with entrenched views against fencing consistently spoke against all such measures and, as a result, development of an effective standard was delayed for nearly 4 years.

This highlights the problems associated with a consensual model for the development of effective standards in areas of dispute. The absence of a performance criteria for safety in the standard, such as that it should protect most children, permitted publication of a safety standard that did not address the single most significant safety issue, the location of the fence, and in fact gave standards endorsement to a dangerous and unacceptable measure.

The Need to Get the Intervention Right

The regulatory requirements for fencing pools were for many jurisdictions and for a long period below the threshold of effectiveness. Although early regulation often mentioned the measures which were demonstrated to be effective, such regulation did not require them. Later legislation that repeated this mistake was drafted in the face of the available evidence. As well as being deficient, this legislation misdirected householders by implying that the major risk was to outside children.

New South Wales (NSW) also serves as a sterling example of this failure. Having deficient legislation in place, it acted to provide effective legislation and then repealed it before it could have full impact. This experience highlights the significance of ensuring that the intervention is manageable in a political and social sense. In hindsight a requirement that extended the time over which pools had to comply could well have prevented this situation.

The Need to Act Before the Hazard Builds

A central lesson from the Australian experience with pool drowning is the significance of timely action and of the penalty of inaction. The easiest pools to regulate are new ones, and action to require fencing of existing pools is both more difficult and more likely to be resisted. By the time the major Australian states acted, the new pools being built represented about 3% of the hazard. Conversely, if the Queensland State government had permitted the 1977 City Council Ordinance to stand then Brisbane is unlikely to have become the "drowning capital of the world".

The Need to Consider Lesser Interventions for Tactical Reasons

Both the NSW and the Queensland experiences indicate the potential value of interventions that do not represent best practice, particularly after the hazard has grown. In NSW it is thought that requiring best-practice isolation fencing for the large number of existing pools was a key factor in the over-turning of regulation in which best-practice requirements for new pools were lost.

In Queensland the reluctant acceptance by advocates of a lesser standard requirement for existing pools, in which a barrier with child-resistant door-sets were permitted, was the tactical step that allowed regulation of all domestic swimming pools. The particular efforts used by public health officials and advocates to win the debate they had lost 15 years earlier and to make the measures work are worthy of separate study.

In analysis of what requirements are acceptable, the risk of falling below the threshold of effectiveness, also needs to be taken into account.

The Need to Pay Attention to Analysts and Advocates

A strong lesson from the pool fencing experience is that the interventions that were later to be demonstrated to be effective were identified very early. If the requirements mentioned but not required in the South Australian regulations in 1972 or the advice proffered by the Australian Consumer Association in 1977 had been followed, then it is likely that two out of three toddler pool drownings in the next 15–20 years could have been prevented.

The Need for Continuing Effort

The final lesson from this experience is that the issue is not over. The Queensland drowning figures have shown that pool drownings continue. Current indications are that around 40% of current drownings occur because of poor maintenance (failure of fence or gate) or poor practice (propping open gate). Compliance checks and continuing education efforts with householders about the need for protective maintenance are required.

Experienced researchers and public health officials such as Pitt and Cass [1] attribute the failure to institute effective and uniform regulation at least partially to the absence of national data collection and collation mechanisms and strongly advocate their establishment to enable scientific analysis to build on existing success.

Further Reading

Milliner N, Pearn J, Guard R (1980) Will fenced pools save lives? A 10-year study from Mulgrave Shire, Queensland. Med J Aust 2:510–511

Nixon J (1994) Swimming pools and drowning, Editorial. Aust J Publ Health 18:3

Nixon J, Pearn JH, Petrie GM (1979) Childproof safety barriers. Aust Paediatr J 15:260–262

Pitt WR, Balanda KP (1991) Childhood drowning and near-drowning in Brisbane: the contribution of domestic pools. Med J Aust 154:661–665

Pitt WR, Cass DT (2001) Preventing child drowning in Australia. Med J Aust 175:603–604

Queensland Injury Surveillance and Prevention Program (undated) Toddler pool drowning in queensland. http://www.qisu.qld.gov.au/pools01 (accessed January 2004)

Standards Australia (1993) Swimming pool safety. Part 2: Location of fencing for private swimming pools, AS 1926.2 (Interim)-1993

Thompson DC, Rivara FP (2002) Pool fencing for preventing drowning in children (Cochrane Review). The Cochrane Library 1, Oxford, Update Software

This chapter is based on a more detailed publication: Scott I (2003) Prevention of drowning in home pools – lessons from Australia. Inj Control Saf Promot 10:227–236.

3.7
The Vigilance of Beach Patrols

ANDREW HARRELL

Since 1990 the Center for Experimental Sociology of the University of Alberta has maintained an ongoing program based on observations of lifeguards and swimmers in public facilities in Edmonton and Calgary, Alberta [1, 2]. Observations have been carried out on more than 80 indoor aquatic centres, approximately 300 lifeguards and over 20,000 children (infancy to 16 years) and adults (over 16 years). In addition to the Alberta observations, data have been gathered at outdoor lakes and ocean beaches in Florida, South Carolina and California.

A major focus in this 13-year program of research has been to chronicle the care taken by parents and lifeguards in safeguarding very young swimmers and in the prevention of drowning. A secondary focus has been to investigate the efficacy of warnings and regulatory signage in prohibiting dangerous activities that could lead to drownings.

A central issue in the program has been the determination of the adequacy of scanning swimming areas by lifeguards as a procedure for locating possible drowning victims. While various approaches to scanning are advocated in the training of lifeguards in North America, we have concluded that scanning itself is an inherently subjective act on the part of lifeguards. Only the lifeguards themselves truly know whether or not they are watching swimmers when they are scanning. It is not possible to get inside the mind of the lifeguard. The research has not attempted to measure this subjective act through lifeguard self-reports because of the obvious self-serving bias: lifeguards are unlikely to report lapses in scanning. Instead, we have relied on relatively crude external or behavioural expressions of scanning, such as head turns or duration of gaze at a given area of a swimming pool, lake or ocean. The validity of such measures as indices of visual vigilance have been found to be acceptable.

Based on the physical measures of scanning, it was found that the typical lifeguard spends a relatively small proportion of time actually observing the water or swimmers. Scanning activities often compete with other activities such as clean up or custodial work, talking to other lifeguards or attending to the needs and requests of swimmers. Major deficiencies in scanning are also likely to occur at the opening and closing times for aquatic facilities, at the end of lifeguard shifts, on weekends, and at certain times of the day, notably during late afternoon [3]. Scanning tends to deteriorate with lifeguard fatigue after 30 min.

Duration of scanning is highly predicted by principles of information theory and is a non-linear function of the number of at-risk swimmers, such as young children. In other words, scanning by lifeguards tends to increase as the information processing requirements increase with greater numbers of children. Scanning is also highly sensitive to the ratio of adults to children in the water, with more scanning taking place when ratios are low [3].

In practice, lifeguards virtually never implement some of the scanning approaches recommended in most lifeguard training courses and manuals such as by the Royal Life Saving Society of Canada [4]. For example, lifeguards rarely carry out head counts of swimmers as a way of checking on the safety of swimmers. The information processing demands of this procedure are too burdensome. Experienced lifeguards come to rely on schemas or cognitive shortcuts that simplify the task of vigilance. Thus, lifeguards will often pay less attention to groups of children, relying on the assumption that there is safety in these groupings. As the dispersion of swimmers increases over a pool or beach area, reducing the size of groupings, lifeguards tend to increase their scanning.

Lifeguards also make assumptions about swimmer safety that decreases safety. They assume that children over the age of 5 are less at risk and less in need of scrutiny than younger children. Lifeguards are less inclined to scan those areas of a pool or beach where adult caretakers such as parents, teachers or swimming instructors appear to be in close physical proximity to young swimmers [1].

Lifeguard vigilance is also strongly impacted by the presence of other lifeguards. Rather than increasing vigilance because of a division of labour between a number of lifeguards working as a team, it is more often the case that multiple lifeguards watching the same pool, lake or ocean engage in social loafing or the diffusion of responsibility. Lifeguards working as teams often assume that others will provide backup scanning or redundancies in scanning that compensate for lapses. Often studies have found that lifeguards have not been trained as a cooperative team. Each individual lifeguard assumes incorrectly that his fellow lifeguards will be scanning more than just their own zone so that they can relax their vigilance. It was often observed that where there are signs of a swimmer in distress, multiple lifeguards may wrongly assume that other team members will deal with it, or that the absence of rescue behaviour from other team members signifies that the emergency is less serious than it might be. Lifeguard manuals or training programs do not recognise these group dynamics and these dynamics are not built in procedures that minimise their impact.

Finally scanning is strongly impacted by the physical positioning of the lifeguard. Lifeguards who are placed in towers are more likely to scan, in part because they are less inclined to engage in competing social activities, such as talking to swimmers, or clean up and maintenance activities. Lifeguards in towers, however, are less likely to sanction negatively minor rule violations by swimmers because of the costs of implementation; to reprimand a violator or to remove him from the facility, they may have to descend from the tower and abandon scanning [3].

It has been the observation of the studies that the majority of aquatic facilities lack adequate signage that may be necessary to regulate swimmer's conduct. Signs are frequently absent altogether, improperly placed, and lacking in signal words or pictorials that highlight the hazards for swimmers.

References

1. Harrell WA (1995) Risky activities and accidents involving children in public swimming pools: the role of adults and lifeguard supervision. In: Proceedings of the 38th Annual Meeting of the Human Factors Society, Santa Monica, CA. The Human Factors and Ergonomics Society, p 933

2. Harrell WA (1999) Lifeguards' vigilance: effects of child–adult ratio and lifeguard positioning on scanning by lifeguards. Psychol Rep 84:183–197
3. Harrell WA (2001) Does supervision by a lifeguard make a difference in rule violations? Effects of lifeguards' scanning. Psychol Rep 89:327–330
4. Royal Life Saving Society of Canada (1993) Alert lifeguarding in action. Royal Life Saving Society of Canada, Ottawa, ON

3.8
Swimming Abilities, Water Safety Education and Drowning Prevention

RUTH BRENNER (COORDINATING AUTHOR), KEVIN MORAN, ROBERT STALLMAN, JULIE GILCHRIST and JOHN McVAN

Competence in swimming and water safety are important life skills, especially since exposure to the aquatic environment can threaten human life. However, the relationship between swimming ability and drowning risk is unclear. The purpose of this chapter is to focus attention on specific topics for drowning prevention that should be included in swimming instructions.

3.8.1
Swimming Ability and the Risk of Drowning

Based on current literature, the relationship between swimming ability and drowning risk is unknown [1]. Some studies suggest that proficient swimmers are at lower risk of drowning while others fail to support this claim. In fact, some have suggested that proficient swimmers might actually be at greater risk of drowning due to increased exposure to the water and specifically increased exposure to high-risk situations. For example, a skilled swimmer might be more likely to swim alone or in an unguarded remote location. Research on the effects of swimming ability on drowning risk has been challenging for a number of reasons including the lack of a clear definition of swimming ability and the need to account for varying exposures to water and other contributing factors.

Currently, there is no universally accepted definition of swimming ability, particularly as it pertains to drowning prevention. Determination of what constitutes swimming ability and how much of it is necessary to prevent drowning has proved problematic. Hogg, Kilpatrick and Ruddock highlight two essential aspects of swimming: flotation to permit breathing and propulsion to provide mobility [3]. Clearly the possession of such attributes could be life-saving in many, but not all, drowning scenarios with flotation allowing maintenance of the airway and propulsion providing a means to return to safe refuge. One working definition of swimming is the ability to perform "a recognisable stroke and breathing in such a manner as to permit a reasonable distance to be covered" [3]. Such a definition is consonant with worldwide practice of swimming instruction where swimming ability is frequently evaluated in terms of distance swum, stroke used and time taken. With respect to drowning prevention, this definition is problematic. First, the ability to swim a given distance under one set of conditions, of calm water, does not translate to the ability to swim the same distance under different conditions with currents. For young children the distance yardstick is particularly troublesome. A child may be an excellent swimmer in a controlled environment; however, the same child may not perform as well in a panic situation, for example when the child falls fully clothed into a swimming pool. Further, in this all too common scenario, it is not clear that the ability to swim a predetermined distance would be the most relevant survival skill. Interestingly, some more progressive agencies include swimming with clothes fairly early in their programs, specifically to prepare for this situation. Even among older children and adults, the ability to swim a predetermined distance may not be the critical skill. For example, a British study reported that 55% of open water drownings occurred within 3 metres of a safe refuge and many of the victims were supposedly good swimmers [4]. Unfortunately, the reliance on a distance measure has probably lead to too much emphasis on the development of these skills at the cost of de-emphasising other important water safety skills. There are notable exceptions, however, and many organisations do not rely on distance swum to measure swimming ability.

Stallman has emphasised that, from the viewpoint of drowning prevention, measures other than the ability to swim a recognisable stroke for a given distance are needed. He identifies eight motor skills that may be important in the prevention of drowning including ability to level off from vertical to horizontal position, swim on the front and on the back using any type of stroke, roll over from front to back and back to front, change direction both on front and back, rhythmic breathing appropriate for chosen stroke, stop and rest with minimal movement, simple surface diving and underwater movement, jump or dive into deep water [6]. Importantly, these eight skills have been embraced by organisations in a number of countries as the set of skills that should be used to define swimming ability.

Few would argue that under identical circumstances, a proficient swimmer is more likely to possess the skills to assure his survival than is a non-swimmer. However, examination of the relationship between swimming ability and drowning risk is complicated by the need to account for differential exposures to water between swimmers and non-swimmers and other confounding factors that may be related to both drowning risk and swimming ability, such as age. Additionally, varying water conditions, such as the presence of currents, cold water temperatures, and wave splash can also alter the relationship between swimming ability and drowning risk [2]. More proficient swimmers are likely to swim more often and in higher risk situations as in unguarded or remote sites, providing this group with more opportunities to drown. Overconfidence in abilities may lead to underestimation of conditions and failure to take reasonable precautions. For example, a proficient swimmer may be less likely to wear a life vest when boating than a non-swimmer. Should the boat capsize the non-swimmer with the life vest would probably be less likely to drown than the proficient swimmer without the vest. Failure to account for these differences in use of protective equipment, risk taking, exposure to water and other confounding factors can lead to erroneous conclusions regarding the relationship between swimming ability and drowning risk.

3.8.2
Swimming Instruction and Development of Water Competence

Parents and others commonly measure the transition from unsafe non-swimmer to safe swimmer by the ability to propel oneself through the water for a certain minimal distance. As noted above, this view is inadequate when evaluating the skills needed to prevent drowning. Furthermore, swimming skills per se, are but one aspect of a wider field of human aquatic endeavour that has been identified as water competence and traditionally referred to as watermanship [5]. Water competence is the sum of aquatic motor skills, cognitive knowledge and affective dispositions that contribute to a person's competency and confidence in the aquatic environment.

To date, much attention has focussed on the physical skill base for water competency. Familiar fundamental motor skills include water entry, leg kick, arm action, breath control and flotation. Self-rescue techniques are an additional important, yet often neglected, component of the physical skill base. These skills, which are often a very natural part and extension of the most elementary skills, should be an integral part of swimming instruction. Just as the teaching of fundamental swimming skills needs to be tailored to the developmental level of the student, so too does the teaching of survival skills. For example, an important survival skill of a beginning swimmer might include the simple act of turning from face down to face up position. As swimmers become more advanced, teachers need to facilitate in-water survival skill exploration through positional postures (supine, prone and vertical) as well as exposure to skill combinations (changing position, finding a position of maximal buoyancy) that might better address survival across multiple aquatic environments (pools, open water) and challenges (waves, currents). As noted above, aquatic motor skills achieved in one setting (a swimming pool) are not always transferable to another (sea, lake or river). Where possible and appropriate a lesson in the natural environment should be included so that students gain a proper understanding and respect for these environments.

Cognitive skills have received far less attention in traditional swimming courses. Just as there is little known about the relationship between aquatic motor skills and drowning risk, data regarding the role of water safety knowledge in reducing drowning risk are also lacking. Still, it seems reasonable to include water safety rules as one component of swimming courses, as this is unlikely to cause harm and may prove to be beneficial. Teaching of safety rules needs to be sequential and developmentally appropriate. Whenever possible, parents and caregivers of young children need to be included in that part of the swimming lesson where safety rules are discussed or promoted. Young children might be taught simple rules: always asking permission before going in the water and never swimming alone. Older children and adults might be taught how to recognise hazards, such as rip currents, dumping waves, offshore winds, outgoing tides, and the effect of alcohol on balance, coordination, perception and judgement.

The final component of water competence relates to the social domain and includes the development of sound water safety attitudes that are informed by the skills and knowledge acquired from the motor and cognitive domains. The establishment of healthy attitudes, especially during the formative years of childhood and young adulthood, may lead to safer behaviours in and around water throughout the lifespan. Whilst attitudes, and therefore behaviours, can also be influenced by other social factors such as perceived norms, self efficacy, perceived benefits of the action, and peer pressure, the potential contribution of instructor, teacher, and parent in developing positive water safety attitudes can be great. Modelling and teaching of positive attitudes towards water safety during swimming instruction can begin the process of lifetime development of safe affective dispositions when in or around water. Examples of teaching, modelling, and reinforcing positive behaviours might include requiring children to ask if it is OK to enter the water at the beginning of the lesson rather than the instructor telling the child to enter the water. The child who independently asks if it is OK to enter could be praised in front of the group. Parents and instructors can model positive behaviours for adolescents as well, refraining from drinking alcohol when in or around bodies of water and by wearing a life vest when boating.

Importantly, in the past, courses have promoted the notion that with proper instruction, a person could be made drownproof. There can be little doubt that children or adults, young or old, can never be considered drownproofed either as the consequence of swimming lessons or accumulated experience and wisdom. Water competence, whether expressed as swimming ability, water safety knowledge or experience, can never proscribe all the risks posed by the aquatic environment. What it can do is make people aware of their limitations in a medium that can offer much, but take entirely.

With this background, we offer the following research needs and recommendations.

3.8.3
Research Needs

- Continued development and dissemination of a concise definition of swimming ability as it relates to drowning prevention
- Increased understanding of those movements in the water that are protective in potential drowning situations so that survival skills can be more concisely defined
- Studies evaluating the relationship between self reported swimming ability and observed aquatic motor skills
- Examination of the transference of skills learned in one aquatic environment (swimming pool) to skills in other water environments (sea)
- Studies examining the relationship between aquatic motor skills and exposure to water and attitudes regarding water safety

- Examination of the relationship between water competence, including aquatic motor skills, water safety knowledge, and affective dispositions and the risk of drowning

3.8.4
Recommendations of the Authors

- That the concept of swimming ability be replaced by the more encompassing notion of water competence with regards to drowning prevention
- That swimming ability be promoted as a necessary component of water competence, but with the understanding that swimming ability alone is not sufficient to prevent drownings
- That developmentally appropriate self-rescue techniques be an integral part of swimming instruction at all levels
- That water safety encompassing the acquisition of knowledge, attitudes and behaviours be promoted as a part of the critical mass of water competence
- That the term 'swimming lessons' be replaced by the term 'swimming readiness lessons' when referring to the pre-school age group
- That the concept of drownproofing be removed from the vocabulary of aquatic professionals' especially those promoting swimming lessons for young children

At the World Congress on Drowning, the following recommendation was made:

All individuals, and particularly police officers and fire fighters, must learn to swim.

Knowing how to swim is a major skill to prevent drowning for individuals at risk. International organisations such as WHO, IRCF and ILS, and their national branches must emphasise the importance of swimming lessons and drowning survival skills at all levels for as many persons as possible. The relationships between swimming lessons, swimming ability and drowning in children needs to be studied. In addition, certain public officials, such as police officers and fire fighters, who frequently come in close contact with persons at risk for drowning must be able to swim for their own safety and for the safety of the public.

References

1. Brenner RA, Saluja G, Smith GS (2003) Swimming lessons, swimming ability, and the risk of drowning. Injury Control Safety Promot 4:211–216
2. Golden F, Tipton M (2002) Essentials of sea survival. Human Kinetics, Champaign, IL
3. Hogg N, Kilpatrick J, Ruddock P (1983) The teaching of swimming; an Australian approach. Landmark Educational Supplies, Drouyn, Vic
4. Home Office (1977) Report of the working party on water safety. HMSO, London

5. Langendorfer SJ, Bruya LD (1995) Aquatic readiness: developing water competence in young children. Human Kinetics, Champaign, IL
6. Stallman R, Junge M, Blixt T (2002) A conceptual model of the ability to swim; drowning prevention revisited. Book of Abstracts. World Congress on Drowning, Amsterdam 2002

3.9
National and Community Campaigns

ELIZABETH BENNETT (COORDINATING AUTHOR), PETER BARSS,
PETER CORNALL, KATRINA HADDRILL, REBECCA MITCHELL,
LAURIE LAWRENCE, JOHN LEECH, MARILYN LYFORD, KEVIN MORAN,
LUIS-MIGUEL PASCUAL-GÓMEZ, PALOMA SANZ, BLANCA BARRIO,
SANTIAGO PINTO, FRANK PIA, LINDA QUAN, MONIQUE RIDDER,
MARCIA ROM, GREG TATE and ANDREW WHITTAKER

Around the world communities are developing campaigns to prevent drowning. The programs featured here are based on data and are strategically focused. These 14 national and community level programs focus on a variety of age groups, special populations, water sites and risks. There are however common themes, which are also reflected in the final recommendations of the World Congress on Drowning:

- Drowning prevention campaigns must use multiple strategies and target specific age groups, cultural groups or water sites and risks based on data and assessments of environmental factors, policy factors, behaviours and beliefs.
- Collaboration among consumer groups, research institutions, manufacturers and retailers, organisations, agencies and national, state and local government is essential.
- Environmental measures, policy change and equipment design must be considered along with education and training.
- Evaluation is needed to identify successful programs.

Each program description includes a website at the end for more information. All of the authors welcome your questions and further interest in their programs.

3.9.1
National Surveillance-Based Prevention of Water-Related Injuries in Canada

PETER BARSS

In the early 1990s, the Canadian Red Cross implemented a national drowning surveillance database. This was developed with collaboration of public health injury prevention professionals, all provincial coroners, and other water-safety organisations including the Coast Guard and Lifesaving Society. The database was funded to provide a sound research basis for national water-safety programs, by monitoring the incidence and circumstances of all water-related injury deaths in Canada on an annual basis. It relies upon structured reviews of the mandatory coroner and police reports for all water-related deaths and includes information from 1991 to the present [1].

On the basis of information from the surveillance database, national water safety standards, a new water safety and swimming manual [2] and water-safety programs were developed using modern principles of injury control. These principles include a structured approach to assessing and managing the most important personal, equipment, and environment risk factors for pre-event, event, and post-event phases of potential injury incidents. Surveillance, programs, and training are centred on major activities. These include boating, aquatic activities such as swimming and wading, bathing, walking and playing near water and on ice, and land and ice transport.

The new training materials and programs were introduced to Canadian Red Cross staff and volunteers and are used in nearly all communities. Media publicity began in 1994 and release of the new water safety manual in 1995. Since then, annual visual surveillance reports, and periodic special reports on drowning of children, boaters, and swimmers, have been distributed to staff, and summaries to students, parents, and others. The national surveillance database is also used as a guide to programmatic activities by other organisations such as the Canadian Coast Guard and Lifesaving Society.

During the first 5 years of new surveillance-based programs, marginal savings (such as decrease over baseline) in lives were highly significant and included 25 infants, 120 toddlers, and 215 persons aged 5 and older. Assuming average direct and indirect costs of $1 million for a drowning death in the 0- to 4-year age group, marginal benefits of providing a surveillance basis for prevention programs for this age group were $145 million, for an investment of $200,000 in surveillance and research. While it is not feasible to prove a causal relationship for surveillance-based national programs, the observed decrease in the rate of toddler drowning was significantly greater than in the nearest neighbouring country without national surveillance based-programs, the United States.

National prevention programs for water-related injuries should, wherever feasible, be based upon good national surveillance data on incidence and risk factors for specific water-related activity categories and risk groups. Surveillance and prevention categories should be congruent. Program materials, training, and public policy should be regularly updated and evaluated using incidence data, and revised accordingly.

For more information visit: www.redcross.ca

References

1. Canadian Red Cross (2001) National drowning report: an analysis of water-related fatalities in Canada for 1999. Visual Surveillance Report 2001, Ottawa, ON, Canada, pp 1–124
2. Canadian Red Cross (1995) Swimming and water safety. Mosby-Year Book, St. Louis, USA, pp 1–308

3.9.2
Child Drowning Deaths in Garden Water Features –
A Concerted Campaign to Reduce the Toll

Peter Cornall

Throughout the 1990s many TV gardening design programs included ponds and water features. The number of water features in gardens increased throughout the UK. A study by the University of Wales College of Medicine, RoSPA and the Royal Life Saving Society showed the number of garden pond deaths rose from 11 in 1988/89 to 21 in 1998/99.

There were 90 fatal drowning incidents involving children aged 5 and under between 1992 and 1999 related to the following water features:
- 62 in garden ponds
- 18 in swimming and paddling pools
- 10 in other water containers

Those most at risk were boys aged 1–2 years old with most deaths occurring during July and August. Perhaps, most surprisingly, accidents were three times more likely to happen in someone else's garden.

RoSPA noticed a worrying trend in garden related deaths in the mid 1990s from its own collection of statistics and started to raise awareness of the problem. The situation was confirmed by the study mentioned above and another commissioned by the Department of Trade and Industry (DTI). Every summer since 1996 RoSPA issued press releases during Child Safety Week warning parents of the dangers.

In 1996, RoSPA staffed a stand at the BBC's Gardeners' World national gardening exhibition giving garden safety advice including pond safety. In 1999 a garden pond fact sheet was produced giving safety information and pond security design advice. This went on-line in 2001. The national press in 2000, primarily the Daily Mirror, supported the campaign. Following its research the DTI consumer safety unit produced the 'Safer Ponds by Design' safety leaflet that was launched by a Government minister.

Awareness of the problem has been raised and the message has reached the very top of government. When a new pond was being built in the garden of No. 10 Downing Street, RoSPA was called in to advise on safety. By installing a child-safe pond the Prime Minister led by example and the surrounding media interest raised awareness further. This campaign has also been supported by leading TV gardening presenters, who include safety advice when featuring garden ponds. We have not stopped such drownings but in the last 2 years the annual incidence has levelled off.

Our campaign snowballed because of a combination of the following:
- Providing clear and practical advice
- Our ability to respond to media requests for comment after each drowning
- Good accurate data being available
- Academic research being published
- Media interest

— The cause being championed at a high level and supported by media personalities

For more information visit: www.rospa.com

3.9.3
SafeWaters Water Safety Campaign in New South Wales, Australia

KATRINA HADDRILL and REBECCA MITCHELL

At both national and state levels in Australia the prevention of drowning have been highlighted as priority areas for injury prevention activities. On average around 300 people drown in Australia each year, around 87 of whom drown in New South Wales (NSW).

Public education campaigns can be a powerful prevention strategy when they are combined with other prevention measures that are ongoing. A public awareness campaign, entitled *SafeWaters*, was devised to raise water safety awareness in NSW on beaches, inland rivers, lakes and dams, and general water safety. This campaign was screened on television during the peak summer swimming season in NSW and during the Easter holiday weekend from 1998/1999 to 2002/2003. The campaign aims to increase the awareness of water safety issues and appropriate safety precautions in the general community in NSW and is coordinated by the NSW Water Safety Taskforce.

The key messages of *SafeWaters* include:
— Learn to swim and survive
— Always supervise children near water
— Never swim alone
— Only swim between the red and yellow flags at the beach
— Fence swimming pools
— Beware of fast flowing water, submerged objects and deep water

An evaluation of the *SafeWaters* campaign was conducted in 2001–2002, using pre- and two post-population-based telephone surveys. A key finding of the evaluation was an increase in the recall of water safety messages between the pre-campaign survey and the first post-campaign survey. Prompted recall of key water safety messages from the *SafeWaters* campaign revealed a significant increase in the recall of seven out of the eight key water safety messages in the first post-campaign survey.

Perceptions of risk in relation to water safety were generally high during all three surveys and two most common safe behaviours practised in all three surveys in relation to water safety were: ensuring that young children were constantly supervised when they were in the water; and swimming between the red and yellow flags at the beach.

Factors that contributed to the lessening recall of the Easter campaign during April included: that the campaign screened for 1 week as opposed to 3 weeks in the December-January period, other campaigns highlighting water safety messages were run during the December-January period and uncharacteristically the campaign did not coincide with the school holiday period in April.

It can be concluded that television is an effective medium for improving awareness of water safety, especially during peak aquatic usage times during summer and school holidays.

The *SafeWaters* campaign continued in 2003–2004, including a particular focus on people from culturally and linguistically diverse backgrounds, with an investigation of water safety messages that have significant meaning to the Chinese community in NSW.

For more information visit: www.safewaters.nsw.gov.au

Acknowledgements. The authors acknowledge assistance from the NSW Water Safety Taskforce.

3.9.4
Community Campaign in Australia
Targeted Towards Parents and Children

LAURIE LAWRENCE

Drowning is the greatest cause of accidental death in the under-5 age group in Australia. Every year, one child drowns each week. The *Kids Alive – Do The Five* program, sponsored by safety gate hardware company D&D Technologies, educates the public on the steps to take in reducing the risk of drowning. The program, started in Queensland, is now being promoted nationally through a Web site, children's pantomime, media and public appearances. The program can be summed up by its five-point message:
- Fence the Pool
- Shut the Gate
- Teach your kids to swim, it's great
- Supervise: watch your mate
- Learn how to resuscitate

For pool owners, owning a swimming pool is a big responsibility. It is up to owners to make sure young children are always safe in the pool. Despite the introduction of pool fencing legislation (barrier codes) in April 1992, children under the age of 5 years continue to drown in backyard pools and spas. Many of these accidents occurred because the pool fences did not comply with legislation. About a third of children who drown in pools in Australia access the pool through a gate with a faulty latch or a gate that has been propped open. Inadequate fencing or no fencing increases drowning risk as does the following:
- Lack of gate security
- Lack of effective water safety skills
- Inadequate supervision
- Lack of resuscitation skills
The message is:

- Be sure that your pool gate and doors leading to the pool and other water areas are self-closing. Do not forget to check any dog or cat doors
- Always shut the gate, make sure it latches properly and never prop it open
- Check the latches and hinges regularly and fix them immediately if needed
- Fence and gate security is not enough. Always keep your pool fence well maintained
- The fence is only as good as its weakest point: the gate
- Do not leave objects leaning against the fence that could be used to help a child climb over

For more information visit: www.kidsalive.com.au

3.9.5
The Approach to Promoting Water Safety in Ireland

JOHN LEECH

Ireland is an island nation with an extensive network of inland waterways. In recent years it has generated considerable income and growth as a nation and with this wealth a corresponding growth in water related sports and activities. In addition, the population of Ireland has increased and emigration decreased. A census was conducted last year and our population is now at its highest level since 1871. The promotion of water safety was first addressed by our Government in 1945 when the provision of swimming and lifesaving was formally arranged under the umbrella of the Red Cross by volunteers.

Regrettably 185 people drown in Ireland every year as a result of accidental, undetermined and suicide drowning. An average of 84 were accidental drownings, 85% were male, 15% were female, and 42% occurred at sea, while 58% occurred in inland waterways. In all, 30% of victims had consumed alcohol. Ireland is ranked 19th in the world, by the World Health Organisation (WHO) for accidental drownings.

Irish Water Safety (IWS) was established in 1999 by statutory instrument to achieve the following objectives:
- The promotion of public awareness of water safety
- The promotion of measures, including the advancement of education, related to the prevention of accidents in water
- The provision of instruction in water safety, rescue, swimming and recovery drills
- Such other services relating to water safety as the Minister may from time to time require, direct or determine

It is financed partly by the government through the Department of Environment and Local Government (DELG) and receives voluntary contributions from local authorities each year for the services which are provided to them and sponsorship from state and private concerns. There are local area committees (LAC) based in each county and for the Defence and Police Forces. They are comprised of volunteers who manage the work.

IWS is governed by a council, which is appointed by the minister for the DELG every 3 years. The council comprises 12 members appointed by the Minister, five of whom will have been elected by the volunteers nationwide and the other seven by the minister himself. The full time permanent staff located at the national office implements their policy. The Association aims at being interactive with all members of the public, state and non-governmental agencies involved in aquatic based activities, sports and employment in an effort to reduce the level of drownings and accidents throughout the country.

For more information visit: www.iws.ie

3.9.6
Community Campaign in Remote Aboriginal Communities in Western Australia

MARILYN LYFORD

Despite the attention to indigenous health issues over the past decades, there has been little overall change, with the health of indigenous Australians being described as poor. Drowning is ranked the second most common cause of injury death and is three times higher than other Australian children aged 0–14 years. In remote communities, deaths have been reported to occur in aquatic surroundings including rivers, waterholes and dams.

As part of a State Government Environmental Health intervention, the Department of Housing and Works has built swimming pools in the remote Aboriginal communities of Burringurrah, Jigalong and Yandeyarra in Western Australia. The Royal Life Saving Society is managing the aquatic facilities and is committed to providing a service that will enhance the overall health status of the community. Whilst the provision of swimming pools may alleviate many health problems, community members need to be aware of not only the benefits in and around aquatic environments, but also of the associated risks of drowning and non-fatal drowning.

Strategies to address this include the implementation of a number of programs designed to encourage active community participation within the aquatic facility, providing a strong social focus for the community. Recreational, educational and social programs are being implemented and include water polo, learning to swim and survive, resuscitation and cadet and traineeships. In particular, the *Swim and Survive* program of the Royal Life Saving society provides a broad, balanced program of swimming, water safety and survival skills in preparation for a lifetime of safe activity in and around water. Resources include an educational video 'Watch out for the Kids' for community workers to educate parents and carers on the prevention of drowning and injury in and around aquatic environments.

With community involvement and appropriate management this project has the potential to enhance the overall health status by addressing the physical, social, emotional and cultural health needs of each community. Health checks conducted by the Telethon Institute for Child Health Research indicate a reduction of ear and skin disease and a general improvement of health. Furthermore, it presents a real agenda for action for the reduction of drowning and the improvement of Aboriginal health throughout Australia.

For more information visit: www.rlss.org.au

3.9.7
Community Campaigns in New Zealand

KEVIN MORAN

With more than 11,000 kilometres of coastline extending over ten degrees of latitude, high exposure to the aquatic environment is inevitable in an island nation such as New Zealand. Death by drowning in New Zealand has been consistently among the highest recorded in developed nations and, with an unintentional drowning rate of 4.4/100,000, New Zealand compares poorly internationally, with drowning rates more than double that of close neighbour Australia and five times that of the USA [1].

At a national level, Water Safety New Zealand spearheads water safety education through public awareness campaigns and by supporting over 20 education programs in conjunction with other water safety organisations. Boating, the leading cause of unintentional drowning in New Zealand, is currently the focus of a major advertising campaign entitled *Boatsafe* that addresses issues of skipper responsibility including checking conditions and ensuring boats are well maintained and carrying appropriate safety equipment. Another campaign entitled *Riversafe* addresses the fact that more people drown in rivers than in any other aquatic environment in New Zealand. Because children and youth under 18 years old are over-represented in the river drowning statistics, the resource is targeted at high school students and focuses on river risk identification and crisis management skills. *Riversafe* is promoted as a school-based activity via pool and classroom teaching and schools are encouraged to include an experiential component of river-based activity during outdoor education camps.

At a regional level, Watersafe Auckland Incorporated conducted a community awareness campaign entitled *Safe Summer 2002/3* that capitalised on the heightened interest in water recreation associated with the second New Zealand defence of the America's Cup in Auckland. The campaign, aimed at both local residents and visitors, promoted key water safety messages for use on Auckland's extensive harbours and surf beaches. Among its more novel approaches was the use of positive policing by on-water police and coast guard authorities during Cup racing who gave out confectionary rewards to those demonstrating good boat safety behaviour. The same organisation has also piloted a local community initiative to combat toddler drowning entitled the *Water Hazard Mapping Project* that includes innovative use of geographic information system (GIS) technology to map water hazards such as storm water drains, home swimming pools, and tidal waterways. The location of the hazards is disseminated via coloured laminated maps to the public predominantly through early childhood centres, libraries and community centres. Initial results suggest an increased awareness of water safety amongst the community, and a reduction of the number of hazards as a consequence of improved local authority interventions.

For more information visit: www.watersafe.org.nz

References

1. Langley JD, Warner M, Smith G, Wright C (2000) Drowning related deaths in New Zealand: 1980–1994. Injury Prevention Research Unit, University of Otago, Dunedin

3.9.8
Community Campaigns *Blue Ribbon Pool* and *Enjoy Your Swim, Sure!* in Segovia, Spain

LUIS-MIGUEL PASCUAL-GÓMEZ, PALOMA SANZ, BLANCA BARRIO and SANTIAGO PINTO

Thousands of public swimming facilities (PSFs) exist in Spain, the most important being leisure resorts, only surpassed by beaches in terms of numbers of users. According to WHO, between 70 and 150 people drown in Spain each year, 80% in pools and most of them are aged under 4 years. Statistics show that at least one serious water-related incident and two medical emergencies occur per 2,000 users in the province of Segovia (55,000 inhabitants, total province population: 125,000) every year.

During 2000, the Segovia Lifesaving School (ESS), inspired by the European program *Blue Flag Beaches* (www.blueflag.org), carried out the investigation project *Blue Ribbon Pool 2000* in Segovia (approximate cost: 2000 euros). ESS analysed the overall quality standards, lifesaving service, first aid equipment and facilities and satisfaction of users of 59 PSFs, including all state-owned pools. The conclusions highlight the most important factors regarding PSF quality standards:

- Efficient management
- Age, condition and maintenance of facilities and services
- Performance, duties, responsibilities and available resources of lifeguards, including first aid equipment and facilities
- Customer service

As a result, during 2001–2002, the local public health department applied stricter opening requirements and sanitary inspections criteria (sign-posting, professional requirements of lifesavers and first aid equipment) to PSFs in the province of Segovia. In 2002, one PSF which was over 30 years old was denied an opening licence on the grounds of these new criteria. Four other PSFs, among those with the lowest standards according to the investigation, had to undergo major changes in terms of facilities and services.

With regard to PSF users, two apparent conclusions arose from the research projects:
- Users are generally uncritical of PSF overall quality standards
- Users are unaware of the importance of prevention and self-protection in water activities in order to avoid drownings and other related incidents

Consequently, during 2001 and 2002, ESS launched the campaign *Enjoy your swim, Sure!* (approximate cost: 3000 euros) throughout the PSF network in Segovia based on the following awareness-raising programs:
- On-the-spot educational programs by certified swimming instructors with all age groups in 45 PSFs
- 15,000 leaflets, 500 posters and two local television programs
- 150 lifesavers were provided with official identification T-shirts in an attempt to highlight their professional role
- Educational program specifically targeted towards 6- to 12-year-old school children in Segovia, with an overall participation of approximately 2000 children from eight different schools

The program reached 95% of PSF users and 100% of our swimming learners, particularly those under 6 years. The results show that this type of local, low-budget campaign seems to be effective in terms of data collection and awareness-raising actions towards drowning prevention ('Think global, act local') and easy to adapt in other countries or areas. Furthermore, these campaigns have also provided ESS with a successful communication system towards drowning prevention in our province.

For more information visit: www.sossegovia.com and www.blueflag.org

Acknowledgements. Mr. Jesus Pascual-Gomèz is acknowledged for translation of the manuscript.

3.9.9
The Reasons People Drown

FRANK PIA

'The Reasons People Drown' is a powerful videotape used in children and adult community drowning prevention and education programs. The videotape and accompanying discussion materials shed light on the causes and misconceptions about drowning by showing actual film footage of drownings, non-fatal drownings and rescues captured by a camera situated on the most active lifeguard's chair at Orchard Beach, Bronx, New York. Viewing the instinctive drowning response of the patrons being rescued by lifeguards, dispels many of the myths the general public has about drowning.

Viewers come to understand that drowning persons are unable to call out or wave for help, and often look as though they are playing in the water, when they are actually drowning. Contextual information illustrating that drowning is a year round risk is provided. Using the classification of the National Safety Council for drowning: swimming, non-swimming, and boating related fatalities – viewers learn that drowning is a major cause of accidental death and injury in the US for ages 1–44. The causes of diving related spinal injuries and infant and toddler drownings are also depicted. The role of alcohol and other drugs in drowning is discussed and viewers learn that only time, not going into the water, will cancel out the effects of alcohol in the bloodstream.

After viewing the program and participating in a discussion, viewers are able to:

- Dispel common misconceptions about the behaviour of a drowning person
- Recognise a drowning person
- Identify the three drowning classifications
- List 20 rules for reducing swimming, non-swimming, and boating related drowning fatalities
- Identify various non-swimming rescue techniques
- Understand how alcohol causes drowning
- Describe the characteristics of the instinctive drowning response
- Understand the dangers of immersion hypothermia
- Identify the various types of personal flotation devices (PFD)
- Understand the risks of headfirst diving into above-ground backyard pools

Anecdotal data from lifeguards, camp counsellors and camp directors, public health sanitarians, and participants in employee safety programs have credited 'The Reasons People Drown' with helping them identify and rescue drowning persons when parents, bathers, and onlookers, who did not recognise the signs of drowning, were nearby.

For more information visit: www.pia-enterprises.com

3.9.10
Washington State Drowning Prevention Project and the *Stay on Top of It* Campaign

LINDA QUAN and ELIZABETH BENNETT

Drowning is the second leading cause of unintentional death among children and adolescents in Washington State, USA. The majority of drownings occur while swimming, boating or playing in lakes or rivers. A comprehensive drowning prevention program focused on increasing the use of Coast Guard-approved lifevests.

Stay on Top of It was developed by Children's Hospital and Regional Medical Center in 1992. Telephone surveys indicated that swimming ability and the age of a child guided the need for life vests but many parents were unaware of their usefulness. To increase use, parents suggested education, laws, trade-ins and loan programs. The main campaign message was: children, teens and adults should use life vests while boating, playing and swimming in open water, and when on docks, beaches or river banks. Additional messages addressed adult supervision, learning to swim, and water safety.

The campaign included: working with a coalition, educational resources, discount coupons, media, publicity and a life vest loan program for pools and beaches. Social marketing, social cognitive and protection motivation theories guided development. A pre- and post-telephone survey showed significant increases in life vest use and ownership among families exposed to the campaign.

In 1994, regional coalitions across the state defined needs based on local data and resources. Community indicators for education, policy, surveillance and community mobilisation were developed. Program elements included working with newspapers, life vest signs in English and Spanish at boat ramps, a *fotonovela* to educate the Latino community and a preschool kit. Loan programs were extended to boat rental shops, apartment pools, marine patrols, marinas and boat ramps. A state law requiring life vest use by children in boats was passed in 1999. Life vest observations showed significantly increased use on small boats between 1995 and 2000. Community indicators showed increasing programs and resources.

Using a teen advisor and youth groups, an adolescent program was developed in 1998 based on developmental assets, including decision-making and dealing with peer pressure and a risk and protective factor model. In focus groups, adolescents were aware of the risks of not wearing life vests and of drinking alcohol. They were unaware of the risks of swimming in lakes and rivers. The primary message was: Know the Water. Know your Limits. Wear a Life Vest. The program included a media campaign, posters, and an educational program with a life vest fashion show. Information was given to families leaving the emergency department. The loan program was adapted for adolescents. Community indicators specific to teens increased. When telephone surveyed, almost all families rated receiving drowning prevention education in the emergency department useful; 42% of families said they would buy a life vest. A state-wide drowning prevention network prioritised adolescent drowning for future activities.

For more information visit: www.kindveilig.nl

Acknowledgements. The authors acknowledge the contributions of Washington State Department of Health and the Washington State Drowning Prevention Network.

3.9.11
Community Campaign in the Netherlands by the Consumer Safety Institute

MONIQUE RIDDER

In the Netherlands drowning is the leading cause of injury death among children aged 0–4 years. Each year about 24 children drown. Another 120 children are treated in hospitals. The estimation of the numbers of children that drown is at least ten times higher. Children of immigrants are considered a risk group.

The Dutch campaign *Be Water Wise* (May 2002–March 2004) concentrated on the most vulnerable group: children aged 0–4 years. They drown in bathtubs (15%), garden ponds (19%), open water (25%) and (public) swimming pools (34%). In most cases, the children were playing in or near the water and were not adequately supervised.

The campaign raised awareness of the risk of drowning. Parents often do not know that drowning happens very quickly and silently and that continuous supervision is needed at all times. The campaign also stimulated parents to create a safer environment and to teach their children swimming and safety skills.

The campaign was a mass media campaign with television commercials, radio commercials and a website combined with personal education. Nurses at child health care centres gave parents safety information by means of leaflets available in Dutch, English, French, Arabic and Turkish. A course of group sessions was developed for immigrants. The campaign was introduced to nurses and health workers by mailings and workshops. Public swimming pools distribute leaflets and, in 2003, 250 public demonstrations were given at swimming pools. Parents were taught to play safely in the water with their children. This event 'Splash' was a joint venture of the Dutch organisation for swimming pools and sponsored by several companies. In addition, the campaign motivated local government to make water safety in neighbourhoods a part of their policy.

In October 2002 we had already reached 65% of the target group. Altogether, 80% of the health workers participated and more than 400,000 leaflets were distributed throughout the Netherlands. The Dutch government has stated that drowning will remain a major issue in the coming years and therefore the campaign will continue.

On a European level the European Child Safety Alliance (ECSA) launched a European Drowning campaign in 2003. In the EU drowning is the second cause of death for young children. The main goal of the European campaign is to raise awareness and to influence European and national policy makers to enforce water safety policies across Europe. ECSA supports individual countries with background information, prototypes of leaflets and an English television commercial.

3.9.12
Preventing Drowning in Alaska:
Float Coats and *Kids-Don't-Float*

MARCIA ROM

Two campaigns to prevent boating-related drownings are ongoing in Alaska. One is a *Float Coat* project targeting rural adult boaters, primarily natives in Alaskan villages which are only accessible by boat or plane in the summer. The second, *Kids Don't Float*, is a personal flotation device (PFD) loaner program, targeting children in boats throughout the state in both urban and rural areas.

Most drowning fatalities in Alaska occur in open skiffs or canoes. Over 90% of fatality victims did not wear a PFD. In 1997, 22% of boating fatality victims were less than 19 years old. And over half of all Alaska drownings occur on lakes and rivers.

Both the *Kids Don't Float* and the *Float Coat* projects are designed to increase usage of PFDs among boaters in Alaska, thereby reducing fatal drownings throughout the state.

Communities throughout the state set up standardised *Kids Don't Float* boards near boating and swimming areas. Through multi-agency collaborations, volunteers and corporate sponsorship, PFDs in a variety of sizes are hung on pegs on the boards. They are available for boaters to borrow and then return to the board. The program also includes an educational component with high school peer teachers, manuals and curriculum.

In an observational study 75% of boating children under 17 wore PFDs at *Kids Don't Float* sites. Only 50% wore PFDs at non-*Kids Don't Float* sites. We found that rural areas where boating is the primary activity had lower losses of PFDs than those in urban multi-use areas.

The *Float Coat* project primarily targets rural adult boaters. The goal is to increase float-coat use by rural Alaskan boaters. A coalition was set up including rural Native members and an Indian Health Services Injury Prevention Specialist. They designed a marketing strategy to promote float-coat use including: finding a quality product; customising it for the local culture; carefully designing a targeted distribution program; marketing incentives to encourage people to purchase them (such as sales and discounts); publicity and public education about the drowning problem and the possible solutions; as well as methods to evaluate success or failure of these programs.

Village residents then ordered PFDs from the Tribal Corporation at wholesale cost.

Float-coat usage increased from an average of 53% to 91% during the evaluation phase of the project.

Both of these programs are ongoing and easily replicable.

For more information visit: www.hss.state.ak.us/dph/chems/injury-prevention/kids_don't_float.htm

3.9.13
Evaluation of the *Keep Watch* Media Campaign

GREG TATE

An evaluation was conducted to assess the impact of the Royal Life Saving Society's state-wide media campaign *Keep Watch* and to assess the reach of Royal Life Saving Society programs in disseminating the *Keep Watch* message to parents and caregivers with children aged 0–4 years.

Two different types of television advertisements were used during the summer months. In 2000, two advertisements utilising 'fear appeals' were aired and a 'softer' approach advertisement using a swimming celebrity was aired in the following year. Additional public education strategies included the delivery of the *Keep Watch* message through existing Royal Life Saving Society programs to home pool owners, resuscitation participants and parents through infant aquatic programs.

A computer-assisted telephone survey was conducted for the purposes of the study in both years. A post questionnaire was developed in the year 2000 and both pre and post questionnaires were developed in 2001 to determine awareness of toddler drowning and recall of the *Keep Watch* message. Open-ended questions were included to determine the effectiveness of the message.

Evaluation demonstrated that there were high levels of awareness amongst the target group of the major issues related to both *Keep Watch* campaigns. However, the television advertisements in 2000 (using a fear appeal) had a greater recall and were rated as more effective than the 2001 advertisement (using a swimming celebrity).

The use of Royal Life Saving Society programs significantly increased the dissemination level of the *Keep Watch* message. The evaluation for 2000 indicated that 66% of the target group had accessed infant aquatic programs endorsed by the Royal Life Saving Society.

Television is an effective medium to promote awareness of toddler drowning amongst the target group. However, the type of advertisements and message delivered can impact the overall effectiveness of the campaign. The use of additional public education strategies can further enhance the retention of the message within the target group.

For more information visit: www.rlsaa.org.au

3.9.14
Community Campaign in Victoria, Australia

ANDREW WHITTAKER

Between 1998 and 2002 there was a comprehensive and intensive water safety campaign, known as *Play it Safe by the Water*, to create a water safety culture and reduce drowning and water related incidents.

It was a joint project between the State Government of Victoria and all elements of the aquatic industry. This was crucial to the structure of the campaign involving coordinated planning and cooperation between the major players. It was recognised that government involvement was necessary to provide the basic funding as drowning was a social and community issue and the main water safety organisations were needed to deliver the programs and services.

A range of different target groups were identified through analysis of drowning statistics, water related incidents and rescues. These covered a complex matrix of age groups, types of activities and environments. Three main environments were used as the basis for promoting key water safety messages:
- Beach: 'Always Swim between the Flags'
- Inland waterways: 'Check it's OK to swim'
- Home pools: 'Never take your eyes off'

These messages were supported by an extensive range of educational resources to all schools, pools and community organisations, including teacher resources, video, student booklets. This was in conjunction with a high profile media campaign using television advertising, newspaper supplements and radio. Schools and educational institutions were seen as crucial to changing behaviour over the long term.

Water Safety Week was a major event that provided many opportunities to promote water safety. The launch of the *Water Safety Week* presented opportunities to generate media coverage and provide political benefits to government. It was also the start of the advertising campaign which was supported by a wide range of promotional material such as stickers, T-shirts, caps, posters, water bottles, and 'Sink or swim' booklets.

A comprehensive media and public relations plan was developed to increase public awareness and understanding of the water safety messages and topics.

Although the messages needed to be simple, the planning was complex and sophisticated, combining media and public relations with education, risk management and participation strategies. Its success is reflected in a 31% drop in drowning since the campaign began in 1998, and a high (78%) recognition rate of the water safety messages.

For more information visit: www.vaic.org.au

Task Force on Rescue – Organisational Aspects: Rescue Planning, Training and Preparation

TASK FORCE ON RESCUE
Section editors: ROB BRONS and CHRIS BREWSTER

Task Force Chairs

- Chris Brewster
- Rob Brons

Task Force Members

- Tom Griffiths
- Jim Howe
- Gabriel Kinney
- Andrew Short
- Peter Wernicki
- Klaus Wilkens
- Mike Woodroffe
- Rick Wright

Other Contributors

- Stathis Avramidis
- Veronique Colman
- Mike Espino
- Julie Gilchrist
- Ralph Goto
- John Long
- Jerome Modell
- Luis-Miguel Pascual-Gómez
- Margie Peden
- Ulrik Persyn
- Richard Ming Kirk Tan
- Slim Ray
- Harald Vervaecke
- Wiebe de Vries
- Ann Williamson

4.1
Overview

CHRIS BREWSTER AND ROB BRONS

The World Congress on Drowning 2002 focused on three specific areas involving drowning: prevention, rescue and treatment. It was widely agreed that the most effective way to prevent death or injury from drowning is by prevention. Through public education, water safety training, proper design of aquatic areas, and other similar means, a large number of people can be protected in a relatively inexpensive and efficient manner. On the other hand, the least effective way to prevent death or injury from drowning is through treatment of drowning victims, because this necessarily takes place after an event that has already done some damage to the victim – damage that is sometimes irreversible regardless of the quality of treatment.

The effectiveness of rescue, as a method of preventing death or injury falls in the middle of prevention and treatment. A properly skilled and equipped rescuer, who recognises the distress of a person in the water or who is dispatched to the area in time, can successfully interrupt the drowning process. Tens of thousands of rescues occur each year throughout the world. In Southern California alone, for example, lifeguards report over 40,000 rescues from drowning in a typical year.

Most rescues stop the drowning process before the victim sustains injury. Some rescues even take place before victims are aware of the peril facing them. Victims in such cases are typically able to walk away without any medical treatment. In other cases, some degree of injury may be sustained, which can either be treated onshore with basic first aid procedures or which necessitates a trip to an advanced medical facility.

Rescuers, such as lifesavers, are not only responsible for rescue itself. Most rescue organisations provide preventive services, both off-site and on-site. Lifesavers may, for example, lecture schoolchildren, organise junior programs, or distribute brochures at special events. When people arrive at an aquatic area, they may find signs, flags, or other devices to encourage them to pursue recreational activities in the safest possible manner. While swimming, lifesavers may move swimmers away from hazardous areas into safer areas, for example. This is often called proactive lifesaving or, more typically, preventive lifesaving.

Lifesavers are not the only aquatic rescuers who practice prevention. So do coast guards, harbour patrols, marine patrols, and other groups responsible for promoting boating safety. Since drowning is the primary source of death from boating accidents, preventing these accidents from happening and promoting use of safety devices, like lifejackets, is critical. It provides the victims a longer survival time and gives rescuers a greater opportunity to respond to reports of distress before serious injury occurs.

In many cases, those who respond to the call for a water rescue are not specialists in this discipline. They may be firefighters, police officers, or park rangers for example. In areas under their purview, where they know aquatic accidents are likely, these people should also promote prevention. For example, in areas where ice related accidents happen with regularity, local law enforcement and firefighters may instruct the populace in how to avoid falling through the ice into the water.

Preparing organisations and the individuals of which they are composed to effectively provide aquatic rescue services is a critical task for any society. Drowning is one of the leading causes of accidental death and injury worldwide, eclipsing death from fire in many countries. Thus, response preparations should be seen as no less important than crime or fire prevention. Likely locations and circumstance that might cause drowning should be identified, organisations developed, personnel trained and equipped, and plans put in place to effectively and efficiently address likely circumstances. In short, communities should prepare themselves effectively to prevent, respond to, and treat drowning.

Rescue is the subject of two sections of this handbook. This expanded treatment addresses the many types of circumstances that require rescue, the myriad techniques involved, the wide array of equipment used, and the different organisational approaches. The World Congress on Drowning 2002 brought together experts in water rescue from a very broad array of disciplines. These sections reflect their contributions. Utilising the information in these sections, effective lifesaving organisations can become even better at what they do, and those beginning to provide lifesaving services will have a roadmap at their disposal, drawn by some of the most respected experts in the field of aquatic rescue worldwide. In this section, we focus on organisational issues that can help prevent accidents and improve outcomes when accidents occur. In the next section, we will focus on specific tools and knowledge disciplines for effective drowning prevention.

Rescue organisations can be made up of volunteers, paid personnel, or a combination of the two. ▶ Chapter 4.3 provides an overview of these approaches, based on discussion at a highly attended expert session at the World Congress.

Whether volunteer or paid, funding lifesaving services requires justifying the need, as well as the cost, to those in positions of authority. An extraordinary document on this topic was produced by the Centers for Disease Control and Prevention (Atlanta – USA). It discusses the effectiveness of lifeguards at preventing drowning and is intended for use by decision-makers who are considering beginning, enhancing, or even terminating lifeguard programs. An overview can be found in the ▶ Chapter 4.4

Part of the effective organisation of lifesaving work includes occasional reviews of the work that is conducted; ▶ Chapter 4.5 provides some recommendations in this regard.

Perhaps the first step in developing an effective approach to rescue is evaluating the need. ▶ Chapter 4.6 details a method for identifying beach (and water) hazards and assessing risk that can be used to determine when, where, and in what magnitude resources should be devoted to drowning prevention. This program has been effectively applied in several areas of the world.

To prepare for aquatic rescue, personnel must of course be properly trained. Several of our chapters address training. The development of appropriate, general standards for training is covered in ▶ Chapter 4.7. There are a variety of specialised circumstances in which lifesaving organisations are needed. Flood rescue is addressed in ▶ Chapter 4.8. An approach to training that involves the latest technology is described in ▶ Chapter 4.9.

Considering the importance of measuring and demonstrating the work done by lifesavers, collecting data is essential. A review of ▶ Chapter 4.10 will yield some valuable recommendations for lifesaving organisations around the world.

Training is one area that can involve special types of risk. ▶ Chapter 4.11 is devoted to this subject. In addition to training, lifesaving work also has inherent risks. Managing those risks and limiting liability are important elements of lifesaving. An excellent overview can be found in ▶ Chapter 4.12.

Can lifesaving training be considered an academic pursuit? In some areas of the world, this is clearly the case, as described in ▶ Chapter 4.13.

Whether the rescue organisation is made up of paid personnel or volunteers, adequate funding is critical. ▶ **Chapter 4.14** provides some new ideas and insight into a particularly effective fund-raising campaign used by the German Lifesaving Federation (DLRG).

Some 97% of drowning deaths occur in less developed nations. Clearly, prevention and other lifesaving services are needed in developing countries, just as they are in developed countries. However, the tremendous challenges faced by developing countries may make it much more difficult to organise lifesaving services there. A discussion of this topic, including some staggering statistics, can be found in ▶ **Chapter 4.15.**

In summary, this section provides a wealth of information on organisational aspects related to lifesaving. The careful reader will gain tremendous insight into ways to develop and improve aquatic rescue services. The opportunity is yours.

4.2
Recommendations:
Rescue Planning, Training and Preparation

CHRIS BREWSTER and ROB BRONS

In some areas of the world, there are few, if any people trained, equipped, or prepared to provide timely rescue to people in distress in the water. In other areas, highly advanced rescue services exist. Even these advanced services however, can improve. Therefore, a comprehensive strategy to reduce drowning worldwide must include methods of providing rescue services where they do not exist, and improving the quality of existing rescue services.

Prior to the World Congress on Drowning, the Rescue Task Force was assembled. This group of nine experts was asked to focus attention on eight rescue-related topics and to make specific recommendations. These were reviewed and accepted by the Rescue Task Force and the Steering Group of the World Congress on Drowning. During the Congress, these topics were discussed in further detail and the recommendations were published, in abbreviated form, in the appendices of the Final Recommendations of the World Congress on Drowning. In this chapter, you will find brief synopses, compiled by the Rescue Task Force leaders, of each of the topics addressed by the Rescue Task Force involving planning, training, and preparation. Specific recommendations are also included. For a more thorough explanation of each topic, please read the chapters in this section authored by the named experts.

During the World Congress on Drowning, additional topics with regard to swimming training and scientific investigation of rescue techniques resulted in additional recommendations as a product of discussion among the experts in attendance. These are listed as recommendations 5 and 6 in this chapter. The remaining recommendations 7–10 are covered in ▶ **Chapter 5.2.**

4.2.1
Recommendation 1 – Risk Assessment of Beaches

Task Force Expert: Andrew Short

One of the greatest challenges to drowning prevention faced by governments and private businesses which oversee aquatic areas used for recreation, is determining the level of drowning prevention efforts justified by hazards present. Inevitably, this determination will be partially based on factors such as the societal valuation placed on human life. For example, an underdeveloped country battling serious disease or malnutrition will likely see the value of drowning prevention as a much lower priority than a developed country.

These factors aside, creating a meaningful drowning prevention strategy necessarily entails gauging the varying levels of hazard presented at aquatic areas. Specifically, for example, are signs an adequate deterrent? Should the aquatic area be staffed with lifesavers? If so, at what levels, with what equipment available, during what times of day or season?

It is particularly difficult to quantify the need for these services considering the widely varying beach conditions that may exist, as well as attendance levels, the skill level of water users, and so forth. Pioneering work in this area has been conducted for Surf Life Saving Australia (SLSA) by Andrew Short.

According to Short, "The Australian Beach Safety and Management Program ... compiled a database containing the location, physical characteristics, access, facilities, and hazards at everyone of Australia's 10,685 beach systems ... SLSA has also used the above system to develop a Beach Management Plan and more recently incorporated it into a Coastal Safety Auditing Program. The former provides a flow chart for the lifesaver to determine both the modal and prevailing beach hazard rating, thereby providing a standard and quantifiable measure of hazard on each and every patrolled beach. The chart goes on to suggest the level of water safety resources (personnel and equipment) required to mitigate the level of risk. The latter is a national auditing process that uses the beach safety rating in combinations with other factors to develop a holistic approach to the development and maintenance of a safe coastal environment." (▶ **Chapter 4.6**)

Rescue recommendation 1:

It is recommended that the work of Andrew Short be considered as a basis for developing a worldwide standard for the evaluation of hazard presented at beaches and for developing appropriate drowning prevention strategies.

4.2.2
Recommendation 2 – Training Personnel for Flood Rescue

TASK FORCE EXPERT: SLIM RAY

Inland flooding, whether from river floods or flash floods, is the top weather-related killer worldwide. Floods inflict thousands of casualties, in many years more than wars, terrorism and revolutions. Surprisingly though, as Rescue Task Force member Slim Ray points out, "… while many countries have large and lavishly-equipped anti-terrorism units, specialised flood rescue units are rare. In fact, few local and national emergency services worldwide possess even the most elementary training and equipment for flood rescue. Unfortunately it is common to see firefighters, police, and military personnel out in flood waters in their service uniforms and fire fighting protective gear, bravely trying to improvise rescues on the spot with inadequate and inappropriate equipment. Often rescuers pay for their unpreparedness with their own lives." For example, in a recent case in the US, in which 52 people died, 10% of the flood fatalities were rescue workers. (▶ Chapter 4.8) This topic is also mentioned in ▶ Section 11.

Rescue recommendation 2:

Communities throughout the world, which can expect to face flooding, must prepare themselves, and the emergency workers they designate, to effectively respond to flood rescue. This includes planning, along with proper equipment and training. Training must be realistic and conducted on moving water. Rescue units must have an effective incident command structure. Plans should call for them to be deployed early enough in the event to make rescues rather than body recoveries. They should be supported by other emergency responders trained locally.

4.2.3
Recommendation 3 – Training Standards for In-Water Rescue

TASK FORCE EXPERT: RICK WRIGHT

Throughout the world, the many organisations which train persons to rescue others in the water have developed training standards which they consider appropriate to the expectations placed upon the lifesavers. Typically, these are based on anecdotal evidence of appropriate minimum training standards, or historical experience. These standards, while in some cases roughly comparable, are as diverse as the number of organisations in existence. However few, if any, scientific studies have been made to objectively determine the minimum levels of training required to adequately prepare one human being to save the life of another in the water. (▶ Chapter 4.7)

Rescue Recommendation 3A:

Scientific study should be undertaken to form a basis for determining the skills required to rescue another human in an aquatic emergency. Such a study should ascertain whether there is a link between the actual biomechanical and physiological performance of in-water rescue and the training and assessment mechanisms that qualified the human to perform such a rescue. Furthermore, the study should seek to determine whether the resulting condition of the patient would be different as a result of the skills or knowledge of the rescuer.

Rescue Recommendation 3B:

Based on the results of the study, the International Life Saving Federation should evaluate its current recommended minimum competencies for lifesavers, making any appropriate modifications.

4.2.4
Recommendation 4 –
Fund-Raising for Aquatic Lifesaving Organisations

Task Force Expert: Klaus Wilkens

Lifesaving organisations of the world must continually seek funds to ensure adequate working capital to provide necessary levels of resources to carry out their mission of drowning prevention. While some are government funded, others rely exclusively on donations and similar sources of income. Both non-government and government rescue organisations can benefit by effective fund-raising programs. Unfortunately, despite the fact that the services they provide have tremendous appeal, lifesavers are not always effective fundraisers. Some aquatic rescue organisations have developed highly advanced fund raising mechanisms. Others suffer greatly for lack of resources. (► **Chapter 4.13**)

Rescue Recommendation 4:

An international study of fund-raising activities by aquatic lifesaving organisations should be commenced to identify the most effective methods. The results of this study should be shared worldwide, with the ultimate benefit of helping these organisations generate necessary working funds to help them reduce the incidence of drowning worldwide.

4.2.5
Recommendation 5 – Swimming Training

Knowing how to swim is a critical skill to prevent drowning for individuals at risk.

Rescue recommendation 5A:

International organisations such as the World Health Organisation (WHO), International Red Cross and Red Crescent (IRCRC) and the International Life Saving Federation (ILS) and their national branches must emphasise the importance of swimming lessons and drowning survival skills at all levels for as many persons as possible.

Rescue recommendation 5B:

The relationships between swimming lessons, swimming ability and drowning in children needs to be studied.

Rescue recommendation 5C:

Certain public officials such as police officers and fire fighters, who frequently come in close contact with persons at risk for drowning must be able to swim for their own safety and for the safety of the public.

4.2.6
Recommendation 6 – Rescue Techniques

Most of the current rescue techniques have evolved by trial and error, with little scientific investigation.

Rescue Recommendation 6:

Rescue organisations such as the International Life Saving Federation (ILS), the International Lifeboat Federation (ILF), the International Red Cross and Red Crescent (IRCRC) but also the International Maritime Organisation (IMO) must be encouraged to evaluate the self-rescue and rescue techniques in their training programs in accordance with current scientific data on effectiveness and efficiency. Based on the data, the best rescue techniques must be selected for education and training programs.

4.3
Rescue Organisations: Paid or Volunteers?

MIKE ESPINO and CHRIS BREWSTER

At the World Congress on Drowning 2002, a full expert session was devoted to the topic: *Rescue Organizations: Is There a Difference Between Volunteers and Professionals?* The session was well attended by representatives of volunteer and professional rescue organisations and many comments were received. It was agreed at the beginning that volunteers can actually be considered professional with respect to the manner in which they carry on their work. Therefore, the subject of the discussion was refined to the differences between rescue organisations composed of paid (compensated as workers) and volunteer (providing services with no salary involved) lifesavers. This chapter is an effort to reflect comments and sentiments expressed during the session. As used in this book, the term 'lifesaver' applies to a person who assumes a responsibility to protect, rescue, and resuscitate others in an aquatic setting, whether formally titled lifesaver, lifeguard, or by some other term.

Aquatic protection and rescue services have evolved differently in different countries. In some countries, such as Australia and Germany, there is strong emphasis and reliance upon volunteer lifesavers, with a smaller number of paid lifesavers. In others, such as the US, there is strong emphasis on paid lifesavers, with very few volunteers. As one participant pointed out, the drowning victim does not care whether the rescuer is paid or volunteer. Nevertheless, there are significant differences between the systems.

The public is not always aware of whether the lifesaver is paid or volunteer, but when this is known, public perceptions of the two systems can differ. Paid lifesavers may be viewed positively by the public they serve as being highly professional in their training and conduct. It is often presumed that if someone has been hired and trained to do the job, and if they do it for a primary source of income, they are likely to be very good at it. On the other hand, some people, whether fairly or unfairly, view public employees with a degree of disdain. Volunteer lifesavers may also be viewed very positively because they are donating their time for the good of the community. Some though, may view them as hobbyists, rather than professionals.

Funding sources for paid and volunteer systems are typically different. Paid lifesavers are usually compensated, whether directly or indirectly, by governments or corporations. People are perhaps less inclined to donate money to these organisations. They expect the services rendered to be funded through public sources, such as taxes and fees. Special fund-raising events may be conducted to augment primary sources of income and some paid organisations do so quite effectively. Volunteer organisations are usually funded by donations, corporate sponsorships, memberships, and fund-raising events. The altruistic nature of their work leaves people more inclined to offer funds to support them. In addition, these groups may be more likely to be allowed to engage in unusual types of fund-raising not normally permitted. For example, some Australian lifesaving clubs are legally permitted to allow forms of gambling and serving of alcohol in their clubs as a means of raising funds. Some volunteer organisations contract their services to public or private organisations, receiving compensation to support the costs of conducting lifesaving work.

Retaining volunteer lifesavers in adequate numbers requires an environment which encourages continued participation and service. Some will remain involved regardless, due to strong ties to the organisation. Others will require incentives, like special events, funding of competitions and travel, and special recognition. These costs must be borne by the organisation. The most effective volunteer systems have strong national structures, which help attract and retain members, and work through local club systems supported by the national organisations. For paid lifesavers, simply maintaining an adequate salary level and employee benefits is typically enough to ensure longevity of service. Even so, a seasonal, paid lifesaver may work only a few years until finding full time employment elsewhere, whereas a volunteer may continue to contribute leisure time to lifesaving for decades.

Paid lifesavers can generally be expected to be more reliable than volunteers with respect to issues like arriving to their assigned work location on time and working designated hours. This is primarily due to the fact that the income of paid lifesavers is dependent upon retaining employment by following work rules. In volunteer organisations, this may be encouraged through minimum requirements expected of all volunteers. However, enforcement is difficult since there is no economic incentive. The ultimate penalty for the paid lifesaver is loss of a job, whereas the penalty to the volunteer is loss of an opportunity to participate and contribute as a lifesaver.

Minimum standards and duty of care for paid and volunteer lifesavers should be the same when they are assigned the same duties. Generally, the training levels of paid lifesavers, whether it be minimum or advanced, are higher than those of volunteers. This stems, in part, from the fact that volunteers have only so much time available and may only be willing to train to a certain degree. Paid lifesavers can be required to undergo extensive training, so long as the employer can afford to provide it or can require it as a condition of continued employment. While higher aggregate training levels in a volunteer organisation come with little cost, typically limited to training supplies and perhaps paid trainers, they are more difficult to achieve. Some volunteer lifesaving organisations attempt to overcome this by staffing higher numbers of volunteers and depending upon a team approach to emergency responses.

More volunteer lifesavers are needed to provide the same staffing level as provided by paid lifesavers. Volunteers can only devote a limited amount of their free time to lifesaving, while paid lifesavers have full or part time employment. Volunteer programs therefore require that far more people be trained. A smaller corps of paid lifesavers, who work more frequently, can be expected to be more familiar with current practices and procedures. They may also know one another better since a limited number of lifesavers work more hours. This may help them work as a team more effectively.

Depending on longevity of employment, paid lifesavers may have either more or less aggregate experience than volunteers. In an organisation where paid lifesavers stay with the profession for a short period of time, but volunteers continue for many years, the volunteers may be more experienced. They may also be older and more mature. On the other hand, in organisations where paid lifesavers continue their employment for many years, the aggregate experience they gain may far exceed that of volunteers.

The number of paid lifesavers is limited to available budgets, and paid lifesaving organisations are more likely to be affected by changing budgetary priorities and circumstances of governments. Volunteer lifesaving organisations are not usually impacted as significantly by variations in local government budgets, since without labour costs, the costs of conducting their lifesaving work is minimal. Even in poor economic times, it may be possible for volunteer lifesaving organisations to maintain consistent levels of service.

In countries and in organisations with a combination of volunteer and paid workers, there can be tension between the two for a variety of reasons. These include different training levels and different work standards, among other reasons. This creates a management challenge. In an organisation where a core paid staff is augmented by volunteers, the responsibility is on management to ensure that volunteers are valued and respected. Conversely, in organisations where volunteers are regarded as the predominant providers of lifesaving, management may need to take steps to ensure that paid staff are also valued.

Regardless of the relative merits of paid versus volunteer lifesaving, some countries simply cannot afford to pay lifesavers, or at least not all lifesavers. In Australia, where a large proportion of lifesaving services are provided by volunteers, a sweeping change to a paid system might be too expensive. Nevertheless, Australia has steadily increased its percentage of paid lifesavers (who are known as lifeguards in Australia). This change is occurring over time. As the responsibilities and expectations of lifesavers grow, the percentage of paid staff can be expected to increase in comparison to volunteers.

In developing nations, it may be difficult to maintain volunteer lifesaving organisations. This is because leisure time, the period during which volunteer lifesaving is usually practised, is extremely limited, if not completely unavailable. Therefore, while developing nations may have the greatest difficulty allocating funds for paid lifesaving services, paid services may be the only viable alternative.

4.3.1
Summary and Conclusions

Based on the discussion in our forum, it would appear that if budget is not a significant obstacle, the paid approach to providing lifesaving services has several advantages. Paid lifesavers can be held to higher standards, be better trained, be more reliable, be more accountable, and be better prepared to act independently. Because of lack of leisure time to volunteer, the paid approach may be the only feasible one in some developing nations. Few areas of the world, however, have the level of resources required to pay the number of lifesavers desired for optimum levels of safety. Thus, where an adequate number of volunteers can be relied upon to meet acceptable minimum standards and to make themselves available when needed, volunteer systems have proven viable. In volunteer systems, it appears that having a core paid staff to work with and help coordinate activities of the volunteers is ideal.

4.4
Lifeguard Effectiveness

RALPH GOTO

The Centers for Disease Control and Prevention (CDC), the American Red Cross, and the United States Lifesaving Association (USLA) routinely respond to inquiries regarding the efficacy of lifesaving services in preventing drowning. Some of these inquiries are from communities and local government officials facing decisions about whether to begin, retain, or discontinue lifesaving services. In response to these inquiries, in 1998, the Centers for Disease Control and Prevention (CDC) Division of Unintentional Injury Prevention conducted a meeting of a panel of experts to discuss the effectiveness of lifesavers in preventing death and injury. This effort was lead by Christine Branche, Director of the Division of Unintentional Injury Prevention. A report, entitled *Lifeguard Effectiveness: A Report of the Working Group*, was issued by the CDC in 2001 and is available at: http://www.cdc.gov/ncipc/lifeguard/lifeguard.htm. The report discusses methods of evaluating the efficacy of lifesaver services, communicating information about the efficacy of lifesavers, and the sources of information about the efficacy of lifesavers, including data, resources, and case studies.

The lifesaver effectiveness report is the result of the efforts to assemble a panel of experts in the US to discuss these issues and to review data on the efficacy of life guarding services. The purpose of the report is to describe the efficacy of lifesaver services for the prevention of drowning. It was also the intent of the group to have the report serve as a tool for local government officials in making decisions about the provision of lifesaver services in their areas. The objective of the report was to provide a balanced overview of the costs and benefits of providing lifesaver services to prevent drowning and water recreation-related injuries. The document was well received in the US by organisations such as the American Red Cross and the USLA.

In June of 2002, an expert meeting at the World Congress on Drowning in Amsterdam was convened to introduce the report to the international community. The Experts Meeting at the World Congress on Drowning provided a forum for the report to be presented to the international lifesaving community. The focus of the report was on effectiveness rather than efficacy. The report should be used as a "model to bridge the gap between lifesaving and science," and it could be used as a reference in the ongoing debate on whether it is best to provide paid professional lifesavers versus volunteer lifesavers, which is addressed elsewhere in this section (see ▶ **Chapter 4.3**). Comments from participants at the World Congress on Drowning were generally favourable towards the report, as most agreed that the document will be of tremendous value when justifying the provision of lifesaving services. Discussion included relevance of the report on an international level, considering the differences in each country's lifesaving system, but the consensus of the group was that the report had global implications and value.

The following is the executive summary contained in the report:

"Each year, about 4,000 people die from drowning in the United States. Drowning was a leading cause of unintentional injury death among all ages in 1998, and the second leading cause of unintentional injury death among children ages 1–14 that same year. Approximately 50%–75% of drownings occur in open water such as oceans, lakes, rivers, and ponds. About 60% of drowning deaths among children occur in swimming pools.

Many organisations, including the Centers for Disease Control and Prevention (CDC), routinely respond to inquiries regarding the efficacy of lifesavers in preventing drownings. Community and local government officials facing decisions about whether to begin, retain, or discontinue life guarding services typically want to know whether lifesavers are truly effective in preventing drowning and other aquatic mishaps, and whether the value of providing lifesaver protection outweighs the costs. Most drownings are preventable through a variety of strategies, one of which is to provide lifesavers in public areas where people are known to swim and to encourage people to swim in those protected areas. Some estimates indicate that the chance of drowning on a beach protected by lifesavers can be less that one in 18 million. There is no doubt that trained, professional lifesavers have had a positive effect on drowning prevention in the United States.

The significance of the patron surveillance and supervision that lifesavers provide is emphasised by understanding how people drown. Many people assume that drowning persons are easy to identify because they exhibit obvious signs of distress. Instead, people tend to drown quietly and quickly. Children and adults are rarely able to call out or wave their arms when they are in distress in the water, and can submerge in 20–60 seconds. For these reasons managers should never assign lifesavers duties that distract them from keeping an eye on the water, such as selling admission tickets or refreshments. In addition, the presence of lifesavers may deter behaviours that could put swimmers at risk for drowning, such as horseplay or venturing into rough or deep water, much like increased police presence can deter crime.

When making decisions about using lifesavers and other means of increasing public safety in aquatic settings, policy makers should use available local evidence. This evidence includes:

- The effects that lifesavers have had on patrons' safety and attitudes
- The number of people using the facility or beach area during the past years
- The incidence of water-related injuries and drownings at the facility or beach area during those time periods
- Data on the number of water-related injuries and drownings at pools and beaches in the local area or state with and without lifesavers, for comparison, and
- The level of lifesavers provides (number of lifesavers per number of persons using the facility)

In addition to these factors, policy makers should consider public attitudes about lifesavers and legal issues related to using lifesavers.

4.4.1
Website

- http://www.cdc.gov/ncipc/lifeguard/lifeguard.htm

4.5
Quality Assessment and Risk Monitoring of Lifesaving

Rob Brons

In 1993 the Dutch government introduced the concept of the safety chain to establish national policy on safety and security. This concept is now used by all police and fire services in the Netherlands. Some local and regional services have adopted this concept as a guiding template to organise their fire service. The fire service of the Hague has implemented the safety chain not only for the fire service but also for lifesaving activities on the beaches of Scheveningen (the Hague, the Netherlands). This chapter introduces how the concept of the safety chain can be implemented for lifesaving services.

4.5.1
The Safety Chain for Firefighters

The safety chain is composed of links which are aimed at the monitoring of safety and security in the community. Once the elements of each link in the safety chain have been identified, it is important to make each link as strong as possible. The five links of the safety chain are:
- Pro-action
- Prevention
- Preparedness
- Response
- Recovery

Within the safety chain the *target care system* is used. For firefighters, the target care system means the most adequate response time to arrive at the potential incident sites, according to the state of prevention and the activities that take place at the site. Level of training and size of the teams and their equipment are determined accordingly. For example, depending on these aspects, the response time of the first fire truck has to be within 5, 8, 10 or 15 min. The target care system applies equally to buildings, industrial plants and non-urban areas.

The safety chain interrelates with the target care system. When there is a large number of persons located at the potential incident site, there is greater need for prevention because response and recovery may become problematic. Prevention is also emphasised when the people in the area are mentally disabled people, children, prisoners or other groups who run extra risks. When prevention measures are well developed (a strong prevention link in the chain), the response time may be longer than when prevention measures are poor or absent.

The target care system also allows checks and balances by other public authorities and government bodies or politicians. The system provides information about which level of safety has been selected for potential incident sites and allows government bodies or politicians to consider whether this level is acceptable or not. In case a higher level is requested by the public authorities, the safety link concept and the target care system make it possible to formulate how the fire service has to be organised to reach this higher level and to calculate the expected costs.

4.5.2
The Safety Chain for Lifesavers

There are many similarities between the skills of firefighters and lifesavers and between the responsibilities of the two organisations (☐ **Table 4.1**). Using the safety chain for lifesaving activities is therefore also a useful tool to plan, execute and check the quality and monitor the risks of lifesaving organisations.

During the planning and implementation of the safety chain concept for lifesaving, additional natural and human factors need to be considered. Examples of natural factors include wind (speed, direction), tide (low, high), waves and temperature changes. Human factors include physical capacities (young age)

☐ **Table 4.1.** Similarities between lifesaving services and fire services

Chains	Lifesaving service	Fire service
Proaction	Infrastructure	Building and infrastructure
	Planning of locations	Reachability of emergency services
Prevention	Patrol by foot, boat, car	Fire prevention advice
	Signs and flags	Building planning advice
Preparation	Planning of personnel/equipment	Planning of personnel/equiment
	Education, training	Education, training
	Response criteria	Risk assessment
Response	Emergency response	Emergency response
Recovery	Personnel and drowned persons	Personnel and victims
	Evaluation	Evaluation

and psychological aspects (fear, courage and handling of dangerous situations). The same five steps in the safety chain can also be identified for the organisation of lifesavers..

Pro-action means 'to step back' and look to the aims and responsibilities of the organisation. How can lifesaving tasks be implemented or improved? Pro-action is the opportunity to think about infrastructure. Examples of pro-action are the manipulation of natural factors, the design a lifesaving station, the identification of areas of high risk and safe swimming and the indication of these areas by signs and flags.

Many questions need to be solved for an appropriate pro-active link. Such questions include: How can natural factors be influenced? Can the natural or man-made environment be changed to reduce hazards? Is it possible to make a risk assessment for beaches? Can unsafe beaches be closed down? How and when can drowning victims reach the nearest hospital? These, and other, questions are very relevant when planning a lifesaving service at a beach.

Prevention helps to avoid rescue, injury or death by drowning. Good and sufficient manpower and mitigation of risks are possibilities for prevention. Examples of prevention are patrol schedules in areas where problems might occur, as well as informing the public about potential dangers.

An adequate lifesaver patrol can provide safe beaches by warnings and anticipating dangers. An understandable warning system can support prevention. The use of positive information is better than the use of negative information. Shields that indicate dangers will challenge certain persons to act in an unsafe way. Pointing out safe areas is therefore better than pointing out unsafe areas. The research and development of warning systems with uniform pictograms are useful for lifesaving activities.

Recognition of certain indicators help lifesavers to focus on times and places where problems are likely to happen. Local statistics for beaches in the Hague revealed that these indicators are days with a light wind, some sunshine, few swimmers, as well as days when the tide turns to flood. When large numbers of people are pursuing recreational activities, social control provides a higher level of safety. These data help to identify the moments that higher levels of risk should be anticipated.

Preparedness can be divided into two parts: subject and object preparedness. Subject preparedness determines the way lifesavers are able to do their job. Education and training are essential elements of subject preparedness. Object preparedness is achieved by preparation of lifesaving material. Examples are the purchase of the most reliable material and procedures to check and double check material.

Preparedness for objects and subjects will reduce unsafe bathing and swimming.

The geographic planning of the locations of lifesaving stations is also part of the preparedness link because the location is essential for good supervision of the beach. This is shown in the following example: The location of the lifesaving stations of the Hague (total beach length 12 kilometres, or 7 miles) was historically based on the rowing distance between each station. According to the target care system, the new aim is that lifesavers arrive at the incident site within

3 min. Since, however, the sun shines from the south in the afternoon and creates a glare that shines in the eyes of the lifesavers looking in that direction, the stations are located at locations from where rescues can occur within 3 min and where one third of the patrol area is to the south and two thirds to the north.

Object preparedness also improves when each station is installed with the same equipment and rescue material and when this material is located at the same point in each station.

The preparedness of lifesavers can also be influenced by good standards of recruitment. In the Hague, every member has to pass tests before he or she may serve as a lifesaver. These tests are based on the daily skills of lifesavers: the requirements include being able to swim 100 meters in 1.55 min, swimming for 15 min, 50 meters transportation swimming and 25 meters under water swimming, as well as running 800 meters within 4.15 min. Practical skills in first aid and basic life support also have to be demonstrated. Because all lifesavers have to pass these tests each year, every lifesaver on duty is confident about his own safety skills, but also about the safety skills of his or her colleagues. Periodic and realistic training is planned and this is essential to keep lifesavers in good physical condition. Quality of equipment and the number of personnel also improve the quality of the lifesaving activities.

Response is the way a lifesaver reacts after an emergency call. It is also closely related to the way a lifesaver sees, feels and believes in lifesaving and for that reason response is the most appealing aspect for lifesavers. The response by lifesavers is also the most eye-catching link of the safety chain for visitors of beaches. Nevertheless this aspect is only one aspect of the safety chain. Adequate response needs a delicate mix of personnel, equipment and organisation. It also needs awareness of potential dangers, alertness and the right amount of adrenalin. In addition to this, the best equipment, good education, frequent training and tight organisation are needed for the best response.

As this book points out, most drowning victims die within 5 min under water. Enabling lifesavers to rescue a victim within this time frame is a very demanding target for the organisation of a lifesaving operation. Not only is the first response essential, but also the link to professional medical help. When a lifesaving organisation is able to save someone from the water and provide basic life support within 5 min, but is unable to get medical treatment or transportation to a medical facility, the preparation link needs improvement.

The last link is *recovery*. Examples of recovery include not only medical care for drowning victims, but also care for the lifesavers themselves, for example in the case of post-traumatic stress syndrome. (▶ **Chapter 5.20**)

It is also important for lifesaving organisations to have facilities within the organisation to deal with post-traumatic stress.

4.5.3
Conclusion

Certainly in some communities, the lifesaver is a local hero due to his response actions. But within the concept of the safety chain, the rescue activity is only one link out of five. All links have to be considered to guard the beach in a professional and reassuring way.

Quality assessment and risk monitoring with the use of the safety chain concept enables lifesaving activities to be improved in a scientific and systematic approach. To develop this concept, data, knowledge and experience needs to be sought and gathered. The application of the safety chain, which has proven effective for police and firefighting organisations, will result in similar benefits for lifesaving organisations.

4.6
Beach Hazards and Risk Assessment of Beaches

ANDREW SHORT

The types of beaches that exist around the world and their associated physical characteristics and dynamics are reasonably predictable using current scientific knowledge of beach systems [4]. With this information it is possible to assess and quantify the associated beach hazards. What is less predictable is the level of beach usage and awareness of people using the beach. It is only with a combination of hazard assessment and a prediction of human knowledge and preparedness, that public risk on beaches can be assessed. This chapter examines the present status in achieving risk assessment of beaches.

4.6.1
Beach Systems

Beaches are wave and tide deposited accumulations of sediment (sand through cobbles and boulders) deposited between modal wave base and the upper swash limit. Beaches are the major route for public access to the sea and oceans. As such beaches are a major site of recreation as well as water access for small craft and boats. The type of beach is a function of the sediment size, the wave height, wave period, tide range and relative tide range (RTR). The latter is the ratio between the spring tide range and average wave height: $RTR = TR/H$ (TR = spring tide range; H = average breaker wave height).

The RTR can be used to divide beaches into three systems: wave-dominated, tide-modified and tide-dominated.
- Wave-dominated beaches occur when the RTR is less than 3
- Tide-modified when the RTR is between 3 and 7
- Tide-dominated when the RTR is between 7 and 15, grading into tidal sand flats when RTR exceeds 15

◻ Table 4.2. Beach systems, types and controls

Relative tide range (RTR)	$\Omega = Hb/WsT$	Beach type	Beach hazard rating in Australia[a]
Wave-dominated			
<3	<1	Reflective	1–2
<3	2–5	Intermediate[b]	3–7
<3	>6	Dissipative	8–10
Tide-modified			
3–15	<2	Reflective and low tide bar	2–4
3–15	>2	Low tide bar and rips	2–4
3–15	>6	Ultradissipative	2–3
Tide-dominated			
7–15	<1	Beach and sand ridges	1
7–15	<1	Beach and sand flats	1
>>15	<<1	Tidal sand flats	1–2

Hb: breaker wave height (m); T: wave period (s); Ws: sediment fall velocity (ms^{-1}); Ω: fall velocity (dimensionless).

[a] Ratings vary in different wave environments between 1 (=low risk) to 10 (=high risk).

[b] There are four intermediate types (long shore bar and trough, rhythmic bar and beach, transverse bar and rip, low tide terrace) all dominated by rip channels and rip currents.

Within each system there can be considerable variation in sediment size, wave height and period. This variation is accommodated in the dimensionless term fall velocity (Ω), which is a function of the wave height, wave period and sediment size, measured by its fall velocity in water. Based on the variation of the fall velocity, the three systems can be divided in nine beach types. Each of the nine beach types is the product of the interaction of shoaling and breaking waves and swash acting over the mobile beach sediment, coupled with tidal movement of the shoreline (◻ Table 4.2).

Across each type, a predictable range and sequence of hydrodynamics (shoaling and breaking waves) occurs, together with a predictable combinations of surf zone processes (breaking waves, long shore currents, rip currents, wave set up and down), which in turn may imprint their dynamics on the underlying beach and surf zone (such as bars, channels, troughs, rip channels, rhythmic

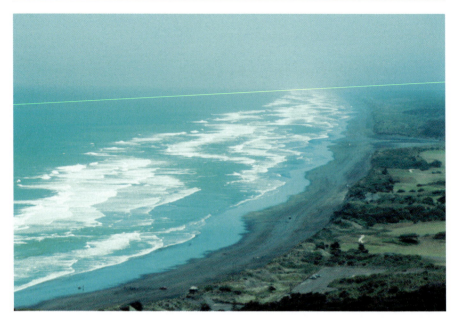

◘ Fig. 4.1. High energy dissipative beach, with a wide double bar surf zone, Muriwai, New Zealand. Beach hazard rating = 9

shorelines, beach cusps). The coupling of the dynamic wave–tide processes and the responding beach shape is termed beach morphodynamics.

In wave-dominated systems when Ω is greater than 6, high energy dissipative beaches prevail (◘ **Fig. 4.1**). Dissipative beaches are characterised by a high surf and 200–500 m wide low gradient multi-barred surf zone. When Ω is between 5 and 2, rip-dominated intermediate beaches occur in situations which are characterises by alternating bars and deeper rip channels and currents dominate the surf zone (◘ **Fig. 4.2**) [7]. When Ω is less than 1, lower energy reflective beaches occur. Reflective beaches have no surf, with wave breaking as they surge up a relatively steep beach face (◘ **Fig. 4.3**).

A similar gradation occurs in the tide-modified and tide-dominated beach systems. However, the increasing tidal range and dominance leads to a wider, flatter intertidal zone, with rips only occurring at low tide on the higher energy tide-modified beaches. The tide-dominated beaches tend to have a steep reflective high tide beach fronted by wide low gradient dissipative intertidal zones.

Therefore, in each of the beach systems there is a gradation from more reflective to more dissipative systems, together with their extensive low gradient intertidal zones which at low tide may reach hundreds of meters in width.

Knowledge of the morphodynamics of each beach type enables the prediction of the associated nature, location and variation in beach hazards, namely the height and type of the breaker, deep water, variable water depth (bars and troughs) and surf zone currents, particularly rip currents [7]. Based on this knowledge each of the nine beach types has been allocated an average or modal beach hazard rat-

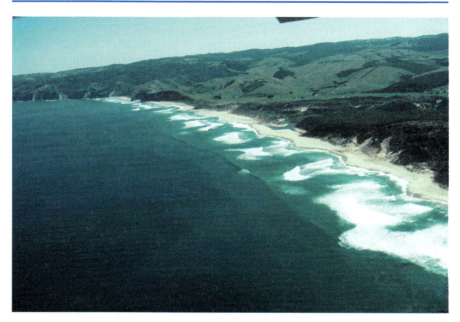

■ **Fig. 4.2.** An intermediate beach with well developed transverse bars and rips. Johana Beach, Victoria. Beach hazard rating = 6

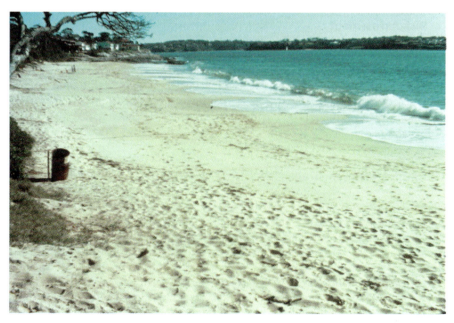

■ **Fig. 4.3.** A low energy reflective beach at Jibbon, near Sydney, with waves not breaking till the shoreline. Beach hazard rating = 3

ing between 1 (low hazards) and 10 (high hazards). Local factors, such as headlands, rocks, rock and coral reefs, inlets, structures (groynes, seawalls) all affect wave height and can change wave direction and may generate additional currents. All of these influence the morphodynamics of each beach and may increase the hazard rating by 1 or 2. Finally, the prevailing beach hazard rating at any particular time will depend on the actual or prevailing wave, tide and wind conditions. Based on all the above both the modal (time averaged) and prevailing (instantaneous) beach hazard rating can be readily determined for any beach at any time.

4.6.2
Beach Usage

The other side of the risk equation is the level of beach usage. While the number of users is a good indicator, it is not the whole story. Beside the actual number, which will fluctuate daily, at weekends, weekly and seasonally, factors such as the age, sex, nationality, beach experience, residence and socio-economic background, will all influence the level of beach awareness and consequently the risk to both individuals and groups of users. Unfortunately such information is difficult and expensive to obtain. Instead estimates of the number of users or samples of the types of users must be used.

4.6.3
Risk Assessment

As both hazards and usage vary in time and space, so too will risk. Beach risk assessment requires knowledge of both the type and level of hazards on an average and prevailing basis, as well as type and level of usage in the same time dimensions. Only with this information can risk be accurately assessed. Risk assessment (R) is a function of both hazard (H) and usage (U), such that $R = f (H \times U)$

4.6.4
Application in Australia

The Australian Beach Safety and Management Program (ABSMP), a joint project of SLSA and the University of Sydney between 1990 and 2004 compiled a database containing the location, physical characteristics, access, facilities, and hazards at Australia's 10,686 beach systems, in addition to publishing books on the beaches of each State [2, 3, 5, 6]. SLSA has also used the above system to develop a Beach Management Plan [1] and more recently incorporated it into a Coastal Safety Auditing Program. The Beach Management Plan provides a flow chart for the lifeguard to determine both the modal and prevailing beach hazard rating, thereby providing a standard and quantifiable measure of hazard on each patrolled beach. The chart suggests the level of water safety resources (personnel and equipment) required to mitigate the level of risk. It is designed to assist, not direct, the lifeguard in making decisions relating to the beach patrol and resources. The latter is a national auditing process that uses the beach hazard rating in combinations with other factors to develop a holistic approach to the development and maintenance of a safe coastal environment.

The procedure for assessing beach hazards and risks developed by ABSMP has been utilised to date by the following organisations: In New Zealand by Surf Life Saving New Zealand in undertaking their Coastal Survey; in Great Britain by Surf Life Saving Great Britain and subsequently by the Royal National Lifeboat Institute in developing their Beach Risk Assessment program; in Brazil by the Universidade de Itaji in developing the Brazilian Beach Safety and Management Program; and in Hawaii by the Hawaiian Lifeguard Association as the basis of their Hawaiian Ocean Safety Survey. With appropriate modification the ABSMP procedure can be used in any beach environment.

During the World Congress on Drowning it was agreed that:

The existing standard for evaluation of hazard presented at beaches should be implemented as the world-wide standard to enable the development of appropriate drowning prevention strategies at beaches.

References

1. Leahy S, Short AD, McLeod K (1996) Beach management plans. Surf Life Saving Australia, Sydney
2. Short AD (1993) Beaches of the New South Wales coast. Australian Beach Safety and Management Program, Sydney
3. Short AD (1996) Beaches of the Victorian coast and Port Phillip Bay. Australian Beach Safety and Management Program, Sydney
4. Short AD (1999) Handbook of beach and shoreface morphodynamics. Wiley, Chichester
5. Short AD (2000) Beaches of the Queensland coast: Cooktown to Coolangatta. Australian Beach Safety and Management Program, Sydney
6. Short AD (2001) Beaches of the South Australian coast and Kangaroo Island. Australian Beach Safety and Management Program, Sydney
7. Short AD, Hogan CL (1994) Rips and beach hazards, their impact on public safety and implications for coastal management. J Coastal Res 12:197–209

4.7
Training Standards for In-Water Rescue Techniques

Rick Wright

This chapter will discuss the following basic question: What skills, knowledge and personal attributes are being assessed as the criteria to effectively save the life of another human being in an aquatic environment by different lifesaving organisations and why are these different approaches taken?

4.7.1
Background

The origins of people rescuing people in danger of drowning can be traced back many centuries. As aquatic recreation and sun bathing became popular, small groups of experienced or goodwill-minded people began to organise into bodies to help people who needed rescuing from an unfamiliar environment. Mention can be made of China's Chin Kiang Association for the Saving of Life, which was established in 1708 to rescue sailors in distress. Similar societies and organisations were established as early as the late 1700s and early 1800s in the Netherlands, England, and the US.

As rescue groups became more organised, training began to evolve equipping these people with common skills and knowledge. With the growing popularity of recreational swimming, governments began to recognise the need to provide safety and preventative processes for people pursuing recreational activities in lakes, rivers and open water, and constructed swimming facilities. During this period various national lifesaving societies began to form, particularly in Commonwealth countries associated with the UK. In these countries, relatively consistent national lifesaving standards were introduced. In other countries, such as the US, less consistency was evident, due to local control over lifesaving services and their paid nature. The volunteer and the paid lifesaving services put different imprints on the level of training considered necessary for their regions.

Due to these evolved standards, which vary from country to country, it is now appropriate to discuss the relationship among the training standards being used by the various lifesaving bodies.

4.7.2
Current State of Affairs

While the various rescue societies and organisations all have one common goal to prevent the loss of loss of life through drowning, they all jealously protect their autonomy to self regulate the standard and level of training for in-water rescue. It is this common humanitarian value, to prevent drowning, which unites these societies and organisations around the world.

The International Life Saving Federation, a global confederation of over 100 national lifesaving federations of the world, has developed recommended minimum competencies for the training of livesavers in various environments. These recommendations are based on an evaluation of various training standards from major lifesaving organisations of the world and can provide a baseline for the development of training programs in a range of aquatic environments.

The International Life Saving Federation recommended minimum competencies include a recommended minimum international standard for a pool lifesaver of being able to swim 300 metres in 6 min or less. For inland and open water lifesavers or surf lifesavers, the minimum competence is to swim 400 metres in 8 min or less, all of these without the use of aids. At the same time, ILS has emphasised that local conditions may require higher standards and therefore member organisations are autonomous in the implementation and controlling of standards within their respective boundaries.

The United States Lifesaving Association (USLA) recommends that a still water or surf lifesaver be able to swim, at a minimum, 500 meters in 10 min or less. But in the US, some employers require 1000 meters in 20 min or less and some require a standard below the 500 meters in 10 min. In Australia, surf lifeguards are required to swim 400 meters in less than 9 min to gain a Surf Life Lifeguard Certificate (Bronze Medallion) which qualifies them to become an active volunteer lifeguard and 800 meters in less than 14 min to gain a an Advanced Lifesaving Certificate (Gold Medallion) qualifying them for paid lifeguarding duties.

The European Union is presently investigating common vocational standards that would allow the free flow of lifeguards across different European countries. Perhaps this should be a goal across all international boundaries. This would enable international humanitarian organisations concerned with drowning to call on the resources of tens of thousands of lifesavers around the world, all similarly skilled and knowledgeable as a result of a single international training and assessment standard.

4.7.3
The Foundation of In-Water Rescue Training Standards

Anecdotal evidence has been used as the premise for the development of rescue techniques for over 100 years. All lifesaving organisations successfully function according to a set of lifesaving standards that are seen as the necessary requirements to perform rescue duties, and strict tests are conducted to ensure members achieve these standards.

Introductory lifesaving training around the world has a common thread to assess initiative, judgement, fitness and knowledge about self-preservation with the ability to save another in an aquatic environment. Specialist training in such areas as first aid, advanced resuscitation, defibrillation equipment, rescue boat operation, scuba diving and specialist rescue disciplines are available to lifesavers to address the perceived needs of the in-water rescue situations served and decisions of the organisation as to the roles that will be performed by lifesavers.

Training is fundamentally developed for the environment in which in-water rescue is performed (this includes pools, lakes and rivers, surf and ocean). For those bearing the responsibility of supervising on-duty lifesavers, further training and qualifications appropriate to the level of responsibility accompanying a supervisory position are usually required. Such a mix of categorisation divides training regimes between and within organisations. As a result rescue techniques rarely change in modern times outside of changes in rescue equipment or the use of rescue equipment.

4.7.4
Evaluating the Standards

Considering the many different adopted training standards used to assess the standard of lifesavers by the various countries, the question is now posed: Why is there no scientific evidence to support which are the best skills to rescue another human in an aquatic emergency? Is there an innate function in humans allowing them to effectively save the life of another? Is there a link between the actual biomechanics and physiological performance of in-water rescue and the training and assessment mechanisms that qualified the human to perform such a rescue? Even more importantly, would the resulting condition of the victim be different as a result of the skills or knowledge of his rescuer?

International training standards for in-water rescue must recognise that the foundation of lifesaving training in each country is based on different training cultures and regimes developed by government, educational institution or organisation themselves. The availability of resources, the management of training and assessment, and the vocational outcomes available to candidates will also need to be taken into consideration.

The International Life Saving Federation has commenced research into this topic in an endeavour to determine the fitness and vocational standards of lifesavers.

4.8
Training and Equipping Rescue Personnel for Flood Rescue

SLIM RAY

Inland flooding, whether from river floods or flash floods, continues to be the top weather-related killer worldwide. In Venezuela, Central America, Mexico, Bangladesh, China, Vietnam, Mozambique and elsewhere, floods account for thousands of victims worldwide, in most years more than wars, terrorism, and revolutions. Unfortunately, little attention is devoted to this problem, and most emergency response agencies are not very well equipped to deal with it.

Before describing specific problem areas, some comparisons of the relative losses of life in other disaster situations are in order. In 1999, for example, the Yugoslav government crackdown against the Albanians in Kosovo, which eventually triggered international intervention, is now estimated to have killed less than 10,000 people; yet in the same year in Venezuela an estimated 50,000 were killed by floods in that country alone. A year earlier, in 1998, hurricane-induced floods in Central America are estimated to have killed over 10,000 people (with an equal number missing); those in Bangladesh and India over 20,000. In the cyclone of 1970 an estimated 500,000 people died in Bangladesh, most of them by drowning (see also ▶ **Section 10**).

What about terrorism, a subject that causes a great deal of concern? According to the US State Department, terrorist groups killed just under 10,000 people (9,255) worldwide in the entire decade between 1980 and the end of 1999, or an average of about 465 people a year. In 1998, by comparison, nearly 100,000 people perished in floods worldwide. Yet while many countries have large and lavishly-equipped anti-terrorism units, specialised flood rescue units are rare. In fact, few local and national emergency services worldwide possess even the most elementary training and equipment for flood rescue.

Unfortunately it is quite common to see firefighters, police, and military personnel braving flood waters in their service uniforms and firefighting protective gear, trying to improvise rescues on the spot with inadequate and inappropriate equipment. One wonders what the reaction would be to photos of firefighters attacking a structural fire in wetsuits, or to police making arrests in lifejackets instead of bullet-proof vests. Offshore lifesaving services are often pressed into service to handle inland flood rescue, with mixed results, since the requirements for inland rescue are quite different than those for offshore rescue.

Often rescuers pay for their lack of preparedness with their own lives. A large number of flood fatalities, perhaps as many as a third, are would-be rescuers: both professional and ordinary citizens trying to rescue family and neighbours. In the 1999 hurricane-induced floods in North Carolina (US), in which 52 people died, the Centers for Disease Control and Prevention estimated that fully 10% of the flood fatalities were rescue workers.

In order to function effectively in inland flood waters, rescue personnel need to understand the unique hazards of moving water, and how inland floodwaters differ from offshore waters and surf. Moving water is extremely powerful. A current of only 14.5 km/h (9 mph) generates a force against the body of over 1.3 kN (302 lbs), and the force rises not in a linear fashion, but rather as the *square* of the speed. Thus a current twice as fast will generate four times the force. It is therefore very easy for both boats and rescuers to be pinned against an obstacle and trapped.

Some acts that seem intuitive in moving water are, in reality, very dangerous. For example, trying to stand in moving water may cause foot entrapment. The person's foot is jammed into a crevice and cannot be dislodged because of the force of the water, leading to drowning. Rescue from this situation is difficult and dangerous.

Another common, but ill-advised, practice is to tie the rescuer to a rope. If the rescuer then loses footing, the rescuer will be forced under water, and the force of the current will prevent release from the tethering line (with likely fatal consequences), unless a special harness is used that is designed to release under pressure.

Rescuers must be properly equipped with personal protective equipment (PPE): a personal flotation device (lifejacket), thermal protection, helmet, gloves, and foot protection. This equipment must be designed for use in turbulent, moving water. Safety equipment designed for use in offshore applications is seldom suitable, as it tends to be too bulky. Each rescuer should also have a knife (capable of one-handed operation), a whistle for signalling and a light for night operations. Some rescuers also choose to carry a small waterproof radio.

Rescuers must also have basic rescue equipment. The most useful device is a simple throw bag with 18–21 meters (60–70 feet) of floating polypropylene rope, which is also quite inexpensive. Most units will also want to carry various tech-

▣ Table 4.3. Swift water training aspects

Shallow water crossings

Self-rescue swimming

Throw-bag practice

Swimming over a simulated strainer in the current

Various rope rescue evolutions

nical items usually associated with high angle rescues, such as long 50- to 90-meter (165–295 feet) nylon rescue ropes, karabiners, ascending and descending gear and a casualty litter with associated gear.

Inflatable boats are usually the best choice for rescue craft. Since motor failure is always a possibility in debris-laden floodwaters, any boat should have the option for paddle as well as motor propulsion. Handling a boat on moving water is different than on flat water or offshore ocean applications and requires special training. A common mistake is to rely too heavily on expensive, high-tech gear like helicopters and hovercraft. These are useful tools, but there are seldom enough of them and helicopters are subject to operating restrictions (weather, darkness) that often limits their use. The crews and rescue personnel also have to have special training and equipment suitable for moving water.

All training has to be realistic, and it is absolutely essential that it be conducted on moving water. It is impossible to appreciate to power of moving water unless one has actually experienced it. Normal swift water training aspects are included in ▣ Table 4.3.

Probably the most important aspect of this training, however, is to make rescuers comfortable in moving water. Students must develop both an abstract, "classroom" knowledge of river hydrologic features like eddies, hydraulics, holes, standing waves, and the like; as well as a practical knowledge derived from actually being in the water. In addition, student rescuers must learn about special river hazards like strainers, reversals and low-head dams or weirs.

Rescue units must have an effective incident command structure and should, when possible, be deployed early enough in the event to make rescues rather than body recoveries. Because of the large number of victims, flood rescue units should be supplemented by other suitably trained local emergency responders. Probably the greatest need, however, is for governments to realise that flooding, and flood rescues, are inevitable, and to make the appropriate commitment to train and equip an effective flood rescue force in advance of the need for them (▣ Fig. 4.4).

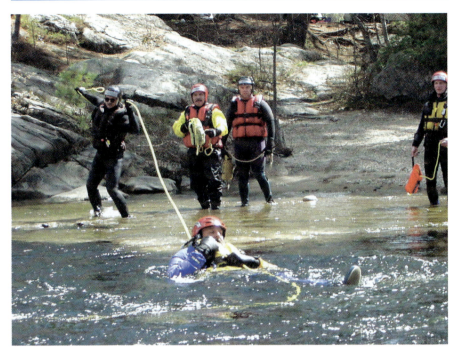

■ **Fig. 4.4.** Flood rescue training

4.9
Learning from Computer Simulations

WIEBE DE VRIES

This chapter overviews the role and requirements of computer simulations for training lifesavers. Three examples of computer-based simulation are presented that can be of help in learning lifesaving skills.

Learning is a relatively permanent change in behaviour as a result of an experience. Permanent change in behaviour and learning of new skills can be obtained via real life experiences. However, drowning is an activity that does not happen frequently and it is difficult to acquire lifesaving skills only through experience.

The aim of teaching is to achieve a change in behaviour by means of planned experiences. The instructor helps the students to store the new information in their memory in such a way that the information is stored for a long time (retention) and can be remembered when the information is needed (retrieval). Most knowledge and skills necessary for rescue activities require a high retention and quick retrieval from memory.

Mastery learning is an effective method of teaching. During mastery learning, each component of the underlying skill is trained under direct supervision and it is ensured that all components are mastered at the end of the training. During mastery learning students are in direct interaction with an instructor. There is good evidence that mastery learning leads to higher achievement than traditional classroom instruction. Direct interaction with an instructor might sometimes be a problem. A student may have difficulties understanding knowledge at the same time as fellow students, he may not understand the instructor, or is afraid of failure during an assessment.

Simulation of rescue situations is an effective method in which life experiences can be trained using a mastery learning process. Simulations can be offered to students in many forms, such as a computer-based program. Some of the computer simulations can be practised at home or at work while other simulations have to take place in the presence of an auditor (instructor).

Computer simulation uses the benefits of mastery learning and avoids direct interaction with an instructor. Even when an instructor is necessary to guide the computer simulation, a student can manage his own learning process by taking the time he needs to learn or repeat some exercises.

4.9.1
Computer Simulations

Students learn better when they receive feedback about the correctness of the answer and the motivation for the correction of an incorrect answer. This is also true for computer-based learning. For this reason, a program for computer simulation has to provide feedback. This is important to enable the student to make the right decisions, to gain new knowledge and skills in a stimulating way and to remain on a stable course in the process of learning [4].

To achieve all of this, computer simulation should have links that direct the student to the correct page after decisions are made. This means that the program has no linear structure, such as in a book, but hides the items that, at that moment, are not necessary or not relevant for the student to know. The student does not to find the relevant items (such as new information, questions to answer, videos with demonstrations) by turning over pages, but by clicking a button. Depending on which button is clicked the student achieves interactive feedback. The design of the program enables a step-by-step approach, thus allowing a mastery learning method without the need, and costs, of an immediately available instructor, or in such a way that the instructor can use his time effectively and therefore be an efficient assistant in the learning process of the student. Most computer simulations that are designed to teach new knowledge and skills with the help of games, randomly present the student with several scenarios in the games. In this way, the student does not know beforehand which scenario he has to deal with and he will learn more each time from the different scenarios.

Learning is also more effective when new knowledge can be connected to existing knowledge of the student. A good computer simulator for lifesavers has to fit in the experience of lifesavers. When the student recognises the situation, he will more easily retrieve existing knowledge from earlier experience during learning or in real practise. Computer simulation can be designed in such a way that students recognise the situations which allow them to retrieve already existing knowledge and skills.

An additional advantage of computer simulation is that it is safe. The student can make mistakes without people getting hurt or life being lost. It is possible to practice over and over again, without putting lives in danger until the student has learned how to save a life.

Computer simulation is a powerful learning tool. It helps students to become competent and act calmly when necessary. Students learn that they can trust themselves, they gain confidence and know for sure what they have to do when they have to act. Confidence is an important factor to bring into practice what has been learned, especially in stressful situations [2]. The final result of learning with computer simulations is that the student lifesaver acts immediately and effectively in a real situation and does not waste time thinking or discussing what to do.

During the World Congress on Drowning, three examples of computer-based simulation were presented:

'Wet'n'Wise' [7] is an education-focused prevention program that aims to save lives by teaching children how to have fun and be responsible in various aquatic environments. As the name suggests, Wet'n'Wise has a dual focus: 'wet' programs to promote water safety practice, and 'wise' programs to promote water safety knowledge.

The simulation program is focused on primary school children. A kit that contains a CD-ROM, a manual for the instructor, classroom posters and a board game (◘ Fig. 4.5).

'Learn First Aid Fast' [6] is a simulation program to improve first aid knowledge among students. The students are confronted with eight realistic accidents and their responses to the situations in the scenarios are crucial in determining whether the injured persons will survive or suffer permanent injury. The scenarios of each incident change at random.

As in real life, the first few minutes are of vital importance. After the scenario is finished, the student receives an evaluation of his decisions and reactions. The debriefing system provides detailed feedback, as well as an overview of all the results of the student thus far (◘ Fig. 4.6).

The 'DiaboloVR' simulation program [3] presents an almost unlimited variety of emergency disasters. The student 'walks around' with his joystick and special glasses for 3D effect in a virtual environment. He, or she, informs the instructor about the decisions he will take in view of the situation. Based on these decisions, the instructor can influence the course of the scenario.

The action of the student can be reviewed immediately after the exercise. Advanced action analysis features enable detailed student feedback, as well as benchmarking by analysis of group results (◘ Fig. 4.7).

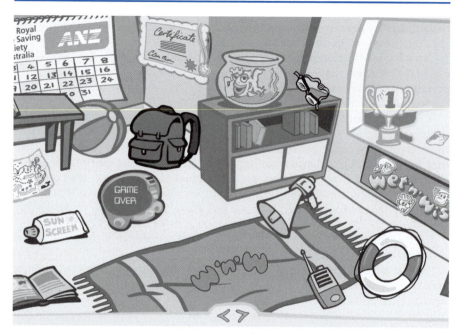

■ **Fig. 4.5.** 'Wet'n'Wise'

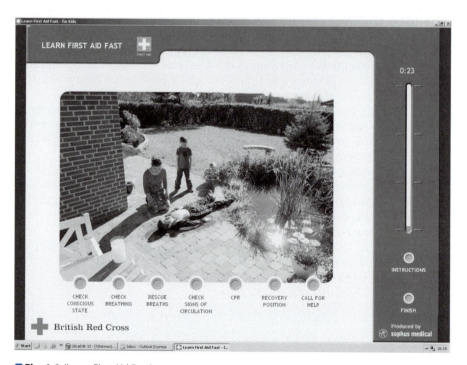

■ **Fig. 4.6.** 'Learn First Aid Fast'

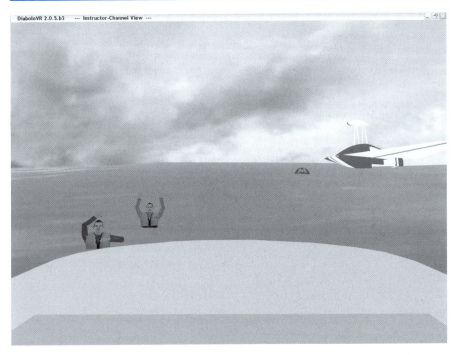

DiaboloVR 2.0.5.b3   --- Instructor-Channel View ---

Fig. 4.7. 'DiaboloVR'. During the computer simulation, the student looks over the bow of a rescue boat to the drowning victims

4.9.2
Curriculum Development

As most knowledge and skills necessary for rescue activities require high retention and quick retrieval from memory [1], an ideal computer simulation for life-savers should contain several instruction methods, such as presentations (video fragment in the program), answering questions (multiple choice, true-false questions), interactive games, puzzles and self-construction tasks (positioning something in the right position). To achieve high retention and quick retrieval at least three different instruction methods are necessary [5].

To develop or purchase a computer-based program for lifesavers the following steps are useful:

- Establish the learning goals or competencies of knowledge, skills, attitude and behaviour to be achieved
- Define, together with experts, the topics that should be part of the program to achieve the desired results
- Draw up a plan of the sequence in which the topics should be presented. Sometimes the sequence is dictated by priority of actions (treat first what kills first), and sometimes by the easiest way to learn new knowledge and skills

- Organise the course content by bringing the topics together in bigger parts, for instance themes or groups, and define the instruction techniques (multiple choice questions, movie parts) in which the topics should be presented
- Test and analyse the format on didactic aspects such as feedback features and randomisation of facts
- Revise the program accordingly after learning results and expert appraisals have been evaluated

Before deciding to develop, or purchase, any computer-based program, the education officer has to be assured that the program corresponds to the goals of the existing curriculum for lifesavers.

4.9.3
Websites

- The Royal Life Saving Society Australia and ANZ: www.wetnwise.com
- The Orange Cross: www.ehbo.nl
- E-Semble: www.e-semble.nl
- www.eric.ed.gov

Acknowledgements. The author would like to thank Andrew Whittaker (Australia), Justin Scarr (Australia), Ulrik Juul Christensen (Denmark) and Martijn Boosman (The Netherlands) for their participation during the workshop on computer simulation at the World Congress on Drowning and their comments on this article.

References

1. Anderson JR (2000) Cognitive psychology and its implications, 5th edn. Worth, New York
2. De Vries W, Alem AP van, Vos R de, et al (2005) Trained first-responders with an automated external defibrillator: how do they perform in real resuscitation attempts? Resuscitation: 157–61
3. Anonymous (2002) DiaboloVR [computer software]. E-Semble, Delft
4. Glassman M (2001) Dewey and Vygotsky: Society, experience, and inquiry in education practice. Educ Res 30:3–14
5. Nuthall GA (2000) The anatomy of memory in the classroom: understanding how students acquire memory processes from classroom activities in science and social studies units. Am Educ Res J 37:247–304
6. The Orange Cross (2002) Eerste hulp; leer het ook [Learn First Aid Fast] [CD-ROM]. Sophus Medical and The Orange Cross, Copenhagen/The Hague
7. The Royal Life Saving Society Australia and ANZ (2000) Wet ,n'Wise; Water Safety Resource Kit [curriculum package]. Banking Group, St. Kilda, Australia and New Zealand

4.10
Data Registration for Lifesaving Organizations

ANN WILLIAMSON and JULIE GILCHRIST

Aquatic environments are very diverse; each with its own risks. For example, there are swimming pools with diving boards, lakefronts with uneven terrain, and oceanfronts with waves and currents. Collecting information on the number, circumstances (where, when, how, and why) and outcomes of water safety incidents is an essential part of developing strategies for preventing them. Interventions to promote water safety should be targeted to the specific risks of the specific local environment. Additionally, the potential for comparisons between aquatic areas is also desirable.

Some countries already collect and report statistics on drowning deaths and drowning victims who are admitted to hospital, but survive. This is very useful for understanding the size of the problem, but such statistics usually include little or no information on the circumstances in which the drowning occurred. Also, many victims who are successfully rescued from drowning do not attend hospital and are therefore not included in the statistics. Lifesaving organisations can collect this sort of information, and can thereby play an important role in compiling and reporting the key information regarding water safety incidents, which can help shape prevention strategies.

Lifesaving organisations need to consider a number of issues prior to establishing a useful data registration and collection system. In order to maintain quality of information collected, the organisation needs to ensure that the data system will collect the same information in the same way over the same time period. Additional considerations include:

- What is the purpose of the collection? Is it to simply find out how many drownings occur or how many rescues are performed, to look at trends or to evaluate the effectiveness of different water safety activities?
- What kinds of incidents should be included in the data? Should it be only information on drowning incidents (whether or not death results) or should information be collected on rescues performed and even on preventive action taken by lifesavers?
- What sort of information should be collected about the circumstances of the incident? Do you collect information only on the incident or on the person involved as well?
- How often should the data be collected and who should collect it? Should it be continuous throughout the year, or only for short periods in peak times? Should it be collected by all lifesavers or only by specific representatives such as supervisors?

The discussion below will address some of these points.

4.10.1
What Is the Purpose of the Data Collection?

Different information will be collected for different purposes. For example, if the data collection is needed to demonstrate that there is a problem, it might be sufficient to simply collect data on the number of drownings (fatal and non-fatal) or rescues over a period of time. If the purpose is to understand how drowning might be prevented, information will be needed on the characteristics of the person involved and the circumstances in which the drowning occurred. If the purpose is to track the effectiveness of a water safety activity, then information will be needed that is relevant to the outcome expected from the activity.

4.10.2
What Kinds of Incidents Should Be Included:
Drowning Deaths, All Drownings, or Rescues?

As a primary function of lifesaving organisations is to perform rescues, it is sensible that the data they collect should be based primarily on rescues. Information on whether death was the outcome of the drowning could also be collected, if available. Information collected should be defined clearly to ensure that all information is collected uniformly. Considerable progress has been made in developing a definition of drowning (▶ **Chapter 2.3**: the definition of drowning), but the definition of the term 'rescue' is less clear. For example, does a rescue include activities where a lifesaver simply tells someone to move to safety, or must it include some physical contact with the person in danger? The United States Lifesaving Association (USLA) has for decades reported data on rescues and preventive actions, with the term 'rescue' including all incidents in which physical assistance is provided to a person in peril. In New South Wales, Australia, a similar data registration system, but one which includes two defined types of rescues, was recently tested successfully. Its categories are as follows:

- Major rescue: any rescue where more than one lifesaver or a member of the public rendered assistance *or* where the rescued persons had to be resuscitated *or* where another agency, such as rescue helicopter or ambulance, had to render assistance
- Rescue: any rescue where a person was physically assisted or supported to return to shore or other place of safety. This includes retrieving a person in difficulty
- Preventive action: any water safety advice provided to the public. This includes asking people to swim between the flags and the use of whistle

4.10.3
What Information Should Be Collected
on Circumstances of the Water Safety Incident?

In determining what information should be collected on each rescue it is important to keep in mind the purpose of the data collection and the question that needs to be answered by the data. The aim might be to make simple counts of the numbers of rescues, or of different levels of rescue such as in the NSW data collection trial. Often, however, data collection is an opportunity to collect information that might guide the organisation's practices. For example, information on the day of the week or the sea conditions may assist in deciding the numbers of lifesavers needed at particular times or under certain conditions. Typically water safety incident data collections could include information about the timing and conditions around the time of the rescue, details of the rescue and, where possible, details of the person involved.

Information about the timing and conditions could include: date, day of the week and time of the rescue, air temperature, wind conditions and wind direction, weather conditions (rain or fine), tide details (low, rising, high, falling tide), sea surface conditions (calm, choppy, rough seas), estimated wave type and height and presence of rips and rip type.

Details of the rescue could include: the person's activity just before the rescue (swimming, fishing, paddling), type of rescue performed, type of equipment used (rescue board, rescue water vehicle), distance from waters edge, distance from lifesaver station, involvement of first aid, involvement of ambulance. Another potentially useful piece of information is the primary cause of the incident, such as rip current, surf, drop-off. By gathering this information, USLA has been able to determine that approximately 80% of rescues at surf beaches in the US are due to rip currents.

Details of the person could include: age, gender, details of place of residence (urban, rural, zip code, postcode, resident, visitor), estimated swimming ability (weak, average, strong), outcome of the rescue (drowning, non-fatal drowning).

It may not be possible to collect all of the types of information listed above in all settings. Some of the types would need to be defined further for the specific circumstances. For example, it may not always be possible to collect information from rescued people as they may leave the scene very quickly or there may be too many people rescued at the same time. It may, however, be possible for lifesavers to estimate some items, such as age, gender, and swimming ability. Also, there are potential problems in collecting other information, such as wave height due to difficulties of where on the wave to measure, or for air temperature if each lifesaver position does not have a thermometer. Above all, the information to be included in data registration and collection systems needs to be clearly defined and able to be collected reliably by all of the collectors. If there are routinely problems in collecting a particular item, it should be modified (actual age to estimated age group) or discarded, rather than to have poor quality information collected.

4.10.4
Who Should Collect the Information and How Often?

There is no clear answer to the question of how the data should be collected as it really depends on the particular circumstances for the lifesaving organisation and the aim of the data registration system. In all cases, the more information to be collected, the more resources are required. A very simple collection involving the number of major rescues, for example, could involve all lifesavers reporting and could cover all times the lifesavers are working. On the other hand, a busy lifesaving post would have difficulty with a collection that seeks information about the conditions and circumstances of the rescue and details of the person rescued for all rescues.

It may be possible to increase the amount of information collected by delegating specific people to collect the data in each lifesaving point, although this will have obvious staffing and cost implications for the lifesaving organisation. Another alternative to collect a large amount of information about each rescue may be to take a sampling approach by collecting at specific intervals, say for 4 days per month throughout the summer season. The disadvantages of this are that it is difficult to decide how often and when the collection should occur. There are also problems with this approach as it only produces estimates of the numbers of rescues and the estimates are likely to be influenced by the conditions during the times of the data collection.

No matter how simple or complete the data to be collected, the time required can be minimised by thoughtful development of data collection instruments. Minimising text fields that require writing information can ease the data collection burden. This can be accomplished by using tick boxes for common choices in activity (such as walking, swimming, fishing), location (the name of each beach if there are only a few), day of the week and time of the day.

4.10.5
How Is the Information Gathered Together?

The final issue in setting up a data registration system is determining how information from lifesaving stations is sent to a centralised data registration point. The potential solutions range from oral reports by telephone from lifesaving stations for very simple data collections, or paper and pencil forms which can be faxed or posted for collections with a larger number of items. Computer-based solutions are also possible and include methods such as computer-based forms or records that can be emailed or could be on the website of the lifesaving organisation. The decision to move to more technologically oriented approaches depends on the scale of the information collected and on the budget available to establish the data registration system set up and maintain it. It may be that the most technologically-based methods, such as a web-based system, are the cheapest in the long term since the only ongoing costs involve maintenance.

In summary, the best way of resolving some of the issues raised in this chapter is to conduct a trial data collection and evaluate the results. The problems with data collection can become very clear, very quickly and modifications can be made to the system to make it as effective as possible from the start. This will also allow the organisation to pilot templates for data reporting to ensure that the data collected meets the needs of both the organisation as a whole and the data collectors who have provided the information.

Further Reading

Brenner RA, Trumble AC, Smith GS, et al. (2001) Where children drown: the epidemiology of drowning in the United States. Pediatrics 108:85–89
Kemp A, Sibert JR (1992) Drowning and near drowning in children in the United Kingdom: lessons for prevention. BMJ 304:1143–1146
Mackie D (1999) Patterns of drowning in Australia. Med J Aust 171:587–589

4.11
Risk Management in Training of Rescue Techniques

RICHARD MING KIRK TAN

This chapter raises awareness of risk management in the training of rescue techniques. Risk management in the training of rescue techniques involves an understanding of the legal liability risks that may confront a rescue instructor and the adoption of measures to manage and control those risks. Unfortunately, for many people, the issue of risk is only addressed after an incident has occurred and when it may be too late. However, the law can affect many aspects of the duties and responsibilities of rescue instructors, and this chapter deals mainly with some aspects of their legal liability risks under the law of tort in Singapore and the management of such risks [2]. The risks under other areas of the law, such as criminal law, are generally not covered. Nonetheless, they should also be considered if a comprehensive risk management program is to be formulated. While the laws of other countries are not generally dealt with, there is some degree of similarity in the risks involved and it is hoped that some of the ideas in this chapter will also be useful to other countries. This chapter is only intended to give a general understanding of the legal issues addressed. It is not intended to provide comprehensive legal advice.

According to law, *tort* means a wrong in which the wrongdoer is under a legal obligation to compensate the injured party. There are many different types of torts, but in the context of rescue instructors the most important is probably negligence. Another tort which instructors may be involved with is that of battery.

Negligence as a tort involves the breach of a legal duty of a defendant that results in injury or damage to the plaintiff. The basic requirements of negligence include: (a) proof of a duty of care, (b) breach of that duty, and (c) foreseeable damage suffered by the victim as a result of that breach. When it can be shown that two people are put in a position whereby the first person owes to the second person a duty to be careful and to take all reasonable care to ensure that his conduct will not cause injury to the other, the law will impose upon the first person a duty of care to the second person. Rescue instructors and their students will be in such a position. It is interesting to note that in the context of teaching resuscitation, it has been said in a paper, published by the Resuscitation Council of the United Kingdom that there is a potential liability for those who train rescuers in resuscitation techniques to third parties who suffer as a result of a negligent resuscitation [1].

Battery is a tort of trespass against the person. In law, it is the intentional and direct application of force against another person. Therefore, if in the course of teaching or training rescue techniques, an instructor deliberately hits a student as a punishment or in anger, an act of battery is likely to have been committed. This may render the instructor liable to legal action for damages for any head and other injuries that the student may suffer as a result of the battery unless his prior consent had been obtained.

The teaching and training of rescue techniques is an activity where the student relies heavily on the knowledge and ability of the instructor. However, knowledge and expertise may not be enough and it will be prudent for the instructor to also have a risk management program in place. A good risk management program includes common sense with some control measures, keeping abreast of the latest developments and continuing education. Some risk management measures are mentioned below for instructors to consider when planning their own program. These measures are not exhaustive and may need to be modified to suit particular circumstances.

- Ensure students are medically eligible: Since the training of rescue techniques can be a strenuous physical activity, it may be desirable to require the student to be certified fit by a medical doctor before allowing him to start training. In addition, if the student shows any signs of being unwell in the course of training, it would be prudent to stop his training to prevent any serious condition from developing.
- Screen students: Notwithstanding the fact that a student may be certified fit for rescue training, the instructor may still wish to reject him because of certain facts. For example he is a small-sized child or person wanting to join a class of adults. Since an instructor is normally not under a legal obligation to accept every student, he may well want to exercise his judgement to reject certain students or ask them to join a more suitable class.
- Remove students with unacceptable behaviour or performance from class: Even after accepting a student, the instructor will still want to pay attention to his performance. This is especially so for younger students, but could equally apply to adults because each person's physical, emotional and intellectual maturity may vary and may not correspond to his biological age. Therefore, if a student is not meeting an acceptable standard, either academically or in practice or behaviour, then that student should not be allowed to continue as he may be a danger to himself and others. He may need to be placed in a special class or require more personalised remedial training.
- Use indemnities, releases and exemption clauses: Although these may be restricted by the law, they serve as useful notices and may be used to the extent that is legally possible.

- Follow recommended policies, guidelines, standards and procedures: These represent the standard to be attained and the instructor should ensure that he keeps up to date with them and follows them.
- Always be prudent, cautious, alert and vigilant and exercise due care and attention: Although this is important always, it is especially important in the case of water skill and contact rescue training, whether in enclosed or open water.
- Always follow a systematic progression in teaching, training and practice: Therefore, a student should not be allowed to progress to the next stage of training without demonstrating proficiency in the basic or prerequisite skills. Imagine how disastrous the situation could potentially be if an instructor assigned a student who had missed the session on defences and releases to face a victim assigned to grab him in a training session.
- Keep proper records, including attendance registers: This will help the instructor remember any details should the need arise. Furthermore, the attendance register will help remind the instructor if a particular student has missed any session and therefore should make up that session before being allowed to proceed to the next stage of training.
- Seek prior consent whenever possible: It is important to obtain the relevant prior consent whenever possible and where minors are involved, their consent alone would usually not be valid and therefore it is best to also obtain the consent of their parent or legal guardian.
- Obtain insurance: Instructors should also consider obtaining such insurance policies whenever available so that there may be compensation available if required.
- Seek legal advice early: This is intended to ensure that the instructor gets the maximum benefit of the law to which he is entitled.

The training of rescue techniques can be hazardous if not carried out properly due to the nature of the activity. This chapter should raise awareness of some of the risks involved for rescue instructors and may help instructors to face claims for liability concerning their training activities. Instructors should be prepared and take steps to manage those risks so that rescue training will be a safe and meaningful experience for everyone concerned. Putting in place a risk management program involves time and money but is worth the effort. A successful risk management program not only reduces the possibility and severity of any loss that may arise but also improves the professionalism of the rescue instructor.

References

1. Colquhoun M, Martineau E (2000) The legal status of those who attempt resuscitation. Resuscitation Council United Kingdom, London
2. Tan RMK (2003) Lifesavers, the law and risk management. Singapore Life Saving Society, Singapore

4.12
Lifesaving as an Academic Career: International Perspectives

VERONIQUE COLMAN, STATHIS AVRAMIDIS, LUIS-MIGUEL PASCUAL-GÓMEZ,
HARALD VERVAECKE and ULRIK PERSYN

To stimulate the mobility between the countries of the European Community and the recognition of professionals in the sport-related professions within the European member states, a five-level training and qualification structure has been proposed by the European Network of Sport Science, Education and Employment (ENSSEE) in active co-operation with governmental and non-governmental bodies [13]. The structure was based on directives from the European Community in 1989 and 1992 [3, 4] and referred to a decision of the European Ministers Council for Education regarding the recognition of vocational training and qualification in 1985 [2].

Mobility and recognition of professionals in any employment within the member states concerning the three highest levels in the structure are defined as follows:

- Level 3: "... Activity involves chiefly technical work which can be performed independently and/or entail executive and co-ordination duties"
- Level 4: "...It does not generally require mastery of the scientific bases of the various areas concerned"
- Level 5: "... complete higher education ... entailing a mastery of the scientific bases of the occupation"

The three highest levels in the structure include university as well as non-university training, with accessibility for highly qualified professionals as well as for unpaid volunteers. The structure has been applied for the sport-related professions and more specifically for the sports coaching professions (◻ Table 4.4). The education commission of the International Life Saving federation (ILS) agreed that it was also appropriate for lifesaving, and this not only for the sport oriented aspects of lifesaving but also for the humanitarian oriented aspects of lifesaving.

For level 3 education, the ENSSEE set up a general questionnaire about sport-related professions, including lifesaving and, more recently in co-operation with ILS, a more specific questionnaire about lifesaving [27]. Almost all member states of the European Community returned one or both questionnaires.

Due to the present transition towards bachelor and master degrees in European higher education, it was too early to set up a questionnaire for level 4 and 5 education. Therefore, no inventory exists on higher and academic education in lifesaving in Europe. Also information from other continents is not available.

The current initiatives and perspectives with respect to level 3, 4 and 5 training in Greece, Spain and Belgium are described in this chapter.

□ Table 4.4. European structure of levels 3–5 proposed for training of coaches

		Level 3	Level 4	Level 5
Keywords for tasks and activities	Execution	X	X	X
	Co-ordination	(X)	X	X
	Teaching		X	X
	Research		(X)	X
	Management		(X)	X
	Supervision			X
	Strategic planning			X
Minimum duration		300 hours	600 hours	2400 hours
		2 years practical experience	2 years practical experience	1200 hours of basic education in sport sciences
				1200 hours of specific education in the chosen sport discipline
				2 years practical experience

◘ **Table 4.5.** Examples of academic studies on lifesaving in Greece

Title	Author (year)
Epidemiology of drowning in Greece	Alexe D (2002) [1]
Influence of biomechanical parameters on the straddle entry that is used in lifesaving	Avramidis S (2001) [5]
Competitive anxiety levels between lifesavers and swimmers	Avramidou E (2002) [7]
Initial findings of the 4W model of drowning and lifesaving	Avramidis S (2004) [6]

4.12.1
Greece

Graduates in sport sciences and physical education play a formal role in professional lifesaving. All graduates in sport sciences have had no formal training in lifesaving or passed relevant examinations. Nevertheless, they are entitled to be professionally active in lifesaving and to work as beach lifesavers. All graduates in sport sciences specialised in any aquatic sport are also entitled to train beach lifesavers and are the only legally appropriate persons for directing private schools for lifesaving.

Lifesaving is not an academic specialisation in Athens but plans are at hand to organise a national academic curriculum as a collaboration between the European Lifeguard Academy of Greece and the Department of sport sciences and physical education at the University of Athens.

Limited research has been done at university level [5–7]. Some researchers have published on the epidemiology of drowning [1] (◘ **Table 4.5**).

4.12.2
Spain

At this moment, there is no national curriculum for lifesavers in Spain. The first regional lifesaving regulation was implemented in Madrid in 2002 and this 80-hour training program is expected to become the national standard for the minimum requirements for lifesavers in Spain. Lifesaving is not included in the academic curriculum. The 3-year curriculum for students of physical and sport management (TAFYD) includes 120 hours on the theoretical and practical aspects of first aid, CPR and aquatic rescues, but this does not qualify these students to become professional lifesavers.

Initiatives to develop level 3, 4 and 5 training for lifesavers are made by the Segovia Life Saving School (ESS) and the Lifesaving Federation in Galicia (FESSGA).

◘ Table 4.6. Examples of academic studies on lifesaving in Spain

Title	Author (Year)
Life saving surveillance techniques	Pascual LM (1996)
Location of surveillance posts in pools	Llorente L, Pascual LM (1998)
Professional profile of lifesavers in Segovia	Barrio B, Pascual LM (1998)
Attention and concentration in lifesaving	Barrio B (1999)
Audio-visual aids in lifesaving instruction	Pascual LM (1999)
Requirements in professional lifesaving	Pascual LM, Barrio B, Sanz P (2002)

Studies supported by the ESS have demonstrated that the physical, psychological and theoretical qualifications and skills of professional lifesavers should be much more than those currently required. The ESS promotes the program from Madrid and has adopted the requirements but their training program takes 120 hours. The training program also includes psychological and physical tests at three instances:

- Pre-course enrolment: a physical test and interview with psychologist
- During the course: written time-limited tests on physical and psychological topics and lifesaving techniques
- At the end of the course: assessment of the acquired skills, interview with psychologist and employment orientation

The ESS has started to develop a specialisation in lifesaving within the national academic curriculum for students who have completed the secondary education period. Important elements in the curriculum will be water skills and techniques, psychological aspects, selection of students and assessment of acquired skills.

In addition, in December 2002, the ESS signed a cooperation agreement with the Faculty of Psychology of the University of Segovia to develop combined research programs for the qualitative and quantitative analysis and assessment of the psychological factors involved in the selection of students, learning and training strategies and professional performance of lifesavers.

Since 2001, the Lifesaving Federation in Galicia (FESSGA) provides level 3 programs for lifesaving. This program includes sport, instruction and management.

The post-graduate education in sport sciences at the University of la Coruña and Barcelona includes a course in lifesaving. This post-graduate course for graduates in sport sciences is oriented to instructors wishing to train and educate students for a level 3 qualification and to the development of research programs in lifesaving.

Most research is carried out by academically trained people, but often without formal academic support (◘ **Table 4.6**).

Table 4.7. Examples of academic studies on lifesaving in Belgium

	Topic	Reference
Master thesis	Accidents and accident prevention in pools (pool infrastructure, law)	[9, 10, 14, 18, 20, 22, 24, 26, 28, 31–37]
	Comparative studies on lifesaving certificates	[27, 30, 39]
	Training, testing of reanimation and defibrillation skills	[8, 11, 19, 21, 29, 38]
	Water lifesaving skills (humanitarian, competitive)	[12, 23, 25, 42]
Article	Movement analysis of water lifesaving skills	[15–17, 40, 41]

A bi-annual ESS and FESSGA convention contributes to the academic development of lifesaving in Spain. The presentations at these conventions are published and available on CD-ROM.

4.12.3
Belgium

At the Faculty of Physical Education and Physiotherapy of the University of Leuven, a course to obtain a professional lifesaver degree (level 3) is incorporated in the academic curriculum of all students. In addition, an academic specialisation in lifesaving is offered. The career of these level 5 trained professionals is primarily directed at the instruction of candidates for a level 3 qualification in the humanitarian as well as in the sport-oriented courses.

Every 4 years since 1970, a satellite meeting of the International Congress of Biomechanics and Medicine includes topics of interest for international experts in lifesaving. In the European Master's Degree in Swimming, the University of Leuven presents a module on the kinesiological aspects of lifesaving.

Almost 40 research theses and articles have been produced about accidents and accident prevention in pools, testing of reanimation and defibrillation skills and lifesaving competitive skills (□ Table 4.7). The kinesiological aspect of the research by the University of Leuven is oriented to provide swimmers and lifesavers movement and on-land diagnosis and advice [8, 9].

4.12.4
Conclusion

There is a need for an academic and scientific basis for lifesaving activities. At present, it would appear advisable for the ENSSEE and ILS to be informed about the current presence of level 4 and 5 lifesaving training on each continent. First, in which countries and universities is a specialisation in lifesaving offered. Furthermore, which topics are involved in the training program and which type of research is undertaken, related to management, biomedical and sport science aspects. And finally, if there is a need for an international academic curriculum, what are the objectives?

Coordination should be initiated when several initiatives are concurrently set up within one country. In countries where no level 4 or 5 training in lifesaving exists, national initiatives should be taken to develop a specialisation in lifesaving within the academic curriculum. This curriculum should then be based on uniform minimal international requirements.

4.12.5
Websites

- www.sossegovia.com
- www.ensshe.lu/documents/cahiers [13]
- www.ela.pre.gr

References

1. Alexe D, Dessypris N, Petridou E (2002) Epidemiology of unintentional drowning deaths in Greece. Abstracts World Drowning Congress, Stichting Foundation drowning, Amsterdam, p 90
2. Anonymous (1985) Council decision 85/368/EEC of 16 July 1985 on the comparability of vocational training qualifications between Member States of the European Community. European Union Official Journal, Brussels
3. Anonymous (1989) Council Directive 89/48/EEC of 21 December 1988 on a general system for the recognition of higher-education diplomas awarded on completion of professional education and training of at least three years' duration. European Union Official Journal, Brussels
4. Anonymous (1992) Council Directive 92/51/EEC of 18 June 1992 on a second general system for the recognition of professional education and training to supplement Directive 89/48/EEC. European Union Official Journal. Brussels
5. Avramidis S (2001) Influence of biomechanical parameters on the straddle entry that is used in lifesaving. Master Thesis, Leeds Metropolitan University
6. Avramidis S (2004) Initial findings of the 4W model of drowning and lifesaving. In: Avramidis S, Tritaki J, Avramidou E (eds) 1st International Lifeguard Congress, Greece. European Lifeguard Academy, p 15
7. Avramidou E (2002) Competitive anxiety levels between lifesavers and swimmers. BSc dissertation, Leeds Metropolitan University
8. Baert L (1989) Knowledge of resuscitation techniques in the Belgian population. Master Thesis, K.U. Leuven

9. Benoit J (1985) Accidents and security organization in the Flemish public pools. Master Thesis, K.U. Leuven
10. Bongaerts B (1984) Accidents and accident prevention in pools: incidence, kind and prevention. Master Thesis, K.U. Leuven
11. Caluwé K (1998) Development of an observation protocol to evaluate the cardiopulmonary resuscitation. Master Thesis, K.U. Leuven
12. Christiaens K (1996) Basic steps for a kinesiological evaluation of life saving competitors. Master Thesis, K.U. Leuven
13. Claude R, Gaugey JP, Persyn U (1999) European structure for the 5 levels of coaches training. Cahiers of ENSSEE (European Network of sport science, education and employment) (http://www.ensshe.lu/documents/cahiers/)
14. Cloetens B (1984) Accidents and security organization in the public pools of East-Flanders. Master Thesis, K.U. Leuven
15. Colman V (1995) Techniques from life saving competition in school. In: Delecluse C (ed) Postgraduate course for PE-teachers, Leuven: ACCO, pp 89-92
16. Colman V, Persyn U, Zhu JP, Vervaecke H (1996) Diagnosis and advice for life saving technique using video and PC. Abstracts of International Water Safety conference, Durban South-Africa, p 21
17. Colman V, Persyn U, Zhu JP, Ungerechts B (1997) Movement analysis and computer animation in swimming and life saving. In: Daniel K, Hoffmann U, Klauck J (eds) Kölner Schwimmsporttage. Sport Fahnemann, pp 68–73
18. Cox A (1972) Qualitative approach of the pool infrastructure. Master Thesis, K.U. Leuven
19. Custers A (1999) Defibrillation education of life savers. Master Thesis, K.U. Leuven
20. Demets B (1998) Accidents and security organization in the public pools of West-Flanders and their infrastructure. Master Thesis, K.U. Leuven
21. Demunter G (1983) The ABC of the resuscitation: teaching and evaluating the basics in 14–17 year old youngsters. Master Thesis, K.U. Leuven
22. Dhondt G (1998) Accidents and security organization in the public pools of Antwerp and their infrastructure. Master Thesis, K.U. Leuven
23. Dumon H (1978) Carrying techniques in life saving: some swim technical dimensions. Master Thesis, K.U. Leuven
24. Gils J (1984) Structure of the lifesaving services in public pools of Limburg. Master Thesis, K.U. Leuven
25. Govaerts A (1982) Releasing techniques in lifesaving: study of some technical aspects. Master Thesis, K.U. Leuven
26. Gysemans L (1974) Aspects of pool hygiene Master Thesis, K.U. Leuven
27. Hubregsen W (2000) Comparative study on lifeguard certificates in Europe; proposal of a European pool-lifeguard certificate. Master Thesis, K.U. Leuven
28. Moons K (1998) Study of accident prevention of public pools in Limburg. Master Thesis, K.U. Leuven
29. Neven S (1978) The development of pulmonary resuscitation. Master Thesis, K.U. Leuven
30. Pollefeyt E (1999) Comparative study of certificates of coast lifeguards Master Thesis, K.U. Leuven
31. Saeys J (1984) Study of accident prevention of public pools in Antwerp. Master Thesis, K.U. Leuven
32. Van Couillie B (1975) Description of the actual situation of the sea pollution. Master Thesis, K.U. Leuven
33. Van Gelder C (1985) Study of accident prevention of public pools in West-Flanders. Master Thesis, K.U. Leuven
34. Van Impe J (1998) Accidents and accident prevention in public pools in East-Flanders and the Vlarem II law. Master Thesis, K.U. Leuven
35. Van Raemdonck V (2001) Study of the evolution of the security services in Flemish pools. Master Thesis, K.U. Leuven
36. Van Zeebroek B (1998) Accidents and accident prevention in public pools in Flemish-Brabant. Master Thesis, K.U. Leuven

37. Vanderkrieken P (1979) Prevention of and actions after accidents in the water. Master Thesis, K.U. Leuven
38. Vandorpe R (1972) Life saving techniques and resuscitation methods after drowning. Master Thesis, K.U. Leuven
39. Verstraelen R (1992) Comparative study of certificates of pool lifeguards. Master Thesis, K.U. Leuven
40. Vervaecke H, Persyn U (1979) Effectiveness of the breaststroke leg movement in relation to selected time-space, anthropometric, flexibility and force. University Park Press, Baltimore, pp 320-328
41. Vervaecke H, Crombez K (1993) Survival swimming. In: Buekers M (ed) Postgraduate course for PE-teachers, Leuven: ACCO, pp 143-175
42. Wybaillie J (1977) Comparative study of the duck-dive. Master Thesis, K.U. Leuven

4.13
Fund-Raising for Lifesaving

KLAUS WILKENS

In view of the increasing scarcity of funds, lifesaving organisations must find new and innovative ways to ensure future funding of their many tasks and goals At the same time lifesaving should become better known and appreciated by the general public. Fund-raising is an expression used in social marketing and means "raising funds, taking measures to find sources of funds for non-profit organisations". This covers all areas such as sponsoring, charity events, merchandising, and advertising for new members and donations. Non-profit organisations generally need money to finance science, special projects and information programs. Fund-raising is the best marketing instrument for getting it.

All this was and is taking place in a selective manner within organisations, aligned only to a certain extent towards the joint objective. Up to now in most lifesaving organisations there has been no reliable donor basis offering clearly reliable long-term donations for the future.

Successful non-profit organisations are as concerned about marketing techniques and their ability to prepare wise marketing plans as any profit making corporation. The non-profit or social purpose organisation must look critically at itself to value its worth, to examine its mission, to determine whether this statement of mission is being interpreted properly through measurable objectives and meaningful programs, and to evaluate overall impact on the market area. There are existing diverse fund-raising instruments and concepts. Their variety depends on:

- The country, density and structure of the population
- Level and structure of income
- Allocation of income (particularly higher income)
- Regional differences
- Size and structure of lifesaving organisations (for instance: central or federalist structure, independent versus non-independent local clubs, competitiveness of suborganisations)
- Kind of instruments

Fund-raisers need to plan by analysing the total market potential after judging gift ability within each market segment.

A variety of fund-raising strategies should be considered:

- Fees
- Donations via direct mailings, house and street collections, lottery
  - Cash
  - Equipment
- Telephone call/solicitation
- Benefit events
- Recruiting donors online
- Legacies and capital campaigns
- Foundations
- Investment funds
- Material collection and trading (such as clothes, paper, metal)
- Partnerships circles of friends and supporters
- Sponsoring
- Governmental supports
- Trading and merchandising

All of these fund-raising strategies are successfully used by the German Life Saving Society (DLRG). One of them, the DLRG direct mail campaign, is introduced here as an example.

In view of financial constraints, which are becoming tighter and tighter, DLRG decided in 1997 to utilize professional fund-raising, in order to ensure the various tasks and aims of the federation for the future and at the same time to make DLRG better known and inform the public intensively about its important work. DLRG developed, together with SAZ Marketing AG – a professional partner for social marketing – a concept which seeks to acquire a large number of German citizens as regular donors by means of direct mailing (donation letters) to select target groups.

The project "donation fund" was founded on a common initiative of the DLRG Board and its branches and local clubs. The main aim was to generate a great number of donors, as many as possible, via direct mailing activities within a period of 3 years. It was anticipated that in the first years, costs would not be offset by donations received, but that in future years, as the donor list was refined to target the most likely donors, income would cover the costs of the program and yield a significant income above these costs. As expected, the first 2 years were a clear investment period in which costs were greater than donations received. The break-even point was reached in the year 2000 and the fund is now making a profit (120% of the distribution for the year 2001, according to the opening budget of every club involved).

In the meantime DLRG has been able to generate more than 200,000 donors with a donation income of 5 million euros per year.

4.14
Lifesaving in Developing Countries

MARGIE PEDEN and JOHN LONG

Drowning is a significant cause of death in many countries around the world. Unfortunately, detailed routine data on drowning is not gathered in many areas, particularly in low- and middle-income countries. Even in high-income countries, where some data on drowning is gathered, there still appears to be significant under-reporting of this major public health problem.

4.14.1
Who Drowns Where?

The World Health Organization Global Burden of Disease (GBD) study provides the most comprehensive global data on all diseases and injuries, including drowning. According to the GBD 2000 data, an estimated 449,000 people drowned worldwide (7.4 per 100,000 population) and a further 1.3 million disability adjusted life years (DALYs) were lost as a result of premature death or disability from drowning. Of these drownings, 97% occurred in low and middle-income countries. Although 38% occurred in Western Pacific regions, Africa had the highest drowning mortality rate (13.1 per 100,000 population).

Males had higher drowning mortality rates than females for all ages and in all regions. Children under the age of 5 had the highest drowning mortality rate for both sexes in all of the WHO regions except for Africa, where children aged 5–14 years had the highest mortality rate. Worldwide, for children under the age of 15 years, drowning accounted for a higher mortality rate than any other cause of injury.

4.14.2
What Should be Done?

At the World Congress on Drowning, an expert meeting focused on lifesaving efforts in developing countries. During this meeting, it was agreed that drowning prevention efforts must be broadened beyond the training and placement of qualified lifeguards at large bodies of water where drownings are common. It was agreed that lifesaving efforts in these countries should involve a heavy emphasis on prevention and include:
- Antenatal education
- Teaching swimming to adults and children
- Inventive floatation devices
- Supervision of children around water by responsible adults
- Vessel safety
- Teaching bystanders rescue breathing

- Courses for first responders
- Training in lifesaving skills

The expert meeting concluded that in order to improve drowning safety in developing countries the following should be addressed:
- Improvement of health care systems to deal with victims of drowning
- Further research on the impact and cost of drowning in these countries as well as an evaluation of interventions in different contexts
- Cross-organisational cooperation
- Additional funding for this critical aspect of injury prevention

4.14.3
Lifesaving Efforts in Developing Countries

Lifesaving efforts are being conducted in developing countries. The International Life Saving Federation (ILS) is one international organisation working to address this issue. The ILS Development Commission aims to identify areas of the world needing assistance in developing or improving lifesaving services and to coordinate assistance to those areas. The greatest focus of the Development Commission is underdeveloped countries where the incidence of drowning is high. In some areas, the Development Commission partners with the Royal Life Saving Society (RLSS), which is closely allied with ILS.

Member federations of ILS exist in over 100 countries. Lifesaving aid is primarily provided by individual ILS member federations and regions, working independently or in concert to assist countries in need. The Development Commission helps to identify and target places in need, as well as to coordinate aid. The Development Commission also works with similar groups in other world bodies, such as the Red Cross and Red Crescent. Information and requests for services can be facilitated through the ILS website (www.ilsf.org) or by contacting the ILS headquarters at Gemeenteplein 26, 3010 Leuven, Belgium.

The goals of the ILS Development Commission are to improve the level of skill, knowledge, and understanding of water-safety practices, resuscitation, and lifesaving. The aims of such programs are:
- To reduce the number of deaths by drowning throughout the world
- To increase the number of sustainable lifesaving organisations and active lifesavers worldwide
- To encourage life saving organisations in developing countries to become members of ILS and thereby to benefit from the expertise, materials and training potential that those world organisations have to offer

Although it can be challenging to organise drowning prevention and lifesaving services in developing nations, a number of areas of the world have benefited from these efforts. For example, public safety workers in Bolivia were recently trained in lifesaving and flood rescue by ILS volunteers. In the Caribbean a regional lifesaving organisation has been formed to meet particular needs of the many islands in that part of the world. Within Europe, a lifesaving school in Sozpol in

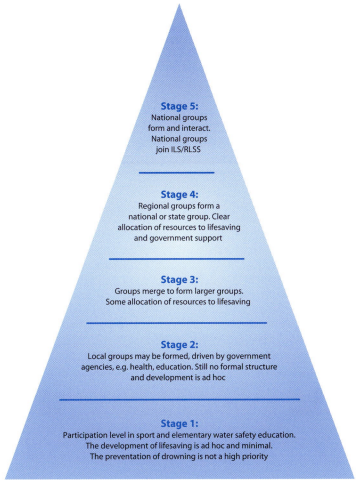

■ **Fig. 4.8.** The stages of development are outlined in the triangle and represent a progressive development

Bulgaria now runs a full range of lifesaving and lifeguarding courses to address the needs of the European nations. In Africa and Asia Pacific similar lifesaving development programs have resulted in national lifesaving organisations being formed in both large and small countries. Through the development of lifesaving organisations, ILS expects to train lifesavers and to educate the general population about drowning prevention measures.

The stages of lifesaving development are outlined in ■ **Fig. 4.8** and represent a progressive development model. Development best evolves from countries with water-safety education on an ad hoc or minimal basis to the final formation of a sustainable national organisation that will be encouraged to join ILS in order to receive ongoing support, advice, and credibility.

Task Force on Rescue – Rescue Techniques

TASK FORCE ON RESCUE
Section editors: CHRIS BREWSTER and ROB BRONS

Task Force Chairs

- Chris Brewster
- Rob Brons

Task Force Members

- Tom Griffiths
- Jim Howe
- Gabriel Kinney
- Andrew Short
- Peter Wernicki
- Klaus Wilkens
- Mike Woodroffe
- Rick Wright

Other Contributors

- Wolfgang Baumeier
- Jenny Blitvich
- Chris Brooks
- Günther Cornelissen
- Peter Dawes
- Michael Ducharme
- Peter Fenner
- Ivar Grøneng
- Ton Haasnoot
- Antony Handley
- Ahamed Idris
- Gabriel Kinney
- Germ Martini
- Ruy Marra
- Jaap Molenaar
- Martin Nemiroff
- Joost van Nueten
- Michael Oostman
- Frank Pia
- Rolf Popp
- Michael Schwindt
- Brian Sims
- Carla St-Germain
- John Stoop
- David Szpilman
- Hans Vandersmissen

- Mike Vlasto
- Sip Wiebenga
- Andrea Zaferes
- Edward Zwitser

5.1
Overview

Chris Brewster and Rob Brons

Rescue is the most glorious method of drowning prevention. It is also the most dangerous. Each year extraordinarily courageous acts of aquatic rescue take place throughout the world. Also each year, would-be rescuers become victims themselves and die or are seriously injured in their efforts to rescue others. Some of these people have no training or experience, others are trained rescuers. In any case, although those involved in drowning prevention include a wide variety of disciplines, from epidemiologists to public educators to aquatic area managers to paramedics to doctors, many of whom invest substantially of their time in the effort, it is the rescuers who are most often called upon to place themselves in peril to assist others. The fact that they know of this peril in advance and that they must often thrust themselves into a threatening, intimidating environment, makes their work all the more impressive.

Aquatic lifesaving has been mechanised to a degree. Boats, motor vehicles, and helicopters, for example, are used to expedite rescue services and protect the rescuers themselves. A variety of tools are also employed, like swim fins, rescue buoys, and wet suits. The very existence of these tools demonstrate an important element of water rescue: It often requires rescuers to enter the water to complete the rescue. In fact, most aquatic rescues performed each year around the world involve an elemental struggle by one human being against the forces of nature to rescue another. It is the ultimate struggle of life attempting to triumph over death.

In addition to prevention, rescuers are also involved in treatment of drowning victims. This is an inevitable responsibility, since it is rare that there is a source of advanced medical care available immediately after a rescue, other than the rescuers themselves. According the International Life Saving Federation (www.ilsf.org), all people who assume a responsibility to protect, rescue, and resuscitate others in an aquatic setting should be taught and maintain proficiency in cardiopulmonary resuscitation (CPR) in a course which is approved in their own country and consistent with the most recent Guidelines for Cardiopulmonary Resuscitation. Additional medical skills are also typically part of the training of aquatic rescuers, so that they may be prepared to handle trauma (particularly including spinal injury), hypothermia, and a variety of other medical problems that can be expected in the aquatic environment. Thus, despite the fact that their primary responsibility may be rescue, most aquatic rescuers are also very involved in both drowning prevention and treatment.

Rescue is the subject of two sections of this handbook. This expanded treatment addresses the many types of circumstances that require rescue, the myriad techniques involved, the wide array of equipment used, and the different organisational approaches. The World Congress on Drowning 2002 brought together experts in water rescue from a very broad number of disciplines. These sections reflect their contributions. Utilising the information in these sections, effective lifesaving organisations can become even better at what they do, and those beginning to provide lifesaving services will have a roadmap at their disposal, drawn by some of the most respected experts in the field of aquatic rescue worldwide. In the prior section, we focused on organisational issues that can help prevent accidents and improve outcomes when accidents occur. In this section, we will focus on specific tools and knowledge disciplines for effective drowning prevention.

Understanding the environment in which rescues are made is critical to the well-prepared lifesaver. Some of the most challenging aquatic environments are produced by the existence of waves and surf. ▶ **Chapter 5.3** provides an overview of types of waves, how they form, and how the rescuer can best be prepared for them.

One of the ways lifesaving organisations can help inform the public about known hazards and help them avoid injury is through the use of signs. A number of different approaches have been taken in different regions of the world, each with inherent similarities, but also local adaptations. ▶ **Chapter 5.4** discusses types of signs, design factors, and efforts to help bring about international standards.

Effective preventive lifesaving necessarily involves effective surveillance of an aquatic area. Only through continual vigilance utilising proper techniques can problems be expeditiously identified and properly addressed. ▶ **Chapter 5.5** offers the reader a history of some leading theories, an overview of the current state of the art, and some thoughts about what the future may hold.

There have been many advancements in open sea search and rescue. ▶ **Chapter 5.6** provides an overview of what is new, what has not changed, and what is needed to further improve upon the readiness of the world to respond to open sea rescue.

How has the design of lifejackets evolved over the years? What are some of the latest features? What types of lifejackets are best for different applications and environments? Answers to these questions and others can be found in ▶ **Chapter 5.7.1**.

Lifejackets are not the only way to maintain safety for those who find themselves in or near the water. Survival suits have long been used as a way to maintain both buoyancy and protection from immersion, particularly in cold water. Design elements have changed, but challenges remain to developing an ideal combination of features like donning properties, ergonomics for on-board tasks, compatibility with evacuation systems, in-water performance, and durability. ▶ **Chapter 5.7.2** discusses these and related issues.

▶ **Chapter 5.8** deals with the issue of self-rescue, and ▶ **Chapter 5.8.1** looks more particularly at the scenario whereby a victim suddenly finds him or herself immersed in cold water, and whether self-rescue would be possible in the absence of others to assist? In addition, ▶ **Chapter 5.8.1** provides vital information on what you can expect to experience and how you might successfully extricate yourself from this peril. What if the water is not necessarily cold? Are there other factors to consider? Yes, according to ▶ **Chapter 5.8.2**. This chapter includes basic information on how to deal with rip currents, tidal currents, waves, and a variety of other circumstances.

In the Netherlands alone, some 30 people die each year when their motor vehicles end up in the water. Indeed, these sorts of accidents occur throughout the world. ▶ **Chapter 5.9** discusses the challenges faced in rescues of people from submerged vehicles and techniques that have proven effective.

When people are rescued from prolonged immersion in cold water, they sometimes suffer cardiac arrest due to the method of extrication employed by rescuers. Physiological factors associated with a vertical rescue can seriously stress the body, leading to this outcome. ▶ **Chapter 5.10** explains this issue and how rescuers can avoid handling victims in a way that threatens their survival.

One of the most dangerous challenges to self-rescue and to rescue efforts by professionals is a fall through the ice. For the victim, getting out is an extreme challenge. Even those who are successful face hypothermia after escape from the water. For rescuers, safely assisting a victim can place those involved in the effort in tremendous danger. ▶ **Chapter 5.11** provides advice both for victims and rescuers to help ensure the best possible outcome.

▶ **Chapter 5.12** looks at rescues under difficult conditions. As long as aircraft fly near or over water, there is a certainty that some will crash in water. ▶ **Chapter 5.12.1** provides an overview of these accidents. ▶ **Chapter 5.12.2** on offshore powerboat rescue addresses an unusual, but challenging form of rescue, including common injuries. Rescue tools and techniques are an integral part of this chapter. According to ▶ **Chapter 5.12.3** on the NASA ocean rescue plan for the Space Shuttle: "After the Space Shuttle Challenger disaster in 1986, NASA developed plans for rescue of astronauts in the event of a catastrophic disaster during launch". Needless to say, one of these plans involves ocean rescue.

Aquatic rescue organisations employ a variety of tools. One of these is rescue boats. Traditionally, these had wooden hulls, but later a variety of other types of hulls were devised, including inflatables. ▶ **Chapter 5.13** discusses a hybrid of rigid hulls and inflatables that has been very effectively used in a variety of challenging environments.

The inflatable rescue boat (IRB), sometimes called the inshore rescue boat, has been successfully employed by lifesavers in the nearshore surf environment for many years, since this use was pioneered in New Zealand and Australia. In ▶ **Chapter 5.14** the author discusses some of the serious injuries that have been associated with these relatively light and highly manoeuvrable craft, suggesting approaches that might reduce the potential for injury.

Personal watercraft (PWCs), such as Jet Skis, were once thought of only as aquatic toys. They have since been adapted by lifesaving organisations throughout the world for rescue. In ▶ **Chapter 5.15** this evolution and some current methods of safely and effectively using PWC for rescue are discussed.

In addition to rigid inflatable boats, IRBs, and PWCs, a variety of alternatives to traditional rescue boats have been developed or adapted; these are discussed in ▶ **Chapter 5.16**. More particularly, ▶ **Chapter 5.16.1** discusses the experience of members of the United Kingdom's Royal National Lifeboat Institution (RNLI) in use of hovercraft, which are now used effectively for certain specialised applications. In Australia, another unusual alternative has been employed. In ▶ **Chapter 5.16.2** the author describes development and deployment of jet boats by Surf Life Saving Queensland. Meanwhile, in Brazil, a unique experiment in aeronautics, the paraglider, is described in ▶ **Chapter 5.16.3**. Interestingly, the author describes use of this craft to patrol aquatic areas and effect rescues as needed.

Spinal injuries (▶ **Chapter 5.17**) are a serious problem in the aquatic environment. ▶ **Chapter 5.17.1** discusses the magnitude of the problem and that the incidence of injury can be reduced through awareness, skills and regulation. Despite best efforts to reduce the incidence of these injuries, they will likely be a problem for many years to come and safely extricating those with spinal injuries from the water will continue to pose a significant challenge. Methods to recognise those who may have a spinal injury and to rescue them in the safest possible manner are described in ▶ **Chapter 5.17.2**.

According to ▶ **Chapter 5.18** "Lifesaving requires a unique combination of physical and mental skills with an ultimate goal of saving lives. There is no other occupation incorporating such a mélange of physical challenges and fitness requirements. These same challenges and requirements create an increased risk of injury, illness, or worse". The authors describe risk factors particular to lifesaving, common and uncommon injuries, and techniques for injury prevention.

The author of ▶ **Chapter 5.19** points out that "… responding to a cardiac arrest is a highly stressful … event". He suggests that CPR training should include information to prepare rescuers for the stress that will inevitably occur so that they can better prepare themselves to deliver effective CPR.

Like any emergency care providers, lifesavers are vulnerable to adverse psychological effects after providing care to seriously injured people, particularly in cases of death. ▶ **Chapter 5.20** discusses the importance of caring for rescuers before, during, and after a stressful incident to help them cope with sometimes serious outcomes.

In summary, this section of the handbook provides a wealth of information on rescue from a wide variety of disciplines. The careful reader will gain tremendous insight into ways to develop and improve aquatic rescue services. The opportunity is yours.

5.2
Recommendations

CHRIS BREWSTER and ROB BRONS

Prior to the World Congress on Drowning, the Rescue Task Force was assembled. This group of experts was asked to focus attention on eight rescue-related topics and to make specific recommendations. These were reviewed and accepted by the Rescue Task Force and the Steering Group of the World Congress on Drowning. During the Congress, these topics were discussed in further detail and the recommendations were published, in abbreviated form, in the appendices of the

Final Recommendations of the World Congress on Drowning. In this chapter, you will find brief synopses, compiled by the Rescue Task Force leader, of each of the topics addressed by the Rescue Task Force involving prevention and rescue techniques. Specific recommendations are also included. For a more thorough explanation of each topic, please see the chapters in this section authored by the named experts. During the World Congress on Drowning, additional topics with regard to swimming training and scientific investigation of rescue techniques resulted in further recommendations as a product of discussion among the experts in attendance. Four of the topics covered by the Rescue Task Force and these two additional topics can be found in ▶ **Chapter 4.2**. Here you will find the remaining topics (7–10) and recommendations.

5.2.1
Recommendation 7 –
Surveillance Techniques for Drowning Prevention

TASK FORCE EXPERT: TOM GRIFFITHS

One of the most critical functions of a lifeguard is water observation to detect victims in distress. It has been shown by Frank Pia that victims rarely call for help, thus the importance of surveillance to detect distress is paramount to preventing drowning. Unfortunately, this is one of the least studied areas of lifeguard performance. Most training appears to be based on anecdotal information, passed on over the years within lifesaving organisations, and little research in this area is available to guide the training of lifeguards to minimise boredom and increase vigilance. As Rescue Task Force member Tom Griffiths points out, a need for quality research in this area clearly exists, because if better preventive actions could be identified and utilised by lifeguards on duty, accident prevention could be enhanced and ultimately many lives saved. In addition, lifeguard retention may be improved by identifying methods to reduce boredom and lessen the stress of missing a rescue (see ▶ **Chapter 5.5**).

Rescue Recommendation 7:

Further research is needed in the area of surveillance, scanning and vigilance by lifeguards from a physiological and psychological perspective to determine the best methods of instruction and practice. This body of knowledge is desperately needed in order to save lives. Whatever methodology used, scanning systems and strategies should be studied objectively by working lifeguards on duty.

5.2.2
Recommendation 8 –
Advantages and Limitations of Personal Watercraft in Aquatic Rescue

TASK FORCE EXPERT: JIM HOWE

Personal watercraft, also known by the trade name Jet Ski, have been successfully utilised in aquatic rescue in a variety of environments. These include surf, off-shore, flood rescue, inland waterways, and other areas. Despite initial resistance by some aquatic rescue agencies, personal watercraft have proven themselves to be effective rescue tools in a wide variety of environments. In coming years, personal watercraft can be expected to be an increasingly common tool for aquatic rescue. Unfortunately, there are no consistent standards for the training of aquatic rescuers in use of personal watercraft as a rescue tool (see ▶ **Chapter 5.15**).

Rescue Recommendation 8A:

All aquatic rescue agencies should consider personal watercraft for rescue work, but further research should be undertaken to identify appropriate uses of the PWC in aquatic rescue.

Rescue Recommendation 8B:

The International Life Saving Federation should develop minimum training and certification standards for aquatic rescuers who will be tasked in the use of personal watercraft for rescue.

5.2.3
Recommendation 9 –
Current Trends in Sea Rescue and Open Water Search Techniques

TASK FORCE EXPERTS: MICHAEL WOODROFFE and GABE KINNEY

The number of persons involved in activities that could place them at risk in the aquatic environment is steadily increasing. With that increase comes a concurrently expanding need for preparedness to respond to aquatic emergencies.

It is widely accepted that vessels and aircraft have a duty to provide assistance to other vessels, aircraft or persons in distress, without regard to location, nationality or circumstances. To coordinate search and rescue, the, *International Aeronautical and Maritime Search and Rescue Manual* (IAMSAR) has been developed. It has been accepted as the National Search and Rescue (SAR) Manual of the several countries.

Meanwhile, a wide variety of advances in open water search techniques based on new technologies and equipment have been developed, such as computer search applications, night vision equipment and VHF direction finding (VHF/

DF) systems. The internationally accepted Global Maritime Distress and Safety System (GMDSS) facilitates communications practices for search and rescue. In future, distress communications will migrate towards satellite systems and cellular technology, and solutions must be found to meet the challenges they present. Also, new technologies are emerging in rescue craft, such as use of personal watercraft (Jet Skis) for inshore cases, jet propulsion systems, improved navigation methods, and better hull and lifesaving appliance design. In addition, more advanced rescue aircraft use state-of-the-market systems in airframe and avionics design, distress location and recovery technology.

The International Maritime Organisation's crusade to establish worldwide Maritime Search and Rescue Regions for the world's oceans was a significant achievement, but there must be full implementation. The challenge now is to put in place communications and SAR assets wherever they are needed throughout the world (see ▶ **Chapter 5.6**).

Rescue Recommendation 9A:

The International Aeronautical and Maritime Search and Rescue Manual should be reviewed and incorporated by the sea rescue organisations of all of the nations of the world to ensure a coordinated and effective approach to maritime emergencies.

Rescue Recommendation 9B:

Rescue communications must provide dependable, robust, integrated, and effective command and control for all involved segments of the response system, not simply point to point communications.

Rescue Recommendation 9C:

Sea rescue providers should ensure that their rescue craft keep pace with available technology, evaluating and embracing effective new types of surface rescue craft and air rescue craft.

Rescue Recommendation 9D:

The Incident Command System, which has been developed to allow for effective oversight and organisation of emergency responses, should be adopted by all aquatic rescue organisations worldwide.

Rescue Recommendation 9E:

The priority now must be to ensure there is a search and rescue response in areas around the world where there is significant maritime traffic, whether it be cruise liners, cargo ships, fishing boats or leisure craft. Those nations with well-established SAR organisations must help those just embarking on providing such facilities to cover their sea area of responsibility. Those with many years expertise in SAR will need to train and counsel those just starting out to fulfil the SAR requirements now demanded by all countries that are signatory to the Safety of Life at Sea (SOLAS) and Search and Rescue (SAR) conventions.

5.2.4
Recommendation 10 –
Spinal Injury Extrication from the Aquatic Environment

TASK FORCE EXPERT: PETER WERNICKI

One of the most challenging circumstances an aquatic rescuer faces is a victim in the water with an apparent or suspected spinal injury. In the view of Peter Wernicki, the rescue is the first and possibly the most important link in the chain of care of spinal injuries. The primary goal is to remove the person from the aquatic environment for further treatment in a manner that does no further harm than the initial injury. This challenge can be compounded by conditions such as currents and wave action. Several different approaches to spinal injury extrication from the aquatic environment have been developed, but none have been scientifically tested to demonstrate their effectiveness.

Some aquatic related spinal injuries are not immediately debilitating and the patient is able to walk up to the lifesaver, complaining of spinal pain, with a history of a mechanism of injury that could produce spinal injury. In these cases, spinal immobilisation is also needed (see ▶ **Chapter 5.17.2**).

Rescue Recommendation 10A:

Considering the devastating consequences of spinal injuries and the tremendous challenge of effective extrication of persons with suspected spinal injuries from the aquatic environment, it is recommended that scientific research be conducted on each of the existing methods recommended by the various lifesaving organisations of the world to firmly establish the best possible methods of extrication.

Rescue Recommendation 10B:

Research by Peter Wernicki has identified three spinal immobilisation techniques which appear to be effective. While different terms may be used for these techniques, they include the vice grip, body hug, and the extended arm grip. It is recommended that until scientific testing can be conducted on these and any other methods in existence, lifesavers be taught at least two of these three methods, as each has advantages and disadvantages in various situations. The vice grip and the extended arm grip appear to be the best two of the three.

Rescue Recommendation 10C:

Differing terms for spinal injury immobilisation techniques creates potential confusion in rescue. It is recommended that common terms for these techniques be adopted by all lifesaving organisations and that the terms should be vice grip, body hug, and the extended arm grip.

Rescue Recommendation 10D:

All lifesavers should be taught the standing backboard technique, to allow for immediate stabilisation of the spine of a person who walks up to the lifeguard complaining of spinal pain post trauma.

5.3
Patterns of Wave and Surf

EDWARD ZWITSER

Everyone has heard of them, almost everyone has seen them and many have actually felt them: waves! They are such a self-evident part of the sea that the theories regarding their origins and effects are seldom thought of or discussed. These theories are discussed below.

5.3.1
Five Different Types of Waves

The waves drawn by children do not actually exist. Perfectly rounded waves, standing still in time, with ships at their peaks, like those one sees in cartoons and the drawings of children, are little more than a product of an active imagination. In reality, waves are in a state of constant movement. In fact, waves actually originate in movement. Based on their origins, five different types of waves can be distinguished.
- Ripple Waves
  Ripple waves are so small that most people do not even consider them waves. Ripple waves are the visible sign of an extremely weak wind along an almost smooth water surface. The air flows along the surface of the water, moving extremely small amounts of the water in its path. The surface begins to ripple, signalling the start of movement in the sea. As the wind increases, real waves develop.
- Wind Waves
  As the wind increases in strength, ripple waves turn into wind waves. The ripples increase in size as the wind increases in strength, which in turn gives the wind a larger surface to grip. As the surface gripped by the wind increases, the height of the waves increases. The height of the waves is determined by a combination of wind speed, the length of the period in which the wind

endures and the fetch, which is the length of the water surface over which the wind exerts an influence. In other words, the free distance in the open sea, from the windward or luff side, over which the wind blows.

- Pressure Waves
  In most cases, pressure waves are caused by seismic activity, underwater volcanic eruptions, or by large pieces of land falling into the sea. Although these waves start out small, they can reach gigantic heights.

- Bottom Waves
  Bottom waves are waves that change in terms of profile in response to changes in the bottom of the sea. As the waves reach an area with a water depth less than half of the length of the waves (the wave length is the distance between the deepest points of two waves), the waves start to 'feel' the bottom of the sea and change in response to what they feel. As the water depth decreases, the length of the wave also decreases. Because the water mass remains the same, the wave height increases, as does the steepness of the waves. If the speed of the wave crest also increases by more than the propagation speed of the wave, the crests break.

In shallow water, the waves break far more quickly and harshly than they do in open sea. At sea, the water from the breaking crests runs back down along the wave in a relatively smooth movement. In shallower water, however, the waves virtually trip over themselves. Sailing in such weather conditions is extremely dangerous.

- Cross Waves
  As two rows of waves run in different directions, they cross paths at a certain point, resulting in wave heights that exceed the average height of the original waves. These waves, which form very quickly and unexpectedly, have the shape of a pyramid. Although these waves look extremely dangerous, they disappear almost as quickly as they appear.
  Waves do not necessarily have to be cross waves to reach above-average heights, however. According to statistical measurements, one in 23 waves reaches twice average height, one in 1175 waves reaches three times average height and one in 300,000 waves reaches four times average height. In stormy weather, keeping a good lookout for these 'green waves' is advisable.
  Most waves are caused by wind, although other factors, such as the ebb and flow of the tide, can also play an important role. If the tide runs in the same direction as the wind, the sea remains relatively calm, but if the tide runs against the wind, waves develop. These waves are short and steep.

5.3.2
Energy

To the naked eye, the water in a wave appears to run in tune with the propagation movement of the wave, but this is not really the case. In fact, the water itself stands still, while the wave moves. What that means is that waves are not actually a movement of water, but a movement of energy, caused by the external factors mentioned above. The energy moves vertically, beneath the water. This concept can be illustrated using a float. Waves do not take floats with them in the direction that they propagate. Instead, the float moves up and down, but remains in its original position.

Even after the wind dies down, the effect of the energy that it generates continues for long periods. The wave movements originally started by the wind continue even after the wind has died. This movement is called heaving. Even in wind-still weather, ships in the open sea can be confronted with heaving waves. These waves are caused in the same way as other types of waves, by wind and other external factors, but they are kept alive by energy once the wind and other external factors disappear. The deeper the water, the greater the impact of the vertical energy movement on the surface of the water and, hence, the higher the heaving wave.

There are various types of waves and no one wave is exactly the same as another, which means that skippers must always be ready for unexpected water movements, particularly in stormy weather. The movement can be an extremely high wave, a breaking wave, a pyramid-shaped wave or other type of movement. Unexpected water movements are an integral part of the undying mystery of the sea. They cannot be prevented and they demand a quick, professional reaction on the part of the skipper. To react appropriately, each skipper must have the necessary knowledge, the right equipment and, particularly important, good old-fashioned common sense. Safety at sea starts with respect for the sea.

5.4
Water Safety Signs and Beach Safety Flags

Brian Sims

Public information symbols and safety signs in the field of water safety, and beach safety flags have a primary and important role in preserving human life. In many cases where accidents have occurred one of the first questions usually asked is "What safety information was provided to prevent such an accident?" It is important therefore to establish the basis for the provision of water safety signs and beach safety flags, and to ensure an adequate educational program for users of water-based activities and those who may come into contact with an aquatic environment.

In recent years there has been a growing trend to supplement, and in some cases replace signs which use text alone, with a range of different graphical symbol designs. Also a wide selection of coloured flags has been used to give the public an indication of beach safety factors. This has been driven by an increasing awareness of the need to inform a widening group of users, who may not understand the language of the host country. The recognition of the benefits from easily read and understood graphical symbols and coloured flags are strong, particularly within sport, leisure, and the tourism industries, where a properly designed sign and/or flag can replace a potentially complicated written sign.

Widening use of graphical symbols for preventing accidents has also led to an increasing awareness of the need to make signs and flags compatible with the environment. Graphical symbols are frequently used to quickly convey a message in publications, authoritative documentation, and information leaflets.

The current range of signs and flags in use in some locations, and used to convey certain safety messages may be in need of replacement with clear graphical symbol signs and/or appropriate flag colours.

5.4.1
Water Safety Signs and Graphical Symbols – Design Factors

One of the key factors in the presentation of a water safety sign is the need to place an easily recognisable graphical symbol within a standardised geometric shape with safety colours and contrast colours appropriate to the type of safety sign. This poses an issue within the international standard community as the International Standardisation Organisation (ISO) in ISO 3864 contains a number of National Standards within specific Regulations and the geometric shape of particular types of safety sign differ from that specified since 1984.

As an example, within the European Union a number of Directives are found. One of these is concerned with the geometric shape, colour and design of safety signs and is referenced under Council Directive 92/58/EEC. The specified geometric shapes and colours of safety signs for use in the workplace are the same as those given in ISO 3864: 1984 and ISO 3864-1: 2002. There are five types of safety sign:

- Prohibition signs: The geometric shape is a circular band with a diagonal bar at 45° to the horizontal, top left to bottom right. The circular band and bar are in red. The contrasting colour is a white background. The graphical symbol is black. These signs indicate that a specific behaviour is forbidden.
- Warning signs: The geometric shape is a triangle and the safety colour a yellow background. The contrasting colour of the triangular band is black. The graphical symbol is black. These signs indicate a specific source of potential harm.
- Mandatory signs: The geometric shape is a circle and the safety colour is blue. The contrasting colour is white. The graphical symbol is in white. These signs indicate that a specific course of action is to be taken.
- Safe condition signs: The geometric shape is a square and the safety colour is green. The graphical symbol is in white. These signs indicate a safety action, the location of safety equipment or a safety facility or an escape route.
- Fire safety signs: The geometric shape is a square and the safety colour is red. The graphical symbol is in white. Fire safety signs in ISO 7010 also incorporate a flame determinant. These signs indicate the location or identification of fire equipment or how it should be used.

Examples of safety signs with specific water safety meanings are:
- Prohibition signs: No swimming, No diving, No personal watercraft
- Warning signs: Strong currents, Thin ice, Deep water
- Mandatory signs: Wear a lifejacket

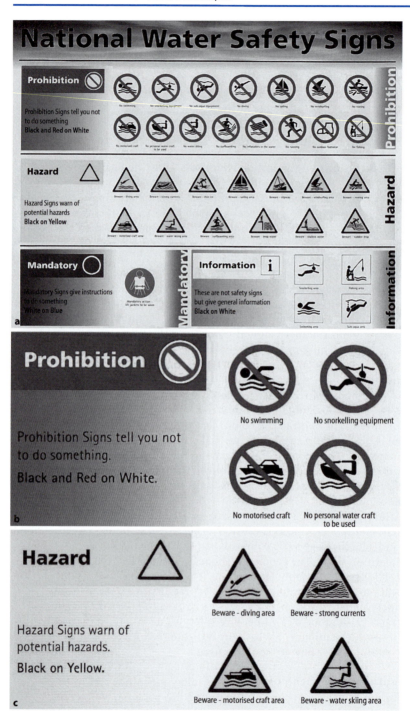

Safe condition signs and fire safety signs may be present in a water activity facility and covered in a general safety standards or regulations. Examples are:
- Safe condition signs: Emergency exit, First aid, Emergency telephone
- Fire safety signs: Fire extinguisher, Fire hose reel, Fire alarm call point

In some countries the geometric shape and colour of particular types of safety sign differ from those described above. Examples of this occur in Australia (AS 2899-2: 1986), also Surf Life Saving Association – State of Victoria (Aquatic signage manual – 2002); Canada – the Lifesaving Society (Safety and warning signs – 1999) (☐ Fig. 5.1); New Zealand – Water safety signage (Draft DZ 8690); and for USA – the United States Lifesaving Association (Standardized Water safety symbols – 1986). It is therefore essential to recognise the current status and regulations that may apply in individual countries and the difficulties that may need to be addressed to achieve an international standards for water safety signs.

Another key factor in the presentation of a water safety sign is to design a graphical symbol, which is easily recognised and understood within an aquatic activity or environment. As an example, the creation of the first British standard for water safety signs (BS 5499-11: 2002) took best practice into account and published references from sources around the world and in particular the extensive amount of work carried out in Australia and New Zealand. The water safety symbols were therefore designed within a consistent style, and in relation to such factors as the size and flow of water, and the balance of the human figure with or without the use of recreational equipment. The water safety signs used the geometric shapes and colours for the particular type of sign specified in ISO 3864-1. Some graphical symbols were used in more than one type of safety sign (for example No diving and Beware-diving area, No sailing and Beware-sailing area). Because the shape and size of the area available for the graphical symbol differed for the different types of safety sign (for example, triangular area compared to a circular area) the final design of the graphical symbol was adjusted so that it was suitable for inclusion in a prohibition or warning sign.

The design of the graphical symbols in particular also needs to take into account the design requirements for small-scale reproduction as used in publications and on safety information leaflets. The use of a short supplementary text may also be needed to give and enhance a positive safety message.

The following subjects and activities have been found to form the majority of graphical symbol needs around the world, and are found within a range of types of safety sign indicating prohibition, warning, and mandatory actions including: swimming; snorkelling; scuba; diving; surfboarding; windsurfing; sailing; water-skiing; rowing; inflatable; fishing; motorised craft; personal water craft; lifejackets; and environmental consideration for deep water; shallow water; sudden drop; strong currents; slipways; thin ice.

The likely locations for erecting water safety signs include swimming pools, beaches, inland open waters, cliff walks, harbours, parks and open spaces.

The problem is one of application for the public and the respective parties concerned to understand, acknowledge, and accept the safety message. The issue of education will therefore play a crucial role in the development of a water safety strategy. This will also be a major factor when a risk assessment is undertaken for a particular aquatic based location.

It has been pointed out above that design differences for water safety signs occur among countries, for example European countries compared to Australia, New Zealand, Canada and the USA, and therefore any attempt to promote a firm international proposal from the meetings held at the World Congress on Drowning were limited to a few generic or specific areas.

As a point of information the UK currently holds the secretariat of the Technical (TC145) at the International Organisation for Standardisation (ISO) for Graphical Symbols.

The route for International Standardisation is more likely to be achieved through ISO, although the advanced work carried out by the International Lifesaving Federation (ILS) is supportive of this process. It had been suggested that it might be useful to expedite this important area of water safety by the provision of an ILS 'best practice standard'. This could be a counterproductive issue and had been heavily debated at the Congress. The outcome was seen as a need to liaise and advances a joint approach as quickly as possible. This is more likely to be achieved within the scope of the graphical symbols. The geometric shape and colour of particular types of safety sign is more likely to be regulated in some countries.

5.4.2
Public Information Symbols – Design Factors

Public information symbols can relate to specific water related activities as well as to general signing of access and other facilities. In the UK, the new British Standard on Water safety signs (BS 5499-11) was developed at the same time as the new British Standard on Public Information symbols (BS 8501).

Those graphical symbols for water related activities were designed to be easily recognised and understood within an aquatic activity or environment. Where a graphical symbol was intended to be used in a public information symbol or a water safety sign, the final design of the graphical symbol was adjusted so that it could be used in different types of safety sign without alteration.

Examples of relevant public information symbols include: showers, boat hire, boat trips, wetlands nature reserve, canoeing, diving, fishing, jet skiing, rowing, sailing, sand yachting, snorkelling, scuba, surfing, swimming, water polo, water skiing, windsurfing, marina, pier-mooring, slipway.

Standardised public information symbols comprise black graphical symbols on a white square background.

Internationally, ISO 7001 covers public information symbols. Currently this standard is being revised by ISO through TC 145.

The inclusion of public information symbols, including those for water safety, will be required for a range of related documents and publications. These are likely to be found in tourist and information centres close to an aquatic centre. Information about relevant public information symbols should also be considered for display at the points of entry to beaches, open water areas and swimming pools.

5.4.3
Beach Safety Flags – Design Factors

A preliminary research project by the ILS sought to identify specifically the range of beach safety flags in use across the world. This identified some variation among a relatively small number, less than fifteen in total, of flags.

At recent meetings of ILS and at the World Congress on Drowning, the issue of a suitable and well-understood flag system was considered. It was concluded that a limited number of flags to identify safety factors, including water and weather conditions, should be promoted.

The flags should be identified under two main groups:

Firstly flags giving an indication of the wind, weather, and water conditions, and include

— Red flag: Danger
   Rough water; powerful dumping waves; surge waves; heavy surf with rip currents; unstable sea-bed; sudden changes in depth near to shore, or unexpected holes and rocks; abnormal weather which temporarily changes placid conditions to those which are life-threatening. The hoist of the red flag indicates all water users should leave the water.

— Yellow flag: Caution
   The water may not be calm; it may vary from heavy swell to breaking surf thus producing varying water depths. Young, the elderly or weak swimmers may not cope and should be discouraged from entering the water.

— Green flag: Calm
   Not necessarily safe conditions and caution should still be exercised especially the young, the elderly, or weak swimmers.

The second group of flags give an indication of aquatic activity control and zoning with criteria to include:

— Red-Yellow (halved) flag: Lifeguarded area
   To indicate that an area usually between two flags is patrolled or observed by lifeguards/s and is likely to be a relatively safe area for swimming only. It is recommended that all swimmers use these designated areas but are still advised to exercise caution.

— Black-white (quartered) flag: Surfing area
   To indicate a zoned area between two flags designated for surfing with boards and other related equipment. Swimmers are advised not to enter these zones.

At this time these flags are seen as best practice and are likely to be taken forward for consideration as an international standard. For this to be effective it will be essential for the beach safety flags to be incorporated within the scope of the water safety signs system, and for further research to be conducted.

It is known that some work has been undertaken to include graphical symbols on coloured flags to emphasise a particular safety message. This system has only recently been promoted and has yet to be taken forward for further research and possible development. Consideration will be give to this concept by ILS.

This initial list of flags is noted only as a guide to those countries who may wish to promote the use of beach safety flags. The designs should be considered as best practice at this time, as further research and development is being carried out particularly in Australia, New Zealand, UK and USA and changes are to be expected in the future. The ILS has now a proposed list of standardised flags under review.

This current system, based on best practice, recognises the definitions used in a number of national publications and standards on water safety issues. Other flags may also be used in addition to identify specific local environmental or marine animal concerns. Also further flags may be recognised for specific needs in some countries.

As noted above for water safety signs, the inclusion of beach safety flags will be required for a range of related documents and publications, and as mentioned these are likely to be found in tourist and information centres close to an aquatic centre. Information about flags should also be considered for display at the points of entry to beaches and open water areas.

It is considered important to have an international standard for beach safety flags. Currently beach safety flags have not been included in international standards, such as ISO standards. This issue will be raised later in this paper.

5.4.4
Role of the International Lifesaving Federation

The ILS seeks to play a leadership role in the development of international standards for water safety signs and beach safety flags through its member federations, which are the national aquatic lifesaving organisations of the world. The infrastructure of the ILS Rescue/Education Commission allows for liaison with ILS Federations and this may offer suggestions for further contact by member Federations to their National Standards Organisations. Some ILS Federation members have already commenced this dialogue and it is known that a number of standards or best practice currently exist, particularly from Australia, New Zealand, the USA and the UK. ILS will continue to play a part in research and development and particularly toward the essential requirement for any testing of signs and flags that may be required across all cultures and nationalities.

Some useful discussions were held on the development of beach safety flags at the World Congress on Drowning with the prime conclusion that an international standard would be ideal. An interesting design factor that emerged during one workshop session was the introduction of a symbolic number added to each coloured flag.

It was considered that this might provide the beach user a greater understanding of a coded system and would particularly benefit those persons who may be colour-blind. A problem with this system is the potential misunderstanding of what the numbers mean (for example the number of the lifesaving stand or the degree of hazard). Another design feature discussed was the inclusion of a graphical symbol on the flag (such as a swimmer in the water, to identify the specific message of the flag signal).

5.4.5
International Standardisation Organisation

As previously mentioned the ISO committee TC 145 is concerned with graphical symbols. It is also concerned with the design principles for safety signs (ISO 3864-1) and with the standardisation of safety signs (ISO 7010) and public information symbols (ISO 7001). The subcommittee SC 1 is responsible for public information symbols and subcommittee SC 2 for safety signs. The committees have formal procedures for the approval of new proposals for public information symbols for standardisation in ISO 7001 and for approval of new proposals for safety signs for standardisation in ISO 7010. Proposals are also submitted by other ISO technical committees or by member National Standards Organisations. In both procedures it is expected that the public information symbol or the safety sign is tested for the degree of understanding by the relevant target audience by testing according to ISO 9186: 2001.

At this time the relevant ISO TC 145 committees have not considered the issue of beach safety flags being within the scope of ISO TC 145. There are formal procedures for consideration and approval of any new work item, as this would also be required for beach safety flags.

5.4.6
Future Developments

During the World Congress on Drowning the opportunity was afforded to any country that wished to display their national standards for water safety signs and/or beach safety flags. A number of countries took up this option and following their presentation some useful dialogue was recorded and placed as a specific recommendation for consideration by organisations such as ISO and ILS.

Formal presentations were then received from the USA for the States of Hawaii and from Florida, and from the UK. A paper from Surf Lifesaving in Australia was also available together with support material from Italy. The research material collated by ILS for water safety signs and beach safety flags was also available for perusal.

As a result of the presentation and the availability of a wide range of support material it was possible to hold a fruitful discussion among the seventeen different nations taking part. This included representatives from governments, lifesaving organisations and consumer groups. In particular, the issue of variations on water safety signs was discussed and this looked at the two aspects of a safety sign, the geometric shape of different types of safety sign and the graphical symbol.

In the first aspect there seemed to be a fairly broad acceptance of the design principles for the prohibition sign, namely red circular band and diagonal negation bar on a white circular background. One exception being the use of an octagonal band with a diagonal negation bar in Canada. The issue of the warning signs is more of a problem. There is a common ground for the safety colour of yellow with a black edge, but the geometric shape is in some countries a triangle (as specified in ISO 3864-1:2002) and in others a diamond.

This is clearly a case where the ISO standard for testing safety signs could be applied. The mandatory sign also had a few minor deviations. However there seemed to be a fairly common approach to the design of most of the graphical symbols for aquatic activities and environments. Even so, some further discussion would be required and once again this could be established through the ISO system.

The beach safety flags also proved to be an interesting subject for discussion with the main aspects being those of a common understanding. In this regard some useful comments were received, particularly from the USA. Suggestions included:

- A plain colour coded system without the visual aid of graphical symbols on the flag depended on an information board with supplementary text to explain the meaning of the warning message
- Beach users in particular expect to be able to see a flag from far away and to understand the message they are deemed to convey without the need to move toward the immediate proximity of the flag. Therefore a symbolic inclusion onto a coloured flag may be a practical solution, although the strength of the wind and its direction may sometimes cause interpretation problems for users of the beach

Therefore some action points or recommendations from the Congress would be taken forward to the ILS in the first instance. This was also to coincide with proposed liaison with the ISO.

It was also recognised that the Congress gave the first opportunity for wide ranging discussion from a broad representation of nations and led to the formations of a number of action points to be taken forward to national organisations and related international bodies. The action points can be summarised as follows:

- That a committee be established, most likely within the ILS Rescue and Education Commissions to examine a common, acceptable and responsive framework to the issue of water safety signs with graphical symbols, public information symbols, and beach safety flags
- That ILS continue their work in this field to advise and implement best practice globally with regard to water safety signs, graphical symbols and flags, and to ensure their member federations are kept informed
- That a core group of graphical symbols be identified for use as water safety symbols by ILS

- That a small group of beach safety flags with a clearly defined safety message be chosen which may be suggested for use by ILS member federations. The possibility of also using a graphical symbol as a component of the flag should also be researched
- That the problem of colour blindness and the challenges posed by a user groups not wearing their glasses or contact lenses be addressed as part of any research process
- That supplementary text is identified as a reinforcement mechanism to water safety signs, graphical symbols and flags
- And finally that ILS liaises with ISO on these matters

It is vital that Congress delegates who wish to participate in this work contact their own Standards organisation and/or their ILS member federation expressing their wish to do so and their support for the work items noted above. If at some time ISO decide there shall be a separate working group for water safety signs, it will require five positive votes from member countries of ISO 145 for this work to proceed and this will require formal ratification at meetings of this committee. The ILS Rescue/Education Commission is currently working toward support for a standard for water safety signs and also beach safety flags.

National Lifesaving and also Standards organisations were invited to support the work undertaken in this Congress and to give all reasonable assistance to those involved in the preventative measures to alleviate the condition of drowning.

Further Reading

International

1. ISO 3864 (1984) Safety colours and safety signs
2. ISO 3864-1 (2002) Graphical symbols – safety colours and safety signs – Part 1: design principles for safety signs in workplaces and public areas
3. ISO 7010 – Graphical symbols – safety signs in workplaces and public areas
4. ISO 7001 – Public information symbols
5. ISO 9186 (2001) Graphical symbols – test methods for judgement of comprehensibility and for comprehension
6. World Tourism Organisation (2001) Tourism signs and symbols. ISBN-92.844.0378.2

European

7. European Council Directive 92/58/EEC on the minimum requirements for the provision of safety and/or health signs at work
8. ILS website www.ilsf.org

United Kingdom

9. BS 5499 – 11 (2002) Graphical symbols and signs. Safety signs including fire safety signs, Part 11: Water safety signs

10. BS 8501 Graphical symbols and signs – Public information symbols
11. Safety on Beaches – Royal Life Saving Society UK

United States of America

12. ANSI Z535 (1998) Safety signs and colour standards
13. USLA (1986) Standardized water safety symbols (Hawaii Region)

Australia

14. AS 2899–2 (1986) Public Information symbol signs. Water safety signs
15. Surf Lifesaving Victoria Inc (Australia) (2002) Aquatic and Recreational Signage Manual

New Zealand

16. Draft DZ 8690 – Water Safety Signage

Canada

17. The Lifesaving Society (1999) Safety and warning signs

5.5
Lifesaver Surveillance and Scanning: Past, Present, Future

PETER FENNER, TOM GRIFFITHS, MICHAEL OOSTMAN and FRANK PIA

5.5.1
The Past (Early 1900s–Mid 1990s)

The recommendations of the World Congress on Drowning in Amsterdam in 2002 include a strong emphasis on prevention: "The vast majority of drownings can be prevented and prevention (rather than rescue or resuscitation) is the most important method by which to reduce the number of drownings" [1]. Today, most water safety experts agree that continuous and effective surveillance and scanning techniques are of paramount importance. But prior to the early 1980s, lifesaving training courses emphasised reactive responses to aquatic emergencies rather than proactive prevention; swimming and rescue skills were stressed more than prevention strategies.

During the late 1960s, based on his filmed observations of actual drowning victims off a flat-water beach in New York, Frank Pia demonstrated that the drowning process can be quick, subtle and silent [2]. Pia contended, that when drowning, non-swimmers will experience an instinctive drowning response. Recognising the objective signs of this instinctive response would help lifesavers effect more timely rescues. This information combined with distinctions between distressed swimmers and drowning victims as well as differences between active and passive drowning, became a helpful component of victim recognition and assessment, particularly for non-swimmers in flat-water environments.

Thereafter, a major thrust toward prevention in lifesaver training began. Rather than waiting for cries for help, lifesavers were now trained to identify active drowning victims by looking for people who were low in the water with the head back and the body vertical, with little or no kick and without forward progress. In addition to their posture and lack of locomotion, the arms remained at or below the surface of the water (low stroke) and the victims could not cry out for help. With the observations by Pia, the grave misconception that drowning victims would create an obvious and noticeable commotion in the water was replaced with the reality that they spend a very brief time on the surface (20–60 seconds) [3]. The American Red Cross incorporated Pia's work into their lifesaving manuals and training programs during the 1980s and 1990s.

During this period, standard-setting organisations for lifeguard training such as the United States Lifesaving Association began to emphasise prevention through the art of victim recognition and assessment [4]. Lifesavers were taught to observe predictive clues both on dry land prior to entry and again after people entered the water. Some of the tell-tale signs of trouble on land were identified as age, body weight, alcohol intoxication, use of floatation devices, improper equipment and attire, and physical disability. Once in the water, signs of trouble included a swimmer facing shore, low head, low stroke, ineffective kick, waves breaking overhead, hair in the face, hand waving, erratic activity, being swept away by a current, along with many others.

Upon realisation of how quickly and quietly the drowning process progressed, lifesaver training agencies became more aware of the importance of faster intervention and protecting the surveillance system from intrusion and distraction [5]. Some organisations attempted to increase lifeguard vigilance by establishing timeframes for scanning. For instance, Ellis and Associates, a US based company, believed that to adequately protect guests at their contracted swimming facilities (mostly waterparks), lifeguards should be expected to scan their zones of coverage in 10 seconds and respond to an emergency, should one arise, within an additional 20 seconds. The rationale for this time requirement is twofold. First, it holds that drowning victims could disappear from the surface in as little as 30 seconds; and second, it provided waterpark lifeguards, for the first time, with an objective scanning parameter. While the 10/20 patron protection rule was adopted as a requirement for Ellis and Associates lifeguards in 1985, others believed that the 10/20 rule was unrealistic for many lifesavers and almost impossible to achieve in heavy surf. Despite differences in scanning recommendations among the lifesaver training agencies during this era, some generally accepted suggestions included:

- Scanning must be continuous
- The head and eyes of the lifesaver must move while scanning
- Rest from surveillance should take place at least hourly
- Scanning high risk patrons, activities and environments could be helpful in predicting problems
- Avoidance of glare and other distractions is important
- Scanning the bottom of the pool should not be overlooked

- Elevated scanning stations were strongly encouraged
- Talking or movement by lifesavers was often discouraged
- Boredom and attention was largely unaddressed

5.5.2
Present (Late 1990s–2003)

After an extensive review of the available literature on visual scanning and attention spans, Peter Fenner wrote about lifesaver surveillance from an Australian Surf Lifesaving perspective. Fenner strongly emphasised that while most lifesaving agencies have their own methods of teaching and conducting visual scanning, few of these have had any scientific basis. Likewise, Fenner urged a more scientific approach to the prevention of boredom, mental lapses, and distractions. Considering the wave action and rip currents experienced in Australia, he also expressed the belief that a 10/20 patron protection rule for pools should be expanded to a more realistic 30/120 goal for surf lifesavers [6].

While the detection and response timeframes proposed in the past were helpful in attempting to keep lifesavers on target, these timeframes were largely untested until recently. To illustrate this point, Ellis and Associates reported having conducted hundreds of trials to determine how long it would take their lifesavers, who were required to meet the 10/20 patron protection rule, to recognise a lifelike manikin on the bottom of the pool. During their time-trials they reportedly concentrated solely on the 10-second detection requirement. This study has not been published in detail or independently reviewed, but according to Ellis and Associates reports, while the lifeguards appeared to be scanning effectively, it took more than 500 lifeguards an average of 1 min and 14 seconds to detect the submerged manikin during the summer of 2001. The following summer (2002) Ellis reported that the study was repeated and the results were only slightly better with the 10-second detection requirement taking an average of 54 seconds [7].

Ellis and Associates concluded that while the lifeguards in this study appeared to be scanning effectively, they were not observing correctly and certainly were not regularly scanning the bottom of the swimming pool. The investigations by Fenner and the Ellis and Associates time-trials produced additional information about vigilance and attention from a variety of surveillance professions. While the vigilance studies were not new to the field of psychology, for the most part, it was new information for water safety educators. At approximately the same time, research findings by Griffiths and his colleagues using thousands of self-reported lifeguard surveys, confirmed that working lifeguards believed boredom while on duty was a major concern. In addition, when asked to specifically describe how they scanned, most lifeguards were unable to do so. Lifeguards in these studies also recommended using movement, mild exercise, talking, cold water and other methods to prevent boredom and increase alertness. Based on this information from lifeguards, along with the available research on vigilance, Griffiths developed the 'Five Minute Scanning Strategy' which utilises the mind and body in addition to the eyes while scanning. Based largely on the scientific premise that increased muscular activity and respiration rate triggers the sympathetic nervous system to increase alertness, Griffiths added physical movement and posture changes to what had been simply an eye and head scanning pattern in order to combat boredom and increase vigilance. Today, 35,000 Ellis and Associates lifeguards worldwide are required to use this arousal 'check and change' every 5 min while on duty. To better define and discuss the scanning process more specifically, Griffiths also suggested differentiating between sweeping (one visual trip through the zone of coverage) and scanning (repeated sweeps through the zone) [8].

It is now becoming accepted that as serious as the lifesaving profession is, for some, perhaps many individuals this work quickly becomes a tedious, sedentary job leading to monotony and boredom, particularly in the absence of critical incidents. Hence, the current interest by water safety professionals in the area of vigilance. At the turn of this century, more attention was directed to the published findings about vigilance [9–14]. A brief summary of findings of this recent interest includes:

- Vigilance drops significantly after just 30 min for some surveillance tasks.
- As temperatures rise, vigilance drops. Vigilance can decline as much as 45% when the temperature reaches 30° Celsius (86° Fahrenheit)
- Individual circadian rhythms (one's own biological clock) affect lifeguard alertness during the day. Many lifesavers experience a drop in alertness when they have the largest crowds to watch
- Background music may reduce boredom and this enhance vigilance on slow days, but maybe a distraction, and this hinder vigilance, during busy periods
- Talking to others may help lifesavers keep alert, but eyes must remain on the water
- Mild exercise, such as stretching and walking, stimulate the sympathetic nervous system opening the attentional gates of the cerebral cortex
- The length of time scanning and the number of patron interventions during that time can effect scanning effectiveness
- Experienced lifesavers can detect and predict problems much faster than novice lifesavers; mentoring or „buddy teaching" of scanning comes highly recommended
- Lifeguard stress negatively affects scanning. Stress can be caused when the surveillance area is too large or there are too many people in the zone. Conversely, low swimmer volumes and a lack of aquatic activity or need for lifesaver intervention leads to boredom and inattentiveness
- Hydration with water increases lifesaver alertness
- Continual training and in-service is paramount to success
- Challenging lifesavers with random, unannounced tests helps attentiveness

While vigilance studies are not new to the field of psychology, for the most part they are new to water safety educators. At a workshop held in conjunction with the World Congress on Drowning, Pia, now a cognitive psychologist, presented research findings that delineated the visual and cognitive processes underlying surveillance and lifesaver scanning [13].

5.5.3
The Future

With the advent of the 21st century came the introduction of high-tech computers and video systems *underwater* that could assist in drowning detection. Several companies are now marketing this victim detection equipment for use in swimming pools and waterparks, asserting that it will be more reliably vigilant than lifesavers. They base their assertions, in part, on the fact that drownings still occur with lifesavers on duty. Independent testing of the efficacy of the equipment, however, has yet to be conducted. One controversy predicted for the future is whether this technology will be used to assist or replace lifesavers.

As Fenner suggests, from a perspective of prevention, scanning is the most important part of a lifesaver's job. There are many factors which affect vision, scanning, and attention particularly as environmental conditions change. Effective scanning does not come naturally, nor does it come with experience alone. Scanning techniques must be taught and learned before carefully attempting to apply them in a practical manner. This is particularly true for those lifesavers who must work alone without back-up support. Balancing these factors may be the best approach:

- Scan large water surface areas quick enough to cover the entire area but slow enough to detect potential problems. One approach may be to scan more generally at first and then more specifically and effectively during repeated sweeps
- Scan outside the primary area of coverage to predict problems with rips, jetties and people on land without detracting from scanning those inside the primary zone of coverage
- Scanning is most effective from elevated stations, particularly in surf conditions, but foot and boat patrols should be considered when conditions and personnel permit

It is clear that many different theories exist with regard to lifesaver surveillance, scanning, and vigilance. They are taught and employed throughout the world. What is lacking is hard facts based on peer reviewed research involving accepted norms for scientific study. The 2002 World Congress on Drowning demonstrated the existence of great interest in surveillance, scanning, and vigilance to reduce drowning deaths. The Congress, which hosted a diverse forum on scanning and surveillance, also illustrated that effective scanning and surveillance was not solely a lifeguarding concern. The need for effective scanning and improved attention spans was also sought by other rescue and emergency personnel. Navy, coast guard, fire, police and rescue personnel alike expressed interest in better defining and studying the scanning process.

At the World Congress on Drowning it was stated that:

Further research is needed in the areas of surveillance, scanning and vigilance by lifeguards from a physiological and psychological perspective to determine the best methods of instruction and practice [1].

Fenner, who endorses the need for a scientific basis for defining and studying the scanning process, specifically recommends that future research should include the study of individual circadian rhythms of actual lifesavers on duty, the effect of nocturnal sleep and daytime naps on lifesavers alertness, the ingestion of different nutrients and their affect on alertness, biofeedback monitoring of working lifesavers using different scanning strategies and the analysis of new technology to assist lifesavers in surveillance. Finally, a more appropriate and specific globally-accepted definition of scanning is needed to reduce drownings at guarded aquatic facilities. The lifesaving profession has and will continue to be an evolution of new ideas, techniques and technologies as evidenced by the multiple and diverse sessions conducted at the World Congress on Drowning in Amsterdam in June of 2002.

References

1. Anonymous (2002) Recommendations from the World Congress on Drowning, Amsterdam 26–28 June 2002
2. Pia F (1970) On drowning. Water Safety Films, Larchmont, New York
3. Pia F (1974) Observations on the drownings of non-swimmers. J Phys Educ July-August:164–167
4. Brewster CB (ed) (1995) The United States Association Manual of Open Water Lifesaving. BRADY/Prentice Hall, Englewood Cliffs, NJ
5. Pia F (1984) The RID factor as a cause of drowning. Parks and Recreation. June:52–67
6. Fenner P, Leahy S, Buhk A, Dawes P (1999) Prevention of drowning: visual attention scanning and attention span in Lifeguards. J Occup Health 15:61–66
7. http:www.poseidon-tech.com/us/lifeguarding.html
8. Griffiths T, Steel D, Volgelsong H (1999) Lifeguard behaviors and systematic scanning strategies. In: Fletemeyer J, Freas F (eds) Drowning: new perspectives on intervention and prevention. CRC Press, pp 267–279
9. Anonymous (2001) Lifeguard vigilance bibliographic study. Paris, France, at http://www.poseidon-tech.com/us/vigilanceStudy.pdf
10. Griffiths T, Ratner J, Yukelson D (2002) The vigilant lifeguard. Aquatics Int May:18–26
11. Thackray RI (1981) The stress of boredom and monotony: a consideration of the evidence. Psychosom Med 43:165–176
12. Ellis and Associates Newsletter (2001) Study of vigilance. 12 December 2001, http://www.jellis.com/news/01news/december/vigilancebyposeidon.htm
13. Brewster C, Fenner P, Leahy S, et al. (1999) Prevention of drowning: visual attention scanning and attention span in lifeguards. J Occup Health 15:208–210
14. Koelinga HS, Verbaten MN, van Leeuwen Th, et al. (1992) Time effects on event related brain potentials and vigilance performance. Biol Psychol 1:59–86

5.6
Trends in Sea Rescue
and Open Water Search Techniques

Michael Woodroffe and Gabe Kinney

Sea rescue is defined, for the purposes of this chapter, as "those mechanisms brought into force to remove a person from a situation of distress in the maritime environment, and deliver them to a place of safety where adequate medical treatment can be provided, as needed". To supplement this definition, distress can be defined as "those circumstances, where unless immediate action is taken, the individual is likely to lose their life". These are closely in line with the internationally accepted definitions used by search and rescue (SAR) organisations throughout the world. There can be many components to this endeavour, and this chapter will explore a number of them.

Sea rescue is unquestionably a global issue that has become the focus of various initiatives within the international community. Many nations throughout the world have recognised a responsibility to provide for the safety of persons that live in, or transit, their territory and areas of influence. There are two specialised organisations of the United Nations (UN) that are particularly relevant to this discussion, namely the International Civil Aviation Organisation (ICAO), and the International Maritime Organisation (IMO). Both are dedicated to encouraging safety within their respective modes of transportation. Both have developed global search and rescue plans, procedures, techniques and training. Both also envision a collection of search and rescue regions (SRR) encompassing the globe with individual countries, or regional alliances, responsible for an assigned SRR.

One of the governing principles of their work states that: "Vessels and aircraft have a duty to provide assistance to other vessels, aircraft or persons in distress, without regard to location, nationality or circumstances". As a result of their close collaborative work, ICAO and IMO have produced an *International Aeronautical and Maritime Search and Rescue Manual* (IAMSAR) [1]. This three volume comprehensive reference is designed to harmonise aeronautical and maritime search and rescue organisation, procedures and terminology. It has been accepted as the National SAR Manual of the US, the UK, Canada, the Netherlands and a number of other countries.

In addition to the highly effective procedures described in the IAMSAR Manual, there is a growing trend in the US to implement an organisational structure for specific rescue operations called the incident command system (ICS). This is an all-hazard, all-risk, multi-agency process to bring together all potential responding organisations to address the challenges of a particular situation.

5.6.1
Trends in Rescues

It is particularly important to recognise some trends that could potentially in-crease the numbers of persons in need of sea rescue. The numbers of persons en-gaging in activities that could potentially put them at risk is increasing through-out the globe. Our world has become much more mobile. Commercial and pri-vate aviation are increasing. Maritime commerce is on the rise. Larger merchant ships are being built, and new trade routes are being established. Passenger cruise ships that can carry 6,000 persons on board are coming on line, and the cruise industry is growing at a steady 10% pace each year. An ever increasing number of individuals are engaging in recreation associated with maritime ac-tivities.

There are now approximately 12 million recreational boaters within the US alone, and the number is growing. The experience in other countries appears to be similar. Most of these individuals are taking precious time from their oth-erwise hectic schedules to enjoy the water, which leaves little, if any, time to be devoted to preparation and training in aquatic or maritime safety.

While discussing our potential rescue customers, we are also faced with a universally common mind-set that "it cannot happen to me". In addition, the media has created a very commonly held high public expectation that rescue will be readily available in any circumstance, creating a dangerously false sense of security.

5.6.2
Trends in Search and Rescue Techniques

At the same time, the cost in both time and fuel alone of the sea searches around the world in any given year runs into millions of euros.

For centuries, a sea search has been a difficult task. In the early days of sail, it was so difficult that it was often not even attempted, not least because seamen, certainly in the British Royal and Merchant Navies, were not taught to swim, as this made desertion easier and crew retention was a priority.

In more recent years, for fortunate and well-funded searchers, modern tech-nology has come to the aid of the primary search tool, the *mark one eyeball* (sim-ple visual surveillance).

But for many, simple visual surveillance is and will continue to be for some time to come the only resource and one with limitations. This can be clearly demonstrated by throwing a white football overboard to use as a datum for a search plan. Even when quite close by, in a sea state producing about 1/3 metre (1 foot) waves, the football is not visible from the boat for far longer than it is visible. Using a landlubbers saying, looking for a needle in a haystack is an apt description of the task when searching for people in the water.

Volume III of the IAMSAR manual is carried aboard ships and rescue vessels and contains various tables to assist the searching mariner. Chapter 3 of this volume spells out clearly the procedure for search planning, which is normally carried out by the search and rescue mission coordinator (SMC) and relayed to the on-scene coordinator (OSC). A datum is established, based firstly on the reported position and time of the SAR incident, and secondly, to it is added any supplementary information like actual visual sightings or radio direction finding (RDF) bearings, and lastly the time interval between the incident occurring and arrival of the first SAR facilities.

Next in establishing the datum, it is necessary to estimate the surface movement of the casualty, depending on drift, which has components of leeway and total current. Leeway direction is downwind, and its speed depends on wind speed. Persons in the water incidentally are not affected by leeway. Total water current can be estimated by calculating set and drift at the scene. Drift direction and speed is the vector sum of leeway and total water current.

In surface search, teamwork is paramount, as is matching resource capability to task. Good communications and frequent situation reports are vital for an efficient search.

There are established and internationally recognised search plans, which can be selected to suit the situation. For example, the expanding square search (SS), which is most effective when the location of the object is known within relatively close limits, or the sector search, particularly ideal for a single rescue unit when the position of the search object is accurately known and the search area is small. But can be used by air and surface rescue units with the search pattern radius being usually between 5 and 20 nautical miles for the former and between 2 and 5 nautical miles for the latter. Sea state, visibility and size of the object being searched for, all will be dictating factors for the search speed chosen.

Even in those countries fortunate enough to have computer technology to assist them in searching, rescue co-ordination centre (RCC) staff must still know and be able to use the manual methods. In any case, planning should not get ahead of resources or infrastructures.

Canada, the US, and the UK, along with a number of other countries, are fortunate to have some highly developed computer applications for searching, notably the Searchmaster program, CANSARP, SARIS, SARPC and Computer Assisted Search Planning CASP. These incorporate environmental data and involve highly complicated calculations. Specifically, in the UK, the search planning program used by HM Coastguard, the Search and Rescue Information System (SARIS), allows coastguard search planners to fully utilise all the benefits made available through new technology. The program incorporates the tried and tested HM Coastguard search planning methodology and algorithms, as well as new features such as a graphical user interface, the automatic calculation of tidal information and digital charting. SARIS has been designed so that it can use both automated and manual input of the environmental data used in search planning calculations. The program also has the advantage that it can be run on a personal computer workstation as either a stand-alone or a networked program.

The search planner uses SARIS to calculate the search datum positions and the search area where the target(s) are expected to be at the time when the search units will arrive on scene. This is achieved using the position of the emergency, the elapsed time, the target or targets to be found and the effects of water currents and the wind, which cause the target(s) to move from the initial point of distress to the datum(s). SARIS will then allow for possible errors in the distress position and drift calculations, and calculate the location and size of the search area.

The calculated search planning results and the associated digital chart are then saved. Once saved, other network users are able to access and rework the plan as necessary but, as a safeguard, the original search plan is locked so that it cannot be overwritten.

Phase 2 of the SARIS project will shortly be completed, which will enable the coastguard to automatically allocate search units to their optimum calculated search areas and gauge the quality of the search carried out.

No matter which search resource is used, it is imperative that as much known information as possible is incorporated to maximise the likelihood of success. It is also a fact that often the solution may not be either obvious or logical, such that search planners must think laterally, or perhaps colloquially 'outside the box'. Often, those for whom a search is being conducted defy both logic and known possible survival times, so efforts must continue until all reasonable and practicable means of finding those in distress have well and truly been exhausted. There are documented incidents in which persons in distress have actually removed themselves from search areas through disorientation toward the actual direction of a safe haven.

The RCC dealing with the distress may not be on its own. Often RCCs adjacent or more distant may be able to help and there are worldwide a number of ship-reporting systems, like AMVER, run by the US and perhaps best known of them all. These can speedily reduce the search area in size, and increase the number of searchers, by having a recent position of participating vessels on its database.

In addition to effective resource management, many services are becoming very aware of the value of risk management, though this topic can raise more questions than answers. Questions that should be considered in any rescue case, but particularly ones that involve obvious risk include: Is there a reasonable chance of success? Has everything been done short of launching a rescue asset? Is the potential positive outcome worth the risk to my crew? Is there a back-up plan if something goes wrong? Particularly in difficult cases, the launch decision should rest with a senior authority. No one wants to be faced with two search and rescue cases instead of one.

This leads to one of the difficult management demands being faced by many nations in sea rescue. Most rescue organisations must deal with a growing demand for services, with limited resources. A common and growing requirement among rescue organisations is for localised assessments of the potential rescue need within their area of responsibility based on historical rescue data, current maritime activities, and projected future trends. This information then forms the basis for management decisions on communications systems, infrastructure, equipment type and location, and personnel staffing levels and training. The common practise for rescue services is to carefully consider all available data before deciding on the type and location of rescue stations, boats and aircraft for greatest effectiveness and efficiency. For example, a coastal area with high surf and a commercial fishing fleet may need a 16 metre, self-righting, self-bailing motor surf boat. An area with a large population of small pleasure craft may be better served by a 7 metre rigid inflatable boat (RIB) (see ▶ **Chapter 5.13**).

In recent years technology has come to the aid of the searching mariner or airman, and some of this equipment is not very expensive. A typical good quality VHF-DF unit would cost in the order of 5200 euros. We would say this item of SAR equipment has saved more lives and barrels of diesel oil than any other in the last 15 years. Close on its heels, after a more recent release from the military, has been night vision equipment of both image intensifying and also infra-red varieties (see ▶ **Chapter 12.4.3**). Another even more recent great asset in use by a number of lifeboat organisations, is the electronic chart, onto which one can superimpose the IAMSAR search plans and with automatic pilot, the lifeboat can follow the search plan automatically.

One of the recognised challenges faced in sea rescue is establishing effective communications. The first step is for the person in trouble to alert rescue forces that a distress situation exists. Once alerted, further communication is vital to quickly locate the distress, and coordinate the response forces. The Global Maritime Distress and Safety System (GMDSS) has now been accepted internationally for all vessels within the Safety of Life at Sea (SOLAS) convention, and small GMDSS VHF sets are becoming more readily available for yachtsmen, so they too will be able to be embraced by this system. Certainly in the UK, small craft still operate channel 16 voice and for this reason shore stations in Europe and SOLAS convention ships will maintain a listening watch on channel 16 for several more years to come, possibly past the IMO cut off date of February, 2005. In addition, GMDSS includes space-based as well as terrestrial systems. Many nations are in the process of implementing the shoreside segment of GMDSS.

Other electronics, some of which are part of GMDSS, are also to be found either on the survivor or on his vessel or survival craft. These include emergency position indicating radio beacons (EPIRBs), search and rescue transponders (SARTs), personal locator beacons (PLBs) and automated identification systems (AIS). The AIS operates from a ship by transponder without a human being in the link.

Better lifejacket lights, of both the fixed and strobe types, more capable pyrotechnics and improved radar with better definition of small targets, have also made searching easier.

Faster and more sea-friendly rescue craft with longer endurance and better heights of eye for visual search and similar improvements in airborne search and rescue fixed and rotary wing aircraft have become available.

However, whilst there is a distinct and clear advantage in operating craft designed and built specifically for SAR work, where cost or other constraints does not permit this, other craft can play a dual role, like pilot boats, tugs and harbour craft. This allows provision of a marine SAR service with very little extra cost. Craft can be manned by existing paid hands or by volunteer crews, as in the case of a number of lifeboat organisations like the KNRM, RNLI, US Coast Guard Auxiliary and the Chilean Lifeboat Service.

In conclusion, where do we go from here? It is evident that sea rescue is a growing business, with a growing customer base. More people take cruises, visit remote maritime areas, and engage in extreme water activities, while at the same time the traditional aquatic and maritime activities also increase. More distress communications will migrate toward cellular and satellite systems. Surface rescue craft must keep pace with available technology. This includes the use of personal water craft for inshore cases, jet propulsion systems, navigation methods, and better hull and lifesaving appliance design. Rescue aircraft will need to use state-of-the-market systems in airframe and avionics design, distress location and recovery technology. Rescue communications must provide dependable, robust, integrated, and effective command and control for all involved segments of the response system, not simply point to point communications. Perhaps remote controlled reconnaissance and rescue craft? There is certainly a need for rapid location of locator beacons (EPIRB, PLB), and better performing miniature PLB with GPS. The development of geostationary satellites for using 406 MHz is already underway, and when on line will provide the ability to detect EPIRB transmissions almost instantaneously.

But still one of the most difficult things in SAR is getting someone, particularly if unconscious, out of the water. Not too much of a problem in calm weather, but still very difficult in heavy weather and only marginally better now than in the days of sail. This is an area which we must address and make easier.

5.6.3
Conclusions

The objective of the IMO is summed up in their well known catchphrase "Safer Ships and CLEANER Oceans", but if the magnifying glass is now focused specifically on SAR one could say with equal validity "SAFER Oceans and ALL waters", of every scale, must be the number one international priority for the future.

IMO's crusade, led by Admiral Mitropoulos, to establish maritime SAR regions for the world's oceans was concluded at the end of 1998 and was a significant achievement. However, these are but lines on the chart and the priority now must be to ensure there is an SAR response in areas around the world where currently there is none, yet there is significant maritime traffic, whether it be cruise liners, cargo ships, fishing boats or leisure craft. So those nations with well established SAR organisations must help those just embarking on providing such facilities to cover their sea area of responsibility. Those with many years of expertise in SAR will need to train and counsel those just starting out to fulfil the SAR requirements now demanded by all countries that are signatory to the SOLAS and SAR conventions.

The sea rescue community must continue to apply the organisational will to face the SAR challenges ahead, and make the rescue systems as strong as possible. Rescuers must act now to provide the leadership for the future in global sea rescue so that we can be "Always ready that others may live".

5.6.4
Recommendations

To further support this ambition, several recommendations have been defined during the World Congress on Drowning. Three of these recommendations are:

The International Aeronautical and Maritime Search and Rescue Manual should be reviewed and incorporated by the sea rescue organisations of all of the nations of the world to ensure a coordinated and effective approach to maritime emergencies.

The Incident Command System, which has been developed to allow for effective oversight and organisation of emergency responses, should be adopted by all aquatic rescue organisations worldwide.

Search and rescue response must be ensured in areas around the world where there is significant maritime traffic, whether it be cruise liners, cargo ships, fishing boats or leisure craft.

5.6.5
Website

■ www.imo.org

Reference

1. Anonymous (2002) The International Aeronautical and Maritime Search and Rescue Manual (IAMSAR Manual). International Maritime Organisation, London

5.7
Lifejackets and Other Lifesaving Appliances

5.7.1
Lifejackets

Chris Brooks, Günther Cornelissen and Rolf Popp

Lifejackets have been used since ancient times. For a review of the history of the development of lifejackets, see the textbooks of Nicholl [9], Goethe and Laban [4] and Brooks [3]. The development of any form of lifesaving equipment was severely hampered until the mid 19th century. This was due to the fact that death at sea was considered (and still is, to some degree) as fate or an occupational hazard. Neither was it helped by wrecking (outlawed in 1808) or the Royal Navy (RN) impressments of sailors (outlawed in 1815). Only with the advent of iron ships after 1850 which sank more quickly and thus contributed even more to the terrible drowning statistics, did the world slowly awaken to the fact that something should be done about preventing death at sea from drowning.

The US introduced the first lifejacket legislation in 1852, followed reluctantly by France (1884), Britain (1888), Germany (1891) and Denmark (1892). The loss of 1490 people from the Titanic (1912) shocked the world into forming the International Maritime Organization (IMO) and the Safety of Life at Sea Committee (SOLAS). From this stemmed the first international lifejacket standard (67 N – 15 lbs buoyancy).

Deaths from drowning continued unabated during the First World War – 12,000 British sailors, 10,000 merchant marines and passengers and 5,000 German sailors perished [2, 8]. The situation was unchanged during the Second World War. Macintosh and Pask [6] carried out their pioneering work on the flotation of an unconscious person in 1941. This work published in the open literature in 1960 was the basis for the BSI 3595 standard and every standard produced since then (initially 134 N – 30 lbs buoyancy). Talbot (1946) [11] and McCance (1956) [7] reported on the shocking loss of between 30,000–40,000 British officers, men and many merchant mariners. This was due to grossly deficient lifesaving equipment and the incorrect policy of providing flotation in rather than out of the water. This precipitated an intense research and development program centred in the UK with collaborative scientific effort from other nations operating in cold waters.

Three more SOLAS conferences were convened (1948, 1960, 1974/1983). They progressively improved the standard by providing a performance specification for clearance of the oro-nasal cavity from the water, an approval process for inflatable lifejackets and introduced the requirement for self-righting. In 1973, the US Coast Guard introduced their personal flotation devices (PFD) legislation (all inherently buoyant) and inflatable PFD (Type 1–Type 5) legislation in 1995. The new European CEN standards became law in 1994. The US Underwriters' Laboratory produced their complementary standards (UL 1123, 1191 and 1517). In addition to these standards, the Federal Aviation Administration (FAA), the Civil Aviation Authority (CAA) and Transport Canada have produced standards specifically for the aviation industry. Currently, there is an ongoing work of standardisation between ISO and CEN to produce worldwide quality standards for different classes of PFDs. In conjunction with this, the IMO is considering the introduction of thermal protection in some lifejackets [1].

Over the last 50 years a whole series of good standards has been developed and these have had a profound effect on drowning statistics. They have never been so low. But why are there still over 140,000 open water deaths each year [5], and drowning statistics of 13.1 per 100,000 people in underdeveloped countries such as Africa? [10] The basic reasons are as follows.

Lack of education is the most important factor, and must include attention to:
- The dangers of sudden entry into cold water, particularly if the temperature is below 15°C. Most people are unaware of the danger of the sudden inspiratory gasp, the severe hyperventilation that occurs within the first 4–5 min of immersion, and with this particularly for older people, the potential danger

of cardiac arrest or an arrhythmia from the massive increase in heart rate and blood pressure. Even if the person survives stage 1 (cold shock), it is still not a well known fact that good swimming ability in warm water is not a good indication of swimming ability in cold water. In addition to the primary purpose of a lifejacket, to keep a person safely afloat, technical features of the PFD which can assist in search and rescue by crew or third party must not be underestimated. Many people die from swimming failure (stage 2) before hypothermia (stage 3) sets in.

- The requirement to wear a flotation device rather than have it available in the boat
- The requirement to choose the correct flotation device for the specific task
- The need to ensure that the flotation device is fitted correctly
- Awareness that alcohol and safe boating do not mix
- Knowledge about where flotation devices are stowed on commercial vessels

The second factor is that eight out of ten recreational boaters who drown do not wear a flotation device. The majority are male and aged between 15 and 45 years old. Education will help this group, but fashion and attention to the ergonomic performance of the flotation devices will improve wearer acceptance.

The third factor is the price of the device. Simply put, the general population and ship owners typically buy the cheapest product, irrespective of performance. This places the manufacturers in a difficult situation because they have to build a product to a price which they know they can sell it for, knowing full well for an additional expense the performance can be improved quite measurably.

Other factors that need further consideration are:
- Mandatory requirements for recreational boaters [1]
- The re-evaluation of how important self-righting is as one of the primary requirements of a flotation device
- The development of a new self-righting test
- The nomenclature of the flotation device (lifejacket versus PFD)
- The requirement for good labelling.

Finally, the addition of a crotch strap is most important in more of the high performance devices. This becomes more critical as more young adults take part in extreme water sports.

Considering that up until 50 years ago there were hardly any standards and there was little national or international resolve to reduce drowning deaths, good progress has been made. Hopefully, if the above factors are addressed, there will be even better improvement in the next 50 years.

The following recommendations on the development and use of life jackets was stated during the World Congress on Drowning:

5.7.1.1
Recommendations

Wearing of appropriate and insulating lifejackets must be promoted.

Without floating aids, a subject generally drowns within minutes due to swimming failure in cold water. Therefore, the development of insulating and safe garments for aquatic activities is needed. Life jackets should always be worn when immersion can occur to prevent submersion in an early stage. When only non-insulating floating aids can be used, the victim should consider whether swimming ashore is achievable.

References

1. Barss P (2002) What we have learned about drownings and other water related deaths in Canada 1991–2000. The Canadian Red Cross, Ottawa
2. Bennett GH, Bennett GR (1999) Survivors: British merchant seamen in the Second World War. Hambledon Press
3. Brooks CJ (1995) Lifejackets through the ages. Hemlock Press
4. Goethe H, Laban C (1988) Die individuellen Rettungsmittel. Koehlers Verlagsgesellschaft, Herford
5. Golden FStC, Tipton MJ (2002) Essentials of sea survival. Human Kinetics
6. MacIntosh RR, Pask EA (1957) The testing of lifejackets. Br J Ind Med 14:168–176
7. McCance RA, Ungley CC, Crossfill JWL, Widdowson EM (1956) The hazards to men in ships lost at sea 1940–1944. Medical Research Council Special Report Series No. 291, London
8. Merchant Shipping Advisory Committee (1923) Report on life saving appliances, training and organizations. HMSO, London
9. Nicholl GWR (1960) Survival at sea. The development, operation and design of inflatable marine lifesaving equipment. Adlard Coles, London
10. Peden MM (2002) The epidemiology of drowning worldwide. Book of abstracts. World Congress of Drowning, Amsterdam, p 255
11. Anonymous (1946) The Talbot Report. Naval Life Saving Committee, London

5.7.2
Personal Lifesaving Appliances Other Than Lifejackets

Ivar Grøneng

A range of personal lifesaving appliances have evolved from the basic lifejacket standards developed post World War II. The thought of merging a lifejacket with a diving suit, allowing the wearer to stay for a nearly infinite period in the water, remains an inspiration for product developers.

The basic assumption behind thermal protection is that cold contributes to drowning death by reducing the period a person is conscious. Lessening heat loss and providing buoyancy have proven to be an important measure in cold water. Experiences from Norway have shown that survival suits are drastically reducing the number of casualties in the fishing industry, especially for incidents involving smaller vessels.

The product range extends from insulated immersion suits for arctic waters, through un-insulated immersion suits for warmer waters, to special purpose protection gear for offshore racing and other leisure activities. Today new material technology allows lifesaving appliances to be built into work clothing and protective gear.

There is a range of international standards for immersion suits (also called survival suits). The International Maritime Organisation (IMO) has standards for immersion suits intended for use in merchant shipping and the offshore industry. International Standardisation Organisation (ISO) has standards for suits and gear for exposed professionals and leisure boating.

5.7.2.1
Why Not a Lifejacket?

A person immersed in water has a heat loss 25 times higher than in dry air. The temperature of seawater is always lower than body temperature and the immersed body will lose heat. The only counter-measure the body has is heat production. Hypothermia is caused by the body's inability to produce enough heat to balance the heat loss.

It is difficult to set a specific critical seawater temperature for development of cold shock and hypothermia. Human response to cold water is highly individual. Laboratory research has shown that individuals develop hypothermia within 2 hours of immersion in water of 20°C [1]. Thermal protection is therefore necessary to reduce the body heat loss.

Thermal protection is provided in two principle ways. Keeping the wearer dry (dry suit) or restricting water flow and the amount of water on the body (wet suit). In addition to this, insulation has to be added according to the temperature difference expected (seawater temperature), as the speed of heat loss increases in colder water. Dry suit insulation is provided by containing air near the skin, either by warm clothing under the suit or by making the suit in an insulating material (or both). Wet suit insulation is provided by making the suit in an insulating material.

As all types of insulation are basically obtained by containing air, buoyancy is added on the whole body by insulated suits and thus the wearer will float on top of the water. This effect gives the wearer of a immersion suit many advantages to a wearer of a lifejacket. Obviously thermal protection is better by far. A suit wearer floating on the water also is easier to spot and locate by rescuers than a person wearing a lifejacket only. And floating on top of the water provides one other great advantage. In wind and waves the wearer is able to avoid mouth immersions and by that the exhaustion process is slowed down.

5.7.2.2
Why Not a Personal Lifeboat?

The intention for lifesaving appliances is to save life after any accident causing persons to enter the water unintentionally. This means that these person have to wear the gear before entering the water, either by always wearing it when exposed to danger or by donning it quickly before entering the water.

On merchant ships personal lifesaving appliances are stored for easy access and quick donning after an emergency situation is established. This is a collective and contingency based approach. Thereby storage and donning performance are important design criteria. People exposed to high risk situations, both in professional and in leisure activities should wear protection at all times. Such gear is designed with a focus on ergonomics and individual user friendliness, allowing the wearer to perform his activities in a safe and efficient manner.

Lifesaving appliances are normally designed on three basic considerations: passing a minimum standard for in-water lifesaving ability, marketing profile, and cost. A risk based approach will show a more complex picture on good design. All risk factors have to be identified and weighed in a logical sequence. An example is the fact that if a person is unable to don the appliance, the in-water performance of the appliance is useless.

Risk based design can be based on the following hierarchy [2, 3]:
- Availability and donning properties
- Ergonomics for on-board tasks
- Compatibility with any evacuation systems
- In-water performance regarding survival in waves, wind and cold water
- Localisation and rescue out of the water
- Maintenance and durability

This approach is intended to demonstrate the need for balancing several contradicting needs. Maximising in-water performance might result in stiff bulkiness. Maximising on-board ergonomics might result in a comfortable work suit. Storage requirements might reduce the maximum allowable storage volume next to nothing. Maximising possible localisation might add costly batteries and transmitters with limited service life.

The perfect lifesaving appliance is a fine tuned balance between positive contribution and negative effects. More buoyancy results in less ergonomics. Better individual fit results in more complicated donning. The big issue is to find international minimum standards that invite designers to be creative and apply new technology to combine contradicting needs (◘ Fig. 5.2).

5.7.2.3
So Why Bother?

The lifesaving appliance is a contributing factor to survival, not a guarantee. Traditionally all outdoor activities in cold climates have been conducted wearing heavy insulated clothing. Consequently any person falling into the water would drown quickly, even wearing a lifejacket. New materials that provide both dry and wet insulation, and buoyancy, are available, so why not take the advantage of that?

The drive should be on how to reduce drowning causalities even further. The focus might be on the following areas:

◻ Fig. 5.2. The perfect life-saving appliance is a fine tuned balance between buoyancy and ergonomics

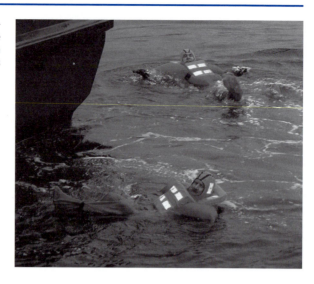

- Providing work and leisure gear with the capability to also function as personal lifesaving appliances
- Providing insulated clothing for cold climates with the capability to also function as personal thermal lifesaving appliances
- Providing simple and cost effective personal lifesaving appliances with thermal insulation for untrained persons on passenger ships and leisure boats
- Teach shipping personnel and inform the public about the extreme risk of drowning in cold water, and how to protect themselves

References

1   Thelma AS (2002) Personal life saving equipment 2002. Cold stress in 20°C and 25°C water. Norwegian Maritime Directorate Report 02-06
2.   Grøneng I (2002) Improved personal lifesaving appliances 2002. Norwegian Maritime Directorate. Report reference 200126794
3.   IMO submissions DE 46/14/1 and DE 45/19/3

5.8
Self-Rescue

5.8.1
Self-Rescue During Accidental Cold Water Immersion

MICHEL DUCHARME

For many decades, cold water immersion death has been primarily associated with the development of hypothermia [4]. This belief has led to the development of the numerous standards and policies related to search and rescue practices, protective clothing use and development, and public safety recommendations. Hypothermia was also reported to be the prime cause of swimming failure leading to drowning [1, 5]. In addition, the cooling rate of swimmers was reported to be 50% higher than that of static people in water [5], and this finding led to the popular recommendation that swimming should not be attempted during cold water immersion [5, 9, 10].

Slowly, evidence from recent studies are supporting an alternative explanation for cold water immersion-related death. A British survey reported that a large proportion of cold water drowning victims perished too quickly for hypothermia to be involved [6]. The results of this survey led some authors to suggest that the first two of the four phases of cold water immersion [3], namely the cold shock and the incapacitation phases, are more relevant in explaining cold water immersion death than hypothermia [12]. Self-rescue is therefore critical during the first 15 min of immersion in cold water.

5.8.1.1
Critical Phases for Self-Rescue

Upon sudden immersion in cold water, the victim will experience a short transitory phase lasting about 2–3 min and characterised by an uncontrollable hyperventilation accompanied by other cardio-respiratory distresses [11]. Unless the situation requires the execution of emergency procedures (as opening a hatch or resurfacing), it is imperative that the victim remains calm and concentrates on regaining control of the breathing pattern before initiating any non-life threatening self-rescue procedures.

Following the cold shock, the next phase, called the incapacitation phase, will develop during the subsequent 20–30 min of immersion. This is the critical phase for self-rescue when the options should be quickly evaluated and a strategy should be developed by the victim based on the situation at hand.

The incapacitation phase is characterised by the progressive diminution of the self-rescue capacity of the victim mainly attributed to cooling of the peripheral tissues, particularly the joints, nerves, and muscles. Manual dexterity and sensitivity, muscle strength, and speed of muscle contraction will progressively deteriorate as peripheral tissues cool, even before the victim develops hypothermia. This incapacitation will render the execution of essential tasks required for self-rescue more difficult and even impossible. It is therefore imperative during this phase to rapidly evaluate the options for self-rescue, keeping in mind that the ultimate objective of the victim is not to preserve body heat, but to move out of the cold water as quickly as possible.

A number of survival measures should be considered. Those include: increasing visibility to optimise the likelihood of rescue (triggering a flare, dispersing dye), deployment of emergency equipment (inflating a life raft or a life jacket, deploying a splash guard or an ice pick in the case of falling through ice, tying a buddy line), righting or climbing over the capsized craft to minimise exposure to water, climbing aboard a life raft, reaching for wreckage, climbing over ice or swimming to shore. The strategy adopted would be based on a number of factors specific to the emergency situation: the chance of being rescued, the state of the sea or ice, the presence of rescue equipment, the presence of a PFD, and the distance to shore.

5.8.1.2
Swimming as an Option

Early studies reported that swimming in cold water in the absence of a PFD could lead to rapid swimming failure due to respiratory distress, lack of coordination between swim stroke and respiration, and early development of fatigue [2, 7]. These findings led to recommendations from public safety authorities such as: "do not attempt swimming," "trying to swim beyond 100 meters is dangerous," and "only if you can get to safety with a few strokes, do so". Those recommendations did not leave swimming as an option for self-rescue.

Since then, studies have improved our understanding of cold shock and its impact on the cardio-respiratory system during the first few minutes of cold water immersion [11]. It is suggested that a significant component of the early swimming failure observed may be attributed to cold shock. Therefore, swimming should not be attempted until the cold shock has resolved and the breathing pattern is under control.

Although hypothermia has been suggested in the past to be a major contributor of swimming failure, recent studies have linked swimming failure to a progressive decrease in swimming efficiency [12] and muscle fatigue primarily due to muscle cooling [8, 13]. Minimising heat loss from the active muscles of the arms is an important consideration since studies have found significant correlations between fat thickness over the arms and swimming efficiency [12] and swimming distance [13].

A recent study performed in a swimming flume found that on average subjects not wearing a PFD could swim in 10°C water for over 1 hour and were able to cover an estimated distance of over 1 kilometre [12]. Other studies performed in the field showed that subjects wearing a PFD could swim a distance of about 900 meters and 650 meters in 14°C and 10°C water, respectively, over a period of 45 min [8, 13]. These results show that once the cold shock has resolved, swimming distance in cold water can be significant and could correspond to about 33% of the normal distance covered in warm water [8]. Opting to swim to shore would improve the chance of survival if the swimming distance is within 1 kilometre and the chance of being rescued is minimum.

The following practical advice should be followed:

- Upon falling in cold water, the effects of cold shock should be expected. The victim should stay calm and wait to regain control of the breathing pattern before initiating any non-life threatening self-rescue procedure
- Once the cold shock has resolved, the potential options for rescue should be considered. The ultimate objective is to get out of the water as quickly as possible
- A number of self-rescue procedures increase the chances of being rescued and should be done during the first 15 min before being incapacitated by the

cold. These procedures include improving visibility, decreasing contact with water by any means and deployment of emergency equipment. Innovative design can play an important role here

- Swimming to shore should be considered if the swimming distance appears to be within 1 kilometre, the chance of being rescued is minimum or absent, and the victim cannot get out of the water by any means

References

1. Dulac S, Quirion A, DeCarufel D, et al. (1987) Metabolic and hormonal responses to long-distance swimming in cold water. Int J Sports Med 8:352–356
2. Golden F, Hardcastle PT, Pollard CE, Tipton MJ (1986) Hyperventilation and swim failure in cold water. J Physiol 378:94P
3. Golden F, Hervey GR (1981) The „after-drop" and death after rescue from immersion in cold water. In: Adam JA (ed.) Hypothermia ashore and afloat. Aberdeen University Press
4. Golden F, Tipton M (2002) Essentials of sea survival. Human Kinetics, Champaign, USA, p 305
5. Hayward JS, Eckerson JD, Collis ML (1975) Effect of behavioral variables on cooling rate of man in cold water. J Appl Physiol 38:1073–1077
6. Home Office Working Party on Water Safety (1977) Report of the working party on water safety. HMSO, London
7. Keatinge WR, Prys-Roberts C, Cooper KE, et al. (1969) Sudden failure of swimming in cold water. Br Med J 1:480–483
8. Kenny GP, Reardon FD, Ducharme MB, Oksa J (2000) Physiological limitation to emergency swimming in cold water. DCIEM Contract report, DCIEM CR 2001-026
9. Royal Life Saving Society of Canada (1997) Hypothermia: the cold wet facts. Royal Life Saving Society of Canada, Ottawa, Ontario, Canada
10. The Canadian Red Cross Society (1995) Swimming and water safety. Mosby Lifeline, Toronto, p 303
11. Tipton MJ (1989) The initial responses to cold water immersion in man. Clin Sci 77:581–588
12. Tipton MJ, Eglin C, Gennser M, Golden F (1999) Immersion deaths and deterioration in swimming performance in cold water. Lancet 54:626–629
13. Wallingford R, Ducharme MB, Pommier E (2000) Factors limiting cold-water swimming distance while wearing personal floatation devices. Eur J Physiol 82:24–29

5.8.2
Survival and Self-Rescue

Anthony Handley

Awareness of the potential dangers of venturing on, in, or near the water can prevent drowning and will at the same time contribute to rescue activities. Children should be taught the risks associated with water and how to deal with this, but in a manner that neither detracts from the pleasures of aquatic activities, nor induces excessive fear. Being able to swim significantly reduces the risk of drowning.

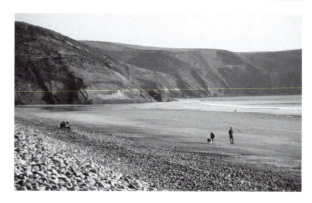

Fig. 5.3. Anyone who intends to visit a site near water should be briefed about the general and local dangers of the area, including such hazards as strong currents, being cut off by the tide and sudden changes in weather condition

5.8.2.1
Before Venturing Near Water

It is important that anyone who intends to visit a site near water should be briefed about the general and local dangers of the area (**Fig. 5.3**). A personal flotation device (PFD) of approved design should always be worn during aquatic activities such as boating, sailing, windsurfing. If the water is anything other than tropically hot, more clothes should be worn than the land temperature would suggest. An ability to swim is no reason to go without a PFD. Fatigue and cold rapidly turn a competent swimmer into a non-swimmer.

5.8.2.2
Falling into Water

If someone falls into water unexpectedly, he or she should tuck their chin onto their chest, put their hands onto the head and protect the face with their forearms. The elbows should be pressed to the sides of the chest, with the knees bent and the feet together. Once in the water, a modified posture should be assumed (**Fig. 5.4**).

It is important to be alert to the effects of sudden entry into cold water: gasping and hyperventilation. Breathing should be controlled as far as possible, keeping the head above water until the cold shock effect wears off (**Fig. 5.5**).

5.8.2.3
Survival Techniques

Above all it is important not to panic. This is easier said than done, but a person is much more likely to survive an immersion accident if able to remain calm. It is important to conserve energy, particularly in cold water. The victim should take a few moments to assess the situation before taking any action and should not start swimming other than enough to stay afloat before deciding whether and where to go. Viewed from near the surface of the water, distances can be deceptively short. Particularly in cold water, everyone's swimming ability is likely

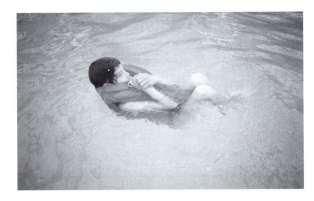

Fig. 5.4. Heat escape lessening posture (HELP). Self-rescue position for when a person falls into water

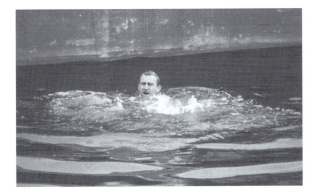

Fig. 5.5. When suddenly entering cold water controlled breathing is important

to be impaired. It may be better to stay where you are, hopefully with a buoyant aid to float, until rescue arrives. This will depend on several factors such as the distance to land, your swimming ability and the temperature of the water (see ▶ **Chapter 5.8.1**). Clothes help prevent loss of body heat and should only be removed if they are dragging the victim down.

5.8.2.4
Special Situations

- Rip current: If caught in a rip current, the victim should swim parallel to the shore until out of the rip, then return to land by swimming through the breaking waves
- Waves: Away from the shore, the back of the victim should be maintained to the waves to help prevent water breaking over the face
- Tidal water: It is important to swim with the tide, moving gradually across it towards your destination; one should never try and swim directly against the tide
- Underwater weed, mud and quicksand: If caught in underwater weed, the victim should move slowly, ideally using a sculling action. In mud or quick-

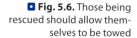

Fig. 5.6. Those being rescued should allow themselves to be towed

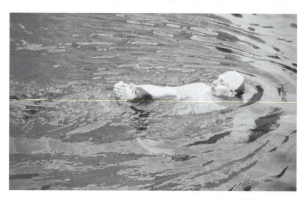

sand, there should be no attempt stand up. The victim should lie flat and spread his weight over as large a surface as possible; moving slowly using arm and leg actions

— Car falling into water: As soon as it is apparent that the car is going to fall into the water, the occupants should unfasten their seatbelts and unlock the doors. An attempt should be made to escape whilst the car is on the surface. As the car sinks, the internal and external lights should be turned on to help the rescuers locate the vehicle. Manually operated windows should be closed, but electrically operated windows left open, as they will fail once the car is underwater. The occupants should take a breath as the car sinks. As the water reaches chin level, an attempt should be made to force open a door. If this fails, a side window should be broken using a glass breaking hammer or similar object – the corner, rather than the centre of the window should be struck (see ▸ **Chapter 5.9**).

5.8.2.5
Being Rescued

Those being rescued from the water should never attempt to grab an approaching rescuer, but rather allow themselves to be towed, even if water splashes over their heads (**Fig. 5.6**). When reaching the edge of the water, the victim should hold on to support until he or she has recovered sufficiently to climb out of the water or be helped out. On reaching dry land, a person who has been rescued should sit or lie down to recover and to prevent any drop in blood pressure, particularly if the water was cold or the period of immersion was more than a few minutes.

5.9
Submerged Vehicle Rescue

JAAP MOLENAAR and JOHN STOOP

Although few in number, accidents involving drowning in submerged vehicles are very serious, causing fatalities among occupants and traumatic consequences for rescue and emergency staff. On average, in the Netherlands annually 750–800 accidents result in vehicles in a flooded ditch or canal, causing about 30 occupants to drown. Considering the severity of this accident type, the Dutch Transportation Safety Board decided to perform a safety study on the issue of drowning in cars, particularly because this type of accident seems to be preventable.

The question was raised as to whether this type of accident represented a trend in modern car technology. No certification standards for prevention of electronic failure regarding ditching are incorporated in vehicle design. A first survey indicated a potential Dutch-specific issue: accidents mainly occurred in rural traffic areas, involving single-sided ditching after uncontrolled skidding of vehicles near curves and slopes [1]. The conditions indicated a potential involvement of black spots in road infrastructure.

5.9.1
Problems Regarding Modern Submerged Vehicles

The increasing level of safety and security for drivers, passengers, cargo and equipment of vehicles may have adversarial effects with respect to escaping from submerged vehicles and places rescue teams in increasing difficulties during rescue operations.

- Electronic system failure: Various types of electronic safety systems in modern cars may easily fail, causing occupants to be trapped inside their vehicle. Since many of these systems also provide security, they hamper access during their failure as well. Examples of these electronic systems are:
  - Automatic locking devices on doors: Above a certain speed these systems serve to reduce the risk of people falling out of moving vehicles
  - Airbag systems: Electronic sensors are provided in the vehicles to activate the right airbag system based on the place of impact and the energy transferred to the body of the people inside the vehicle
  - Electrically powered windows: If modern vehicles are equipped with fully electrically powered windows, escape from the vehicle can be impossible due to failure of the electrical system. If the system is partly manually operated, such as with rear windows, there is still a possibility to leave the vehicle
- Laminated glass: Laminated glass windows are installed in vehicles as a safety measure. Front windshields are already commonly applied with laminated glass. Rear window applications are applied in more expensive cars, but this threshold is declining. The next step is to provide side windows with laminated glass. In case of a regular road traffic accident, laminated glass can

be cracked and removed. After submerging, this is no option because it is not possible for a rescue diver to develop enough force to crack and remove the window. Windows made out of synthetic laminate are unbreakable. The primary goal of using this type of material for windshields and windows is to provide security against burglary and theft. The only way to get these windows removed is to drill a hole in the material and use a special saw to cut the material

5.9.2
Reduced Self-Reliance and Accessibility of Submerged Vehicles

It may be impossible to escape from a submerged vehicle because failure of electronic safety systems may block escapes routes. Secondly, airbag problems must be overcome. Due to the impact several airbags may be activated. After activation and taking the impact of the crash, they will deflate and float through the passenger compartment, causing disorientation and loss of position awareness. Thirdly, problems may occur with submerged vehicles because vehicles sink deep into the mud on the river or canal bottom, while the vehicle may have landed on the side or roof. In summary, self-reliance of occupants and efforts of rescue teams may be hampered by the inaccessibility of modern vehicles due to technological failure, aggravated by an unfavourable vehicle position after submerging.

5.9.3
How Rescue Teams Can Act

Time is very precious since people have limited time to survive in a submerged vehicle. Worldwide research has shown that a submerged person must get full medical treatment within 1 hour. Consequently, an underwater rescue operation must be very efficient. Several standard situations regarding submerged vehicles may be defined.

On arriving at the scene, information should be gathered about the most likely location of the submerged vehicle and confirmation should be obtained about presence of vehicle occupants. While this information is being gathered, rescue divers should prepare to enter the water. After swimming to the presumed location, the diver descents to the bottom and starts searching for the vehicle.

After identifying the vehicle the diver will establish the position of the vehicle, which can be:

- A basic situation in which the submerged vehicle is standing on its wheels on the bottom of the canal/river. The first option is to open one of the doors in the normal way using the handle. The second option is to break the glass by using the back of the divers knife or a special automatic (spring release) centre point. This is only effective with tempered glass. Laminated glass and synthetic laminates will not be damaged. The final option, if these others are ineffective, is to pull the vehicle out of the water as quickly as possible.

- The submerged vehicle has sunk into the mud. Since a diver cannot develop enough force to open the door and move the mud layer away, trying to open the doors is no option. One option, in case of vans and hatchbacks, is to open the backdoor. The second option is try to break the windows. A final option is to pull the vehicle out of the water as soon as possible.
- The submerged vehicle is on its side. Opening the door on top is a possibility but the diver must be aware of the hazard that the door can close again and lock him in. A second option is to enter the vehicle through the back window or the back door. Passengers can be down or float in the passenger's compartment. A final option is to pull the vehicle out of the water as quickly as possible.
- The submerged vehicle is upside down. Orientation problems for the diver may occur inside and outside the vehicle. The car can be entered if doors function properly, otherwise the windows may provide the next option. The final option, again, is to pull the vehicle out of the water as quickly as possible.

5.9.4
Some Practical Advice

In reducing the hazard of drowning in submerged cars, some practical advice may be drawn up:
- Preparation of rescue diving teams focusing on training in various conditions
- Development of new underwater rescue techniques for emergency services
- Development of specific tools promoting self-reliance, such as life hammers
- Improvement of information regarding safety features, such as crash charts, a vehicle manual safety chapter, and instructions for behaviour during various types of incidents
- Stimulate safety certification on a European level, related to drowning in modern vehicles with respect to electronic power and system failures
- Modification of road infrastructure layout and equipment on black spots dealing with drowning hazards.

Reference

1. Anonymous (2002) Cars in the water: escape issues. A safety study. Dutch Transportation Safety Board, The Hague, The Netherlands, December 2002

5.10
Horizontal and Other Rescue Techniques: Practical Aspects

Wolfgang Baumeier and Michael Schwindt

5.10.1
Circum Rescue Collapse

An accident at sea including immersion will almost always lead to accidental hypothermia [1]. Hypothermia has an enormous influence on the physiological functions of the human body. Metabolic rate slows and impairs organic functions. The effects on brain, muscle and circulation functions are of critical importance to successful rescue of hypothermic patients.

Cooling of the brain eventually results in derangement and deceleration of brain function, as well as impairment of consciousness. Even victims who are responsive cannot be expected to be able to help themselves in any way. Cooling of the muscular system results in increasing rigidity, due to muscle stiffness, with considerable impairment of coordinated grasp functions.

Because of the circulatory centralisation into the body core, the cooling process of the body parts close to vital organs slows down. Increased diuresis occurs, with resulting hypovolaemia. Bradycardia and arterial hypotension arise adjusted to the decreased metabolism. The heart, which is particularly sensitive at this temperature, can no longer react adequately to changed circulatory situations, such as that which can occur in case of a change in body position. Even the slightest irritations, due to causes such as this, can result in ventricular fibrillation, which will result in death unless it can be corrected.

Golden [2], in particular, has dealt with circum rescue collapse associated with the rescue of immersion victims. The circulatory collapse can come about as a result of a number of factors. Primary among these are:

- Loss of hydrostatic assistance to venous return
- Re-imposition of the effects of gravity
- Hypovolaemia and increased blood viscosity
- Diminished work capacity of the hypothermic heart and reduced time for coronary filling
- Dulled baroceptor reflexes
- Unfeasible demands to perfuse skeletal muscle
- Psychological stress and pre-existing coronary disease

For these reasons, after an accident in the water, people have often died during rescue operations when they were winched out of the water in a vertical position. Today, it is commonly recognised that a horizontal position during a rescue manoeuvre is not only preferable but seems to be the only safe alternative.

If possible, the hypothermic casualty should be kept in a horizontal position and should not be moved any more than absolutely necessary, either during the rescue operation or afterwards, until the casualty is rewarmed [2].

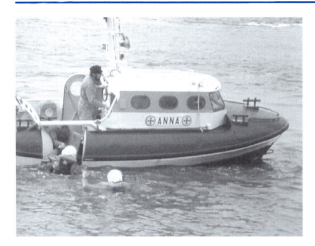

Fig. 5.7. The rescue boats and the daughter boats of the rescue vessels of the German Maritime Rescue Service (Deutsche Gesellschaft zur Rettung Schiffbrüchiger) have side doors close to the level of the water surface to pull in persons nearly horizontally

5.10.2
Horizontal Rescue Techniques

Rescue equipment for removing hypothermic victims from the water can be divided into two broad groups: passive systems which require the survivor to take some action to reach the safety of the deck of the rescuing ship and active systems which are able to recover an incapacitated person. The various transfer measures and techniques include dedicated SAR equipment, such as winch-fitted helicopters, lifeboats, and other rescue craft, recovery nets or scoops, rescue strops, rescue slings, rescue seats, rescue litters, rescue baskets, line-throwers, scrambling nets, Jason's cradle, embarkation ladders, and side doors. Ideal equipment will require little or no activity on the part of the casualty. Recovery of people from the water, even into boats, can be difficult without specific training and equipment. High-sided ships need some sort of lifting aid. In most cases a rescue team member needs to go into the water for assistance. The recovery of elderly, frail, and hypothermic persons without direct assistance is unrealistic. A variety of modern systems will be described.

5.10.3
Boat Side Door

If rescue boats have side doors close to the surface of the water (**Fig. 5.7**), casualties can be pulled into the boat in a more or less horizontal position. This operation is an energy consuming act for two rescuers and often hurts the back of the survivor, especially in rough seas. Some boats use outside platforms at the same level or special life rafts as a sledge to move casualties from the waterline to the deck.

■ **Fig. 5.8.** The Jason's Cradle is a ladder like device which is fixed to one side of the boat. When lifting one end of the cradle the casualty rolls up towards the deck

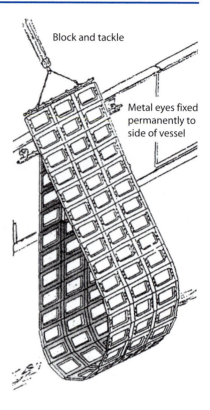

Block and tackle

Metal eyes fixed permanently to side of vessel

■ **Fig. 5.9.** Markus Lifenet. Rescue device for vertical and horizontal lifting

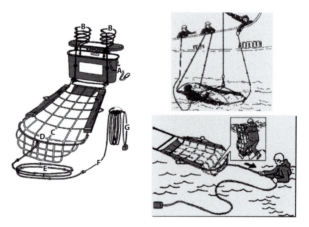

5.10.4
Jason's Cradle

The Jason's cradle (◘ Fig. 5.8) is a ladder-like rescue scoop which can be used to roll persons in a horizontal position into a boat up to a freeboard height of more than 1.5 metres. The cradle is similar to a wide belt, fixed with one end to the side of the vessel. The other end is held with a block and tackle in such a way that the cradle forms a "U" under the waterline, into which the person is floated alongside the boat. As the free end of the device is hoisted upward, the survivor will roll around his longitudinal axis until he reaches the level of the deck of the boat rescue boat. Using this device, one crew member can quite easily recover a 100 kilogram man in water-soaked clothing. To effectively use this device, the casualty must be brought near the side of the ship or the ship must manoeuvred close to him. Sea state is a limiting factor. The rescue procedure using the Jason's cradle requires moving the casualty.

5.10.5
Markus Net

The Markus net is a rescue device that enables one person to react immediately to a man overboard situation, regardless of freeboard of the vessel, thereby increasing the casualty's chance of rescue (◘ Fig. 5.9). The buoyant rescue net has a combined rescue and lifting line of up to 40 metres length, which can either be thrown to the casualty or taken to him by a waterborne rescuer. Once lying on the net, the casualty can be towed to the rescue vessel by lifting two lines with knots. The casualty will be lifted up hanging in the net. The Markus net is manufactured in three versions according to the freeboard height of the rescue vessel. The net structure and functions are the same in all versions, but differ in length of knot lines. Particularly in the case of an unconscious casualty, the rescue procedure requires a well trained rescue team. In order to use the various possibilities the system offers, regular training is required, several times a year.

5.10.6
The Rescue Lifting System (RLS)

The Rescue Lifting System was developed recently at the University of Applied Sciences and Arts in Hildesheim, Germany. The double loop of this device enables rescuers to lift a person out of the water in a deckchair position. The RLS consists of a horseshoe-shaped orange floating loop that is placed under the arms like an ordinary, U-shaped lifebuoy and a horseshoe-shaped sinking loop that is placed behind the thighs. Both loops are connected to a grip ring by straps. After the sinking loop has sunk, its drag anchor function is advantageous for use in rough seas. The survivor uses the only visible U-shaped floating loop like a lifebuoy. A rescue line which can be thrown is fixed at a grip ring, with which the person can be hauled close to the ship's side from the deck. While lifting the rescue system,

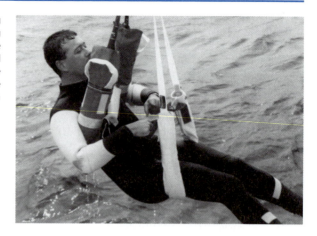

Fig. 5.10. Rescue lifting system (RLS). The floating loop (*grey*) is put under the arms like a horseshoe-shaped lifebuoy. When lifting the sunken loop (*white*) brings the person to a deckchair position

the sinking loop automatically rises from its diving depth under the thighs of the casualty resulting in a nearly horizontal deckchair position (**Fig. 5.10**). In this position the thorax is slightly more elevated than the pelvis of the casualty. The arms and lower legs are hanging down. This position is comfortable, does not compress the thorax, and prevents the person from falling. The conscious rescued person, with head up, feels safe and relaxed and has no desire to move. An unconscious casualty will not slip out backwards, even under rough conditions. No medical disadvantages are known regarding the circulatory system in comparison with a fully horizontal body position [3].

5.10.7
RLS and Open Lifeboats (Type H)

In this variation, the double loops are equipped with special additional hand straps to secure the person with two helpers, who are in the dinghy or in the lifeboat, and pull the person into the boat in a deckchair position (**Fig. 5.11**). This type is for small open boats and small lifeboats with a low freeboard of no more than 1 metre. RLS type H is also equipped with safety straps which prevent rescuers from falling overboard when leaning out of the boat, especially when lifting a heavy person. By using this system no rescuer has to enter the water for assistance, even when an unconscious person has to be rescued.

5.10.8
RLS for High-Sided Ships (Type B)

For high-sided ships, an additional device called a "stopperblock" was developed. This is the ideal connecting device between the heavy steel rope ending at the hook of the crane on board and the buoyant, light rescue line (**Fig. 5.12**). Any crane or davit can be used. At first the rescue line with the RLS double res-

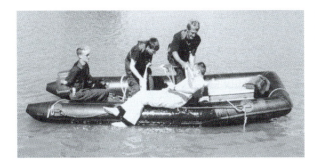

Fig. 5.11. Rescue lifting system (RLS Type H). With this system the casualty can easily be lifted into the boat by hand

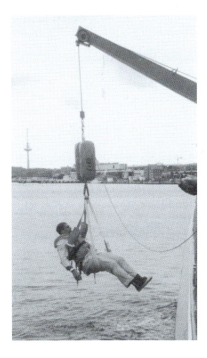

Fig. 5.12. Rescue lifting system (RLS Type B). This device with a "stopperblock" is used for rescue operations from high-sided ships

cue loops can be pulled by hand easily and gently near the "stopperblock" which hangs over the surface of the sea. The rescue line blocks in the "stopper" and cannot slip back. The crane hoists the "stopperblock" and the RLS while the person in a deckchair-position is suspended under the block and hoisted on deck. The system has been tested and proven effective in waves up to 2 metres. For this device, a helpless person needs a rescuer in the water to assist him.

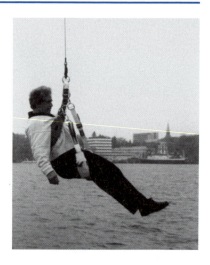

☐ **Fig. 5.13.** Rescue lifting system (RLS Type L). In the first step a floating loop will be closed around the chest with a snaphook. In the second step a special mechanism unties the sinking loop from the chest loop

5.10.9
RLS and Helicopter (Type L)

Another modification of RLS was developed for rescue operations with a helicopter (☐ **Fig. 5.13**). Both loops are stuck together to one loop to prevent twisting of the device in the downwash of helicopters when lowered empty to the water surface. After this loop has been closed with a snaphook around the chest by the casualty or by a rescue team member, the sinking loop can be untied with a simple procedure. If the RLS is now winched up, the person automatically hangs in a deckchair position. Type L can also be used from a high-sided vessel.

5.10.10
RLS and the Helpless Person

Casualties handicapped by cold, physical disability, injuries, or unconsciousness can be rescued with the RLS, both from high-sided vessels and from small open boats. It is a special advantage of Type H that no member of the rescue team on small boats has to go into the water, even in moderate seas.

For assistance a rescuer can lie in the RLS loops when RLS type B or C are lowered to the sea. The rescuer pulls the casualty to his chest and wraps his arms around the chest of the casualty. Both are lifted in a twin position, if the weight of the casualty is tolerable for the rescuer.

For all types of RLS, the person in the water needs no knowledge about the sinking loop or the deckchair position. As soon as the floating loop is put under the arms by the casualty or rescuer, the person is pulled towards the ship with the rescue line by the rescuers onboard. A further development of the systems aims at a U-shaped lifebuoy in which both loops are combined to one. The water drag will cause pressure on the rescue line, so that the sinking loop is released and sinks behind the back of the victim automatically.

References

1. Baumeier W, Bahlmann L, Schmucker P (2004) Accidental hypothermia and the project 'SARRRAH' – first experiences with a multicenter study. In: Oehmichen M (ed) Hypothermia: Clinical, pathomorphological and forensic features. Res Legal Med 31:129–140
2. Golden FStC, Hervey GR, Tipton M (1991) Circum rescue collapse: collapse, sometimes fatal, associated with rescue of immersion victims. J Roy Nav Med Serv 77:139–149
3. Rollnik JD, Witt K, Hänert W, Rix W, Schwindt M (2001) Rescue Lifting System (RLS) might help to prevent death after rescue from immersion in cold water. Int J Sports Med 22:17–20

5.11
Ice Rescue

CARLA ST-GERMAIN and ANDREA ZAFERES

The aim of this chapter is to create an understanding of the typical problems related to ice rescues. Practical guidelines are proposed and the importance of more public awareness is emphasised.

People who actively participate in ice-related activities like walking on or near ice, skating, snowmobiling, or ice fishing, run a constant risk of suddenly and unexpectedly finding themselves in the water, or being placed in a position of attempting to rescue others.

Anyone who will be on or near ice should be fully prepared for unintended immersion. They should travel only on marked areas, obey all warning signs, wear thermal protective buoyant clothing, and carry potentially lifesaving equipment, such as ice picks, a rope, waterproof matches, and fire starters.

Members of public safety agencies in areas with ice are expected to have the skills and equipment to perform ice rescues. Neither individuals nor professionals can afford to wait for a tragedy to occur to learn the fundamentals of ice rescue.

Proper ice rescue techniques allow rescuers to quickly bring others to safety without themselves becoming victims. Unfortunately, the same tragic scenario unfolds many times each winter: Someone falls through the ice and well-intentioned people try to help, but are unable to perform the rescue or worse, become victims themselves. Often professional rescuers lack the necessary training and equipment to save someone's life while staying safe themselves. Proper preparation is essential.

5.11.1
Self-Rescue

People are normally extremely frightened when falling into cold water. The body experiences cold shock, causing gasping and hyperventilation, which typically last between 1 and 2 min. During the cold shock, the main priorities for victims are to maintain buoyancy and to get breathing under control. As soon as possible, victims should attempt to return to the spot where they fell in, since it is known that the ice can support body weight in that location. Victims should kick into a horizontal, floating position and turn the face to the ice in the direction from which they came. Victims should then place their hands or arms on the unbroken ice surface, keep kicking in a horizontal position, and claw their way to solid support. Upon successfully gaining a position on the ice surface, victims should roll away from the ice opening until reaching more solid ice and then crawl the rest of the way to safety.

If these efforts are not successful or feasible, victims must take appropriate action to extend their survival time while waiting to be rescued. Victims should keep as still as possible, since thrashing or swimming will only cause more rapid loss of body heat and energy. Victims should also try to get as much of the body as possible out of the water by laying the arms flat on the ice surface and by leaving them stationary. This step is very important because cold water pulls heat away from the body much faster than cold air. With luck, their arms will freeze to the ice surface and keep victims supported, even if unconsciousness sets in prior to rescue.

If self-rescue from the water is successful, hypothermia remains a serious threat to survival. Victims who are in remote areas must decide whether to stay put and try to find ways to increase body temperature or to go and seek shelter. If shelter is reasonably close (as a general rule: less than 30 min of exposure to the cold), it is best to go. If not, it is best to stay. If the decision is to go for help, victims should keep moving to increase heat production and quickly find shelter where wet clothing can be removed. If the decision is to stay, victims should wrap their bodies in some kind of vapour barrier and insulation. If possible, victims should build a fire. Dry clothing will help significantly. If it is available, victims should change into it. If not, wet clothing should be removed, wrung out, and put back on. A shelter should be built with anything available, particularly if the victims must spend the night.

5.11.2
Bystander Rescue

Those who are on the ice when someone else falls through should immediately, but slowly, lie down, distributing their weight over as large an area as possible, then move away from the area of weak ice by slowly rolling or crawling. If any means is available to summon further assistance, even by yelling to others, it should be done immediately. Rescuers should also don lifejackets or other buoyant objects, if available, for personal protection.

The safest approach for bystanders is to attempt to talk the victim out of the water, using the advice noted under self-rescue. Meanwhile, rescuers should look for objects to throw. Anything buoyant will help. If a rope is available, rescuers should tie a noose so that the victim can loop it around the body. Victims will have little strength or dexterity to hold the rope or tie it around themselves. If no rope is available, rescuers should look for anything that might be available to extend to the victim, such as a tree branch. The least favoured option is to attempt to slide sharp objects, such as screwdrivers or key-sets, across the ice that victims might be able to use to claw their way out of the water.

Rescues involving others can be physically and emotionally demanding for both rescuers and victims. The safety of rescuers is the primary and ongoing concern in a rescue

During any rescue effort, bystanders should wear personal flotation devices and be tethered ashore. If this is not possible, bystanders should seriously reconsider going on the ice or attempting a rescue. If one victim fell through, it is very likely that a second person will fall through, especially since the ice was weakened by the first victim. If rescuers fall through as well, the victim may be left with no source of assistance and there may well be a much more complex situation with two or more victims in a life threatening situation.

5.11.3
Professional Rescuers

Public safety agencies rarely seem to give ice rescue the respect accorded other types of rescue situations. Fire chiefs would never send fire fighters into burning buildings without thorough training and proper personal protective equipment. Search and rescue personnel are not expected to descend a sheer cliff without lines, harnesses, and other high angle tools. Nevertheless, untrained and poorly equipped public safety personnel are all too often allowed to attempt ice rescues. The result is that professional rescuers sometimes become victims and the victims they attempt to rescue needlessly drown.

A properly equipped and trained ice rescue team is needed anywhere there is ice. In addition to the ice rescue team, all members of the public safety departments should be trained at least to the awareness level. That includes training to recognise hazards, to keep bystanders away from hazards, and to perform some initial response duties like calling for appropriate response agencies, securing the scene and setting up the incident command system.

Proper protection of rescue personnel and victims requires an initial acknowledgement that effective training and equipment are mandatory to perform ice rescue operations. This includes equipment like ice rescue suits, harness, lines, and flotation slings, along with training in how to use them. There is also a need for policies that define effective and safe procedures, training, and equipment for ice rescue. Currently there is little consistency in ice rescue procedures and equipment designs are too often poor.

The conditions that necessitate ice rescues can include high winds, weak ice, open water, long distances and deep snow. Victim variables include trauma, body size, weight, panic and level of consciousness. Rescuer variables include body size, fitness, water experience and number of responding rescuers. All of these must be addressed in training and equipment design.

Well-designed rescue equipment is essential but this is often not the case for all commercially available ice rescue gear. An ice rescue suit should fit properly, have inherent positive buoyancy and not obstruct breathing. Many manufacturers however offer two sizes, both of which are very large. Conversely, ideal ice rescue technicians are lightweight people for whom these suits are often much too big. The gloves are sometimes so large that rescuers cannot grip ice awls. Their feet come out of the boots and the suits easily flood at the face opening. The feet of rescuers in these suits float to the surface unless ankle weights are worn. The rescue suits may have face flaps that fully cover the wearer's mouth and nose, thus obstructing the rescuer's breathing during exertion. It is very difficult for rescuers to move efficiently in the water when wearing protective ice rescue suits.

Rescue procedures must be designed and practised for negatively buoyant, very weak, cardiac-fragile, slippery victims being saved using the suits that will be used in actual rescue. A proven technique is to have the rescuer lay face down and approach the victim from the side to decrease the chance of breaking supportive ice. The rescuer clasps the wrist of the victim and applies a flotation sling to establish independent victim positive buoyancy (IVPB). The goal should be to accomplish this application within 10 seconds of contact. The more commonly taught rear approach places rescuers in the water and in a position in which they are more likely to pull the victim off the supportive ice before IVPB is established.

Another commonly taught rescue technique is to have a rescuer grab a victim, put a rope around the victim and use the suit of the rescuer for victim buoyancy. Sometimes the rescuer uses the victim for support while attempting to submerge the feet or change location in the water and accidentally pulls the victim under water or away from supportive ice. This technique sometimes works in training sessions, because mock victims wear buoyant ice rescue suits, but it is not effective in actual rescues.

Some transport devices designed to bring rescuers out and victims back work well in ideal conditions such as strong ice, no wind, and cooperative victims, but become difficult or risky to use in realistic, weak ice conditions. Recommended transport device features are listed in ◘ Table 5.1. Recommended ice rescue standards that allow safe and effective ice rescues are summarised in ◘ Table 5.2. The device should be usable with both adult and child victims, in states that range from aggressive to unconsciousness, including those with spinal and other trauma.

Equipment and training should allow for a properly prepared team to arrive on scene, dress one or two rescuers, reach a victim 70 metres out, gently establish IVPB, and gently transport the victim back to shore, in well under 10 min.

◘ Table 5.1. Features of good transport devices

Low wind susceptibility

Single rescuer operation

Easy righting if flipped in water

No assembly at scene

Padded edges

Two-victim capacity

Allowance of initial establishment of IVPB

Easy portage across difficult land conditions

Efficient crossing from ice to water and back on very weak ice

Simplicity of use

Usable with both adult and child victims

Usable with aggressive to unconscious victims

Usable for victims with spinal and other trauma

◘ Table 5.2. Ice water rescue standards

Minimum rescuer fitness levels

Minimum equipment and training levels for different kinds
of ice operations

Gentle and horizontal patient transport procedures

Definitions of "no-go" incidents

Annual drill requirements

Scene organisation

Incident command system officer duties

Proper incident documentation

Post-operation procedures

5.11.4
Lack of International Standardisation

The lack of international standardisation, and in many nations the lack of national standardisation, presents a significant problem. Additional research and discussion is badly needed in ice rescue to ensure consistency, safety, and effective methods for accomplishing this dangerous work.

5.11.5
Summary

Ice is never 100% safe. The best advice is to stay off it. Bystanders should use tremendous caution in attempting rescues, avoiding becoming victims themselves. Public safety organisations in areas where there is ice should be trained, prepared, and equipped to quickly and safely effect rescues using techniques that are thoroughly tested in real-life conditions. Regular drills are essential to maintain proficiency.

5.11.6
Websites

- www.teamlgs.com
- www.rip-tide.org
- www.lifesaving.ca

Further Reading

1. The Royal Life Saving Society Canada (2003) Ice, the winter killer: a resource manual about ice, ice safety and ice rescue. The Lifesaving Society, Ottawa
2. Hendrick B, Zaferes A (1999) Surface ice rescues. Fire engineering/PennWell, Tulsa
3. Hendrick B, Zaferes A (2003) Ice diving operations. Fire engineering/PennWell, Tulsa

5.12
Rescues Under Difficult Circumstances

5.12.1
Plane Crashes

MARTIN NEMIROFF

Data on submersion or immersion accidents following aircraft crashes in water is derived from areas where these crashes occur with regularity (◘ **Fig. 5.14**). One such area is the US State of Alaska, where the road system is minimal and much

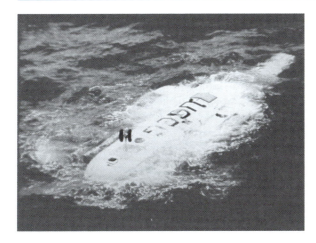

Fig. 5.14. Submerged fuselage of an aircraft crashed in ice-cold water

travel for recreation and business is conducted by air. It is not uncommon to have one air crash a day in certain areas, due to the volume of traffic and the inclement weather.

By nature air crashes in Alaska occur without much warning and mostly in remote areas. Because of the northern latitude much of the winter months are dark, leading to poor visibility. The suddenness, darkness, cold, and the water environment make these accidents difficult to survive, hard to find, and makes victim treatment very challenging.

5.12.1.1
Discussion

Survival factors that are normally considered in cold water near-drowning cases are:
- Age: the younger the age, the better the survival
- Underwater time: the shorter the better
- Water temperature: the colder the better
- Quality of cardiopulmonary resuscitation: major breaks in technique or omissions reduce survivability
- Amount of struggle: the less struggle the better the survival
- Water quality: better survival in clear water (translucent) than in swamp, mud, or other fluids
- Other major injuries: other injuries markedly reduce survival regardless of injury (blast, burn, head or long bone trauma)
- Suicidal intent: victims seeking suicide by drowning do less well than matched victims of accidental submersion [1]

We have used these factors to evaluate survivability of an air crash in the water. These crashes by their nature lead to panic, struggle, and problems in egress. The victims have a reduced survival rate compared to pure water immersion and submersion accidents. Water entry in non-acclimatised victims is associated with gasping, aspiration, and rapid onset of hypoxemia. This milieu makes the air crash in water deadly. Victims are rarely wearing appropriate floatation, and find themselves trapped in the aircraft. If the wreckage is not floating, water submersion commonly leads to drowning fatality.

If cardiac arrest occurs in the water there is much difficulty in performing adequate cardiopulmonary resuscitation without access to a solid surface. Some say it can only be done successfully on small children cradled in your arms while giving mouth to mouth breathing. This also necessitates some form of personal floatation.

Negative acceleration injuries associated with the aircraft striking the water may in and of themselves cause death. Striking the instrument panel, or being struck by flying debris in the cabin can cause injuries hampering normal survivability in water. Long bone fractures and closed head injuries commonly seen in such accidents decrease the survivability compared to victims with water submersion alone. Burn or blast injuries are especially lethal when added to this type of water accident.

Reference

1.   Nemiroff MJ (1992) Near drowning. Respir Care 37:600–608

5.12.2
Offshore Powerboat Rescues

Joost Van Nueten

Offshore powerboat racing has made an evolution as a very high-tech sport with a great concern for the safety of the pilots. The pilots are competing at speeds as high as 170 nautical miles (250 kilometres) per hour, quite against the laws of nature, and its unpredictability. Briefly, it is not the wind, but the washes of the waves, which are the most important risk factors for accidents to occur (◘ Fig. 5.15).

As in the history of all motorised sports, accidents result in attention by organisers and boat constructors to the importance of safety. The safety of the pilots could be optimised by introducing technical innovations such as mandatory carbonate safety cockpits.

There are, however, still many rescue problems for which better solutions have to be found. Knowledge of accident mechanisms during powerboat racing is critical for all rescuers to understand, including the risks that can be expected during rescue. All accident mechanisms can be combined with drowning. In these situations, the injured pilot needs to be rapidly extricated to prevent death by drowning.

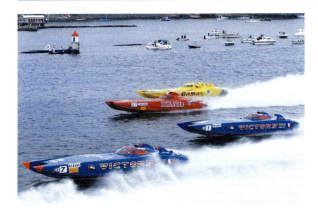

■ **Fig. 5.15.** Power boat pilots compete at speeds of up to 170 nautical miles per hour against the laws of nature

5.12.2.1
Each Time a Different Approach

The different types of water (open sea, lakes, or rivers) where powerboat racing occur have consequences for rescue activities. Most races take place offshore in open sea. The approach to a crash in open sea can be very difficult because of the current. Rescue divers should be dropped as close to the accident as possible, but still at a safe distance near the victims, to avoid separation. It should also be considered that escaping fuel can spread out very easy over a large area, especially when there is a strong current. Sudden fires over a large area result in a dangerous situation for rescue workers and victims.

The distances within the race circuits are very important towards rescue intervention times, so rescue boats always have to be placed at very strategic places.

5.12.2.2
Extrication of Trapped Pilots

Pilots in powerboat racing are principally strapped with a five-point safety belt with an unlock-system. All race pilots must fulfil an annual test in a simulator cockpit in open water to free themselves from a situation where the boat ends upside-down in the water (a 'turtle'). Most competitive powerboats have an emergency tank with compressed air. If a boat becomes inverted, the conscious pilot can use a mouthpiece to breath freely for approximately 10 min.

Some of the boats have an open cockpit, which means the pilot can be freed easily. For closed cockpits, it is a requirement that the rescue teams check the opening facilities in advance.

Despite extensive safety preparations the rescue team must often assist in the extrication of a pilot because the pilot is unable to free himself. If a pilot is unconscious or panicking, it is impossible for him to open the cockpit from the inside. The pilots express the experience as: "You are drowning in your helmet with visibility zero".

◘ **Table 5.3.** Common injuries in powerboat racing

Neurotrauma

Thorax and facial trauma

Cervical trauma

Penetrating injuries

Burns

Hypothermia

Neurotrauma

Rescue divers must work under extremely circumstances. Whenever there is a boat upside down with one or two unconscious pilots inside, the divers must divert their visual approach. In offshore powerboat racing there is an additional problem. Both pilots must swim away from the centre of the boat, otherwise they will be trapped under the 4- to 5-meters wide centre of the boat and drown. New techniques, like an escape hatch at the underside of the boat increases the possibility of an easy self-rescue by the pilots, but are hard to use by the rescuers in an emergency situation with injured pilots, because both victims have to be extricated together in a very short time to prevent them from drowning.

Once the victim is in a safe environment the treatment is not much different from the treatment of a victim from a road traffic accident or motor vehicle accident.

5.12.2.3
Use of Special Equipment

Stretchers used for the immobilisation and evacuation of multi-trauma victims in powerboat accidents should float. The stretcher must also be capable of being pushed easily under the water surface to scoop the victim in a stable, horizontal and completely immobilised way.

At races with large distances, the use of a rescue helicopter with special trained medical rescue divers on board should be considered. The divers can jump out of the helicopter on the accident site and immediately intervene. When a victim is winched out of the water, there is a risk that this worsens the injuries.

5.12.2.4
High Speed Water Racing Accident Mechanisms

The most common injury mechanism in powerboat accidents is deceleration trauma. The body of a powerboat pilot receives high G-forces during an accident.

The kinetic energy appearing in powerboat accidents with a sudden deceleration mechanism can be enormous. Collision often results in a multi-trauma victim. Common injuries in powerboat racing are summarised in ◘ **Table 5.3**.

Statistics of deadly accidents during offshore races between 1980 and 1995 show that 61% of the victims who die suffer from a basal skull fracture. Sometimes it is not clear if deceleration is the initial cause of the fracture or if the fracture is caused by contact with a hard rigid object (contact trauma).

The more space the pilot has in the cockpit, the higher the chances for neurological injuries. A helmet can never guarantee 100% safety at heavy impact accidents. Neurotrauma can cause different kinds of intracranial bleeding such as acute subdural hematoma and epidural hematoma. Concussion is very common in powerboat accidents. Scalp injuries have to be taken very seriously because this can result in a serious traumatic hemorrhagic shock.

5.12.2.5
Thorax and Facial Injuries

When a boat makes a nose-dive ('stuffed') it is possible that due to the collision with the water, the hood will break in several parts, resulting in facial injuries or thoracic injuries such as tension pneumothorax, pneumo-hemothorax or multi-rib fractures with a flail chest. The immediate insertion of a chest-tube can be lifesaving, even if this means an intervention on a rescue boat.

5.12.2.6
Cervical Trauma

During a race the head has to turn freely within limits, making the risks of injuries evident. A powerboat accident can cause serious cervical trauma and the risk of a serious whiplash injury is high. Every powerboat victim should be considered to have suffered from a cervical trauma. He must be treated according to the appropriate standards, until it has been proven otherwise. Extensive training by rescue divers is required to maintain the skill of stabilising the neck and applying a cervical collar in a proper way while both victim and rescuer are still in the water.

5.12.2.7
Penetrating Injuries

Penetrating injuries are fairly uncommon, and most likely caused by loose parts of the cockpit after a collision. The primary problem is to free the pilot who is struck in the shortest possible time without removing the penetrating object, to avoid heavy, uncontrollable bleeding. The rescue-workers should have all necessary equipment to extricate victims.

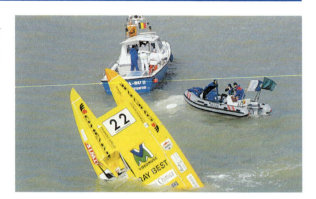

◘ Fig. 5.16. Rescue, extrication and resuscitation of power boat pilots can be extremely complicated

5.12.2.8
Burns

Although pilots wear fireproof clothing, serious full-thickness burns can occur. Rescue workers must start an IV fluid reanimation on-site as quick as possible. A rapid sequence intubation (RSI) must be considered in case of burning in the face, because of the risk for serious inhalation injuries.

5.12.2.9
Hypothermia

Offshore powerboat races are partly organised in countries with weather circumstances where hypothermia can occur. In most situations a short intervention time prevents the pilots from staying in the water for such a long period that the body temperature drops below 30°C.

In some situations, however, it takes a considerable length of time to reach and rescue the pilots and hypothermia occurs in these situations.

If drowning is combined with fast hypothermia, the chances of successful reanimation of the victim will increase. In these situations it is also considered to be important that the victim is removed from the water horizontally. A victim who is hypothermic should only be pronounced dead if there is no response to resuscitation after the corporal body heat has been increased gradually during CPR in a trauma centre.

5.12.2.10
Ventricular Fibrillation

Ventricular fibrillation can occur due to immersion hypothermia. When the body temperature is below 30°C it seems to be useless to defibrillate immediately. The victim must be warmed, both intra- and extra-corporally, before the medical team can defibrillate.

Experience has shown that fibrillation also occurs in powerboat accidents with non-hypothermic pilots, probably due to the high endogenous adrenaline discharge and the sudden contact with cold water. In these situations it has been demonstrated that defibrillation on board of a rescue boat can be successful and several pilots who have been defibrillated on board have been discharged from the hospital.

5.12.2.11
Conclusions

Extensive experience, technical knowledge, and a perfectly oiled, advanced approach system are mandatory for the successful rescue of powerboat victims (◘ Fig. 5.16). Both drowning and injuries can be life threatening. Rescue skills must continuously be reviewed and improved. The challenge to save lives after powerboat accidents is a delicate and often unequal battle against nature [1].

5.12.2.12
Website

━ www.powerboat-rescues.be

Reference

1. Van Nueten J (1996) The medical safety and approach of accidents in powerboat racing. RN-Thesis, Antwerp, p 70

5.12.3
The NASA Ocean Rescue Plan for the Space Shuttle

AHAMED IDRIS

The space industry is one of the most high tech, high profile, and high-risk enterprises existing in the world market. There are a wide variety of activities associated with the launch and landing of spacecraft including designing, construction, and vehicle testing. The tasks range from the routine to the very hazardous including handling toxic and highly reactive fuels. Astronauts are exposed to the most dangerous situations, including the possibility of catastrophic failure of the spacecraft during launch and landing. NASA has developed a detailed emergency medical rescue plan to enable a robust response to many of the known hazards that can occur during launch and landing operations of the space shuttle. This chapter will discuss briefly the space shuttle, its purpose, the hazards of space flight, and the emergency medical response plan in case of potential drowning.

5.12.3.1
Space Transportation System or the Space Shuttle

The space transportation system (STS) consists of four components: two solid rocket boosters, a main fuel tank, and the orbiter, which contains the crew compartment and the cargo bay. The space shuttle generates 7.3 million pounds of thrust during launch and it accelerates to 17,000 mph in 8 min, at which time it is in orbit around the earth. The combustion gases from the rocket engines are 3315°C (6000°F) and exit at 6000 mph.

5.12.3.2
Space Shuttle: Missions and Operations

The space shuttle has many important missions that have an impact on life on earth. The space shuttle carries telecommunications satellites into space and places them in orbit. Astronauts conduct scientific experiments on board the shuttle, send scientific probes into earth's orbit or send them into deep space for exploration and have conducted highly successful missions to repair satellites while in orbit. In addition, a few spectacular missions accomplished satellite repair by capturing satellites the size of a bus while in orbit, placing it in the shuttle cargo bay, and bringing it back to earth. At the present time, the shuttle is involved in constructing the International Space Station, which will be a base for scientific experimentation and a launch platform for human missions to mars and other planets.

All launches and most landings of the space shuttle take place at Kennedy Space Center (KSC) on the east coast of Florida where 12,000–16,000 workers are employed, including scientists, engineers, technicians, and other support personnel. They design, build, test, launch, and land spacecraft and their tasks range from the routine to the hazardous.

5.12.3.3
Hazards and Deadly Incidents at Kennedy Space Center

The myriad causes of injury during space flight operations include traumatic injury from explosion and high-speed crash on landing, burns, and the possibility of toxic exposures at KSC is abundant, severe, and sometimes deadly. Since 1983, there have been 1227 incidents in which workers sought medical care. Occasionally, some of these incidents have been fatal.

- 1967: Apollo 1 fire kills three astronauts during routine testing while on the launch pad. Following this disaster, 100% oxygen is no longer used for breathing in any space vehicle
- 1986: Challenger disaster, seven astronauts die. Cold and stiff O-rings in the solid rocket booster were implicated in this event
- 1995: Inhalation of nitrogen gas kills two European Space Agency technicians while working in a closed compartment
- 1996: Explosion of the Chinese Long March 3B booster kills hundreds, 1000 injured. This disaster occurred in China, not at KSC

- 2003: The Space Shuttle Columbia burns up during re-entry into the atmosphere. All astronauts on board are killed. An investigation panel blames foam and ice falling from the main fuel tank and striking the leading edge of the left wing during launch. The strike opens a small gap or hole in the wing that allowed 3000°C plasma gases to enter and melt the internal airframe of the wing during re-entry

5.12.3.4
Toxic Hazards

A variety of highly reactive and toxic fuels are used in various engines in the space shuttle. The fuels used in the three main engines of the shuttle are cryogenic propellants: liquid hydrogen (–257°C; –423°F) and liquid oxygen (–183°C; –298°F). A number of smaller engines for manoeuvring and attitude control use hypergolic propellants: hydrazine and nitrogen tetroxide. These highly reactive fuels explode on contact with air. The fumes are similar to breathing nitric acid and produce severe lung and CNS damage. The solid propellants used in the solid rocket booster release nitric acid-like compounds after burning. Rescue personnel are always deployed upwind of the launch pad to avoid contact with these fumes. The shuttle also contains liquid nitrogen and ammonia used for refrigeration and cooling.

A number of potential disasters (contingencies) have been identified and plans, called modes, have been developed to respond to these contingencies.

5.12.3.5
Prelaunch and Landing Contingencies

- Mode I: Unaided egress/escape
- Mode II: Aided egress/escape by closeout crew
- Mode III: Aided egress/escape by pad rescue team
- Mode IV: Aided egress/escape by pad rescue team, closeout crew on station
- Mode V: Unaided egress/escape after landing
- Mode VI: Aided egress/escape after a landing mishap on or near shuttle landing facility runway
- Mode VII: Unaided egress/escape, remote area
- Mode VIII: Unaided egress/escape in flight

5.12.3.6
Triage Sites

Rescue and medical forces are positioned at designated sites before launch or landing. The site is declared approximately 9 min before launch and is always placed upwind of the shuttle (◘ **Fig. 5.17**).

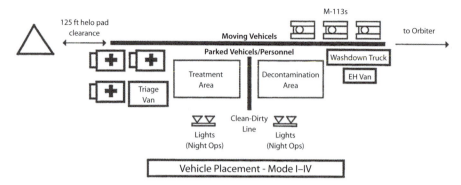

■ **Fig. 5.17.** Kennedy Space Center convoy configuration. The design for a triage site and triage site vehicle placement. M-113s are armoured personnel carriers. Vehicles identified with a cross are ambulances, the Washdown Truck is for decontaminating personnel. The EH Van is responsible for environmental control. The triage sites are designated areas. Equipment is brought to a triage site only after it has been designated 9 min before launch to ensure it is located upwind of the shuttle. The Clean-Dirty Line is the transition between the decontamination area and the medical care area. Only those who are uncontaminated with toxic substances or who have been decontaminated may cross to the clean side

5.12.3.7
Ocean Rescue Plan (Mode 8 Rescue)

After the Space Shuttle Challenger disaster in 1986, NASA developed plans for rescue of astronauts in the event of a catastrophic disaster during launch. In such a contingency, the shuttle is still flyable but lacks sufficient energy to achieve a runway landing. The shuttle is placed in controlled gliding flight after the solid rocket boosters are expended and jettisoned along with the main fuel tank. Each astronaut wears a pressurised space suit during launch and landing. The suit contains a parachute, and water wings and a life raft that automatically inflate on contact with water. The manoeuvre begins at an altitude of 40,000 feet (12,121 m) and starts with the shuttle slowing to approximately 200 knots. Next, the cabin is vented to obtain near-atmospheric conditions and the port hatch is jettisoned using explosive bolts. From 25,000 feet to 5000 feet (7575–1515 m) each crew member attaches his lanyard to a telescoping escape pole and tumbles out of the hatch. The telescoping escape pole was designed and tested following the Challenger disaster and will direct the crew member to fall under the shuttle wing. The parachute of the astronaut is automatically deployed when the lanyard reaches the end of the pole. After splashdown in the ocean, the astronaut is located and rescued by a US Department of Defence medical helicopter with a physician and paramedic-jumper on board. The helicopter is then directed to a triage site or to a hospital depending on the condition of the astronaut.

5.12.3.8
Summary

The space shuttle has been in operation since 1982 and has performed many important scientific and commercial missions. Between 1982 and 2003, there have been 113 launches and two catastrophic disasters. No unplanned ocean rescues have occurred but a medical disaster plan to deal with this and other possible contingencies have been prepared.

5.13
Rigid Inflatable Boats

HANS VERSMISSEN and TON HAASNOOT

From the early 1970s the (British) Royal National Lifeboat Institution (RNLI) and the Royal Netherlands Sea Rescue Institute (KNRM), have been developing a new concept of lifeboat design, the rigid inflatable boat (RIB). An RIB is basically a power boat with a fast 'deep-V' planing rigid hull and inflatable tubes as bulwark all around. Especially waterjet propelled RIBs have proved to be excellently suitable as lifeboats for the coastal environment of the Netherlands, where shoals over sandbanks, strong tides and, especially in strong northwesterlies, heavy surf dominate the scene. An abundance of yachts and traditional charter vessels with large crews in summer and of fishing craft all year round, further made fast lifeboats, with the excellent manoeuvrability of a waterjet RIB, a logical choice. In the 1980s the KNRM decided to further develop the RIB as their standard type of lifeboat.

The relatively light and fast RIB is a far cry from the old salt's conviction that a good seaboat should have 'a lot of wood in the water'. Indeed, the RIB owes its seaworthiness and usefulness as a lifeboat largely to their unprecedented agility, the deep-V bottom's soft ride in heavy seas and the significant contribution to stability of the bulwark tube. The energy absorbing traits of the tubes come to the fore when steep seas are encountered as well as in coming alongside casualties, especially not very robust ones, such as yachts. The tubes certainly protect lifeboat and crew when coming alongside very robust structures in heavy seas.

With over 15 years of experience with RIBs, the crews are convinced that the larger all weather units (47-foot and 62-foot) are under all circumstances faster and more responsive than the old self-righters of 1960s vintage; that the smaller craft (35-foot and 21-foot) are faster, safer and easier to launch than the old beach-launched double enders of pre-war Danish design; and that the currently used RIBs are great tools for lifesaving in Dutch coastal waters and river estuaries.

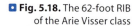 **Fig. 5.18.** The 62-foot RIB of the Arie Visser class

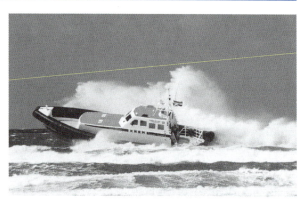

5.13.1
Demand for Fast Lifeboats

Throughout the two centuries history of lifeboat development, the increase in seaworthiness of lifeboats has seen an increase in the number of calls that could be answered. When in the early 20th century pulling boats were pushed into the museum by motor lifeboats, these could brave heavier weather and were consequently launched for services that would have been impossible under oars. When the third wave of improvement, self-righting motor lifeboats, appeared, a similar increase in calls answered and dangers to be braved occurred, despite the fact that merchant and fishing vessels were getting bigger and safer, so that fewer ran into trouble.

After the Second World War, dramatic changes on the 'client side', especially from the 1960s, made a fourth generation of lifeboats necessary. The proliferation of series produced glass reinforced plastic (GRP) yachts with affordable diesels and electronic navigation aids, brought relatively inexperienced yachtsmen in open waters. Ever increasing air traffic with jetliners and helicopters for the offshore industry, and mushrooming car-ferry services, made lifeboat services aware that disasters might occur many miles from the coast, involving large numbers of casualties with a short life expectancy in cold water. Clearly faster lifeboats would be needed and were tried by other lifeboat institutions. With conventional designs, however, speed and seaworthiness tended to be inversely proportional.

5.13.2
Developing and Funding of the Waterjet RIB

In 1973 the KNRM ordered its first *Atlantic 21* RIB, developed by RNLI. The 32 knots 180 nautical miles range craft, powered by twin 50 hp outboards, proved extraordinarily seaworthy, capable of keeping its speed for a relatively long period of time and very practical in coming alongside smaller craft. The experiences were so promising that larger waterjet driven types were developed.

The new building program took flight when, during the 1990s, the KNRM enjoyed a handsome increase in the size of bequests and dividends on its own assets, allowing an impressive investment program. RIBs with waterjets became the mainstay of the fleet.

Fitting out an entire fleet of 28 large (35-foot, 47-foot and 62-foot) and 31 smaller, relatively expensive fast RIBs obviously absorbs huge amounts of money. Also exploitation of fast craft is inherently more expensive than running a similarly sized fleet of conventional craft, mainly because of higher fuel consumption and a higher risk of material failure. Stocks of spare parts for each type must therefore be larger and more reserve craft are needed. However, these adverse effects are largely compensated by the fact that just five different types of RIB have replaced a fleet of 11 different types of conventional craft, including nine expensive 70-foot self-righting motor vessels.

5.13.3
Characteristics of RIBs

The KNRM's 47-foot all weather *Johannes Frederik* class and 62-foot long range *Arie Visser* class RIBs (◻ **Fig. 5.18**) have aluminium alloy hulls with many watertight compartments, the longitudinal and athwart bulkheads of which further add to the hulls' stiffness and impact resistance. The tubes consist of an outer tube made from closed cavity foam and a number of air-filled inner tubes. If the outer tube is damaged, only part of the enclosed air may escape. The 35-foot beach launched *Valentijn* class also has a 'boxed' aluminium alloy hull but a tube made of a thick foam plastic inside and a hard plastic outside. The smaller craft have GRP hulls, similarly divided in watertight boxes. In the event of an RIB hull being ripped open, for instance by hitting a container in the water at 32 knots, the tube will have sufficient buoyancy to keep the entire craft above water. With their buoyancy the tubes have proved to be very effective bulwarks against capsize.

Apart from the 'in hull' boxes, the 47-foot and 62-foot classes have six watertight compartments: forepeak, storage, two completely separated engine rooms, jetroom and wheelhouse. The wheelhouse offers the only 'inside' accommodation for crew and casualties, and is the 'air pocket' that will right the boat after capsize. As soon as the boat lists more than 90°, the engines are shut off automatically. The weight of the engines, above the waterline in inverted position, further helps the air pocket in the wheelhouse to right the boat. In the 35-foot *Valentijn* class, with open conning position, the air case in the double 'wheelhouse' roof does the righting job. From 2000 onwards a slightly bigger version of the *Valentijn* was introduced, mainly with more working space aft.

A capsize in the open RIB is more likely to throw all the crew off, which would make automatic self-righting dangerous, because the righted craft could easily be swept beyond the reach of the swimming crew. Here the coxswain must pull the trigger that inflates the inflatable bag on top of the roll bar, once he is convinced that all crew have got hold of the boat. In a larger RIB, with enclosed wheelhouses, at least the helmsman will remain on board after a capsize and he may be able to reach crew and/or casualties who may have been thrown off. Recovering people from the water with less than three men on board may however present problems. Some main particulars of the RIBs are summarised in ◘ Table 5.4.

5.13.4
Recovery of Drowned Persons with an RIB

To recover people from the water the 35-foot, 47-foot and 62-foot craft have hinged stern platforms, which normally act as vertical bulwarks, but in lowered position form a platform very near to the waterline and facilitate scooping up bulky bodies. The 47-foot class units for deployment in northern ports do without this arrangement because it decreases reserve buoyancy aft, which would be unhelpful in the heavy seas typical of the area. They have an 'A'-shaped outrigger, which swings outboard, with the lifting rope of the recovery net rove through its top-sheaf. The foot of the net is tied to the tube of the boat. The casualty can be floated into the net and horizontally recovered by pulling the rope and lifting the frame. Also, on the smaller RIBs recovery nets are used, one side tied to the inner-side of the tube, to roll the casualty on board. Although this method is far from ideal in circumstances with fractures, it enables the crew to get the casualty on board quite easily and, as needed in case of hypothermia, in a horizontal position.

5.13.5
Casualty Handling

On a smaller open RIB, casualty handling will often be restricted to improvising shelter against wind and spray. Resuscitation is only possible at reduced speed. In any case, the needs of patients must be the decisive factor for the throttle of the helmsman. Casualties should be kept aft in the boat, especially with their head, to minimise suffering from pitching.

Several modifications have been made in the 47-foot and 62-foot classes to allow stretchers to be carried into the wheelhouse without undue lifting by the crew or danger for the casualty by protruding bollards. Once in the wheelhouse, there is not much difference between a big RIB and other lifeboats, apart from the stresses that higher speeds may cause. The ability, however, to keep pace with the worst of waves in the North Sea, is an advantage that the lifeboat coxswain may deploy to alleviate the suffering of severely wounded patients. He may decide to call at a downwind port at a greater distance rather than persevere in the teeth of a storm.

Table 5.4. Main particulars of the hard core RIBs used by the KNRM

	Arie Visser	Joh Frederik	Valentijn	Harder	Atlantic 21	Atlantic 75
Overall length	18.80 m	15 m	10.60 m	9 m	6.5 m	7.5 m
Beam	6.10 m	5.20 m	4.10 m	2.94 m	2.64 m	2.49 m
Draught	1.03 m	0.90 m	0.75 m	0.52 m	0.79 m	0.81 m
Main engines	2×1000 hp	2×680 hp	2×430 hp	2×250 hp	2×70 hp	2×75 hp
Speed	35 knots	34 knots	34 knots	32 knots	32 knots	32 knots
Endurance at full speed	16 hours	8 hours	5 hours	5 hours	2.75 hours	3 hours
Displacement	28 tons	15 tons	10 tons	3.8 tons	1.4 tons	1.4 tons
Crew	6	5	4	3	3	3
Casualties	120	90	50	20	19	19

5.13.6
Personnel

Fast boats move more violently than conventional craft and hence need younger volunteer crews, aged 21–45. They will have to spend more time for the lifeboat than their conventional forebears, since the extended capabilities of the lifeboat imply that they will be called out more often. The dynamic behaviour of the lifeboat, increased technical complexity and often high exposure to the marine environment, also make higher levels of training compulsory, both intellectually and physically.

During courses, trainees are expected to get to grips with the intricacies of modern waterjet propulsion, radio communications, electronic navigation, radar and boat handling. There is a fuzzy interface to battle drill training: those aspects of lifeboat work in which the crews should best learn to act instinctively, such as survival in heavy weather, boat handling alongside casualties, retrieving and restarting the boat after capsize, and emergency medical treatment of casualties. The increased numbers of calls and courses imply that increasingly young crews find it difficult to combine a serious job ashore with their work for the lifeboat. Contrary to what had been hoped, the complexity of the RIB made professional coxswains necessary for the larger units (47-foot and 62-foot). Approximately 35% of the KNRM's coxswains now have a nautical background. For a beach launched Atlantic 21 or *Valentijn* a hardened yachtsman or windsurfer, trained for lifeboat duties might also be a good, or even better, alternative.

5.13.7
Navigation

Conventional chartwork is utterly impossible because at high speed, there is little time left for navigation and decisions must be taken rapidly, in a less than ideal environment. As it is often impossible to plan the voyage beforehand, modern lifeboatmen must be able to use their navigation system straight away, 'playing by ear', and the composition of the system must be geared to such use.

The KNRM puts emphasis on instruments that enhance the perception of the crew of their surroundings but do not construe the signals. Devices such as automatic radar plotting aid (ARPA) are therefore shunned because in the view of the KNRM it gives a false feeling of safety. Fast lifeboat crews need raw data and not already interrogated and interpreted data because these can lead to a wrong decision. More specifically and notably, the relative course instability of the RIB might cause the ARPA system to give wrong information.

Radar and electronic chart displays, whether or not with position plotters, are indispensable but it is difficult to find electronic equipment made for hard slamming in a wet environment. The 35-foot *Valentijn* class has an entirely watertight dashboard.

In its course bridge resource management (BRM), the KNRM trains crews to digest and interpret information from electronic sources as well as from what is actually happening outside, and to cooperate and share crucial information. In the often turbulent and noisy environment of an RIB in action, implicit trust in the judgement and actions of fellow crew members is crucial for success.

Whatever the level of sophistication of instruments might be, however, there is nothing that beats local knowledge as a sound basis on which to interpret all information, either from the sensory perception of the crew or from their electronic wizardry. Lifeboats operate in a relatively small sea area around their station and constantly upgrading local pilotage information is a crucial goal of exercises, in which the crews also train in old-fashioned seamanship, such as boat handling and deck work, at times under exceedingly difficult conditions.

RIBs are small craft and the skills needed to operate them safely are often underestimated. Reaction times are short; safe navigation therefore requires participation of the entire crew in looking out and sharing information about their observations with coxswain and helmsman. If there is any doubt about the safety of the waters ahead, speed must be reduced.

At high speed, the helmsman should concentrate on driving the RIB; other tasks such as navigation and radio communication fall necessarily to other crew members. The coxswain will preferably keep his hands free for leading the crew and not steer the craft himself. He must be able to concentrate on processing information, to command and act where needed, rather than be bound by the wheel.

5.13.8
The Value of the RIB to Rescue from Drowning Under Extreme Conditions

A heroic service to a German yacht, grounded on the dangerous northern mole of IJmuiden's outer sea harbour on September 4th 2001, proved the talents of the RIB.

After several days of northwesterly gales, IJmuiden's 47-foot RIB *Christien* and nearby Wijk aan Zee's beach-launched 35-foot RIB *Donateur* were alerted at 15.28, after a life-raft had been sighted on the mole. Not knowing what to expect, *Christien* left port immediately and *Donateur* was launched soon after, in a severe northwesterly gale with 18-foot waves. With help from the shore, both RIBs sighted a German yacht on the mole only when they had come to within a cable's distance. The coxswain of the *Donateur* put his craft stern first against the yacht, which was washed further up the big, square concrete blocks of the mole with each 18-foot breaker. The three crew members of the yacht, however, remained apathetic in the cockpit and only after a second run in, stern first, head to the atrocious seas, was one crew member retrieved with extreme difficulty. During the third run in a man was spotted in the water. While *Donateur* manoeuvred alongside the casualty to take him on board, *Christien* moved between lifeboat and yacht to retrieve the third, motionless man, at which point one crew member jumped in the water to rescue him. With *Donateur* very close astern – and by then two men in the water, one crew member having been pulled overboard by the overweight yachtsman – and the wreck, concrete blocks and swimming crew

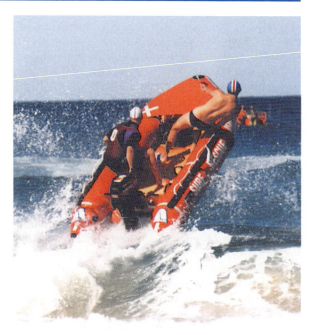

■ **Fig. 5.19.** The IRB is the most important rescue craft for lifesavers in Australia and injuries can occur during rescues

in front of him, the coxswain of the *Christien* had to keep his boat on station. Finally the *Donateur* crew recovered their two men and *Christien* moved in, bow first, to pull crew and the remaining yachtsman free. Both men were hit once by the 15-ton lifeboat but were eventually recovered alive. By 16.20 both lifeboats had delivered their patients to IJmuiden.

In a conventional boat this action would have been utterly impossible, with vulnerable propellers in danger of getting fouled on the wreck, on the rocks or in the rigging, which was adrift all over the place, and with insufficient power and manoeuvrability to steer clear of the casualties and the treacherous mole in 18-foot breaking waves.

5.14
Inshore Inflatable Rescue Boat Injuries with Implications for New Designs

PETER FENNER

The inshore inflatable rescue boat (IRB or 'rubber duck') is probably the most important rescue craft for surf lifesavers in Australia (■ Fig. 5.19). Due to its speed and manoeuvrability, it is used for up to 75% of rescues. However, injuries occur to both crew person and driver during such rescues. It was found that the standard IRB did not have sufficient speed and was susceptible to rollovers while operating in the larger surf or dumping surf, which is often the cause of swimmers encountering difficulties and requiring rescue.

IRB competition was used by Surf Life Saving Australia (SLSA) to promote skill in both drivers and crew persons, but as competition became increasingly fierce, boats and engines were developed which made the craft faster and faster with crews attempting more dangerous manoeuvres at speed. The escalating injury rate eventually caused the SLSA insurers to insist on a review of procedures that culminated in the total cessation of current IRB racing whilst other formats were developed [1]. Investigations into cause and effect through an epidemiological study of injuries in patrol and rescues were assessed. SLSA insurance claim forms and injury report forms from competition injuries were reviewed.

Epidemiology research at Queensland Institute of Medical Research (QIMR) investigated and published data on the incidence, type, and location of injuries of Queensland surf lifesavers for WorkCover (Queensland Workers Compensation insurance scheme) [2]. WorkCover injuries were documented for one season and suggested an estimated incidence of injury of 1.2%. Injury forms from Surf Life Saving Queensland showed that these injuries showed a substantial rate of morbidity and it was believed that a considerable number of injuries occurred that were not reported to WorkCover for various reasons [3]. Their statements confirmed witnessed events at the start of the biomechanical investigation.

The data showed that 62% of the injuries occurred to the right side of the body and of these injuries, 68% were to the lower limbs. The most prevalent injury types were fractures and fracture-dislocations where 75% occurred to the lower limbs, and that the crew person sustained 86% of the injuries. Also, the majority of injuries took place when the IRB was travelling out to sea in medium sea conditions at medium to slow speeds in overcast conditions when hitting spilling or plunging waves. It was suggested that the possible cause of these injuries identified related to driver inexperience or immaturity, and the faults in the design of the IRB.

5.14.1
Biomechanical Study

The Queensland University of Technology, hoping to explain why the injuries were occurring and to propose changes for prevention or reduction, undertook an investigation of the biomechanics of the boat and crew person. The objective of the biomechanical project was to identify causes and to propose processes that might reduce the instances and severity of injury to surf lifesavers during the operation of IRBs in patrol work and competition.

They identified common injuries; sites of injury and the epidemiology were then linked to a mechanical engineering design using biomechanics and a computerised model (◘ Fig. 5.20). An analysis of the craft design was then performed whilst various accelerations and forces applied to the crew in the IRB were investigated through experimentation [4].

IRBs encounter waves that cause large decelerations of the boat. Evidently, the causes of IRB injuries are closely related to problems resulting in motor vehicle

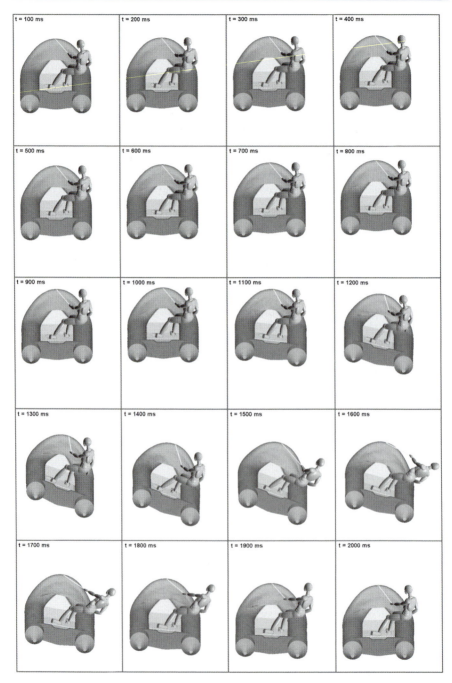

🔲 **Fig. 5.20.** The biomechanical model used to identify injuries that can occur during IRB rescues (courtesy of the School of Mechanical Manufacturing and Medical Engineering at the Queensland University of Technology, Australia)

injuries, where energy is transferred from the vehicle to the occupant. However, the injuries that occur in motor vehicles are due to vehicle crashes, unlike IRB injuries, which generally occur during normal operation of the boat.

Four key areas studied were:

- Variability of strap design and placement on the floorboards in all IRB models in use
- Measurement of the mechanical properties of the boat relating to the position of the hinge in the floorboard, inflation pressure, and model type
- Development of a mathematical model of the IRB and crew in three-dimensions to show the physical characteristics of the boat and personnel
- Measurement of the accelerated movement of the IRB in use to establish the ride characteristics of the IRB, as well as the movements and forces encountered by the crew

This analysis showed the IRB foot strap pattern and position were directly related to the patterns of injury seen. Early results in craft set-up and altered or adjusted crew positions have been encouraging and further work continues in this area. Analysis also showed that increasing foam thickness a little reduced impact, but after a critical point no benefit was observed. Variation in density in thin foam was very beneficial, whereas this effect was less noticeable in thicker foam.

Another major development has occurred with the assessment of other types of IRB including the new Gemini IRB. This is a catamaran craft that has a small pontoon under each side. This construction gives a smoother and softer ride than the conventional keeled IRB and the Gemini IRB rides the water flatter than the current IRBs. This is evident when punching waves which results in it coming down softer and more comfortably for the crew. It is also more stable than existing IRBs, allowing greater movement on the Gemini IRB without affecting the trim of the craft, and does not require the crew to move to compensate the trim. It has different turning capabilities, is more responsive, and can be turned relatively sharply.

The Gemini IRB also offers two crewing positions: the usual crew position on the pontoon, but also the option of sitting inside the boat, securely on the floor. The bow rope has been positioned further around to the port side of the craft to ensure better centre of gravity. Finally the flow-through transom ensures that the craft does not take water when going through the break. SLSA is currently working on alternative techniques for the drag and launch of the craft, as it is somewhat heavier than the usual IRBs.

5.14.2
Skeletal Maturity, Strength and Technique

The 'Bronze Medallion' is an award that can be gained at the age of just 15 years. Until recently part of the Bronze Medallion syllabus included a section of training as an IRB crew person; however, at 15 lifesaver trainees usually have insufficient strength and have not reached skeletal maturity, thus making them more prone to injury. IRB skills have now been removed from the Bronze Medallion training regime and the minimum age for an IRB crew person has been raised to 16, whereby physical strength, development, skeletal maturity must still be taken into account, as well as the presence of any pre-existing physical characteristic predisposing to possible injury. Others, especially those having been previously injured, may have a medical biomechanical problem that affect safe lifting practices with any task.

Medical and occupational health data has been used to produce guidelines to ensure that physical characteristics and growth maturity can be assessed by qualified personnel prior to training for many SLSA awards, including the IRB crew person's certificate.

References

1. Ashton LA, Grujic L (2001) Foot and ankle injuries occurring in inflatable rescue boats (IRB) during surf lifesaving activities. Orthop Surg (Hong Kong) 9:39–43
2. Fairfax R (1998) Ergonomic evaluation of inflatable rescue boat operation. WorkCover Techsource, WorkCover NSW (unpublished)
3. Bigby KJ, McClure RJ, Green AC (2000) The incidence of inflatable rescue boat injuries in Queensland surf lifesavers. Med J Aust 172:485–488
4. Ludcke JA, Pearcy MJ, Evans JH, Barker TM (2001) Impact data for the investigation of injuries in inflatable rescue boats (IRBS). Australas Phys Eng Sci Med 24:95–101

5.15
Development and Use of Personal Watercraft in Aquatic Rescue Operations

Jim Howe

The use of small boats in aquatic rescue is well documented, beginning with the use of dories or shoreboats. These small oar-powered rescue boats were standard equipment for aquatic rescuers from the 1840s through the 1960s.

In 1848 the US Congress appropriated funds to build eight small lifeboat stations on the Eastern Seaboard of the Continental United States. The typical method for rescuing the occupants of ships which had foundered was the use of lifeboats, launched through the surf [3].

The introduction of motorised inflatable rescue boats (IRB) in Australia in the late 1960s changed the way rescue of recreational swimmers was managed: "The potential of the craft for Australian conditions was recognised in 1969 and in the very short time since has become the modern-day reel, line, and belt" [2].

The initial introduction of the personal watercraft (PWC) to the surf rescue community was undertaken by PWC manufacturers in Southern California in the 1970s. The first PWCs were designed for operation by a single driver in the standing position. They were developed to combine the elements of small craft size, manoeuvrability, and an active ride. These first PWC proved less desirable than the already established IRB. Hull instability, lack of carrying capacity, and the high potential for operator and patient injury led to the concept being dropped.

PWC designs changed dramatically in the mid 1980s, from the single person stand-up style craft to a sit-down craft model designed for one- or two-person use. These redesigned craft, which had larger capacity and a more stable hull design, were commercially successful. The industry responded by developing even larger, more stable crafts, which can now accommodate two, three, or four people.

In early 1989 ocean rescue IRB operators on Oahu, Hawaii, began to experiment with the use of sit-down PWCs. IRBs, which were successfully deployed in Hawaiian surf conditions up to heights of 4 meters since 1985, had proved to be unreliable for use in surf conditions any larger. The IRB did not have sufficient speed and was highly susceptible to overturn while operating in the larger surf (surf heights routinely reach 6–8 meters in Hawaii and regularly reach heights of 20 meters). Flip-overs, in most cases, put the craft out of operation.

PWC proved to be faster, less susceptible to flip-over, and in the event of a flip-over, could go immediately back into operation. These craft characteristics, coupled with the simultaneous development of a specialised rescue sled towed by the PWC, allowed rescue operators to perform rescues quickly and safely in surf and ocean conditions the IRB could not safely handle.

The PWC and rescue sled (PWC-RS) system was extensively field tested in the Hawaiian Islands. During the 1990–1991 Hawaiian winter surf season the system proved its reliability in limited trials. At the end of the high surf season the trials were further expanded. The PWC-RS system proved to be effective in a wide variety of ocean conditions and aquatic rescue applications. This system outperformed the IRB in every situation during the trial period.

In 1991, PWC-RS was introduced to the world aquatic rescue community at the Powered Surf Rescue Experience in New Plymouth, New Zealand. Since that time the use of PWC-RS has spread to the aquatic rescue community worldwide.

The PWC-RS provides the craft operator with a stable, high-speed, exceptionally manoeuvrable vessel, which can operate under the most extreme aquatic conditions. Its shallow draft, compact size, and relatively low weight allow for quick launching and operation in environments inaccessible to propeller-powered craft. The rescue sled adds additional stability, a platform to carry rescue and safety equipment and other rescuers, and the ability to pick-up, transport and treat single or multiple patients (◘ Fig. 5.21).

In addition to its main mission of assisting and rescuing recreational swimmers, PWC are now routinely used for the towing of disabled craft, such as kayaks, sailboards, sail kites, surfboards, and small boats of all varieties up to 30 feet. Of special note was the use of a single PWC to rescue multiple boaters in distress during Hurricane Iniki from Lahaina Harbour moorings in 1992. Cliff and rock stranding rescues, ocean cave rescues, search and recovery missions, and aircraft crash responses have also been documented.

As the use of the PWC-RS has spread beyond Hawaii, it has been adopted for use in other aquatic environments and rescue scenarios. The Hood River (Oregon) Fire Department successfully developed a PWC response team for the

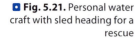 **Fig. 5.21.** Personal water craft with sled heading for a rescue

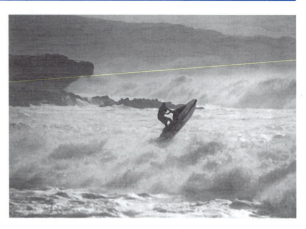

rescue of windsurfers, boaters, and kayakers in the area popularly know as 'The Gorge' located on the Columbia River in 1995.

In 1993 and again in 1997 the San Diego Lifeguard River Rescue Team responded to major flooding situations in the Tijuana River Valley and in Sacramento, California. In both cases PWC and IRBs were utilised. In situations where barbed wire fencing and other flood debris presented puncture and entanglement problems for IRBs, the PWC became the craft of choice. PWC were used to assist in evacuation efforts and to transport feed to stranded livestock.

PWC have been specially adapted for use in a number of other aquatic safety applications. Craft have been modified to carry a foam spray cannon, mounted on the bow, which allows for quick response to and suppression of small boat gasoline fires on the waterways. PWC are being used by the military for man-overboard situations at sea, shore landings, and ordinance disposal missions. They are also being extensively used for aquatic safety in television and film industry projects, aquatic-sporting events, underwater and near-shore construction projects, and in oil spill mitigation efforts.

Having enumerated the benefits of PWC use, it is also prudent to note limitations. Operator skill and proficiency training has been noted by the US National Transportation Safety Board as an area of concern. Their 1998 Safety Study on Personal Watercraft quotes a Centers for Disease Control analysis that, "... the rate of PWC related injuries requiring emergency medical treatment was 8.5 times higher than the rate of injuries from motorboats" [1].

The report goes on to state that the most prevalent type of accident (46%) was vessel collision. The estimated speed at the time of accidents in 49% of cases was between 21 and 40 mph. In 84% of cases, the operator of the craft reported having no training in the use of the PWC. For operators with more than ten experiences operating the craft, the accident rate was reduced to 18%.

Of equal concern is the area of operator and patient safety during rescue missions. The PWC allows the craft operator easy access to highly dynamic and inherently hazardous aquatic environments. The PWC system quickly and efficiently moves a rescuer to the scene of person(s) in distress and back to shore. In the event of craft failure under hazardous conditions the operator and the mission can be put at substantial risk. In such cases, mission safety will be dependent upon the aquatic skills of the craft operator independent of the craft.

Additionally, PWC use puts the operator, crew, and patient in close proximity to the water. In cold-water environments, this can be problematic. PWC use requires a high degree of operator reflex and motor skill coordination. The effects of cold, in its slowing of reflex and motor skills, must be considered when deciding on the use of a PWC-RS system.

To date, the PWC-RS system has proven to be an effective method to move professional rescuers to persons in distress in numerous aquatic environments and situations. Given the speed, manoeuvrability, and access advantages the system offers there is little doubt use will continue to expand. In 1998 PWCs accounted for more than one-third of new recreational boat sales, at more than 200,000, with more than 1 million in current use in the US.

At present, there are no studies available for accident rates during rescue operations. Anecdotal evidence, based on 10 years of daily operations of four PWC-RS system teams on the Island of Oahu, indicates that the majority of injuries to operators and crews occur in the first 6 months of assignment to craft operations.

All persons who will be engaging in rescue operations utilising PWCs need to complete training programs designed to develop adequate craft handling and riding skills prior to rescue skill training. Of equal importance is rescue skill training, with and without the PWC-RS system, specific to the aquatic environment where the craft will be operated.

It is clear the PWC-RS system is a tool of significant value in many aquatic rescue applications. There are numerous indications that the use of this system will continue to grow and variations on proven applications will be undertaken. At the present time there is a lack of recognised training standards for PWC operations.

Further research is necessary to identify appropriate uses of the PWC in aquatic rescue. Minimum training and certification standards are needed if the full potential of the PWC is to be realised in the aquatic rescue field.

References

1. National Transportation Safety Board (1998) Personal watercraft safety, NTSB/SS-98/01, Washington, D.C.
2. Surf Lifesaving Association of Australia (1986) Inflatable rescue boat training examination and operations manual, 3rd edn.

5.16
Alternatives for Rescue Boats

5.16.1
Hovercraft

MICHAEL VLASTO

The vision of the Royal National Lifeboat Institution (RNLI) is to be recognised universally as the most effective, innovative and dependable lifeboat service. As part of this quest, the RNLI has kept an eye on many forms of transport. Recent developments in power plant design enabled a reduction in the size of diesel engines on hovercrafts and allowed a fresh look at the potential of small hovercrafts as search and rescue (SAR) vehicles.

The current situation is that there are probably a dozen lifeboat stations throughout the UK and Northern Ireland where there is a history of mud rescue and where the RNLI has been unable to reach casualties. In such cases, HM Coast Guard or Fire Brigade mud rescue teams need to be deployed with great difficulty from the shore, or helicopters are deployed to effect rescue. Also at some estuary locations, lifeboats have to take large detours in order to circumnavigate sand and mud banks to reach casualties at low water.

With a target of otherwise inaccessible tidal areas of our coastline in mind, hovercraft should prove to be a positive asset to our search and rescue capability (◘ **Fig. 5.22**).

5.16.1.1
Phase 1

In 1999, a small group was given the task of sourcing an "off the shelf" hovercraft to meet the needs as defined by the RNLI Operational Requirements for an inshore rescue hovercraft (IRH) for evaluation purposes.

The findings of the group showed that hovercraft may have a role to play in the SAR operation of the RNLI, and the group therefore recommended that the operational requirements be re-examined and a suitable commercially available hovercraft be obtained, tested and reported on.

5.16.1.2
Phase 2

The operational requirement was duly revised and the necessary budgetary considerations made to purchase a Griffon 450TD hovercraft. The only changes made to the original specification of the manufacturer was to replace part of the rigid side deck with an inflatable section (sponson) to allow the craft to conform with the requirements of the UK Road Traffic Act when being towed on its trailer. Additional to the basic specification was the fitting of a Furuno Radar, a Northstar GPS Chart plotter, and a blue beacon.

The Griffon 450TD was delivered in December 2000 and pilot training was carried out at the beginning of January 2001.

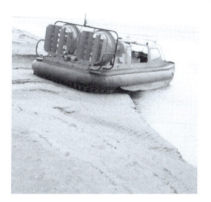

Fig. 5.22. The inshore rescue hovercraft makes the transition from water to land

The following objectives were laid down prior to the commencement of the trial:

— To establish the operating limitations with respect to terrain, weather, sea state, visibility and darkness
— To compare the efficacy of the hovercraft with the "D" Class for afloat casualties within the operating limits
— To assess environmental obstacles
— To establish the amount of training required to achieve an adequate level of competence for pilots and crew
— To determine whether a hovercraft can safely approach a casualty without causing added distress such as spraying or blasting the casualty with mud, sand or water, with a technique for achieving this under diverse conditions to be developed during trials
— To determine the time-to-readiness and the clean-up-time
— To determine how effectively a hovercraft can recover a casualty vessel to a place of safety (towing capabilities)
— To determine whether a hovercraft would be more effective if fitted with radar
— To determine how well the hovercraft can deal with a medevac (the evacuation of victims)

The craft was put through its paces and tested in various terrains, weather conditions and rescue scenarios and the recommendation was that the hovercraft be modified and further trialled at selected coastal inshore lifeboat stations. For an overview of the criteria borne in mind throughout and an evaluation of the trials see **Table 5.5**.

◘ **Table 5.5.** Key performance issues for rescue craft

Fitness for purpose

Robustness

High availability

Speed to casualty

Safety and survivability of crew

Sea keeping

Communications capability

Navigation capability

Ease of maintenance

Ease of handling

Operation and maintenance compatibility with volunteer crew

Built to appropriate codes and standards

5.16.1.3
Phase 3

Having established that the hovercraft was capable of satisfying the operational requirements, extended coastal trials were conducted during the summer of 2001 where the following objectives were tested:

- To assess whether the maintenance load on the volunteer crew is acceptable
- To assess whether the training requirements of the volunteer crew is acceptable
- To confirm that the hovercraft is suited to the types of coastal terrain in the selected areas
- To expose the hovercraft to true operational scenarios and evaluate its durability

5.16.1.4
Results of the Trials

The terrain limitations and the capabilities of the hovercraft are influenced by the payload. The hovercraft operates well on water, but is limited by weather and sea state.

The hovercraft operates well on sand; considerations are the dryness of the sand and the slope of the surface influencing direction. The maximum slope that the hovercraft can operate on is dependent on the load carried and the length of the slope, as the hovercraft can tackle steeper slopes using momentum to assist.

Mud of any consistency is coped with well by the hovercraft, mud features such as skerries up to a height of 40 cm (16 inches) can be passed down the centre of the hovercraft and vertical steps of up to 30 cm (12 inches) can be tackled with the right amount of momentum. Generally the maximum continuous slope that can be tackled is in the order of 1 in 10.

The hovercraft cannot cope with dry, loose shingle. Shingle mixed with sand can be traversed but the commander must be sure of the consistency of the shingle prior to venturing onto it. It is more prudent to avoid such terrain.

Gullies with steep sides of depths up to 30 cm (12 inches) can be crossed with care, approaching this depth, the skids under the hovercraft cause damage to the banks of the gully.

The type of vegetation encountered during the trials was primarily sea grass. It was found that the hovercraft would be stopped by sea grass of a length of 80 cm (32 inches) if there is no water at the base to maintain a seal around the cushion.

Beyond a wind speed of more than 25 knots, the hovercraft is not controllable and the hovercraft is strictly limited to a 60-cm (2-foot) significant wave height. Whilst the hovercraft hull can cope quite effectively with this sea state, the risk of shipping green water through the thrust fans is too great. The result would be catastrophic failure of the high revving propeller blades with resultant disabling of the craft and potential risk to personnel.

The minimum horizontal visibility required to operate the craft to its full potential safely and effectively is a quarter of a mile. Visibility severely limits night operations.

Environmental Impact

To assess the environmental impact, close liaison with English Nature (EN), the Royal Society for the Protection of Birds (RSPB) and Poole Harbour Commissioners has been maintained, and the Dorset Wildfowlers organisation consulted.

Surface marks on sand and mud are erased by the next tide. Damage is virtually nil and birds were observed to feed in the affected areas soon after the craft had passed. Within the operational limits of this type of terrain, there is no damage to grass and reeds.

Approaching a Casualty

The approach must be slow with minimum revs to maintain cushion and forward movement, in this manner there is no spray or blasting forward and the noise levels are not intrusive. As the casualty is drawn alongside the craft, the weight disposition of the crew ensures that any air escaping from the cushion (causing spray) is expelled on the opposite side of the craft.

Time-To-Readiness and the Clean-Up-Time

The time to clean the craft after a normal training sortie was 1 hour for two people and after mud rescue sortie was 2 hours for four people, including the mud rescue equipment.

With appropriate post operation checks, cleaning and routine maintenance, the craft is typically ready to deploy within 2 min of the commander reaching the craft kitted out in personal protective equipment.

How Well Will the Hovercraft Deal with a Medevac?

It has been proven that the carriage of a stretcher-borne casualty poses no problems but any ongoing treatment whilst on board may be limited by the requirement to maintain trim.

5.16.1.5
Results of Extended Coast Trials

In general, location selection for hovercraft should be based on terrain type; large areas of shallow water, tidally exposed sand and mud. Site familiarisation will become an important part of the successful use of hovercraft and will help to keep skirt and hovercraft damage to a minimum.

The hovercraft can approach casualties over sand banks in a more direct line, saving time.

The presence and location of steep-sided sandbanks should be reconnoitred during exercises.

Mud flats, usually featuring gullies, can usually be negotiated but experience and familiarisation will minimise the possibility of getting stuck.

On completion of the trials at each of the four RNLI stations, questionnaires were distributed to all those involved. All responded positively with 100% acceptance of the training, maintenance and post sortie cleaning requirements. Approximately 40% of the respondents experienced weather and sea state limitations but none of the respondents experienced terrain limitations.

Also, none of the respondents experienced any problems with the public and all respondents saw a future for the hovercraft within the RNLI.

5.16.1.6
Conclusions

- A hovercraft is not a lifeboat in the conventional sense, but what it can do, it can do very well. Beyond its narrow band of capability it is ineffective by comparison
- Payload is critical with hovercraft and therefore any equipment that is added must be both essential and of minimum weight
- The areas of competence of the hovercraft are confined to the inter-tidal margins in areas where banks have a relatively shallow gradient and smooth profile
- With respect to the environmental aspects, the hovercraft does virtually no damage in those areas where it is capable of operating. There is a perceived problem with noise, however, measurements have shown that noise levels are acceptable (less than 85 dB) outside a radius of 15 metres
- Casualties can be approached safely and without adding to their discomfort or distress
- Clean-up time depends on the nature of the sortie and typically will vary between 1 and 2 hours

- Hovercraft should not be used as a towing vessel
- Bearing in mind the operational limitations of hovercraft and the concentration required of the commander, radar would not enhance the capability of a hovercraft in this role

5.16.2
Jet Boats

Peter Dawes

For an organisation dedicated to the saving of lives the suitability and reliability of the equipment it uses is vital.

Surf Life Saving Queensland has developed a craft with a waterjet propulsion system based on more than 20 years of experience. The craft is used for patrolling extensive beach areas in Queensland. The operational environment includes high seas, shallow waters, and river mouths where the jet system provides a high level of performance (◘ Fig. 5.23).

5.16.2.1
The Craft

After extensive evaluation of other craft used by rescue organisations around the world Surf Life Saving Queensland settled on a package that includes an aluminium hull with a Volvo TAMD 42 marine diesel engine coupled to a Hamilton model 212 waterjet.

The craft has excellent shallow water running and inshore capabilities combined with a longer range than the existing inflatable rescue boats (IRB) that have been available to Surf Life Saving Queensland (◘ Table 5.6).

In addition, design features of the craft deliver the following benefits:
- Flat profile with shallow draft suitable for operations across shallow sandbanks
- No propellers or underwater appendages to hit debris or patients
- High power to weight ratio. This means high speed and high manoeuvrability
- Option of recovering patients, divers, or rescuers via a transom door and platform at the rear of craft
- Engine box covered with a surf mat. This is a floating mat capable of being detached as a rescue and survival aid
- Excellent towing capability for the size of craft
- Capable of limited night operations

Surf Life Saving Queensland operates jet rescue boats as part of a total service concept incorporating: beach patrols, powercraft, 4WD vehicles, helicopter surveillance and communications systems. The organisation currently operates four jet rescue boats in SE Queensland each performing 1200–2000 hours of operations each season.

◘ **Fig. 5.23.** A jet boat

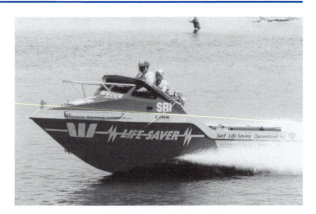

◘ **Table 5.6.** Specifications of the SLS Queensland jet boat

Length	5.9 metres
Beam	2.3 metres
Draught	100 mm
Displacement	1.8 tons
Construction	Hamilton 212 waterjet
Engine	Volvo TAMD 42, 170 kW at 3800 rpm
Speed	35 knots
Weight of craft (all up)	2 tons
Fuel tank capacity	200 litres
Range of craft	10 hours at 35 knots at 3500 RPM
Average fuel consumption	17 litres per hour
Capacity	3 crew and up to 6 patients

The Surf Life Saving Australia crew training provides for three levels of crew: jet rescue boat crew, jet rescue boat driver and jet rescue boat skipper. All candidates for training are required to have an extensive background as patrolling surf lifesavers prior to commencing training.

5.16.2.2
Future Design Considerations

While the existing craft have proven successful, continued improvement in jet units – in particular with the increasing popularity of PWCs and advances in potential construction hull materials such as light weight, stronger composites – will no doubt lead to improvements in design options.

5.16.3
Paraglider

RUY MARRA

5.16.3.1
Para Life Rescue Tool

The invention of a paramotor (a paraglider with an engine behind the pilot) was not originally considered for use as a potential rescue tool. It seemed to fit into sport and entertainment activities. However, in 1997 this reality changed when Ruy Marra (two-time Brazilian champion of paragliding) was flying under the sponsorship of a multinational company with a team of ten paramotors. He observed a woman drowning and flew above her. He dropped his life preserver to her and performed the first para-lifesaving act in the world. The technique has since been used successfully on different beaches in Brazil and para-lifesaving was responsible for 85 rescues in a 3-month period. The lifesavers are satisfied with the Para Life Support and both teams work together connected through radios, which reinforce the importance of humans and technology working towards lifesaving.

5.16.3.2
The Operation

The paragliders begin the day by strapping on 30 kilograms of lightweight equipment that folds up to the size of a knapsack. Equipped with life preservers, binoculars, radios, and a small motor that allows for rapid ascent or descent, the pilot takes off on foot.

A pilot can stay airborne for 3 hours and consumes roughly 3 litres of gas per hour. In Rio de Janeiro, three teams of two pilots each work on Saturday, Sunday, and public holidays during a 3-month high season (which corresponds to the summer months of the southern hemisphere). Each team flies twice daily, for 1 hour each time, as long as the winds are below 30 km/h.

The flight coverage is focused on high-risk areas, which are easily identified by the pilot. Rip currents, which are responsible for the higher number of drowning victims, have a different colour when seen from above. For the pilot, it is much easier to identify these areas than a lifesaver standing at the beach.

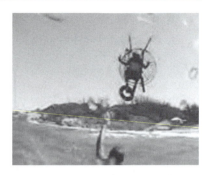

◘ Fig. 5.24. The paraglider passes the rescue equipment to the victim

Once a victim is detected the first step is to communicate to the lifesaver for prompt assistance. Flying against the wind to reduce flight speed, the pilot hands the life preserver to the victim and stays flying above the victim until the lifesaver has completed the second phase of the rescue procedure (◘ **Fig. 5.24**).

5.16.3.3
Maintenance and Support Team

In order to guarantee pilot and victim safety it is essential that the paraglider receives daily maintenance. Each team must rely on well trained mechanics and adequate spare parts to support a successful operation.

5.16.3.4
Paid by Sponsor

Pilots are not remunerated by municipal authorities, but instead earn their pay from corporate sponsors who communicate their brand on the bright and visible 10×10 meter sail. The social impact and the brand exposure transform this lifesaving tool into a valuable marketing tool for companies who wish to position themselves as socially responsible and interested in protecting the lives of consumers.

5.16.3.5
Website

▬ www.paralife.com.br

5.17
Spinal Injuries: Prevention, Immobilisation and Extrication from the Aquatic Environment

5.17.1
Prevention of Spinal Injuries

Jenny Blitvich

Worldwide, injury sustained as a result of diving into shallow water makes a significant contribution to the incidence of spinal cord injury (SCI), ranging from a reported low of 2.3% of all traumatic SCI in South Africa to a high of 21% in Poland [2]. The true incidence is underestimated, as some deaths attributed to drowning occur as a result of an unidentified SCI, and hence are not included in these figures.

The typical SCI casualty is an athletic male, aged 15–29 years [8]. His diving skills are usually self-taught, and he is unaware of both the potential dangers associated with diving into shallow water and the skills required to perform low risk dive entries. Alcohol consumption has been associated with 50%–80% of diving SCI [6]. The most common resultant injury is fracture or dislocation of C_5 or C_6 vertebrae [1].

At the University of Ballarat (Australia) the velocity of in excess of 600 dives performed by recreational and competitive swimmers has been measured [3–5]. In all dives, velocity at maximum depth was greater than that considered sufficient [10] to dislocate cervical vertebrae, while in more than 99% of dives the velocity was greater than that required to crush cervical vertebrae [10]. Hence, every dive has the potential to result in catastrophic injury. Alarmingly, analysis of more than 300 dives performed by recreational swimmers showed that in 18% of all dive entries, swimmers pulled their arms backward in a breaststroke-like arm action. This dangerous action leaves the head and neck completely unprotected.

While many authors highlight the importance of preventing diving SCI, until recently, prevention programs reported in the literature have been based primarily on increasing awareness of the risk of diving SCI [2, 7]. Increased awareness is important, but alone it is insufficient. A multifaceted approach, targeting skills, the structural aspects of public regulations and awareness, is necessary to decrease the incidence of diving SCI.

5.17.1.1
Skills

Providing recreational swimmers with the skills required to perform safer dives is vital to diving injury prevention. Many recreational swimmers do not maintain the arms in an extended position beyond the head, nor do they use steering-up techniques to minimise dive depth [5]. Without these skills, the risk of injury is increased. A short intervention program of *safe diving skills* (seven 10-minute sessions), conducted with recreational swimmers identified as having poor diving skills, successfully increased the safety of dives of participants. The intervention program emphasised locking hands together to avoid them being forced apart upon water contact ('lock hands'); locking arms tightly against the head to prevent lateral movement of the neck ('lock head'); and steering-up skills so that the underwater pathway minimised depth and distance at depth ('steer-up'). Almost half of the skills sessions focused on gliding and steering-up in shallow water without head first entries. [4]. Post-intervention, dives were shallower and participants protected their heads by locking their extended arms beyond the head. Follow-up investigation of dive performance 8 and 20 months later showed strong retention of safer diving skills [5].

5.17.1.2
Regulation

Appropriate government or council regulations can help provide the public with safer environments for swimming. Publications such as the Royal Life Saving Society Australia *Guidelines for Safe Pool Operations* [9] can provide guidance, but must be based on scientific research rather than tradition. Factors to be considered to minimise the risk of diving SCI include: pool depth markings; bottom markings to assist depth perception; demarcation between deep and shallow water; diving block and diving board design and placement; pool tile colour; ,No Diving' signage; adequate depths in areas where diving is permitted; sufficient lighting; appropriate landscaping and fencing; and supervisory or lifeguarding requirements. Signage and regulation without enforcement will not be effective. It is crucial that a safety culture is established, which requires proactive guarding and supervision. Home pool owners should also be competent in the conduct of SCI management procedures.

Additionally, learn-to-swim teachers and competitive swim coaches should be adequately educated in teaching safe diving skills, and learn-to-swim curriculum must include instruction in and revision of safe diving. Accreditation in teaching safer dive entries, such as the AUSTSWIM Teaching Safer Diving modules conducted in Victoria, Australia, is an important step in injury prevention. As most injured divers had self-taught diving skills, the risk of injury could be reduced if learn-to-swim teachers have adequate preparation to ensure all learn-to-swim participants successfully achieve the skills required for low-risk dive entries.

5.17.1.3
Promotion

Increased awareness of the potential for injury is still required. The importance of checking that water depth is sufficient for head-first entries, and that water is free of submerged obstacles, is crucial. This is necessary in every aquatic environment. The cues "Lock hands; lock head; steer-up" provide recreational swimmers with pertinent prompts of the skills necessary for safer dives. They also serve as reminders to parents when supervising their children. Swimming teachers and coaches should take every opportunity to reinforce safety issues in diving. Media campaigns, highlighting the risk of SCI injury ('Feet first is using your head'; 'When diving, lock hands; lock head; steer-up'), can provide an avenue to reach the target age group.

5.17.1.4
Conclusion

Diving is a high risk activity, but this risk can be reduced with awareness, skills and appropriate regulations. The likelihood of successful diving injury prevention is maximised through the implementation of a multifaceted approach.

References

1. Bailes JE, Herman JM, Quigley MR, et al. (1990) Diving injuries of the cervical spine. Surg Neurol 34:155–158
2. Blanksby BA, Wearne FK, Elliott BC, Blitvich JD (1997) Aetiology and occurrence of diving injuries: a review of diving safety. Sports Med 23:228–246
3. Blitvich JD, McElroy GK, Blanksby BA, Douglas G (1999) Characteristics of ,low risk' and ,high risk' dives by young adults: risk reduction in spinal cord injury. Spinal Cord 37:553–559
4. Blitvich JD, McElroy GK, Blanksby BA (2000) Risk reduction in spinal cord injury: teaching safe diving skills. J Sci Med Sport 3:120–131
5. Blitvich JD, McElroy GK, Blanksby BA (2003) Retention of safe diving skills. J Sci Med Sport 6:155–165
6. Branche CM, Sniezek JE, Sattin RW (1991) Water recreation-related spinal injuries: risk factors in natural bodies of water. Accident Anal Prevent 23:13–17
7. Damjan H, Turk P (1995) Prevention of spinal injuries from diving in Slovenia. Paraplegia 33:246–249
8. Gabrielsen M, Spivey M (1990) The etiology of 486 case studies with recommendations for needed action. Nova University Press, Ft. Lauderdale, FL
9. Royal Life Saving Society – Australia (2001) Guidelines for safe pool operation. RLSS-A, Melbourne
10. Stone RS (1981) A rationale for rating pools with diving boards. (Arthur D. Little Study No 4). Arthur D. Little, Cambridge, Ma

5.17.2
Immobilisation and Extraction of Spinal Injuries

Peter Wernicki, Peter Fenner and David Szpilman

"A spinal injury happens in an instant... it lasts a lifetime".
(Tom Gregor)

The effects of spinal cord injury can be devastating and the aquatic environment is a common location for these injuries. Lifesavers and other emergency professionals should therefore expect to be called upon to rescue and manage spinal injury victims in the water. This requires an understanding of the injury, development of protocols, appropriate training, preparation, and availability of proper equipment.

Spinal cord injuries occur with alarming frequency throughout the world and with a frequency of 52 per million population in the US. Although auto accidents account for the greatest numbers, recreational activities may be the second leading cause, with aquatic accidents causing the majority. Most of these are due to diving injuries. In fact, in some areas more than 60% of all sports and recreational spinal injuries are diving related. They can occur in the open water or pool environment. Their causes may involve striking bottom in shallow water, striking underwater objects, being twisted or thrust to the bottom by surf, or watercraft accidents. Spinal cord injuries usually occur in young people with the average age being 28.7 years and the median age just 19. Males comprise 82% of these victims. Consumption of alcohol, horseplay, and poor judgement are often contributing factors. Most injuries occur on summer weekends.

Studies suggest that spinal injures are not an emergency that lifesavers encounter with high frequency [1]. One study in the surf environment evaluated 46,060 rescues and found that 0.009% had some spinal injury. A retrospective survey of more than 2400 drownings with a history of obvious trauma from diving, falling from height, or a motor vehicle accident, found that less than 0.5% had a spinal cord injury.

Circumstances can vary, however, depending on the presence or absence of sandbars, wave action, water visibility, or aquatic activities. Regardless of frequency, spinal injury can have severe outcomes and can be worsened by inappropriate handling. Moreover, it is sometimes difficult or impossible to determine whether someone has sustained a spinal injury without full medical evaluation in a hospital setting. Therefore, it is critical that lifesavers use great caution when spinal cord injury can reasonably be suspected.

The spinal cord runs through bones known as vertebrae, which help protect it from injury. Spinal injuries sustained in the aquatic environment most commonly occur in the neck at cervical vertebrae 5, 6, and 7, due to flexion forces. When fractures, dislocations, or other vertebral injuries occur with significant force, the spinal cord itself can be damaged. This will often lead to permanent quadriplegia (four extremity paralysis), and frequently death, depending on the specifics of the injury. Even when the victim survives a spinal cord injury, the impact can be devastating to the victim and the family of the victim. Future life-long care and tremendous, public and personal, expenditures will be required. Thankfully, many more people suffer damage to the vertebral column without spinal cord damage, thus without nerve damage or paralysis.

The epidemiology of spinal injuries is well known and there is ongoing research with respect to medical and surgical treatment. Unfortunately, the techniques to stabilise and transport victims of suspected spinal injury have been developed rather subjectively, with limited scientific study. No significant studies are available on aquatic techniques. Therefore, further scientific research on the rescue itself, which is the first and possibly the most important link in the chain of care of spinal injuries, is needed.

Treatment of suspected spinal cord injury, whether ashore or in-water, is generally focused on the goal of doing no inadvertent harm. In some cases, an initial trauma to the spine may not have immediately severe consequences, but further manipulation of the spine, by the victim or rescuers, may cause life-long injury or even death. This is the reason why proper handling of these victims by rescuers is so crucial.

Standard protocols for treating suspected spinal injury focus on immobilising the victim in an effort to avoid further injury. During the World Congress on Drowning it became clear that various techniques have been developed for this purpose. Each has specific pros and cons which vary under differing conditions and situations. Lifesaving professionals should use the following information to help develop and evaluate their own appropriate protocols and training programs.

5.17.2.1
Recognition

The first step in treatment of spinal injury victims is recognition. Any neck pain after injury, even trivial, or head trauma should create a suspicion of possible spinal injury. Numbness, pins and needles, or weakness, even if temporary, are all serious signs of possible spinal injury. A person with an abrasion to the forehead may well have sustained it by falling forward or by hitting a sandy bottom after body-surfing. Victims found in the surf or floating in shallow water, or those seen diving prior to an injury, need appropriate precautionary care for possible spinal injury.

5.17.2.2
Initial Treatment

Airway, breathing, and circulation (ABC) should be first addressed. Despite the importance of treating spinal injury, breathing takes obvious precedent. If the victim is not breathing or unable to breath as a result of a face-down position in the water, the face needs to be carefully removed from the water and rescue breathing begun as soon as possible, using appropriate techniques to minimise spinal movement. The modified jaw thrust or jaw thrust manoeuvres are the recommended methods. They will allow the rescuer to maintain the neck in as neutral a position as possible.

The victim is first approached by the rescuer, who should avoid causing unnecessary turbulence. For example, if the victim is close to the edge of a pool jumping or diving should be avoided. The lifesaver with the highest degree of medical skill should direct the process and take control of the head of the victim. Unless the victim is not breathing, all actions should be taken slowly, carefully, and in unison.

The goal of the rescuers is to stabilise the spine and prevent further motion, maintaining the neck in a neutral straight position or in the position of comfort. Ultimately, this involves use of a backboard, straps, and cervical collar. Then the patient can be safely transferred by ambulance to hospital facilities for definitive care. The interim steps between recognition and transport are where the training and techniques of the rescuers most importantly come into play. Proper immobilisation will protect from further damage, facilitate moving to shallow water, and allow for efficient permanent immobilisation.

The method used depend on several factors:

- Location, such as onshore or offshore, deep or shallow water, surf or still water, distance to shore
- Rescuer size, training, and the number of rescuers available
- Victim size and condition such as: face up or face down, breathing or non-breathing, other injuries
- Equipment and transportation available

5.17.2.3
Onshore Presentation – Standing Backboard Technique

The most common scenario, and the easiest to deal with, is the victim who walks up to the lifesaver onshore complaining of neck pain or injury. Immediate steps should be taken to immobilise the victim and the standing backboard technique should be used.

The lifesaver first advises the victim not to move, explains the importance of immobilising the spine, and simultaneously moves to the rear of the victim to stabilise the head and neck with one hand over the ears on each side. A second lifesaver applies a properly fitted cervical stabilisation collar. A backboard is then slid in between the first rescuer and the victim. While the first lifesaver maintains neck stabilisation, two other lifesavers then stand facing the victim, grasp opposite sides of the backboard through the armpits of the victim, and gently lower the backboard to the sand. Standard protocols are then followed to secure the victim to the backboard.

5.17.2.4
In-Water Presentation

In-water techniques fall into three main manoeuvres and one or more are used by almost all lifesaving organisations throughout the world. However, there are no standard terminologies referring to these techniques and numerous confusing names are used. Instances are even seen where different lifesaving organisations use the different techniques, but the same names. The following three standard names are suggested for each technique. Some are better under different conditions and one may not fit all circumstances.

5.17.2.5
Vice-Grip

The rescuer approaches from the side of the victim, places his or her dominant arm along the sternum (breastbone) of the victim and stabilises the chin with the hand. The other arm of the rescuer is then placed along the spine with this hand cupping the back of the head of the victim. The arms are squeezed together forming a vice which provides stabilisation. If the victim is face down, the victim is slowly rotated toward the rescuer to a face-up position.

This method is quickly and readily applied by any size rescuer to any size victim. It works in deep or shallow water and positions the rescuer well to check respiratory status and carry out rescue breathing. Care must be taken to avoid excessive pressure on the airway.

5.17.2.6
Body Hug

In the case of a face-up victim, the rescuer approaches from behind and partially submerges. The arms of the rescuer are then slid through the armpits of the victim and the rescuer places open hands on either side of the head of the victim and over the ears of the victim, thus providing stabilisation. The face of the rescuer is placed next to the head of the victim. In the case of a face-down victim, the technique is also applied from behind, in a similar manner. After the arms of the rescuer have been slid through the armpits of the victim and the head of the victim grasped, the rescuer rolls the victim into a face-up position.

While this method provides exceptional immobilisation, it is of limited value in shallow water. It may not be feasible if there is a significant size discrepancy between rescuer and victim. A lone rescuer cannot adequately perform rescue breathing without changing grip, although some modifications are used by some lifesaving organisations. Before placing the victim on a backboard, a change in immobilisation, with assistance of a second rescuer, is required.

5.17.2.7
Extended Arm Grip

The rescuer moves to a position at one side of victim and grabs the nearest arm of the victim just above the elbow, using the right hand for the right elbow or left hand for the left elbow. Both of the arms of the victim are then carefully raised above the head of the victim by the rescuer pressing them together against the ears. This immobilises the head and neck of the victim. The head grip can be maintained by the rescuer with only one hand holding the two arms of the victim together. Further stability can be obtained if the rescuer uses two hands to hold the arms together while at the same time using the thumbs of the rescuer to support the back of the head of the victim. A face-down victim has the method applied as above. The victim is then gently glided head first and slowly rolled toward the rescuer, thus positioning the victim on the rescuer's free arm.

This is probably the most unique and complex method. It can allow the rescuer a free hand to support the body or to check for and begin rescue breathing. It can even allow a free arm for side or backstroke to assist in moving the victim toward shore or recovering the victim from a submerged position. It works in deep or shallow water and is arguably the only method for a single rescuer to roll a victim in the turbulent or extremely shallow water. This is done using one hand to apply the overhead arm pressure and the other to roll the hips of the victim. It further allows for easy transition to a backboard. There may be some concerns about the degree of immobilisation provided with this method, especially towards flexion forces.

Other methods are used by some lifesaving organisations, but cannot be recommended at this time. Their levels of immobilisation are not sufficient or equal to those presented here.

5.17.2.8
Deep Water Presentation

If in deep water, once an appropriate stabilisation method is applied, the victim should be carefully moved toward shore or a rescue boat. If necessary, the rescuer can straddle a rescue tube and continue the immobilisation until further help arrives.

5.17.2.9
General Recommendations

Lifesaving organisations are strongly encouraged to make spinal stabilisation equipment readily available to stabilise victims of suspected spinal injury. This equipment, including a backboard, straps, and cervical collar, should be properly maintained. Securing a victim to a backboard cannot be accomplished by a single rescuer and is difficult with less than three. It is helpful to have more. Unless water turbulence or cold water preclude it, the victim should be kept in shallow water until sufficient help and equipment arrive. Specifics on strapping and movement also need to be taught and trained. Movement is usually carried out in a 45–90° angle towards approaching waves or current. Oxygen should be provided to the victim. Lifesaving organisations with this equipment available should have all lifesavers practice coordinated transition from the immobilisation methods described here to backboard stabilisation.

If a backboard is not available to extricate the victim from the water, if in-water, and to stabilise the victim, choices must be made. The best approach, if feasible, is to limit movement of the victim to the barest minimum required to ensure the highest possible level of stabilisation. This may mean, for example, that a suspected spinal injury victim in warm water with little turbulence is left in the water, held immobilised by lifesavers until an ambulance with appropriate spinal immobilisation equipment arrives. In cases where the victim must be removed from the water because of turbulence, cold, ABC priorities, or for other reasons, lifesavers may consider use of a flat rescue board or a unified carry involving several lifesavers with arms laced under the victim. In either case, the move should be as slow as possible, with great care taken to avoid unnecessary movement of the spine.

No single in-water spinal immobilisation technique fits all circumstances. Lifesavers should be trained in at least two water immobilisation methods. Perhaps the vice-grip and extended arm grip are best. These have more versatility and universal applications. There are, however, no scientific studies known which address the benefits of one method over another. There are only anecdotal reports and opinions. What is needed is specific scientific research on neck movement during these manoeuvres. Such studies could help to choose and modify the techniques. For now, however, each lifesaver should learn and practice the various methods. Proficiency will further the ability of the lifesaver to prevent spinal cord injuries with their devastating results.

Reference

1. Watson RS, Cummings P, Quan L, et al. (2001) Cervical spine injuries among submersion victims. J Trauma 51:658–662

5.18
Injuries to Lifesavers

PETER WERNICKI and PETER FENNER

Lifesaving requires a unique combination of physical and mental skills with an ultimate goal of saving lives. There is no other occupation incorporating such a mélange of physical challenges and fitness requirements. These same challenges and requirements create an increased risk of injury, illness, or worse.

Lifesavers can be injured while performing their daily duties, such as rescuing a victim, or from environmental hazards both in the water and onshore [1–5]. Injury can preclude the lifesaver from completing the rescue or carrying out any of the other normal activities of lifesavers, until fully recovered from the injury. Lifesavers may also be injured whilst keeping fit for their occupation through training in swimming, boarding, running and paddling or rowing [6–8]. Competition is an added risk, although participation is encouraged to aid in maintaining fitness.

5.18.1
Unusual Risk Factors

Lifesavers have an increased risk of injury over other athletes for several reasons.
-   They cannot schedule their rescue. Therefore, they usually cannot warm up ahead of time or carry out a stretching regimen in advance of athletic output. They must often jump from a sedentary position to one of sudden strenuous activity. Musculoskeletal injuries may occur due to cold and tightness in the muscles.
-   They usually cannot back off when performing a rescue, even when injured, because the life of another person is on the line.
-   Although they may not feel at their best every day, they are still expected to perform at peak levels, whereas other athletes can skip or modify their training.

5.18.2
Injury Types

Statistics from the San Diego Lifeguard Service (California) show that the most common body area injured is the foot, followed by the back, knee, trunk, shoulder, hand, and face. The vast majority (40%) occur as strains. Others are exposure (12%), contusions (11%), sprains (7%), and lacerations (6%).

- Foot injuries: 79% of lifesavers sustain foot injuries, making this the most common injury. Most are lacerations to the foot from natural or man-made causes including shells, needles, or other sharp objects.
- Swimmer's shoulder: Swimming injuries include swimmer's shoulder, which involves tendonitis of rotator cuff muscles sustained because lifesavers usually use a single stroke in carrying out their activities. Strain is increased when swimming a victim or victims to shore.
- Running injuries: These are often caused on the shore or pool deck where lifesavers do not have the biomechanical protection of supportive shoes and the ground has irregular contours or firmness, with holes present. Significant joint injuries are possible. Overuse running (or over-walking) may cause patellar (knee cap) irritation, shin splints, or plantar fasciulitis (heel spurs).
- Lifeguard calf: This is a unique lifesaver injury, which involves discomfort in the posterior calf muscle (gastro-soleus injury) whilst running and walking in soft sand, jumping from the height of a lifeguard tower, and exacerbated by cold starts.
- Exposure: A common injury of a chronic form is extensive outdoor exposure to the elements, particularly due to the sun and its harmful UV light, especially UVB. Sun exposure causes short-term skin problems such as sunburn, but more importantly long term exposure leads to skin cancers [9, 10]. In the eye, injury from the sun, sand, wind, and water can cause cataracts, pingueculae, and pterygia [11].
- Infectious disease: Exposure to blood from an open wound or lesion, as with any person who provides medical aid, creates potential exposure to hepatitis B, C, or even HIV. Lifesavers are typically less clothed and thus less protected in these encounters than ambulance or hospital personnel, so the degree of exposure is increased. Resuscitation efforts typically involve exposure to saliva, vomit, and possibly blood products. To date, however, none of these diseases is reported to have occurred after work exposure [12, 13].
- Joint injuries: Paddling, kayaking, and surf ski injuries mainly occur to the shoulders, elbows, and forearms with tendonitis, neck, and back strains.
- Rowing injuries: Up to 44% of lifesavers who row regularly will experience some type of injury within a single season. Most injuries are muscular strains, but head injury, fractures, dislocations, and sprains also occur. Up to 20% of these lifesavers may be sidelined for the remainder of the season by the injury.

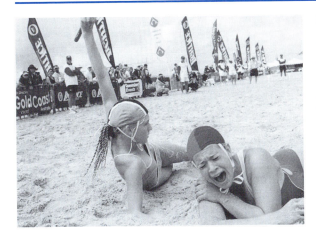

Fig. 5.25. During the finish of a beach flag event, the competitors run down the beach and dive to a flag. It is quite usual that either the winner or the runner up gets hurt by the flagpole or a fellow competitor

5.18.3
Competition Related Injuries

The physical skills that are used during lifesaving are heavily tested during lifesaving competitions. These competitions give a clear view on the injuries that can happen to life savers.

Some 5000 competitors and an equal number of officials and spectators attend the annual 4- to 5-day Australian lifesaving championships. Approximately 100 people a day are treated for a multitude of ailments ranging from minor to severe, during the 5 days of competition. The largest caseload is musculoskeletal injuries, which are usually treated in beach first aid stations. The medical area handles more extensive or serious injuries, including fractures, dislocations, lacerations (both small and extensive, which need suturing), heart attacks, asthma, heat stress, and dehydration, as well as all the common injuries noted previously. The beach flags event, in particular, can result in shoulder injuries (**Fig. 5.25**). Approximately ten cases a year are serious enough to require transportation to hospital.

5.18.4
Rescue Craft Related Injuries

Inflatable rescue boat (IRB) use, mostly from competition, but also in routine patrol work or training, has resulted in a number of serious foot, ankle and knee injuries. This is usually caused by high impact and instability in heavy or unpredictable surf. Fracture dislocations of the midfoot, ankle fracture variants, and tibial shaft fractures occur most often. Other common injuries include sprained knee ligaments, whilst head injuries, various strains, sprains, dislocations and skin injuries occur less often (see also ▶ **Chapter 5.14**).

Regardless of the source or type of injury, until a lifesaver has recovered enough to be able to perform a rescue proficiently, the lifesaver should be assigned to non-rescue duties.

5.18.5
Injury Prevention

Injury prevention can be promoted through consistent attention to the prevailing risk factors.

Lifesavers should undergo an appropriate pre-assignment physical exam with the strenuous level of activity in mind. This examination must include a screening or testing procedure where fitness and skill levels are measured to ensure that appropriate standards are met.

It is also important that lifesavers maintain excellent cardiovascular fitness and strength year-round, and undergo gradually increasing preseason training to avoid rapid increases for the start of the season. Cross-training and maintaining fitness can help prevent overuse injuries.

Before the start of each shift, lifesavers should undergo an appropriate warm-up and stretching routine.

To prevent foot injuries and lower limb injuries, lifesavers should evaluate their workplace on a daily basis looking for natural and man-made hazards. They should fill in holes and remove dangerous material, such as glass or sharp objects from their area. Consideration should be given to using footwear when feasible.

Lifesavers should be fully knowledgeable of the local environment and the hazards it presents to prevent them from placing themselves in unnecessarily harmful situations and should be taught the use of proper ergonomics to help avoid injury in circumstances such as lifting or transporting rescue craft or movable observation platforms.

Observation platforms should be of the correct height and weight with steps or ramps. Rescue equipment, including boats, should be of an appropriate weight and design, and stored in appropriate locations. Rescue boats and the training of those who will use them should be designed to minimise injuries.

Proper training and certification of lifesavers in use of craft and vehicles should be carried out. Wearing of all safety gear including seat belts, helmets and life vests must be mandatory.

Prevention of sunburn and skin cancer requires mandatory use of long sleeve shirts, collars, hats, and sunglasses, all with UV protection. Sunscreen and shade should be provided. Wearing the full uniform, along with regular use of shade and sunscreen, should be mandatory.

Exposure to infectious agents should be minimised by use of barrier devices, gloves and other universal precautions. Vaccinations should mandatorily be provided for tetanus and hepatitis B and for hepatitis A in areas where endemic. Appropriate exposure plans, to include testing and treatment on a timely basis, must be in place in the event of exposure. Lifesaving organisations must be continually aware of the state of water quality, assisting local governments in monitoring and testing, and enforcing beach closures when necessary. In general, lifesavers should avoid swallowing water and should avoid entering the water when they have open skin lesions.

5.18.6
Conclusion

Lifesaving is extremely rewarding. It blends the ability to save lives and help the public with unique physical and athletic challenges. Lifesavers, however, need to be mindful of the hazards and dangers they face. Many of these injuries and other problems can be prevented with appropriate training and instruction. They can be lessened by maintaining necessary fitness levels and avoiding overuse. Employers need to encourage safe daily routines, enforce necessary rules, and foster professionalism. Lifesavers and those who employ them should heed the proactive steps discussed here for injury prevention. The results will be happier, healthier lifesavers with greater longevity, reduced costs and problems for the agencies, and ultimately better care and safety for the general public.

References

1. Dahl AM, Miller DI (1979) Body contact swimming rescues – what are the risks? Am J Public Health 69:150–152
2. Sarnaik AP, Vohra MP, Sturmans SW, Belenky WM (1986) Medical problems of the swimmer. Clin Sport Med 5:47–64
3. Schiff KC, Weisberg SB, Dorsey JH (2001) Microbiological monitoring of marine recreational waters in southern California. Environ Manag 27:149–157
4. Kueh CS, Grohmann GS (1989) Recovery of viruses and bacteria in waters off Bondi beach: a pilot study. Med J Aust 151:632–638
5. Grenfell RD, Ross KN (1992) How dangerous is that visit to the beach? A pilot study of beach injuries. Aust Fam Physician 21:1145–1148
6. McFarland EG, Wasik M (1996) Injuries in female collegiate swimmers due to swimming and cross training. Clin J Sport Med 6:178–182
7. Pen LJ, Barrett RS, Neal RJ, Steele JR (1996) An injury profile of elite ironman competitors. Aust J Sci Med Sport 28:7–11
8. Hickey GJ, Fricker PA, McDonald WA (1997) Injuries to elite rowers over a 10-yr period. Med Sci Sports Exerc 29:1567–1572
9. American Cancer Society (2002) Cancer facts and figures – 2002. American Cancer Society, Atlanta
10. Jeffs P, Coates M, Giles GG, et al. (1996) Cancer in Australia 1989–1990 (with projections to 1995). Australian Institute of Health and the Australasian Association of Cancer Registries, Canberra, Cancer Series No. 5
11. Javitt JC (1994) Cataract and latitude. Doc Ophthalmol 88:307–325
12. Occupational Health and Safety Administration (1991) Occupational exposure to bloodborne pathogens. 29 CFR Part 1910.1030
13. Anonymous (2002) Infection control guidelines for the prevention of transmission of infectious disease in the health care setting (Draft 24 May 2002). http://www.health.gov.au/pubhlth/strateg/communic/review

5.19
Management of Physical and Psychological Responses During Administration of CPR to a Drowned Person

Frank Pia

The current first responder resuscitation-training models for lifesavers blend substantive knowledge acquisition with an emphasis on psychomotor skill performance [1, 2]. Course completion and additional mannequin practice form the foundations for the expectation that effective administration of CPR by a lifesaver to a drowned person will occur under emergency conditions.

While CPR skill acquisition and temporal stability variables will remain important ones for resuscitation research, CPR research needs to be expanded to study the effects of acute stress arousal responses of lifesavers who have no experience administering CPR to a drowned person [11].

From a psychological standpoint, responding to a cardiac arrest is a highly stressful psychophysiological event. In addition to autonomic nervous system responses, the emotional responses by lifesavers while treating a drowned person who has suffered a cardiac arrest, especially if the drowning occurred in the area of responsibility of the lifeguard, can induce debilitating feelings of guilt during the primary survey appraisal process that may delay, interfere, or ultimately render the lifesaver unable to administer CPR.

5.19.1
Review of the Literature

William Cannon, an American physiologist, noted in his classic studies that stress related adrenal gland hormonal discharges that occur during emergencies might induce cardiovascular changes [6]. Selye defined stress as "... the result of any somatic or mental demands on the body". Medical literature notes that despite dissimilar situations, stress induced biochemical changes that prepare the body for flight or fight, are uniform [14].

Selye noted that the goal of stress management was not to eliminate, but rather respond adaptively to stressful situations [13]. Meichenbaum developed the conceptual model underlying the cognitive behavioural treatment procedure known as stress inoculation training (SIT). Stress inoculation developed as an analogous concept to medical inoculation and sought to build cognitive and affective antibodies to stress through a three-phase process: conceptualisation, skill acquisition and rehearsal, and application and follow through [9]. Starr applied stress inoculation concepts to the administration of cardiopulmonary resuscitation and noted "...witnessing a cardiac arrest, even after having completed a course in CPR, remains a highly stressful and emotionally arousing experience...(with)...altered levels of perception, attention, decision making...." [15].

During certification, retraining and in-service CPR training, lifesavers must be instructed that during the resuscitation of a drowned person, rescuers will experience certain natural bodily reactions to stress within seconds after adrenaline enters the bloodstream. When these symptoms occur to a lifesaver during a CPR emergency, these responses to adrenaline must be accepted as natural manageable phenomena. If the physiological manifestations of adrenaline release are misinterpreted as unnatural symptoms, some lifesavers will shift their information processing focus from the external task of administering cardiopulmonary resuscitation, to internal sensations evoked by the discharge of adrenaline into the bloodstream.

In order to operationalise self-efficacy beliefs, lifesavers must understand the physiological effects of adrenaline release into their bloodstreams, so that they are able to make logical connections between the adrenaline release and their physiological reactions to this hormone [3, 4]. The physical effect of adrenaline release during a CPR emergency includes increase in heart rate and blood pressure, rapid shallow breathing, profuse sweating, trembling, and sweaty palms. Without this information, some lifesavers misinterpret their reactions to adrenaline as unnatural and use catastrophic interpretation of their physical responses to reach the conclusion they are not capable of administering CPR.

One of the most serious effects of adrenaline release upon the performance of a lifesaver during CPR resuscitation is the onset of rapid shallow breathing by the rescuer, which may induce hyperventilation. Hyperventilation causes increased alkalinity of nerve cells, decreased carbon dioxide level, and constriction of the brain blood vessels. These physiological effects, particularly decreased blood flow to the brain, can cause a perceptual shift from the external requirement of administering CPR to a drowned person to the internal focus on the bodily sensations of the lifesaver that narrows attention, increases psychomotor errors, and causes memory retrieval deficits.

Once the internal focus on increased sympathetic nervous system functioning occurs, the human information processing of visual, auditory, tactile, olfactory, kinaesthetic, and proprioceptive stimuli shifts from focusing and responding to cues in the external CPR environment, to internal thoughts of unnaturalness, inadequacy, and catastrophic self-defeating thoughts and feelings. Shortly after the onset of the catastrophic interpretation of adrenaline induced physiological sensations, the ability to administer CPR may be further compromised because the erroneous interpretations of the physiological and psychological responses to acute stress generates negative internal dialogue.

Research has shown that the presence of self-defeating thoughts and feelings in individuals experiencing either acute and/or chronic stress may lead to suboptimal performance and dysfunction. Sarason indicated that individuals under stress tend to become self-preoccupied, often displaying a variety of self-defeating and interfering thoughts and feelings [12].

Lazarus found "the degree to which a particular situation elicits an emotional response depends in large part on the organism's appraisal of the situation and his or her ability to handle an event" [7]. Lazarus and Folkman differentiated between primary and secondary appraisal [8]. Primary appraisal is the initial evaluation of the stimuli, condition or performance requirement, while secondary appraisal assesses the perceived capacity to meet stress generated performance requirements. The CPR resuscitation requirement acquires a positive or negative value through the appraisal processes, leads to the formation of performance expectations, and the generation of physiological, cognitive, emotional, and social sequelae.

The work of Lazarus and Folkman can be used to discuss a general four-stage acute stress model, and a specific five-stage CPR emergency response continuum for inexperienced rescuers. The CPR model includes:

- A requirement to immediately administer CPR to a clinically dead person
- Increased sympathetic nervous system responses to this CPR emergency
- Perceptual shift by the inexperienced rescuer from the external emergency situation to increased internal physiological responses to adrenalin
- Catastrophic psychological interpretations of normal psychological responses to adrenaline
- Negative CPR performance expectations

Coping strategies intend to keep the emergency response of the rescuer processes at phases one and two; initiating circumstances (presence of a drowned person) and increased sympathetic nervous system functioning. The work of Bandura illustrated that the development of positive performance expectations is a critical factor and a strong predictor of actual performance [4]. By pre-exposing inexperienced rescuers to normal physiological reactions to a CPR emergency, and providing them with strategies for normalising their reactions, the likelihood that positive performance expectations will be formed and maintained are increased.

The works of Beck and Meichenbaum can be used as the basis for strategies and activities to help lifesavers manage acute stress during a CPR emergency [5, 10]. Practice in normalising acute stress physiological responses and rehearsing positive statements that directly challenge, review, or invalidate negative self talk, can be trained.

During a 1-day pre-conference workshop and an expert meeting during the World Congress on Drowning, the concepts and techniques were presented for helping attendees understand the physical and psychological acute stress reactions that can occur during the first administration of CPR of a lifesaver to a drowned person. The sessions during the World Congress on Drowning focused primarily on the negative consequences of stress, not on the conditions where stress enhances performance. Attention was devoted to delineating internal and external stimuli, such as vomit, that may be cognitively and emotionally perceived or appraised in an emergency, by the lifesaver with valid CPR certification, as exceeding the capacity of the rescuer to administer cardiopulmonary resuscitation effectively.

The conceptual adaptation of SIT hypothesised that lifesavers must be pre-exposed to the physical and the psychological arousal processes that may be present during a CPR emergency which will enable lifesavers to anticipate their acute stress responses, make plans to cope with their physiological reactions, and rehearse effective psychological coping skills was well received by the attendees.

References

1. American Heart Association (1973) CPR for lifeguards. American Heart Association, Dallas
2. American Red Cross (2002) CPR for the professional rescuer: stay well. American Red Cross, Boston
3. Bandura A (19829 Self-efficacy mechanism in human agency. Am Psychol 37:122–147
4. Bandura A, Reese L, Adams NE (1982) Microanalysis of action and fear arousal as a function of differential levels of perceived self-efficacy. J Personal Social Psychol 43:5–21
5. Beck A (1984) Cognitive approaches to stress. In: Woolfolk R, Lehrer P (eds) Principals and practice of stress management. Guilford Press, New York
6. Cannon WB (1935) Stresses and strains of homeostasis. Am J Med Sci 189:1–14
7. Lazarus R (1981) The stress and coping paradigm. In: Eisdorfer C (ed.) Models for clinical psychopathology. Prentice-Hall, Englewood Cliffs, NJ
8. Lazarus R, Folkman S (1984) Stress, appraisal and coping. Springer, New York
9. Meichenbaum D (1977) Cognitive behavior modification: an integrative approach. Plenum Press, New York
10. Meichenbaum D (1985) Stress inoculation training. Allyn and Bacon, Boston, MA
11. Pia F (1998) Managing stress during a CPR emergency. A workshop presented at PRO Aquatics Conference: Parks and Recreation, Halliburton Heights, Ontario, Canada
12. Sarason I (1975) Anxiety and self-preoccupation. In: Sarason I, Spielberger C (eds) Stress and anxiety, vol 2. Hemisphere Press, Washington, DC
13. Selye H (1974) Stress without distress. Lippincott, Philadelphia, PA
14. Selye H (1980) The stress concept today. In: Kutash IL, Schlesinger IB (eds) Handbook on stress and anxiety: contemporary knowledge, theory, and treatment. Jossey-Bass, San Francisco

5.20
Psychological Care After CPR and Rescue

TON HAASNOOT

One of the primary roles of lifesavers is to intervene in life-threatening emergencies in an effort to protect people from death or injury. This responsibility subjects lifesavers to both physical and psychological danger. While the physical dangers are widely understood, the psychological dangers are not as well recognised. They may result, for example, from anxiety over an unsuccessful effort to revive a drowning victim or feelings of guilt after the death of a person in an area under the protection of lifesavers. Lifesavers may feel great responsibility for the death of a person if they fail in an attempted rescue, even if it may be clear to others that the attempt was well executed. Support personnel, such as radio officers, are also vulnerable. Although their work takes place at distance, they may be mentally involved and possibly feel guilty because they think they may have done something wrong during the operation. Especially, rescue organisations are concerned about how to deal with psychological care after CPR.

At the World Congress on Drowning, an expert session was devoted to this subject. Participants included the author of this chapter, as chair, Martin Nemiroff (US Coast Guard – retired), Jan Paul de Wit (Royal Netherlands Navy), Frank van Aalst (Royal Netherlands Navy), Joanne Ravestein (Merkawah Institution), Sip Wiebenga (Royal Netherlands Life Boat Institute), John Leech (Irish Water Safety) and Frank Pia (American Red Cross). This chapter is an effort to reflect the opinions of these experts at that moment (June 2002). Considering a growing understanding of the needs and risks of psychological care, it is advisable to check current opinions in the literature and on relevant websites.

5.20.1
Psychological Aspects of Lifesaving

In maintaining mental health, there are a variety of risk factors. Predominantly they deal with the severity of the event like the death (dying) of a child, unsuccessful lifesaving operations, strong emotions of involved family of friends, and the amount of victims in the case of disasters.

Another factor is lack of experience in dealing with traumatic events. When confronted with a drastic event for the first time lifesavers may not able to keep a psychological distance. In this case they show a habit of looking at all details, rather than ignoring stressful aspects of the event like experienced lifesavers do.

Experience, however, can also pose a danger. Those who have had previous traumatic experiences may find repeats of similar incidents to be especially troubling. For example, a lifesaver who has observed a prior drowning death may experience flashbacks to the previous case upon witnessing another drowning. Recent unresolved life events or trauma in their private lives can also be considered as a risk factor.

To be properly prepared for these possibilities, lifesavers should be informed during their initial training to expect to be involved in serious, life-threatening situations and advised that they might feel great stress or experience mental health problems as a result. When stress overwhelms the lifesavers normal coping mechanisms, post traumatic stress disorder (PTSD) or post traumatic stress syndrome (PTSS) might develop.

However, the absence of a disorder such as PTSD does not imply the absence of disturbances in the adaptation to acute stress or the absence of ongoing health problems. It does not mean that the majority, 70%–80% of rescuers, do not suffer from the consequences of drastic events. A large part of the affected persons at some time experience specific symptoms which interfere with work, such as irritation, sleeping disturbances, fatigue at the workplace and concentration difficulties. Nevertheless, in most cases these problems disappear after some time and the functioning of the person will return to an adequate level.

During lifesaving work, there are several steps that can be taken to limit the possibility of psychological trauma to lifesavers. Where possible, more experienced lifesavers should be assigned to potentially stressful incidents. For example, if a body must be recovered from the water, there is usually an opportunity to add a more experienced person for the task, instead of sending an inexperienced lifesaver alone.

The buddy-system may lessen the chance that a single lifesaver feels uniquely responsible for a traumatic outcome and ensures that there is someone to talk to during the incident. Using a team approach can also be beneficial. For a team it is easier to cope with difficult situations, as they can support each other before, during, and after a rescue attempt.

It is good practice to have an informal meeting after a mission is completed. This should always be done, not only after a potentially psychologically traumatic mission. This is valuable not only for release of stress, but also to discuss ways to better respond to similar incidents in the future. To ease psychological tension, it is important for people to have the chance to talk over traumatic experiences in their own, well-known surroundings, where they feel comfortable discussing such matters. Being used to these informal sessions will contribute to the feeling of comfort after serious incidents, as people are used to talking things over as normal practice. The use of alcohol during these meetings should be avoided, since its use can be counterproductive and may exacerbate the psychological difficulties the person might be experiencing. If the mission was of such significance that there may be serious risk to mental health of lifesavers involved, then a more formal victim-assistance program should be held with a trained facilitator. The informal meetings should not be confused with formal critical incident stress debriefing (CISD), which was not discussed in detail.

Unit leaders and supervisory personnel should be trained to recognise the manifestation of unusual mental stress in lifesavers. Special attention should be paid to changes in behaviour. Examples of subtle changes in behaviour are people who become unusually silent or volunteers who cease attending regular training sessions. More serious indicators include sudden and unexpected wishes to change jobs or difficulties in personal relationships.

If good practices are in place, most issues related to critical incident stress can be adequately addressed within the lifesaving team. In some cases, however, these efforts are not adequate and further help is needed. Therefore lifesaving organisations should develop a plan for providing further mental health counselling. They can do so by consulting with appropriate mental institutes or by seeking assistance from local governmental organisations that specialise in this type of support and expertise. This plan, including use of professional psychologists, is normally implemented only when informal options appear unproductive and the person continues to experience difficulties. It is best to have a good medical advisor, with whom it is easy to speak, for advice on the best course of action and to help determine when a higher level of assistance is appropriate.

The people most likely to feel great stress as a result of a serious injury or death are friends and family members of the victim. Where reasonably possible, support should be provided to them by lifesavers, who should also be prepared to make referrals to further care. Some lifesaving organisations use counselling services for this purpose.

Both victims and lifesavers who themselves survive life-threatening situations sometimes experience a near death experience, which can be accompanied by a panoramic life review. As a result of this, great stress can be experienced afterwards. In these cases, it is crucial that the person involved is provided the chance to talk to others about the experience and that people who are close to the person take the time to listen sensitively. Sometimes people in these situations feel a need to tell their stories again and again. This should be considered normal behaviour after serious experiences and although the listening partner may consider the reaction excessive, it is essential to the good mental health of the person involved that others listen patiently and maintain serious interest.

5.20.2
Conclusion

During the meeting the consensus of the experts was that informal meetings are good practice in dealing with psychological stress. Further professional mental help should be available when needed. While no international consensus has emerged as of yet, lifesaving organisations would be well advised to consult with mental health experts in their area to access the most current advise and choose the best course of action.

5.20.3
Summary of Recommendations
Regarding Mental Health of Lifesavers

- Psychological aspects of lifesaving are a serious issue for which lifesaving organisations should prepare
- This issue should be included in instruction and instructional materials provided to lifesavers
- Lifesavers need to be prepared for the possibility of failure
- As part of the training, a phased approach to levels of stress (which should be as realistic as possible) should be adopted
- It should be a normal and routine practise to discuss matters following an operation or rescue attempt in an informal and comfortable environment
- If the crew leader or senior lifesaver suspects that a person is having difficulty coping, further assistance should be considered
- A plan should be in place for seeking assistance outside the lifesaving organisation when needed

5.20.4
Websites

- http://www.ncptsd.org/
- http://www.nimh.nih.gov/research/massviolence.pdf
- http://www.nimh.nih.gov/council/min102.cfm

References

1. Kleber RJ, Velden PG van der (2003) Acute stress at work. In: Schabracq MJ, Cooper CJ, Winnubst JAM (eds) The handbook of work and health psychology. Wiley
2. Carlier IVE, Voerman AE, Gersons BPR (2000) The influence of occupational debriefing on post traumatic stress symptomatology in traumatized police officers. Br J Med Psychol 73: 87–98
3. National Institute of Mental Health (2002) Mental health and mass violence: evidence based early psychological intervention for victims/survivors of mass violence. A workshop to reach consensus on best practices. NIH Publication No. 02–5138. US Government Printing Office, Washington, DC

Resuscitation

TASK FORCE ON RESUSCITATION
Section editors: PAUL PEPE and JOOST BIERENS

Task Force Chairs

- Paul Pepe
- Joost Bierens

Task Force Members

- Robert Berg
- Leo Bossaert
- Anthony Handley
- Ahamed Idris
- Peter Morley
- Martin Nemiroff
- Volker Wenzel
- Jane Wigginton

Other Contributors

- Steve Beerman
- Alfred Bove
- Christine Branche
- Andrea Gabrielli
- Shirley Graves
- Robyn Hoelle
- Bo Løfgren
- Denise Mann
- Fernando Martinho
- Robyn Meyer
- Jerome Modell
- Luiz Morizot-Leite
- Linda Papa
- David Persse
- Linda Quan
- Rienk Rienks
- Justin Scarr
- Gert-Jan Scheffer
- Paul Sirbaugh
- Luiz Smoris
- Martin Stotz
- David Szpilman
- Andreas Theodorou
- Wolfgang Ummenhofer
- Wiebe de Vries

6.1
Overview

PAUL PEPE and JOOST BIERENS

The Task Force on Resuscitation for the World Congress on Drowning 2002 was comprised of some of the world's recognised experts in resuscitation medicine. Cited at the conference as the Drowning Resuscitation Dream Team, this group of individuals represented multiple continents, disciplines and international organisations.

Task Force members had backgrounds from anaesthesia, critical care, emergency medicine, internal medicine, paediatrics, public health, pulmonary medicine, surgery, general practice and several other disciplines. Most of the members of the Resuscitation Task Force remain currently active as scientific advisors, committee members and consensus developers for several of the major resuscitation and resuscitation research-related organisations including the International Liaison Committee on Resuscitation, the American Heart Association, the Australian Resuscitation Council, the European Resuscitation Council, the International Lifesaving Federation, the International Committee on Resuscitation, the American Academy of Pediatrics, the Royal Lifesaving Society, the American College of Emergency Physicians and the National Association of EMS Physicians, as well as the National Institutes of Health and Centers for Disease Control and Prevention.

The expertise, experience and credibility of this task force are significant and the knowledge elements that they brought to the World Congress on Drowning 2002 were not only based on long-standing personal experience with the challenges of drowning events, but also on the most up-to-date scientific evidence and consensus available.

In that respect, the Resuscitation Task Force had some unique advantages. Much of the scientific data and conclusions from these deliberations could be immediately derived and extrapolated from recent international consensus conferences on resuscitation and the resultant published proceedings. Almost all of the task force members had participated in these conferences and subsequent collation of the information. A key example was the international guidelines on cardiopulmonary resuscitation published recently by the American Heart Association in conjunction with ILCOR in the year 2000. During the development process of those guidelines, the world literature on resuscitation was scientifically evaluated and weighed by international experts, including the available information on drowning resuscitation. This experience helped to expedite the process for the task force and also strengthened and expedited the consensus regarding the final conclusions and recommendations.

6.1.1
Specific Focus of the Task Force

The delegated focus of this task force was the prehospital (out-of-hospital) setting where, of course, most drowning incidents occur, and where, presumably, most resuscitation efforts should take place. The task force was asked to evaluate multiple overlapping issues in drowning resuscitation, including:

- The key role of lay persons and their actions (on-scene CPR)
  Jane Wigginton and Paul Pepe (USA), lead authors
- Basic rescuer actions (basic life support)
  Ahamed Idris (USA), lead author
- Automated defibrillators in the aquatic environment
  Stephen Beerman (Canada), lead author
- Positioning the drowning victim (rescue and spinal considerations)
  Anthony Handley (UK) and David Szpilman (Brazil), lead authors
- Invasive life support (advanced life support)
  Volker Wenzel (Austria), lead author
- The long Q-T syndrome in drowning incidents (prevalence and implications)
  Alfred Bove (USA) and Rienke Rienks (the Netherlands), lead authors
- Paediatric considerations (physiology and anatomy)
  Robert Berg (USA), lead author
- Prognosis and termination of resuscitation (age, timing, physiology and temperature considerations)
  Martin Nemiroff (USA), lead author
- Special resuscitation circumstances (unusual rescue situations)
  Peter Morley (Australia), lead author
- Several case reports of extreme situations (lessons that can be learned)
  Martin Stotz, Wolfgang Ummenhofer (Austria), Gert-Jan Scheffer (The Netherlands) and David Spzilman (Brazil), lead authors

In addition to these primary medical issues, the charge for the group also included the development of a first aid course for the aquatic environment as well as the development of standardised nomenclature and mechanisms for data collection and reporting related to drowning events:

- First aid course for the aquatic environment (recommended actions for bystanders)
  David Szpilman (Brazil), lead author
- Utstein-Style template for drowning (standardised nomenclature and mechanisms for data collection and reporting)
  Ahamed Idris (USA), lead author

It should be noted that the consensus on this priority project (standardised nomenclature and reporting) has now been published as an international consensus in [1] and [2] as well.

In the following chapters, the main findings and conclusions of the task force will be reviewed in detail. But first, we provide an executive summary of these conclusions in the following chapter.

References

1. Idris A, Berg R, Bierens J, et al. (2003) ILCOR Advisory Statement. Recommended guidelines for uniform reporting of data from drowning: The Utstein style. Resuscitation 59:45–57
2. Idris AH, Berg RA, Bierens J, et al. (2003) Recommended guidelines for uniform reporting of data from drowning: The Utstein Style. Circulation 108:2565–2574

6.2
Consensus and Recommendations

PAUL PEPE and JOOST BIERENS

6.2.1
Overview

One of the overall conclusions of this group is that, apart from the need for immediate and rapid resuscitative actions by on-scene bystanders (be they professional or lay persons), data are lacking regarding the optimal resuscitative management for victims experiencing a drowning incident. Therefore, a host of research efforts need to be initiated, starting with the development of standardised definitions and nomenclature for information to be collected and, in turn, standardised reporting mechanisms for these data.

Nevertheless, there is substantial empirical experience with drowning events and given the available data and collective experience of the task force members, the following recommendations should be highlighted for the time being.

6.2.2
Main Conclusions and Recommendations
from the Task Force on Resuscitation

Basic resuscitation skills must be learned by all volunteer and professional rescuers as well as lay persons who frequent aquatic areas or supervise others in a water environment.

The instant institution of optimal first aid and resuscitation techniques is the most important factor to ensure survival after a drowning event has occurred. Professional rescue organisations and other groups involved in the aquatic environment should promulgate this concept and promote widespread CPR training. Resuscitation organisations, and in particular those related to International Liaison Committee on Resuscitation (ILCOR), as well as professional rescue organisations and other groups who frequent aquatic areas, must promote training programs in first aid and basic life support for anyone who frequently visits or is assigned to work in the aquatic or other water environment.

There needs to be uniform use of standardised definitions and nomenclature for data to be collected for drowning incidents, and, in turn, there also needs to be standardised reporting mechanisms for these data.

To increase the understanding of the dying process and the resuscitation potential in drowning, a uniform reporting system must be developed and used for the registration of resuscitation of drowning. International resuscitation organisations, such as ILCOR-related organisations and medical groups, must establish a uniform reporting system, facilitate its use, be involved in the analysis of the data and support recommendations based on the resultant studies.

Consensus process: These conclusions were developed by the Task Force in consensus and then presented multiple times at the World Congress on Drowning in 2002 and later at the 2002 meeting of the European Resuscitation Council (ERC) and the International Liaison Committee for Resuscitation (ILCOR), as well as multiple subsequent relevant national venues and meetings in the US and Europe without any signifivant objection or modification. The recommendation for the standardisation was formally adopted by ILCOR and its member organisations.

6.2.3
The Critical Role of Lay Persons
and Their Actions in Drowning-Related Incidents

6.2.3.1
Conclusions

Several studies now confirm that, most lives are indeed saved by the immediate action of on-scene bystanders (be they lay persons or professional rescuers).

Relatively-speaking, without such immediate first aid and basic cardiopulmonary resuscitation (CPR) techniques, subsequent advanced and invasive life support techniques appear to be of little value in almost all cases.

The data supporting these conclusions were originally derived from two large studies of children, but preliminary information involving adult cases also support these conclusions.

Not enough people know or perform basic CPR, particularly when considering the high incidence of drowning in children less than 5 years of age and the low frequency of CPR performed by parents who witness cardiopulmonary arrest due to drowning of their own child.

6.2.3.2
Recommendations

Additional research and public health initiatives need to be implemented to increase the probability that there will be immediate performance of CPR and other first aid techniques at every drowning incident.

Additional research should attempt to delineate those aspects of CPR that are most effective, be they rescue breaths, chest compressions, variable combinations of these techniques, or other potential interventions by on-scene rescuers.

Subsequent research should examine new techniques for training lay persons in CPR that will be more easily taught, performed and retained as a learned skill.

Consensus process: These conclusions and recommendations were developed by the authors of the relevant study and were then accepted by the Task Force on Resuscitation for presentation to the main body of the World Congress on Drowning. These conclusions were then presented multiple times at the World Congress on Drowning in 2002 and later at the 2002 meeting of the ERC and the ILCOR, as well as multiple subsequent relevant national venues and meetings in the US and Europe without any significant objection or modification.

6.2.4
Basic Life Support for Drowning Victims

6.2.4.1
Conclusions

There is no need to clear the airway, no need to perform the so-called Heimlich manoeuvre, and no need to perform a pulse check if the basic life support (BLS) provider is a lay rescuer. A traditional healthcare provider who checks pulses routinely in their professional activities may do so, but should not focus on this action if other signs of absent circulation are present.

Without oxygen supplementation, tidal volumes provided by bag-valve-mask (BVM) device, mouth-to-mouth or mouth-to-mask (unprotected airway) should be 10 ml/kg or, in most situations, enough to make the chest wall rise.

If supplemental oxygen is being used, however, this tidal volume may be reduced somewhat to 6–7 ml/kg in most cases to diminish the risk of gastric insufflation.

Although chest compressions in those with circulatory arrest should be transiently interrupted to deliver breaths to the patient, every effort should be made to minimise this period of no compressions and every effort should be made not to frequently interrupt chest compressions.

In the situation of circulatory arrest, the number of breaths per minute may be less than currently recommended (15 compressions and two breaths), even in the case of drowning, and particularly with hypothermic conditions.

6.2.4.2
Recommendations

Researchers need to investigate alternative ventilatory techniques such as the active-compression decompression pump and inspiratory threshold devices or other novel techniques that will produce negative intrathoracic pressures such as a phrenic nerve stimulator.

Future research considerations should include an evaluation of appropriate compression-to-ventilation ratios in drowning incidents (and particularly in hypothermic conditions) and they should evaluate optimal tidal volumes for drowning events in view of the unique pathophysiology and alveolar effects of inhaled liquids.

Consensus process: These conclusions and recommendations were developed largely from the previous recommendations of ILCOR and the American Heart Association (AHA) and were accepted by the Task Force on Resuscitation and then presented multiple times at the World Congress on Drowning in 2002 and later at the 2002 meeting of the ERC and the ILCOR, as well as at multiple subsequent relevant national venues and meetings in the US and Europe without any signifivant objection or modification.

6.2.5
Automated Defibrillators in the Aquatic Environment

6.2.5.1
Conclusions

While ventricular fibrillation (VF) is an uncommon complication of drowning, especially in children, it can be a precipitating event on occasion.

VF occurs wherever persons at risk for sudden cardiac death are located and the aquatic environment is a frequented destination for persons of all ages, including such at-risk persons.

Therefore, by being a common gathering place for adults (and adults who supervise children), the aquatic environment is a reasonable target area for planning for the performance of cardiopulmonary resuscitation (CPR) and, in turn, the use of automated external defibrillators (AED), which, today, is considered a key part of CPR.

6.2.5.2
Recommendations

Aquatic areas are important target areas for stationing CPR providers and AEDs, especially if the aquatic locations are distant from responding rescuers or if they are visited by large numbers of persons, be they swimmers or otherwise.

Consensus process: These conclusions and recommendations were developed largely from an ad hoc working group of World Congress participants and the conclusions then presented multiple times at the World Congress on Drowning in 2002 and later at the 2002 meeting of the ERC and the ILCOR, as well as at multiple subsequent relevant national venues and meetings in the US and Europe without any significant objection or modification.

6.2.6
Positioning the Drowning Victim

6.2.6.1
Conclusions

Evidence suggests that the best outcomes occur following drowning events when the recovery position for the drowning victim is one that is horizontal and parallel to the shoreline, especially when there is a significant incline on the beach or shore.

It is unclear whether the left or right lateral position is more advantageous.

6.2.6.2
Recommendations

Future research in positioning needs to delineate the different aspects of positioning, not only in terms of left versus right lateral positions, but also what to do during the various phases of salvage and recovery: during rescue, upon reaching land, during resuscitation and during recovery.

Future research efforts also need to include closer examination of the absolute need for spinal precautions and relative risk stratification under various circumstances.

Consensus process: These conclusions and recommendations were developed largely from the previous recommendations of ILCOR and the AHA and individual research conclusions from the authors. These conclusions were accepted by the Task Force on Resuscitation and then presented multiple times at the World Congress on Drowning in 2002 and later at the 2002 meeting of the ERC and the ILCOR, as well as at multiple subsequent relevant national venues and meetings in the US and Europe without any significant objection or modification.

6.2.7
Invasive (Advanced) Life Support for Drowning

6.2.7.1
Conclusions

Few data support the absolute value of advanced life support (ALS) interventions, but evolving data in the general population of cardiac arrest patients have demonstrated the efficacy of inducing mild hypothermia to improve neurological outcome. These observations have implications for traditional attempts to re-warm resuscitated victims of drowning incidents. Empirically, with some special considerations about ventilatory techniques, ALS interventions targeted for the general cardiac arrest population should be used.

6.2.7.2
Recommendations

Recognising that bystander CPR is now the clear rate-limiting step in recovery and that hypoxia and hypoxemia are the main factors in the pathophysiology of drowning sequelae, extensive research is still needed, particularly in terms of proposed advanced therapeutic modalities such as tidal volumes, positive end-expiratory pressure (PEEP), respiratory rates, vasoactive agents, neuroprotective agents, and therapeutic hypothermia.

Consensus process: These conclusions and recommendations were developed largely from the previous recommendations of ILCOR and the AHA and were accepted by the Task Force on Resuscitation and then presented multiple times at the World Congress on Drowning in 2002 and later at the 2002 meeting of the European Resuscitation Council and the International Liaison Committee for Resuscitation (ILCOR), as well as at multiple subsequent relevant national venues and meetings in the US and Europe without any significant objection or modification.

6.2.8
The Long QT Syndrome and Drowning

6.2.8.1
Conclusions

Long QT Syndrome is a risk for divers and swimmers, largely because of related exertion and other particular factors that may trigger a related arrhythmia in these circumstances.

6.2.8.2
Recommendations

Individuals with documented long QT syndrome (LQTS), even those with an implanted cardioverter-defibrillator, or those who have experienced potentially-related syncope or episodes of ventricular fibrillation should be advised against swimming or diving.

During the medical examination of (aspiring) scuba divers, it is recommended that specific inquiries be made about any potentially related symptoms or the occurrence of sudden death among family members.

Consensus process: These conclusions and recommendations were developed largely from an ad hoc group (comprised of the authors) who then presented these recommendations at the World Congress on Drowning in 2002 without any significant objection or modification.

6.2.9
Paediatric Considerations in Drowning

6.2.9.1
Conclusions

Drowning is one of the most common causes of death for children, especially for those aged 1–5 years.

With the exception of the usual caveats about body size and proportions and increased susceptibility to temperature extremes, there are no significant differences that can be delineated at this time between adults and children in terms of the special circumstances of drowning.

Hypothermia may be therapeutic and thus it deserves further investigation as do concepts of how we provide re-warming.

Efforts aimed at the prevention of drowning deaths are currently weak worldwide as are efforts to promote CPR and its key role in paediatric drowning events.

6.2.9.2
Key Recommendations

There needs to be more prospective, population-based studies of drowning in children looking at the epidemiology, management and outcome predictors for this major public health problem.

There needs to be consideration of special interventions (that is, child-specific, targeted hypothermia techniques) and special pharmacological needs (such as dobutamine) in future research efforts.

There is a need for more focused training and public education about the key role of CPR in paediatric drowning incidents.

Consensus process: These conclusions and recommendations were developed largely from the previous recommendations of ILCOR and the AHA and were accepted by the Task Force on Resuscitation and then presented multiple times at the World Congress on Drowning in 2002 and later at the 2002 meeting of the ERC and the ILCOR, as well as at multiple subsequent relevant national venues and meetings in the US and Europe without any significant objection or modification.

6.2.10
Termination of Resuscitation Efforts

6.2.10.1
Conclusions

Current data about futility of resuscitation efforts are limited, not absolute and the prognosis can be multi-factorial.

Although there are rare exceptions, almost all neurologically-intact survivors, including cold water victims, are resuscitated within 1 hour of the initiating event.

Almost all normothermic adult patients are resuscitated within 25 minutes of the initiation of advanced life support techniques.

Water temperature below 21°C and younger age are correlated with improved prognosis.

6.2.10.2
Recommendations

Future research efforts should attempt to delineate the circumstances and applicable stratifications for the futility of continued resuscitation efforts following drowning incidents.

In addition to demographic information and water temperature considerations, future research efforts should determine maximum time intervals for resuscitation efforts under these various circumstances and stratifications, particularly with any new proposed neuro-protective or resuscitative interventions.

Consensus process: These conclusions and recommendations were developed by the authors of the relevant studies and were then accepted by the Task Force on Resuscitation for presentation to the main body of the World Congress on Drowning. These conclusions were then presented multiple times at the World Congress on Drowning in 2002 and later at the 2002 meeting of the ERC and the ILCOR, as well as multiple subsequent relevant national venues and meetings in the US and Europe without any significant objection or modification.

6.2.11
Unusual Rescue Circumstances, Considerations and Case Studies

6.2.11.1
Conclusions

A special attribute frequently differentiating drowning incidents from most other resuscitation situations is the occasionally odd location of the event (such as buckets, toilets, tubs, pools, floods, storm surges, culverts, lakes, tanks, reservoirs, storm drains, rivers or oceans), all providing unique challenges and often special coordination with other (non-healthcare) professionals as rescuers.

The association of other predisposing illnesses (particularly in the elderly) and also associated sequelae (for example, ensuing or accompanying injuries) also make this a special type of resuscitation event.

6.2.11.2
Recommendations

Whenever and wherever possible, epidemiological studies are recommended that track drowning circumstances, associated illnesses and injuries, and other related sequelae and associated hazards.

There should be anticipation, pre-planning, and follow-up of joint training needs for all potential rescuers in terms of the unique situations that may be encountered and associated with drowning events.

Consensus process: These conclusions and recommendations were developed by the authors of the relevant section materials and were then accepted by the Task Force on Resuscitation for presentation to the main body of the World Congress on Drowning.

6.2.12
Utstein-Style Guidelines for Drowning-Related Incidents

6.2.12.1
Conclusions

Among a myriad of other consensus-based terms, drowning is now defined as a process of experiencing respiratory impairment from submersion/immersion in liquid. Implicit in this definition is that a liquid/air interface is present at the entrance of the victim's airway, thus, preventing the victim from breathing air. A person may live or die after this process has occurred, but all who experience this process have had a drowning incident.

Improved validity, clarity, and data compatibility of future scientific investigations of drowning will improve our knowledge base, improve epidemiological stratification, improve appropriate treatment of victims of drowning and, ultimately, save lives.

6.2.12.2
Recommendations

To increase the understanding of the incidence, epidemiology, demography, risks, sequelae and outcomes of drowning-related events and to better understand the effects and resuscitation potential of various interventions, a uniform reporting system must be developed and used for the registration and study of drowning events.

Resuscitation organisations, and in particular those related to ILCOR, as well as rescue organisations and other groups who frequent aquatic areas, must promote and facilitate the concept that there needs to be uniform use of standardised definitions and nomenclature for data to be collected following drowning incidents. In turn, there also needs to be standardised reporting mechanisms for these data and scientific analysis of these data.

Therefore, all related organisations should adopt the consensus guidelines developed (see previous references).

Consensus process: These conclusions and recommendations were developed by the authors of the relevant publications mentioned previously and were then accepted by the Task Force on Resuscitation for presentation to the main body of the World Congress on Drowning. The special working group involved key members of the Task Force on Resuscitation and Task Force on Epidemiology and other invited specialists from key organisations such as ILCOR, the AHA, the Australian Resuscitation Council and the ERC. These conclusions were then presented multiple times at the World Congress on Drowning in 2002 for feedback and later at the 2002 meeting of the ERC and the ILCOR, as well as multiple subsequent relevant national venues and meetings in the US and Europe without any significant objection or modification. They have now been published in key scientific journals as noted previously.

6.3
The Critical Role of Lay Persons and Their Actions in Drowning Incidents

JANE WIGGINTON, PAUL PEPE, DENISE MANN, DAVID PERSSE and PAUL SIRBAUGH

It has been well-accepted for many years that most victims of critical drowning events will require instant on-scene medical attention such as the immediate performance of cardiopulmonary resuscitation (CPR) techniques by bystanders [1, 2]. However, the relative contribution of those bystander actions in drowning events has not yet been explicitly delineated.

6.3.1
Background

In most day-to-day situations, basic CPR performed by bystanders is considered to be a somewhat effective intervention, but only as a temporising action used to maintain some degree of critical tissue perfusion prior to arrival of a defibrillator in the patient with sudden cardiac death [3]. In other circumstances, it is also accepted as a way to maintain some limited form of circulation while advanced life support (ALS) actions are taken. Therefore, while there may be occasional exceptions, in general, basic CPR is not considered a definitive therapy in itself, especially for the majority of survivable sudden cardiac deaths.

In contrast to sudden cardiac death events, however, defibrillation is rarely needed in drowning incidents, particularly in the case of children [4, 5]. Also, be it for cardiac arrest or drowning, the scientific basis for most ALS interventions has been limited largely to laboratory evidence and some preliminary clinical data [3, 6–8]. Therefore, the role of basic CPR in drowning events has yet to be defined, either as a definitive therapy or as a temporising intervention that is provided as a bridge to ALS.

In addition, it has not been clear whether the key action in drowning is simply rescue breathing. It may also be that chest compressions or some other type of aggressive stimulation is the key intervention. Specifically, it is not known whether chest compressions alone could be efficacious and what the relative contributions of chest compressions should be under various circumstances [9].

The difficulty with answering these questions is that drowning events, particularly those occurring in children, are sudden, unanticipated and emotional events, often occurring in fairly uncontrolled settings. Even the need for full CPR procedures (rescue breathing and compressions) may be more difficult to assess, especially since respiratory arrests usually lead to cardiac arrest and bystanders may not be able to distinguish pulselessness. Not only are the potential witnesses unlikely to recall the exact actions taken and the sequencing of those actions, but even the rescuers themselves may have recall problems and uncertainty about what they actually did. This problem is often compounded by the re-telling of the event to a series of professional responders, perhaps beginning with lifesavers and firefighters as first responders and then continuing on to ambulance personnel and the first receiving in-hospital emergency personnel. Except in certain systems designed to collect data as optimally as possible, the exact actions of the bystanders are therefore unlikely to be well-recorded and the concomitant correlations with outcome difficult to establish.

Recognising these issues, several of the authors of this chapter undertook an initiative to improve data collection and correlation to outcome, particularly as it relates to drowning events in children to solve this puzzle [10]. The prospective, population-based study of paediatric (ages 0–14 years) drowning incidents, conducted in Houston, Texas (USA), between 1990 and 2000 inclusively, provides us with some additional insight into the problem of drowning and the critical role of bystander actions. The results corroborate previous studies in children and are compatible with preliminary studies involving adult as well as paediatric populations [11, 12].

6.3.2
The Houston Paediatric Drowning Data

In an attempt to capture the magnitude of the problem of paediatric drowning and examine elements that correlated with risk and outcome, investigators conducted an 11-year prospective population-based study of drowning incidents in the City of Houston, a municipality of about a 1.8-million resident population and 565 square miles (nearly 1000 square kilometres). The at-risk population (ages 0–14 years) averaged 418,000 during the decade of study. An average of 43 drownings occurred each year, making an annual incidence of 10.3 per 100,000 at risk. Two-thirds of all serious drowning incidents requiring a 9-1-1 (EMS system) response, occurred in the children (0–14 years) and 71% of those occurred in children less than or equal to 5 years of age (annual incidence of 18.3 per

100,000 at risk). In some years, this 0–5 years category accounted for as many as 87% of the paediatric cases.

Of the total number of 473 serious drowning cases in children 0–14 years of age requiring an EMS response, two-thirds of these clearly required some type of resuscitative effort. Of the 300 total cases requiring resuscitation, 101 died and two-third of deaths occurred in those less than or equal to 5 years of age. Also, two-thirds of the deaths occurred following pool incidents.

Perhaps the most impressive piece of information was the impact of bystander CPR. Half of the drownings received CPR by bystanders and 79% of those receiving bystander CPR survived to hospital discharge (97% neurologically intact). Most of the patients responded to bystander resuscitative efforts within a very short period of time to some degree or another and if the patient was still apneic and pulseless when the EMS rescuers arrived, only 5% responded to resuscitation and of these none remained neurologically intact.

Based on data collection projects conducted prior to the current study, there had been suspicion that many children receiving CPR may not have needed that intervention because patients were awakening and pulsing when responding rescuers arrived. This raised the concern that there was overzealous initiation of CPR by bystanders in certain cases for which it may not really have been needed. However, this concern was eliminated by a strict set of criteria in which the patients included as 'requiring resuscitation' had to be those reported by all available witnesses at the scene as clearly being unresponsive, lifeless, apneic, cyanotic or those later found to have chest roentgenogram and laboratory or physiological abnormalities consistent with water aspiration. These reports were obtained by a designated rescuer who conducted intensive follow-up interviews to document the strict criteria. Therefore, this information appears to be quite reliable and the remaining 173 cases of drowning not reported as requiring CPR may have been more serious than previously thought, but simply excluded because the investigators could not document the required criteria to designate these as true resuscitation cases. In essence, this means that survival rates may be even better than the results reported here.

6.3.3
Discussion

This decade-long, population-based study demonstrated most strikingly that bystander CPR appears to be the most definitive action for children with serious drowning incidents requiring resuscitative efforts. Other studies support this conclusion [11, 12]. A previous study from Southern California, by Kyriacou, corroborates the same observations in children [11] and a recent report from Brugge, Belgium, found similar findings in adults [13]. In that Belgian study, Hooft studied 103 drowning incidents occurring between 1991–1996. The mean age of this group was 49 years and among the 26 patients receiving CPR from bystanders, only eight ultimately survived and only five had a good neurological outcome. Of these five, four had return of spontaneous circulation prior to the initiation of advanced life support interventions. Of the 76 patients not receiving bystander CPR, none survived despite the implementation of such advanced interventions in most cases.

Therefore, performance of CPR by bystanders, usually lay persons, appears to be the necessary factor in terms of determining intact survival for the paediatric drowning victim. Relatively-speaking, without such immediate first aid and basic CPR techniques, subsequent advanced and invasive life support techniques appear to be of little value in almost all cases.

6.3.4
The Need for More CPR Training

Although the frequency of CPR is slightly higher in the settings of drowning (usually public places), it should probably be even higher than portrayed in this and other studies. Simply put, not enough people know or perform basic CPR, particularly when considering the low frequency of CPR performed by parents who witness the cardiopulmonary arrest of their own child [4].

Considering that the frequency of CPR training and performance is generally low in most venues, more aggressive campaigns to require CPR training for all persons (for example, required CPR training in the high schools, in the workplace or to acquire a driver's license as they do in some countries) must be conducted. Additional research and public health initiatives need to be implemented to increase the probability that there will be immediate performance of first aid techniques and CPR at every drowning incident. Also, additional research should attempt to delineate those aspects of CPR that are most effective, be they rescue breaths, chest compressions, variable combinations of these techniques, or other potential interventions by on-scene rescuers. In addition, subsequent research should examine new techniques for training lay persons in CPR that are shorter and more easily taught, performed and retained as a learned skill.

References

1. Haynes BE (2000) Near drowning. In: Tintinalli JE, Kelen GD, Stapczynski JS (eds) Emergency medicine. McGraw-Hill, New York, pp 1278-1279.
2. Modell JH (1993) Drowning. N Engl J Med 328:253–258
3. Cummins R, Ornato J, Thies W, Pepe P (1991) Improving survival from sudden cardiac arrest: the chain of survival concept. A statement for health professionals from the Advanced Cardiac Life Support Subcommittee and the Emergency Cardiac Care Committee, American Heart Association. Circulation 83:1832–1847
4. Sirbaugh P, Pepe P, Shook J, et al. (1999) A prospective, population-based study of the demographics, epidemiology, management, and outcome of out-of-hospital pediatric cardiopulmonary arrest. Ann Emerg Med 33:174–184
5. Quan L, Kinder D (1992) Pediatric submersions: prehospital predictors of outcome. Pediatrics 90:909–913
6. Stiell IG, Wells GA, Field B, et al. (2004) Advanced life support in out-of-hospital cardiac arrest. N Engl J Med 351:647–656
7. Wenzel V, Krismer AC, Arntz HR, et al. (2004) A comparison of vasopressin and epinephrine for out-of-hospital cardiopulmonary resuscitation. N Engl J Med 350:105–113

8. Pepe P, Abramson N, Brown C (1994) ACLS – Does it really work? Ann Emerg Med 23:1037–1041
9. Roppolo L, Wigginton JA, Pepe PE (2004) Emergency ventilatory management as a detrimental factor in resuscitation practices and clinical research efforts. In: Vincent JL (ed) 2004 Yearbook of Intensive Care and Emergency Medicine. Springer, Berlin, pp 139–151
10. Pepe PE, Wigginton JG, Mann DM, Persse DE, Sirbaugh PE, Berg RA (2002) Prospective, decade-long, population-based study of pediatric drowning-related incidents. Acad Emerg Med 9:516–517
11. Kyriacou D, Arcinue E, Peek C, Kraus J (1994) Effect of immediate resuscitation on children with submersion injury. Pediatrics 94:137–142
12. Goh SH, Low B (1999) Drowning and near-drowning – some lesions learned. Acad Med Singapore 28:183–188
13. Hooft P (2002) The influence of lay cardiopulmonary resuscitation on outcome after cardiopulmonary arrest due to drowning. Book of abstracts, World Congress on Drowning, Amsterdam, p 164

6.4
Basic Life Support for Drowning Victims

AHAMED IDRIS

The most important consequence of submersion without ventilation is hypoxemia [1, 2]. The duration of submersion and accompanying hypoxemia are the most critical factors in determining the outcome of the victim. Thus, logically, oxygenation, ventilation, and critical organ perfusion should be restored as soon as possible.

6.4.1
Basic Life Support (BLS) Sequence

The first and most important treatment of the drowning victim is immediate mouth-to-mouth ventilation, which has been shown to have a positive effect on outcome [3]. Rescue breathing should be started as soon as the airway of the victim can be opened. Ventilation devices that provide oxygen supplementation should be used as soon as they are available and a call should be made to the emergency medical system (EMS) as soon as possible.

There is no need to clear the airway of aspirated water. Some victims aspirate nothing because of laryngospasm and only a modest amount, at most, is aspirated by the majority [1, 2]. Abdominal thrusts (Heimlich manoeuvre) should not be used routinely because it increases the risk of regurgitation and aspiration and it also delays initiation of ventilation [1].

If signs of circulation are absent, chest compressions should be started immediately [4]. If an automatic external defibrillator (AED) is available, it should be applied to assess the cardiac rhythm of the victim. If a shockable rhythm is present, defibrillation should be attempted [4].

6.4.2
Rescue Breathing Techniques

Recent changes have been made to BLS guidelines for typical cardiac arrests. Among these are modifications in the approach to rescue breathing and bag-valve-mask (BVM) ventilation. Gastric inflation frequently develops during mouth-to-mouth ventilation as air being forced into the oropharynx can travel either down the trachea or oesophagus. Gastric inflation can produce serious complications such as regurgitation, aspiration or pneumonia [1]. If overzealously done, it also can increase intragastric pressure, elevate the diaphragm, restrict lung movement, and decrease respiratory system compliance. Gastric inflation generally occurs when the pressure in the oesophagus exceeds the lower oesophageal sphincter opening pressure. This causes the sphincter to open, so air delivered during rescue breaths may more likely enter the stomach, instead of the lungs. During cardiac arrest, the likelihood of gastric inflation increases because the lower oesophageal sphincter relaxes. Factors that contribute to a gastric inflation during rescue breathing include: obstructed airway (tongue, poor positioning), a short inspiratory time (rapidly delivered breath), a large tidal volume, and a high peak airway pressure (usually brought on by the previous three factors). Therefore, actions that can open the airway more (better positioning, oral airway devices, jaw thrusts, chin lifts), slow ventilatory delivery time (slow steady breath delivered over 2 seconds) and better control over the tidal volume delivered are important as is cricothyroid membrane pressure to compress the oesophagus.

This is most of all important in drowning victims where loss of surfactant and acute pulmonary impairments will lead to a decreased pulmonary compliance.

6.4.3
Tidal Volume Considerations

Recent recommendations for tidal volumes and inspiratory times for ventilation have been modified [4]. A tidal volume of approximately 10 ml/kg (approximately 700–1000 ml for most adult persons) is delivered slowly and steadily over 1.5–2.0 seconds. This usually leads to observation of a well-defined chest rise when mouth-to-mouth breathing or mouth-to-mask breathing is provided without oxygen supplementation (Class IIa recommendation) [4].

However, in view of the unprotected airway and risk for gastric insufflation, when supplemental oxygen is available, a tidal volume of 6–7 ml/kg (approximately 400–600 ml for most adult persons) may be preferable. This breath should be delivered over 1.5–2.0 seconds until a chest rise is observed. This would most typically be applicable when rescuers are using a BVM device or a mouth-to-mask device with oxygen supplementation that provides an inspired concentration of oxygen of 40% or more (Class IIb recommendation) [4]. While these tidal volumes may not be as applicable in the drowning scenario, in which surfactant loss and other physiological sequelae may make alveolar recruitment more difficult, there are no studies that would confirm the need for an alternative approach [1].

6.4.4
Pulse Check

The pulse check has been deleted from the assessment steps performed by lay rescuers [4]. Lay rescuers should check for signs of normal breathing, coughing or movement to determine the presence or absence of circulation. Healthcare providers accustomed to taking pulses can perform a pulse check, but they should do so in conjunction with assessment of signs of breathing, coughing or movement (Class IIa recommendation) [4].

6.4.5
Chest Compressions

The recommended compression rate for one- and two-rescuer adult CPR has been increased to 100 compressions per minute (Class IIb recommendation) [4]. However, in the year 2000, the ratio of 15 compressions to two ventilations was recommended for both one- and two-rescuer CPR for the adult victim with an unprotected (non-intubated) airway (Class IIb Recommendation) [4]. Recommendations for children remained at 5:1, but these practices, both for adults and children, are being re-evaluated.

Although chest compressions in those with circulatory arrest should be transiently interrupted to deliver breaths to the patient during BLS, every effort should be made to minimise this period of no compressions and every effort should be made not to frequently interrupt chest compressions. Although positive pressure breaths may inflate lung zones, they may also increase intrathoracic pressure enough to impede venous return. Also, stopping to ventilate impairs coronary perfusion [5–7]. It may take 10–15 compressions to return to previous levels of coronary perfusion achieved when compressions are interrupted to deliver a breath. Therefore, with current techniques, most of the compression cycles are used to return to the pressure head lost when compressions were halted.

In fact, in the situation of circulatory arrest, the number of breaths required per minute may be much less than currently recommended, even in the case of respiratory impairment such as drowning, and particularly when there are hypothermic conditions due to lower metabolism and less carbon dioxide excretion. More recently, recommendations are evolving and leaning toward a higher ratio of compressions to ventilations such as 50:2 or 30:2 for adults and 15:2 for children [5, 8]. Readers should refer to the most recent guidelines for compression–ventilation ratios which are due to be published in December of 2005. Also, one should differentiate between those with pulses (who will need more ventilation) and those in circulatory arrest. Ventilation should match perfusion.

Chest compression-only CPR has been recommended in certain circumstances [4] such as those in which a rescuer is unwilling or unable to perform mouth-to-mouth rescue breathing (Class IIa recommendation) [4], or those in which dispatchers are providing instructions over the telephone to bystanders on-scene. The simplicity of this modified technique allows untrained bystanders to rapidly intervene (Class IIa recommendation) [4]. For teaching purposes, and during performance of CPR, audio timing prompts may help to achieve the required rate for the performance of chest compressions (Class IIb recommendation) [4].

6.4.6
Relief of Foreign-Body Airway Obstruction

It has been recommended that the guidelines sequence for management of airway obstruction in unconscious adults should not be taught to the lay public [4]. Emphasis should be placed on continued effective chest compression, opening the airway and attempting ventilation (Class IIb recommendation) [4]. The healthcare provider, however, should continue to learn how to achieve relief of foreign body airway obstruction in both conscious and unconscious victims.

6.4.7
Conclusions and Recommendations

Researchers need to investigate alternative ventilatory techniques to inflate lung zones while minimizing the gastric insufflation and maximizing of venous return. Interventions should be examined such as the active-compression decompression pump and inspiratory threshold devices or other novel techniques that will produce negative intrathoracic pressures such as a phrenic nerve stimulator [9].

Also, future research considerations should include an evaluation of appropriate compression to ventilation ratios in drowning incidents, particularly in hypothermic conditions. Future drowning research should evaluate optimal tidal volumes for drowning events in view of the unique pathophysiology and alveolar effects of inhaled liquids.

References

1. Bierens JJLM, Knape JTA, Gelissen HPMM (2002) Drowning. Curr Opin Crit Care 8:578–586
2. Modell JH (1993) Drowning. N Engl J Med 328:253–258
3. Safar P, Escarraga LA, Elam JO (1958) A comparison of the mouth-to-mouth and mouth-to-airway methods of artificial respiration with the chest pressure arm-lift methods. N Engl J Med 258:671–677
4. Idris AH, Basic Life Support Subcommittee (2002) Basic life support and special situations. American Heart Association Guidelines 2000 for cardiopulmonary resuscitation and emergen-

cy cardiovascular care – international consensus on science, August 22, vol 102 (Supplement I), pp 1–384
5. Roppolo LP, Wigginton JA, Pepe PE (2004) Emergency ventilatory management as a detrimental factor in resuscitation practices and clinical research efforts. In: Vincent J-L (ed.) 2004 Yearbook of intensive care and emergency medicine. Springer, Berlin, pp 139–151
6. Koster RW (2003) Limiting ‚hands-off' periods during resuscitation. Resuscitation 58:275–276
7. Berg RA, Sanders AB, Kern KB, Hilwig RW, Heidenreich JW, Porter ME, Ewy GA (2001) Adverse hemodynamic effects of interrupting chest compressions for rescue breathing during cardiopulmonary resuscitation for ventricular fibrillation cardiac arrest. Circulation 104:2465–2470
8. Babbs CF, Nadkarni V (2004) Optimizing chest compression to rescue ventilation ratios during one-rescuer CPR by professionals and lay persons: children are not just little adults. Resuscitation 61:173–181
9. O'Connor RE, Ornato JP, Wigginton JG (2003) Alternate cardiopulmonary resuscitation devices. Prehosp Emerg Care 7:31–41

6.5
Automated External Defibrillators in the Aquatic Environment

Steve Beerman and Bo Løfgren

The use of the automated external defibrillator (AED) has become widely-adopted and has even become part of standard CPR training. This chapter discusses the issues of AED in the modern chain of survival, and, in particular, its potential use in the aquatic environment.

6.5.1
Cardiac Arrest and Defibrillation

Early defibrillation is a key determinant of survival from cardiac arrest due to ventricular fibrillation (VF) [1–4]. Ventricular fibrillation is the initiating event in the majority of adult cardiac arrests out-of hospital and it is the presenting rhythm for about 30%–50% of cardiac arrest victims in the emergency medical systems (EMS) in major developed cities [1–3]. Fast rescuer response intervals increases the likelihood of the cardiac arrest victim having VF at the time of arrival and concomitant rapid defibrillation improves the chances of survival, especially with performance of CPR by bystanders [1–4]. Broadening access to AEDs as well as training in AED use beyond health care professionals can help reduce the time to defibrillation and thus improve survival probabilities [2, 3, 5–14].

While untreated VF is a uniformly deadly event, VF is almost always reversible with the immediate availability and use of a defibrillator [2]. However, since most patients do not have immediate access to a defibrillator, resuscitation to survival may depend on a series of critical interventions being performed. The chain of survival metaphor has been used to describe this sequence of critical interventions [1]. The traditional chain has four interdependent links: early access (notification of emergency response dispatchers), early basic life support (BLS) on CPR, early defibrillation (with AED or manual defibrillator), and early advanced life support (ALS) with medications and advanced airways. However, immediate use within a minute or two of an AED may obviate the need for ALS and even BLS, as patients may even respond and awaken long before traditional professional rescuers arrive [2, 6].

Cardiac arrest associated with VF or ventricular tachycardia (VT) is rare in drowning victims [15–19]. There is very limited case study literature on the use and success of defibrillation in drowning cases. Most of the case reports in the medical literature of defibrillation in the aquatic environment were not related to drowning victims, but rather cardiac arrests from non-drowning causes.

Specifically, many aquatic facilities are associated with large public areas. Cardiac arrest is more probable within high volume public areas [1–3, 11]. As a result, some aquatic facility staff members have placed AED equipment in or near aquatic areas in order to be prepared to respond to cardiac arrests due to VF and VT, not in the water, but at the edge of the water where many people gather, including those at risk for VF or VT.

6.5.2
AED and Defibrillation

Defibrillation is primarily intended to correct problems associated with most sudden cardiac arrest, specifically VF or VT. However, the AED has no positive impact on the outcomes for non-shockable rhythms in cardiac arrest [20]. An AED is a computerised defibrillator programed to recognise and shock either VF or VT. If the machine recognises either VT or VF in the victim, it will charge itself and indicate, usually by voice prompt, that a shock is advised.

When a shock is delivered to the heart, this will momentarily stop all electrical activity in the heart. This may terminate the VF or VT that was occurring. The natural pacemaker of the heart, the sino-atrial node, may then have a chance to take command and begin generating the impulses, which will start the normal pumping action at the heart. Sometimes multiple shocks are required to achieve this sequence of events.

The reliability of the AED is as good as any medical device can be [3]. The identification of VF is better than human interpretation and almost 100% specific [2]. Technological advances have resulted in AEDs that are portable, safe, easy to use and easy to maintain with batteries that can last for years in stand-by conditions. It is logical that as they become less expensive, they are more likely to be placed in areas of public use [3, 11, 12]. Recent studies of defibrillation by the public at the Chicago airport showed remarkable save rates for VF (>75%) at nominal costs per life saved [2].

6.5.3
The AED in the Aquatic Environment

To achieve the earliest possible defibrillation, many organisations such as casinos, stadiums or airlines have created targeted AED training and rapid AED access for security guards and flight attendants, achieving remarkable save rates and hundreds of lifesaving incidents since implementation in the late 1990s [2, 6–10]. In turn, lifesavers and those who live, work and play in the aquatic environment have expressed interest in the use of AED to improve resuscitation outcomes in their targeted setting. Aquatic personnel should still appreciate that an AED is not necessarily a top priority equipment requirement due to the relatively low risk of a VF or VT event at a given site. However, an AED can be an appropriate adjunct to basic water rescue equipment, oxygen equipment, basic first aid and CPR equipment. Again, it is recognised that aquatic environments are a frequent venue for large numbers of people, as are recreation and fitness facilities, and events and activities that invite and attract people who may also be at risk for cardiac arrest. For all of these reasons, individuals and organisations providing supervision to aquatic environments, should have a keen interest in the availability of an AED for the aquatic settings and its environs.

Most drowning victims have healthy hearts that cease to function due to hypoxia. The best approach in treating drowning victims is to prevent prolonged submersion, provide immediate CPR measures, ideally with high flow oxygen, and then, if available, an AED may be used, in accordance with the criteria of the manufacturer and the local response priorities. This may be helpful in the relatively unlikely case that the drowning victim has a cardiac arrest with VF or VT.

In 1999, the Medical Commission of the International Life Saving Federation (see ▶ **6.5.7**) recommended a statement on AED use by lifesavers.

The principles, stated in ◻ **Table 6.1**, are a reasonable starting point for those seeking to prepare for AED use in the aquatic environment. In recent years, many lifesaving organisations have trained, placed and used AEDs in the aquatic environment. A critical appraisal of large cohort data from these initiatives will be extremely useful.

6.5.4
Barriers to AED Use

Early concerns about the use of AED on wet cardiac arrest victims have not been a problem in the field and there has not been any environmental specific risks reported. Although dry surfaces are preferred, this is a relative concern and not a contraindication to the use of AED. A quick drying of the pooled water from the chest prior to application of shock is recommended. At the time of this publication, there has not been one report of dangerous conduction of shock from cardiac arrest victims through the adjacent wet surfaces. Testing by the manufacturers confirms this safety issue. However, the AED is not recommended for in-water application. Nevertheless, it may be appropriate to apply an AED at the earliest convenient moment once the victim is placed on a hard surface.

Use of the AED in the aquatic environment is a concept that is gaining use as the barriers of ideology, priority and economics are being challenged. Perceived liability for rescuers misusing these devices, a near-impossibility, is being replaced by legal exposure for not having these lifesaving devices available. There

> **▣ Table 6.1.** Statement by the International Life Saving Federation, Medical Commission on automated external defibrillator (AED) use by lifesavers and lifeguards
>
> 1. Outcomes from drowning and water-related accidents can be tragic. The principle objective for lifesavers and lifeguards is to prevent, drowning and water-related accidents through education, supervision and rapid rescue response
>
> 2. The principle consequence of drowning is hypoxia. The provision of lifesavers and lifeguards with training and equipment for early recovery of victims from water is the highest priority
>
> 3. All lifesavers and lifeguards should receive training in basic life support (chain of survival, early access to EMS, airway management and CPR)
>
> 4. Early defibrillation in the management of cardiac arrest is effective in cases of VF and VT. When an arrest victim, in VF or VT, has early application of defibrillation, this is associated with conversion to sinus rhythm and to functional survival. VF and VT may be present in some drowning resuscitations when early recognition, speedy rescue and effective CPR with oxygen supplementation, has occurred. Early application of AED may be helpful in these cases
>
> 5. Advanced life support skills (defibrillation, medication and intensive care) may be part of the community response to cardiac arrest. It is appropriate for some lifesaving and lifeguard services to investigate AED use. This review should include investigations of other community AED providers, AED response times, frequency of cardiac arrests, supervision and management of AED, AED license requirements, cost/benefit analysis and outcomes studies. Decisions about the availability, placement, training and use of AED should be a community level decision based on the principles of the "chain of survival", local resources and community priority
>
> 6. Lifesaver and lifeguards may play a role in the delivery of AED if this is consistent with the support and service priorities of that community
>
> 7. If lifesavers or lifeguards will be delivering AED, they must receive appropriate training in the use of AED and the associated issues related to outcomes, stress and grief
>
> 8. National, regional and local lifesaving and lifeguarding organisations may choose to participate in the development of training policies for the use of AED by non-medical personnel, if and when communities choose to implement AED use by lifesavers or lifeguards. Lifesavers and lifeguard services are part of a community risk management and response plan, an integral part of a wider population safety network
>
> 9. Outcome studies of the application of AED by lifesavers and lifeguards in aquatic settings should be encouraged

EMS, emergency medical systems; CPR, cardiopulmonary resuscitation; VF, ventricular fibrillation; VT, ventricular tachycardia.

now exist very sound and well-established principles for decision-making, training, use and reporting of AED, paving the way for their routine use in the aquatic and near-aquatic environment [3, 12, 21, 22]. Most victims of cardiac arrest are from adjacent land-based crowds and land-based associated recreation or fitness activities. The lifesaver or lifesavers may be conveniently located, trained and equipped to provide immediate care. Education about changes in AED and CPR training should be monitored and updated as needed. [22, 23].

6.5.5
Caveats

A significant percentage of cardiac arrest victims do not survive to hospital admission [1]. Unsuccessful outcomes are usually more frequent than successful outcomes, regardless of the equipment available to assist assessment and treatment. Training in resuscitation, with or without adjunctive equipment, should include realistic rescuer expectations and critical incident debriefing education [22].

6.5.6
Conclusion

The AED may become an increasingly common link in the chain of survival within aquatic environments. Shockable rhythms in drowning victims are very rare and uncommonly cited in published drowning cardiac arrest papers and case reports. However, VF and VT may still be more likely to occur in areas adjacent to the water. Beaches, poolsides, lakesides and riverbanks are common attractions for human gatherings and VF and VT cases are more likely to surface wherever humans gather in large numbers. The assessment of the AED impact on outcomes in the aquatic environment and adjacent domains is a research priority.

6.5.7
Website

International Lifesaving Federation – Medical Commission – www.ilsf/med

References

1. Cummins RO, Ornato JP, Thies WH, Pepe PE (1991) Improving survival from sudden cardiac arrest: the chain of survival concept. A statement for health professionals from the Advanced Cardiac Life Support Subcommittee and the Emergency Cardiac Care Committee, American Heart Association. Circulation 83:1832–1847
2. Caffrey SL, Willoughby PJ, Pepe PE, Bedker LB (2002) Public use of automated defibrillators. N Engl J Med 347:1242–1247
3. Weisfeldt M, Kerber RE, McGoldrick RP, et al. (1995) American Heart Association report on the public access defibrillation conference, Dec 8–10, 1994. Circulation 92:2740–2747
4. Hertlitz J, Bang A, Homberg M, et al. (1997) Rhythm changes during resuscitation from ventricular fibrillation in relation to delay until defibrillation. Resuscitation 34:17–19

5. Bunch TJ, White RD, Gersh BJ, et al. (2003) Long-term outcomes of out-of-hospital cardiac arrest after successful early defibrillation. N Engl J Med 348:2626–2633
6. Valenzuela TD, Roe DJ, Nichol G, et al. (2000) Outcomes of rapid defibrillation by security officers after cardiac arrest in casinos. N Engl J Med 343:1206–1209
7. Page RL, Joglar JA, Kowal RC, et al. (2000) Use of automated external defibrillators by a U.S. airline. N Engl J Med 343:1210–1216
8. Wassertheil J, Keane G, Fisher N, Leditschke JF (2000) Cardiac arrest outcomes at the Melbourne Cricket Ground and Shrine of Remembrance using a tiered response strategy – a forerunner to public access defibrillation. Resuscitation 44:97–104
9. MacDonald RD, Mottley JL, Weinstein C (2002) Impact of prompt defibrillation on cardiac arrest at a major international airport. Prehosp Emerg Care 6:1–5
10. O'Rourke MF, Donaldson EE, Geddes JS (1997) An airline cardiac arrest program. Circulation 96:2849–2853
11. Becker L, Eisenberg M, Farhenbruch C, Cobb LA (1998) Public locations of cardiac arrest: implications for public access defibrillation. Circulation 97:2106–2109
12. Nichol, G, Valenzuela T, Roe D, et al. (2003) Cost effectiveness of defibrillation by targeted responders public settings. Circulation 108:697–703
13. Myerburg RJ, Fenster J, Velez M, et al. (2002) Impact of community-wide police car deployment of AED in survival from out-of-hospital cardiac arrest. Circulation 106:1030–1033
14. Watt DD (1995) Defibrillation by basic emergency medical technicians. Ann Emerg Med 26:635–639
15. Monolios N, Mackie I (1988) Drowning and near-drowning on Australian beaches patrolled by life-savers: a 10 year study 1973–1983. Med J Australia 148:165–171
16. Kuisma M, Suominen P, Korpela R, et al. (1995) Pediatric out-of-hospital cardiac arrest– epidemiology and outcome. Resuscitation 30:141–150
17. Sirbaugh PE, Pepe PE, Shook JE, et al. (1999) A prospective, population-based study of the demographics, epidemiology, management and outcome of out-of-hospital pediatric cardiopulmonary arrest. Ann Emerg Med 33:174–184
18. Orlowski JP, Szpilman D (2001) Drowning. Rescue, resuscitation, and reanimation. Pediatr Clin North Am 48:627-646
19. Modell JH (1993) Drowning. N Engl J Med 328:253–256
20. Pepe PE, Levine RL, Fromm RE Jr, et al. (1993) Cardiac arrest presenting with rhythms other than ventricular fibrillation: Contribution of resuscitation efforts toward total survivorship. Crit Care Med 21:1838–1843
21. Kloeck W, Cummins RO, Chamberlain D et al. (1997) An advisory statement from the Advanced Life Support Working Group of the ILCOR. Circulation 95:2183–2184
22. American Heart Association (2001) Fundamentals of BLS for healthcare providers. American Heart Association, Dallas, Texas, pp 37–55
23. Cobb LA, Fahrenbruch CE, Walsh TR, et al. (1999) Influence of CPR prior to defibrillation in patients with out-of-hospital ventricular fibrillation. JAMA 281:1182–1188

6.6
Positioning the Drowning Victim

David Szpilman and Anthony Handley

For centuries, people falsely believed that draining water from the lungs of drowning victims was an essential part of the resuscitation process. In the 18th century, this was the main reason why victims were positioned hanging vertically head down. Even today, many theories about positioning are offered, but few with hard data to back them. In the following chapter, an attempt is made to provide the most logical rationale for positioning based on the available information, recent studies and consensus. In turn, this discussion will focus on issues such as water in the lungs and positioning during rescue (in the water and on-land), and position during resuscitation and recovery for the drowning victim (■ Table 6.2).

6.6.1
Water in the Lungs

Massive aspiration during the drowning process is seldom observed in humans [1]. Placing the victim head down does result in the drainage of some aspirated fluid, mainly after salt water drowning, but the disadvantages outweigh the benefits. In particular, such action does not improve oxygenation of the patient during a resuscitation attempt [2–4]. Although it does not take long, in the usual sense, to drain water from the lungs (1–3 min), such delay before resuscitative efforts is significant as far as outcome is concerned because most of the significant electrolyte and fluid shifts have already taken place [1, 2, 5].

In addition, inappropriate positioning has other consequences that outweigh any theoretical advantage. During prehospital resuscitation, attempts at active drainage by placing the victim in a head-down position increases the risk of vomiting more than five-fold, and leads to a significant increase (19%) in mortality when compared with keeping the victim in a horizontal position [6]. The presence of vomit in the airway can result in further aspiration and impairment of oxygenation by obstructing the airways. It can also discourage rescuers from attempting mouth-to-mouth resuscitation [7, 8].

Although it has been recommended by some, the abdominal thrust (Heimlich manoeuvre) should not be used as a means of expelling water from the lungs. It is ineffective and carries significant risks [9].

6.6.2
In-Water Rescue

If resuscitation is started whilst the drowning victim is still in the water, the chance of survival without sequelae is increased three-fold [10]. Chest compression is not a practical option, but rescue breathing can be undertaken, preferably with support, in deep water (■ Fig. 6.1) or at the edge of the water.

6.6.3
Rescue From the Water

Maintaining the victim in a head-up vertical position during rescue from the water reduces the incidence of vomiting (D. Szpilman, personal observation, 1996) and facilitates spontaneous respiration (■ Fig. 6.2). When hypotension or shock is suspected, the victim should be rescued in a near-horizontal position, but with the head still maintained above body level [11]. Horizontal recovery is

Table 6.2. Recommendations for positioning a drowning victim without suspected spinal injury according to the condition of the victim

Setting	Condition of the drowning victim	
	Conscious victim	Exhausted, confused or unconscious victim
In-water (during rescue)	Position according to the rescue technique chosen	Whenever possible, rescuers should keep the face of the victim out of the water, extend the neck to open the airway and keep it clear during the rescue process (◘ **Fig. 6.1**)
Recovery to on-land	Transport vertically with head up. Keep horizontal if prolonged immersion or immersion in cold water (◘ **Fig. 6.2**)	Transport in as near a horizontal position as possible but with the head still maintained above body level. The airway should be kept open and the victim should be kept horizontal if prolonged immersion or cold water is involved
On-land	Maintain the victim in a supine position with head up	If cardiopulmonary resuscitation is required: place victim supine, as horizontal as possible, and parallel with the waterline (◘ **Fig. 6.3**)
		Unconscious but breathing: Place in recovery position (◘ **Fig. 6.4**)

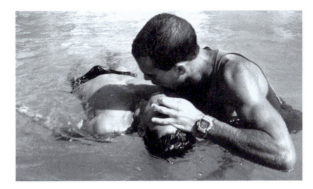

Fig. 6.1. Rescue breathing with support in deep water

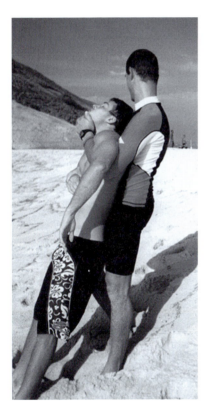

Fig. 6.2. Maintaining the victim in a head-up position during rescue

important after prolonged immersion, particularly in cold water, as a combination of the release of hydrostatic pressure and the effect of the cold may result in severe, sometimes irreversible, hypotension [12].

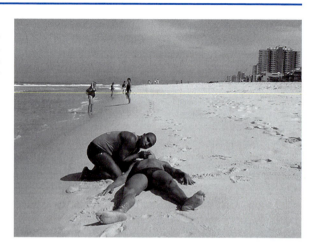

■ **Fig. 6.3.** On sloping beaches, the victim should be placed parallel to the waterline and the rescuer should be with the back to the water

6.6.4
On-Land Resuscitation

All victims should initially be placed in a position parallel to the waterline [6], as horizontal as possible, lying supine, far enough away from the water to avoid incoming waves. During CPR, the brain is most effectively perfused with oxygenated blood if the victim is in a horizontal position [13].

On sloping beaches or riverbanks, rescuers attending the victim should kneel with their backs towards the water so as to facilitate evaluation and CPR manoeuvres, if needed, without falling over the victim (■ **Fig. 6.3**).

6.6.5
The Unconscious but Breathing Victim

On land the airway of an unconscious victim who is breathing spontaneously is at risk of obstruction by the tongue and from inhalation of mucus and vomit. Placing the victim on the side (recovery position) helps to prevent these problems, and allows fluid to drain easily from the mouth (■ **Fig. 6.4**). The person should be placed in a position that is horizontal (parallel) to the shore line if there is an incline. It is not known whether it is preferable to have the left or right side down.

6.6.6
Summary of General Principles

The Basic Life Support Working Group of the International Liaison Committee on Resuscitation (ILCOR) has agreed on six principles that should be followed when managing the unconscious, spontaneously breathing victim [14]:

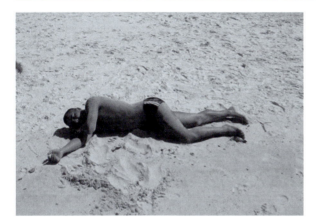

Fig. 6.4. On sloping beaches, the victim should be placed parallel to the water-line in the lateral position during recovery

- The victim should be in as near a true lateral position as possible with the head dependant to allow free drainage of fluid.
- The position should be stable.
- Any pressure on the chest that impairs breathing should be avoided.
- It should be possible to turn the victim onto the side and return to the back easily and safely, having particular regard to the possibility of cervical spine injury.
- Good observation of, and access to, the airway should be possible.
- The position itself should not give rise to any injury to the victim.

References

1. Modell JH, Davis JH (1969) Electrolytes changes in human drowning victims. Anesthesiology 30:414–420
2. Werner JZ, Safar P, Bircher NG, et al. (1982) No improvement in pulmonary status by gravity drainage or abdominal thrust after seawater near-drowning in dogs. Anesthesiology 57
3. Modell JH (1981) Is the Heimlich manoeuvre appropriate as first treatment for drowning? Emerg Med Serv 10:63–66
4. Ruben A, Ruben H (1962) Artificial respiration. Flow of water from the lung and the stomach. Lancet 1:780–781
5. Orlowski JP (1987) Adolescent drowning: swimming, boating, diving, and scuba sccidents. Pediatr Ann 17:2
6. Szpilman D, Idris A, Cruz Filho FES (2002) Position of drowning resuscitation victim on sloping beaches. Book of abstracts, World Congress of Drowning Amsterdam, p 168
7. Manolios N, Mackie I (1988) Drowning and near drowning on Australian beaches patrolled by life-savers: a 10 year study (1973–1983). M J Aust 148:165–171
8. Bierens JILM, Velde EA, Berkel M, Zanten JJ (1997) Submersion in the Netherlands: prognostic indicators and results of resuscitation. Ann Emerg Med 19:1390–1395
9. Rosen P, Stoto M, Harley J (1995) The use of the Heimlich maneuver in near drowning: Institute of Medicine report. J Emerg Med 13:397–405
10. Szpilman D, Soares M (2004) In water resuscitation – is it worthwile. Resuscitation 63:25–31
11. Szpilman D (1997) Near-drowning and drowning: a proposal to stratify mortality based on the analysis of 1,831 cases. Chest 112:660–665

12. Golden FS. Hervey GR, Tipton MJ (1991) Circum-rescue collapse: collapse, sometimes fatal, associated with rescue of immersion victims. J R Naval Med Serv 77:139–149
13. American Heart Association (1992) Guidelines for cardiopulmonary resuscitation and emergency cardiac care, Part 4: Special resuscitations; near-drowning. JAMA 268:2242–2249
14. Handley AJ, Becker LB, Allen M, et al.H (1997) Single rescuer adult basic life support: an advisory statement from the Basic Life Support Working Group of the International Liaison Committee on Resuscitation (ILCOR). Circulation 95:2174–2179

6.7
First Aid Courses for the Aquatic Environment

DAVID SZPILMAN, LUIZ MORIZOT-LEITE, WIEBE DE VRIES,
JUSTIN SCARR, STEVE BEERMAN, FERNANDO MARTINHO,
LUIZ SMORIS and BO LØFGREN

This chapter is based on the expert meeting "Do we need a special first aid course for drowning victims?" during the World Congress on Drowning, in which all authors participated. The authors are responsible for first aid and BLS courses in their country or well informed on the subject.

First aid courses for the aquatic environment involve issues and principles that are not found in typical first aid classes. Some of these principles are unique and specific to aquatics and they are essential to all persons living or working near or around the water. Other principles are more water-rescue specific, and they focus on information and skill training concerning lifeguards or those directly involved in aquatic activities. Therefore, it is recommended that these principles can be best assimilated through a supplemental first aid course for the aquatic environment named 'basic water life support' (BWLS).

The BWLS course is intended to address the information and skills necessary to understand the process of drowning, accompanying problems and water-related incident management. It should include:

- Preventive measures
- Recognition and alarm raising
- Rescue techniques
- In-water life support

Various BWLS courses may have differing depths of information and education based on the level of skill of the participants, the time spent near an aquatic environment, the possibility of witnessing a drowning event and the need to act.

Nevertheless, it is strongly believed that any BWLS course can save lives simply by teaching prevention measures to the public. If organisations choose to provide first aid training for the aquatic environment, consultation with local, regional, national and international resources is advised.

6.7.1
Prevention, Recognition and Raising Alarms

Appropriate measures for prevention, recognition and alerting of professional rescuers, specific for the aquatic incident, can avoid more than 85% of all critical drowning events [1, 2]. Prevention needs to be clarified and highlighted in all regular first aid courses. These can be divided into basic and advanced levels:

- Basic prevention (30−60 min). This topic includes preventive steps to avoid drowning of self and others in and around the water. It should include beach and pool preventive measures. For example: learn how to swim; never swim alone; dive only in deep water; preferably swim in shallow areas; always swim in areas protected by lifeguards and know when they are on duty; know what a rip current is and how to escape from it. Following these tips will help the swimmer to enjoy leisure time and return home safely. Basic prevention should also include how to recognise an incident in the water and the steps to be followed after recognition and how to alarm professional rescuers.
- Advanced prevention (3 hours). Advanced education should include the above mentioned basic prevention concepts and additional information about:
  - The different environments where drowning can occur
  - The behaviour and characteristics of a drowning victim and applicable interventions that might prevent the event
  - Different measures to signal danger such as hand signals, flags, and whistle codes
  - Recognition of dangerous locations in and near the aquatic environment
  - Ways to prevent, and deal with, emergencies at the aquatic environment such as storms, sharks and other water-related incidents such as hypothermia and envenomation
  - Drowning aetiologies

6.7.2
Rescuing the Victim

Removal of the victim from the water is the first step in the chain of events that must occur in a drowning-related emergency (◘ Table 6.3). Rescue techniques can make the difference between life and death for both lay or professional rescuer and the victim. This topic should include:

- Rescue tips (30−60 min). How to rescue a victim without getting in the water yourself. For example by throwing lifesaving devices to the victim or securing the victim with extended reach tools before assisting the victim directly, tips about self-rescue, such as how to save one's own life, survival swimming and floating, how to minimise the loss of body-heat.
- Basic rescues techniques (2−6 hours). Knowledge of how to save a life without becoming a second victim. This topic includes knowledge about:

Table 6.3. Recommendations for a first aid course for the aquatic environment

Basic water life support[a]	Basic	Advanced		Healthcare providers[e]
	Lay person (no AF)[b]	Lay person (with AF)[c]		
		A	B	
Prevention, recognition and alarming				
– Basic	X	X		X
– Advanced			X	X
Rescue				
– Tips	X	X	X	X
– Basic techniques		X	X	X
– Advanced techniques				
Life support for drowning				
– Basic		X	X	X
– Artificial ventilation and oxygen therapy			X	X
– Advanced life support				X
Time recommendation (in hours)[f]	1–2	5–9	9–13	9–13

AF, aquatic familiarisation.

[a] Should have basic life support (BLS) course as a pre-requisite.

[b] A lay person with no AF is a member of the general public with a possible, but less likely, exposure to drowning (such as at schools, childcare centres, hotels, resorts).

[c] A lay person with AF can be separated into subgroups based on the time spent near an aquatic environment or the possibility of witnessing a drowning, indicating more likely a need to act. For example, Group A is comprised of people living in a house with a pool; employees of water parks, condominiums, and hotels; and athletes involved in aquatic sports; Group B is comprised of coaches of aquatic sports, professionals working in and around an aquatic environment, such as security guards, or possibly police officers or firefighters in some cases... Both of these groups can have different approaches based on age (5–7; 7–9; 10–14; and above 15 years).

[d] Lifeguards (Duty to Act) can include pool lifeguards and junior lifeguards (paid or volunteers).

[e] Health care providers, although not the concern of this chapter, should be knowledgeable about the particularities of drowning events. This will help to better ensure that a perfect link will be established between basic and advanced life support.

[f] Indicates the minimum and maximum time in hours suggested to complete each level.

- Entering calm water with a minimum of physical activities (swimming and running)
- What to do in more hazardous aquatic environments such as dangerous places that could facilitate drowning and how to avoid drowning in these situations
- To recognise the persons who present the highest risk of drowning
- Self-rescue and rescue techniques using basic lifesaving equipment.

6.7.3
Medical Support

Medical support for drowning is unique and specific for the aquatic environment. A basic life support (BLS) course including CPR techniques and the use of an automated defibrillator (AED) must be a prerequisite to any BWLS training.

- Basic water life supports for drowning (2–4 hours). BWLS procedures include checking for consciousness level, breathing status and starting artificial ventilation in the water if indicated. It should be reinforced that:
  - Resuscitation that starts in-water (BWLS) can, in some circumstances, save lives three times more often than the resuscitation that starts on the shore or on a pool deck [2].
  - Breathing status should be checked in all unconscious victims, even with the victim still in the water and, if needed, rescue breathing should be provided immediately.
  - The victims at risk for possible cervical trauma should have in-line cervical spine immobilisation performed while he or she is still in the water.
  - Removal of the victim out of the water should be performed according to the level of consciousness, but preferably done in a vertical position to avoid vomiting and further airway complications.
  - In CPR situations, positioning of victim should be performed with the trunk and head at the same level to avoid regurgitation [3].
  - Cricothyroid membrane pressure to compress the oesophagus (Sellick manoeuvre) may decrease the risk of gastric regurgitation and pulmonary aspiration of gastric contents during CPR [4].
  - Even if a submersion time has been 1 hour, the drowning victim still has a chance to survive without sequelae in certain circumstances. This makes drowning resuscitation efforts different from most other medical conditions [1, 5] as outlined in ▶ Chapter 6.11.
  - The severity scales in drowning should be applied (scale 1–6) and the victim treated according the severity scale (see ▶ Chapter 7.11).
  - How to proceed after first medical care (hospital vs. home).
  - The mechanism and treatment of hypothermia deserves special attention.
- Artificial ventilation and oxygen therapy (4–6 hours). Having emphasised that rescue in water may require breathing BWLS should focus on:
  - How to perform rescue breathing and to monitor breathing in and out of the water

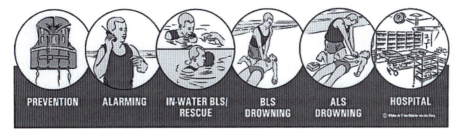

Fig. 6.5. Chain of survival in drowning

- The advantages of using oxygen at the site
- The indications for the use of oxygen
- The different methods of ventilation and oxygen delivery
- How to use oxygen safely according to medical indications

6.7.4
Summary

In summary, BWLS courses are recommended for persons who work in, visit or use an aquatic environment. A basic life support course should be a prerequisite to a BWLS course. All BWLS courses should at least include basic preventive measures, rescue tips and information on the chain of survival in drowning (**Fig. 6.5;** **Table 6.3**). Advanced life support is not the intended focus of BWLS.

References

1. Orlowski JP, Szpilman D (2001) Drowning. Rescue, resuscitation, and reanimation. Pediatric critical care: a new Millennium. Pediatr Clin North Am 48:627–646
2. Szpilman D, Soares M (2004) In-water resuscitation – is it worthwhile? Resuscitation 63:25–31
3. Szpilman D, Idris A, Cruz-Filho FES (2002) Position of drowning resuscitation victim on sloping beaches. Book of abstracts. World Congress on Drowning, Amsterdam, p 168
4. Sellick BA (1961) Cricoid pressure to control regurgitation of stomach contents during the induction of anaesthesia. Lancet ii:404
5. Szpilman D (2002) 22 minutes submersion in warm water without sequelae. Book of abstracts. World Congress on Drowning, Amsterdam 2002
6. Anonymous (2000) Special resuscitation situations. Guidelines for cardiopulmonary resuscitation and emergency cardiac care (ECC). Circulation 102
7. Bierens JJLM (1996) Drowning in The Netherlands: pathophysiology, epidemiology and clinical studies. University of Utrecht, PhD-thesis.

6.8
Advanced Life Support

Volker Wenzel and Paul Pepe

The traditional definitions for advanced life support (ALS) techniques generally have been classified as those interventions and procedures that would require physician orders if not the physicians themselves to deliver [1–6]. These interventions traditionally would include the delivery of intravenous medications and invasive procedures such as intravenous access or endotracheal intubation [4, 5]. While some jurisdictions have allowed non-physicians such as ALS-providing paramedics and nurses to utilize these interventions, most of these providers still do so under physician orders, direction and prescribed protocol [7, 8].

In addition to non-physicians performing these so-called invasive techniques, the traditional lines delineating basic from advanced techniques have blurred with the introduction of use of alternative airways by basic life support (BLS) providers, such as emergency medical technicians, and the use of automated external defibrillators (AED) by lay persons [9–11]. Also, while not necessarily invasive in all circumstances, techniques for therapeutic hypothermia might be considered advanced techniques [12].

This chapter will deal with concepts that are typically more invasive in nature and requiring physician-level authorisation or performance and most notably invasive airway techniques and intravenous medication administration.

6.8.1
Evidence for the Effectiveness of Advanced Life Support

Most of the data regarding ALS techniques, particularly in the prehospital setting, have come from the laboratory or from in-hospital care experience [2, 3, 5, 6, 12]. Preliminary clinical data do suggest the value of several medications such as vasopressin and amiodarone in the prehospital setting [13–15]. However, to date, there are no explicit clinical trials to prove their absolute value on a one-by-one basis [2, 3, 6]. Many investigators have even questioned their use altogether. Even time-honoured interventions such as endotracheal intubation have been questioned, particularly in paediatric resuscitation [16]. More relevant to this discussion is that it has become more and more evident that ALS interventions are still of very little value, if they are of any value at all, if BLS is not provided immediately at the scene by bystanders [17–19], be they lay or professional (see
▶ Chapter 6.3.3).

Nevertheless, there is some evolving suggestion that certain ALS interventions, while extremely effective in the laboratory, have not demonstrated to be effective in the clinical setting [20–22] perhaps because of confounding variables such as uncontrolled and overzealous ventilatory techniques during the trials [23–26]. It has also been made clear that some aspects of ALS must work, considering the number of survivors among out-of-hospital cardiac arrest patients who do not present with ventricular fibrillation (VT) and never receive defibrillatory countershocks [2, 13, 27]. Since these patients do not respond to BLS and are resuscitated after ALS interventions, some aspect of ALS techniques apparently are effective. What is not clear is the specific intervention.

6.8.2
Specific Indications for Advanced Life Support in Drowning Incidents

The indications for ALS techniques for drowning events are even less supported than they are for standard cardiac arrests [17–19]. However, the studies indicating BLS as the rate limiting step in drowning resuscitation does not preclude the need for ALS. Although most survivors usually respond after BLS, particularly children, many survivors still receive ALS techniques following initial resuscitation. It is therefore assumed that such supportive care is worthwhile. In fact, there may be laboratory indications that vasopressin [13] may be somewhat effective in hypothermic states, a common complication of drowning events. Again, the specific interventions are not clear and therefore, until proven otherwise, current ALS techniques for typical cardiac arrest would be recommended [4, 5].

There are some caveats about such recommendations to follow techniques advised for standard cardiac arrest techniques. Drowning is often associated with hypothermia, and sometimes with associated trauma and shock conditions, meaning that even standard rates of ventilation could be harmful [25, 26, 28] and so caution not to overzealously ventilate even though drowning is a primary respiratory event. The main concern is that positive pressure breaths, and continuous positive pressure in particular, can inhibit venous return and significantly compromise cardiac output and coronary perfusion [25, 26, 28]. These effects are exacerbated with obstructive lung disease, reactive airways, hypovolaemia and severe circulatory compromise [25].

The main issue to be considered is the appropriate tidal volume. In general, in the resuscitative phase of a drowning event, tidal volumes in the realm of at least 10 ml per kg are probably useful with placement of an endotracheal tube and no application of positive end-expiratory pressure (PEEP). The pulmonary presentation of drowning in terms of chest röntgenogram, arterial blood gases and response to PEEP, may resemble acute respiratory distress syndrome (ARDS). Therefore, tidal volumes of 6–7 ml per kg may be advocated by some under these circumstances because of recent relevant studies of tidal volumes in ARDS patients [29, 30]. However, such studies were performed in patients in a post-resuscitation phase who had diffuse inflammatory lung disease with heterogeneous distribution and who, for the most part, were also being ventilated with levels of PEEP above 10 cm H_2O. Therefore, such restrained tidal volumes may not be as applicable in the resuscitative phase of the drowning scenario in which surfactant loss and other physiological sequelae may make alveolar recruitment more difficult, particularly in the absence of PEEP.

In other words, in the resuscitative phase, there are no studies that would confirm the need for a low tidal volume approach, especially since the pathophysiology of drowning is probably very different from the typical ARDS case and has a different natural history and response to therapy [31]. Nevertheless, if the patient is hemodynamically stable and can tolerate the application of PEEP (that is, in lieu of other invasive monitoring, there are no obvious effects on blood pressure and pulses), low levels of PEEP may be useful in the field. In turn, if pulse oximetry is operable (good circulation and warmed extremity site), tidal volumes may be reduced accordingly if saturation is maintained above 95%.

The main concern in terms of ventilatory techniques is the situation of shock or circulatory arrest in which PEEP would be relatively contraindicated because of the effects on cardiac output and yet oxygenation is still paramount. Tidal volumes greater than 10 ml/kg and much slower rates would likely be the best recommendations at this time, especially in the face of potential hypothermia in which ventilatory rates should be infrequent.

6.8.3
Recommendations for Future Research

The evidence for ALS in drowning resuscitation is obviously limited, and empiric at best, yet there are promising studies in the laboratory and, preliminary results in the clinical prehospital setting, particularly in terms of vasoactive drugs. Limited re-warming and controlled hypothermia may be of value. The use of other neuroprotective therapies may need to be explored (▶ **Section 8**). The complicated issue of tidal volumes, PEEP application, and respiratory rates in this unique resuscitative situation deserve focus considering that oxygenation is the primary problem in drowning events [32].

References

1. Cummins R, Ornato J, Thies W, Pepe P (1991) Improving survival from sudden cardiac arrest: the „chain of survival" concept. A statement for health professionals from the Advanced Cardiac Life Support Subcommittee and the Emergency Cardiac Care Committee, American Heart Association. Circulation 83:1832–1847
2. Pepe P, Abramson N, Brown C (1994) ACLS – Does it really work? Ann Emerg Med 23:1037–1041
3. Stiell IG, Wells GA, Field B, et al. (2004) Advanced life support in out-of-hospital cardiac arrest. N Engl J Med 351:647–656
4. American Heart Association (2001) ACLS provider manual. American Heart Association, Dallas, Texas, USA, pp 1–252
5. American Heart Association (2000) American Heart Association guidelines 2000 for cardiopulmonary resuscitation and emergency cardiovascular care – international consensus on science. Circulation 102 (Suppl I):1–384
6. Pepe PE (1995) ACLS systems and training programs – do they make a difference. Respir Care 30:427–433; discussion 433–436
7. Eisenberg M, Bergner L, Hallstrom A (1979) Paramedic programs and out-of-hospital cardiac arrest: I factors associated with successful resuscitation. Am J Public Health 69:30–38
8. Pepe PE, Bonnin MJ, Mattox KL (1990) Regulating the scope of EMS services. Prehosp Dis Med 5:59–63
9. Pepe PE, Zachariah BS, Chandra N (1993) Invasive airway techniques in resuscitation. Ann Emerg Med 22:393–403

10. White RD, Vukov FL, Bugliosi TF (1995) Early defibrillation by police: Initial experience with measurement of critical time intervals and patient outcome. Ann Emerg Med 23:1009–1013
11. Caffrey SL, Willoughby PJ, Pepe PE, Becker LB (2002) Public use of automated external defibrillators. N Engl J Med 347:1242–1247
12. Bernard SA, Buist M (2003) Induced hypothermia in critical care medicine: a review. Crit Care Med 31:2041–2051
13. Wenzel V, Krismer AC, Arntz HR, et al. (2004) A comparison of vasopressin and epinephrine for out-of-hospital cardiopulmonary resuscitation. N Engl J Med 350:105–113
14. Kudenchuk PJ, Cobb LA, Copass MK, et al. (1999) Amiodarone for resuscitation after out-of-hospital cardiac arrest due to ventricular fibrillation. N Engl J Med 341:871–878
15. Dorian P, Cass D, Schwartz B, Cooper R, Gelaznikas R, Barr A (2002) Amiodarone as compared with lidocaine for chock-resistant ventricular fibrillation. N Engl J Med 346:884–890
16. Gausche M, Lewis RJ, Stratton SL, et al. (2000) Effect of out-of-hospital pediatric endotracheal intubation on survival and neurological outcome: a controlled clinical trial. JAMA 283:783–790
17. Pepe PE, Wigginton JG, Mann DM, et al. (2002) Prospective, decade-long, population-based study of pediatric drowning-related incidents. Acad Emerg Med 9:516–517
18. Kyriacou D, Arcinue E, Peek C, Kraus J (1994) Effect of immediate resuscitation on children with submersion injury. Pediatrics 94:137–142
19. Goh SH, Low B (1999) Drowning and near-drowning – some lesions learned. Acad Med Singapore 28:183–188
20. Brown CG, Martin DR, Pepe PE, et al. (1992) A comparison of standard-dose and high dose epinephrine in cardiac arrest outside the hospital. The multicenter high-dose epinephrine study group. N Engl J Med 327:1051–1055
21. Callaham M, Madsen CD, Barton CW, et al. (1992) A randomized clinical trail of high dose epinephrine and norepinephrine vs. standard-dose epinephrine in prehospital cardiac arrest. JAMA 268:2667–2672
22. Stiell IG, Hebert PC, Weitzman B, et al. (1992) A study of high-dose epinephrine in human CPR. N Engl J Med 237:1047–1050
23. Pepe PE, Fowler R, Roppolo L, Wigginton J (2004) Re-appraising the concept of immediate defibrillatory attempts for out-of-hospital ventricular fibrillation. Crit Care 8:41–45
24. Menegazzi J, Seaberg D, Yealy D, et al. (2000) Combination pharmacotherapy with delayed countershock vs. standard advanced cardiac life support after prolonged ventricular fibrillation. Prehos Emerg Care 4:31–37
25. Roppolo L, Wigginton JA, Pepe PE (2004) Emergency ventilatory management as a detrimental factor in resuscitation practices and clinical research efforts. In: Vincent JL (ed) 2004 Yearbook of intensive care and emergency medicine. Springer, Berlin, pp 139–151
26. Aufderheide TP, Sigurdsson G, Pirrallo RG, et al. (2004) Hyperventilation-induced hypotension during cardiopulmonary resuscitation. Circulation 109:1960–1965
27. Pepe PE, Levine RL, Fromm RE, et al. (1994) Cardiac arrest presenting with rhythms other than ventricular fibrillation: Contribution of resuscitation efforts toward total survivorship. Crit Care Med 21:1838–1843
28. Pepe PE, Raedler C, Lurie K, Wigginton JG (2003) Emergency ventilatory management in hemorrhagic states: elemental or detrimental? J Trauma 54:1048–1057
29. The Adult Respiratory Distress Network (2000) Ventilation with lower tidal volumes as compared to traditional tidal volumes for acute lung injury and the acute respiratory distress syndrome. N Engl J Med 342:1301–1308
30. Bierens JJLM, Knape JTA, Gelissen HPMM (2002) Drowning. Curr Opin Crit Care 8:578–586
31. Pepe PE (1986) The clinical entity of adult respiratory distress syndrome: definition, prediction and prognosis. Crit Care Clin 2:377–403
32. Modell JH (1993) Drowning. N Engl J Med 328:253–258

6.9
Long QT Syndrome and Drowning

ALFRED BOVE and RIENKE RIENKS

The long QT syndrome (LQTS) is a disease of the cardiac ion channels resulting in a prolonged repolarisation. In the congenital form, gene mutations cause abnormalities of potassium or sodium channels, resulting in impairment of the outward potassium repolarisation current or increase of the inward sodium depolarisation current. The net result is a prolonged repolarisation (□ **Fig. 6.6**). This may cause electrical instability of the cellular membrane and facilitate arrhythmias (□ **Fig. 6.7**). At this time, six types (LQTS 1–6) have been described [1]. LQTS is often associated with sinus bradycardia and individuals with LQTS have a high risk of ventricular fibrillation (VF) and sudden death [2].

6.9.1
Diagnosis and Triggers

The diagnosis of LQTS is made with the electrocardiogram (ECG) and since the QT interval is dependent on heart rate, the measured QT interval has to be corrected (the QTc) to confirm the abnormal prolongation [1, 3]. Females generally have a longer QT interval than males at comparable heart rates [3]. Patients are usually children or young adults who are found to have a corrected QT interval (QTc) in excess of 440 ms. The first presentation of LQTS is often syncope or cardiac arrest precipitated by emotional or physical stress. Events that trigger the arrhythmias include exercise, swimming, loud sounds, electrolyte imbalance and certain drugs. Conspicuously, the trigger for arrhythmias varies depending on the phenotype. In LQTS 1, arrhythmias are triggered mainly by exercise, diving or swimming [5, 6], whereas in LQTS 2, acoustic stimuli and arousal may be the trigger [7]. In LQTS 3, arrhythmias occur mainly at rest or during sleep [1]. The torsade de pointe fibrillation pattern (□ **Fig. 6.7**) is characteristic [4].

6.9.2
Specific Association of LQTS and Drowning Events

Ackerman reported a case of a healthy woman who died suddenly while swimming in a pool. Initially, she was considered to be a drowning victim, but on DNA analysis was found to have a gene that causes the LQTS [5]. These authors published a study involving a series of patients with a similar history of swimming-induced sudden death [6]. These cases were first thought to be caused by drowning, but their identity as LQTS patients indicated that the primary event was VF. A similar report has studied 78 family members of several subjects who died suddenly while swimming [8]. In all, 35 had unexplained syncope or non fatal drowning events. Also QT prolongation during face immersion in children is documented [9]. They suggested that immersion is an independent factor

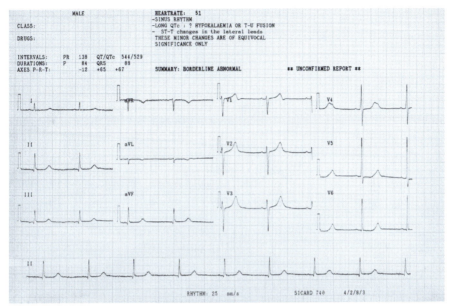

MALE

CLASS:
DRUGS:

HEARTRATE: 51
-SINUS RHYTHM
-LONG QTc : ? HYPOKALAEMIA OR T-U FUSION
- ST-T changes in the lateral leads
THESE MINOR CHANGES ARE OF EQUIVOCAL
SIGNIFICANCE ONLY

INTERVALS: PR   138   QT/QTc   544/529
DURATIONS: P   84   QRS   88
AXES P-R-T: -12   +65   +67

SUMMARY: BORDERLINE ABNORMAL   ** UNCONFIRMED REPORT **

RHYTHM: 25   mm/s   SICARD 740   4/2/8/3

Fig. 6.6. Example of long QT syndrome. The corrected QT interval (QTc) is 529 ms (normal: 440 ms). There is a long iso-electric ST segment, especially notable in the extremity leads and V5 and V6

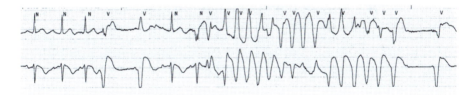

Fig. 6.7. Electrocardiogram tracing from a patient with syncope who developed torsades de pointes type of ventricular tachycardia (VT). The QT interval of the sinus beats is about 0.46 seconds. Normal beats (N) start the sequence on the *left*, and are followed by two ventricular beats (V). The rhythm subsequently deteriorates into the characteristic torsades form of VT (a series of ventricular beats). The rhythm spontaneously reverts to sinus rhythm after the short period of VT

in causing ventricular arrhythmias in these subjects. Ott documented VF in a woman with known LQTS who became unresponsive while swimming. She had an implanted defibrillator that fired and restored her cardiac rhythm [10].

Although many people with the LQTS syndrome are aware of this problem from childhood [11], some patients may only manifest the changes when other factors are present. Swimming and other forms of exercise, electrolyte imbalance, and medications may combine to cause sudden death in these patients. The data from the above-mentioned clinical studies did not include scuba divers. However, the circumstances of exposure (face immersion, cold, diving) are typical of scuba diving and could act as a stimulus for VF in scuba divers as well as swimmers. It is suggested that the incidence of the LQTS gene is about 1:165 drowning cases [12].

6.9.3
Identification of Persons at Risk

Identification of patients with LQTS in the general population is difficult, since the general prevalence is low (1:10,000–15,000) and a lethal arrhythmia may be the presenting symptom. However, patients with LQTS formed 30% of a group of patients with unexplained syncope. Moreover, 60% of patients are identified as a family member of a patient with syncope or cardiac arrest [13]. Thus, in addition to questioning about episodes of syncope, a family history of sudden death should also be addressed during screening. In individuals with a history of unexplained syncope and/or a positive family history of sudden death, an ECG should be performed to exclude LQTS.

There is also an acquired form of LQTS. Causes are manifold and include neurologic pathology, hypothermia and the use of anti-arrhythmic drugs like flecainide and quinidine [14].

LQTS should also be considered in unexplained diving fatalities.

Many (scuba) diving activities are located in areas where antimalarial prophylaxis is necessary and QTc prolongation as well as arrhythmias without QTc prolongation has been described with mefloquine [15, 16]. Of particular interest for scuba divers is the presumed prolongation of the QT interval under hyperbaric circumstances. Although this has been described in animal studies [17], it has not yet been established in humans [18–20]. The result of the use of anti-arrhythmic drugs (for instance to treat atrial fibrillation) or anti-malaria drugs on the QT interval during hyperbaric circumstances has not been established, but is of theoretical concern.

6.9.4
Pretreatment of Those at Risk

Beta-blockers are effective in preventing syncope in LQTS 1 and 2 patients, but may be ineffective in patients with LQTS 3. Also, 25%–35% of patients with symptomatic LQTS are likely to have another event within 5 years while on therapy [21]. Other therapeutic options include pacemaker therapy and the placement of an internal cardioverter-defibrillator [22]. Otherwise, based on the above discussion, persons with documented LQTS who are symptomatic, and particularly those who have had an aborted sudden death event, should avoid swimming and scuba diving.

6.9.5
Resuscitation

Swimmers or divers who suddenly become unresponsive while in water may be victims of a cardiac arrest from VF. These victims may become unresponsive and become submerged with no warning or prior distress. Lifeguards should be suspicious of swimmers who appear motionless or unresponsive. Persons with VF require immediate cardiopulmonary resuscitation and rapid defibrillation to survive, and the usual CPR protocols should be followed. Patients with LQTS respond well to rapid defibrillation. Therefore, immediate defibrillation should be provided after the victim is removed from the water, assuming a defibrillator is available. If a defibrillator is available in a wet environment, precaution should be taken to dry the victim's chest to some degree before shocking. However, experimental data show that a wet environment does not constitute a particular risk for defibrillation using the typical automated external defibrillator (AED) that is able to detect VF and recommend shock in these patients [23].

6.9.6
Conclusions

In cases of unexplained drowning particularly in children, adolescents and young adults, assessment of individual and family history of sudden death, or known long QT syndrome should be documented. Individuals with documented LQTS who have experienced syncope or even episodes of VF or ventricular tachycardia should be advised against swimming or diving because of the potential for increased risk from submersion activities. Individuals with documented LQTS who have an implanted cardioverter-defibrillator (ICD) should be advised against swimming and diving. It is also recommended to inquire about the occurrence of sudden death among family members in the medical examination and screening of scuba divers.

References

1. Schwartz PJ (2000) The long QT syndrome: from genotype to phenotype. In: Aliot E, Clementy J, Prystowsky EN (eds) Fighting sudden cardiac death. A worldwide challenge. Futura , Armonk, NY, pp 301–307
2. Harris EM, Knapp JF, Sharma V (1992) The Romano-Ward syndrome: a case presenting as near drowning with a clinical review. Pediatr Emerg Care 8:272–275
3. Moss AJ (1998) Sudden cardiac death in the long QT syndrome. In: Akhtar M, Myerbyrg RJ, Ruskin JN (eds) Sudden cardiac death. Prevalence, mechanisms, and approaches to diagnosis and management. Williams & Wilkins, Philadelphia, pp 209–214
4. Smith WM, Gallagher JJ (1980) „Les torsades de pointes": an unusual ventricular arrhythmia. Ann Int Med 93:578–584
5. Ackerman MJ, Schroeder JJ, Berry R, et al. (1998) A novel mutation in KVLQT1 is the molecular basis of inherited long QT syndrome in a near-drowning patient's family. Pediatr Res 44:148–153

6. Ackerman MJ, Tester DJ, Porter CJ (1999) Swimming, a gene-specific arrhythmogenic trigger for inherited long QT syndrome. Mayo Clin Proc 74:1088–1094
7. Wilde AAM, Jongbloed RJE, Doevendans PA, et al. (1999) Auditory stimuli as a trigger for arrhythmic events differentiate HERG-related (LQTS2) patients from KvLQT1-related patients (LQTS1). J Am Coll Cardiol 33:327–332
8. Bradley T, Dixon J, Easthope R (1999) Unexplained fainting, near drowning and unusual seizures in childhood: screening for long QT syndrome in New Zealand families. N Z Med J 112:299–302
9. Yoshinaga M, Kamimura J, Fukushige T, et al. (1999) Face immersion in cold water induces prolongation of the QT interval and T-wave changes in children with nonfamilial long QT syndrome. Am J Cardiol 83:1494–1497, A8
10. Ott P, Marcus FI, Moss AI (2002) Ventricular fibrillation during swimming in a patient with long-QT syndrome. Circulation 106:521–522
11. Weintraub RG, Gow RM, Wilkinson JL (1999) The congenital long QT syndromes in childhood. J Am Coll Cardiol 16:674–680
12. Lunetta P, Penttila A, Levo A, et al. (2002) Post-mortem molecular screening for the long QT syndrome (LQTS) in victims of drowning. Book of abstracts. World congress on Drowning, Amsterdam, p 104
13. Moss AJ, Robinson J (1992) Clinical features of the idiopathic long QT syndrome. Circulation 85: I-140
14. Goldstein S, Bayes-de-Luna A, Soldevila JG (eds) (1994) Sudden cardiac death. Futura, Armonk, NY, pp 193–206
15. Davis TME, Demblo LG, Kaye-Eddie SA, et al. (1996) Neurological, cardiovascular and metabolic effects of mefloquine in healthy volunteers: a double-blind, placebo controlled trial. Br J Clin Pharmacol 42:415–421
16. Richter J, Burbach G (1997) Aberrant atriventricular conduction triggered by antimalarial prophylaxis with mefloquine. Lancet 349:101
17. Doubt TJ, Evans DE (1982) Hyperbaric exposures alter cardiac excitation-contraction coupling. Undersea Biomed Res 9:131–145
18. Eckenhoff RG, Knight DR (1984) Cardiac arrhythmias and heart rate changes in prolonged hyperbaric air exposures. Undersea Biomed Res 11:355–367
19. Lafay V, Barthelemy P, Comet B, et al. (1995) ECG changes during the experimental human dive HYDRA 10 (71 atm/7, 200 kPa). Undersea Hyperbar Med 22:51–60
20. Lund V, Kentala E, Scheinin H, et al. (2000) Hyperbaric oxygen increases parasympathetic activity in professional divers. Acta Physiol Scand 170:39–44
21. Moss AJ, Zareba W, Hall WJ, et al. (2000) Effectiveness and limitations of β-blocker therapy in congenital long-QT syndrome. Circulation 101:616–623
22. Moss AJ, Zareba W (2000) Congenital long QT syndrome: therapeutic considerations based on the international LQTS registry. Fighting sudden cardia death. A worldwide challenge. Futura, Armonk, NY, pp 309–321
23. Vance J, Espino M (2002) Automated external defibrillation in a wet environment. Book of abstracts. World Congress on Drowning, Amsterdam, p 169

6.10
Paediatric Considerations in Drowning

Robyn Meyer, Andreas Theodorou and Robert Berg

Drowning is one of the most common aetiologies of out-of-hospital paediatric cardiac arrest [1] and constitutes a major cause of paediatric mortality and morbidity [2]. The basic pathophysiology of drowning is fundamentally the same for children and adults but there are critical physiologic differences that go beyond simple differences in body size. In addition, there are important differences in the epidemiology, and consequently, approaches to prevention. Perhaps the most notable difference is the unique cultural and emotional role of children in society and the unique response of individuals and of society to childhood injury and death. To adequately care for paediatric drowning victims and their families, the distinctive characteristics of the paediatric population must be understood.

In this section, we briefly review the unique aspects of the epidemiology, pathophysiology, and outcome of paediatric drowning, and integrate that information in relation to resuscitation of paediatric drowning victims. We will also discuss what is not yet known about paediatric drowning and suggest research that is needed to improve knowledge and care.

6.10.1
Unique and Relevant Aspects of Epidemiology

While toddlers often enter water unintentionally and during brief lapses in supervision, adolescents tend to endanger themselves by high-risk behaviours, including intoxication with alcohol and other substances of abuse [3, 4].

6.10.2
Unique Aspects of Pathophysiology

Although the basic pathophysiology of drowning is the same for all ages, the paediatric population has unique characteristics that alter the response to asphyxia. Children have less pulmonary oxygen reserves due to smaller residual volumes and they will develop hypoxia more rapidly following apnoea. Hypoxia also develops more rapidly in children due to a higher metabolic rate. On the positive side, however, children are less likely to have a pre-existing illness that may complicate asphyxial injury. Protective effects from icy-water submersions are more likely to occur in children. In contrast to adults, the smaller body size and greater surface area to body mass ratio of a child leads to more rapid core cooling and hypothermia accompanying a drowning injury is common.

Despite the attention that has been paid to dramatic recoveries following prolonged icy-water drowning, the effects of hypothermia are often detrimental as well. Protective effects of hypothermia are dependent upon rapid central cooling with a decline in cerebral metabolism before hypoxic-ischemic injury occurs. This sequence of events occurs only in extremely cold waters, generally less than 0°C [5]. Meanwhile, detrimental effects of hypothermia are common and include arrhythmias, coagulopathy and impaired immune and myocardial function.

6.10.3
Nuances of Resuscitation

Prevention and prompt cardiopulmonary resuscitation (CPR) following a drowning incident are the key life-saving factors for children. There are four distinct phases of resuscitation:
- The pre-arrest phase which includes the precipitating events and the co-morbidities existing before the drowning and arrest.
- The no-flow phase of untreated cardiac arrest.
- The low-flow phase which occurs during CPR.
- The post-resuscitation phase.

Interventions need to be coordinated to the unique aspects of each phase in order to be efficacious [6]. The specific phase of resuscitation dictates the focus of care. Interventions that improve outcome during one phase may be deleterious during another phase.

The pre-arrest phase includes pre-existing conditions (for example neurologic, cardiac, respiratory or metabolic problems), developmental status (for example premature neonate, mature neonate, infant, child or adolescent), and precipitating events (for example trauma at the time of immersion, water temperature or aspiration). It may represent a period of low, normal or high blood flow. Obviously, interventions during the pre-arrest phase focus on prevention. For toddlers, placing barriers, both physical and behavioural, between the child and water is a key preventive measure. Four-sided fencing for residential pools, in which the pool is not only fenced but also separated from the house, clearly decreases drowning rates for children. Pool alarms, pool covers, flotation devices, swimming lessons and supervision may all play some role but none of these measures alone has yet been shown to decrease drowning rates. While adult supervision of young children around water is essential, it is not fail-safe. Children may enter the water during momentary lapses in adult attention. Adults may expect to be alerted by the sounds of splashing or struggling but most childhood drowning events are silent.

Outcome of drowning is closely related to the duration of submersion. Prospects for functional recovery are dismal with prolonged submersion greater than 25 min [7]. Once the child is removed from the water, it is essential to promptly initiate effective resuscitation. Substantial delays for more than 8 min until the arrival of professional rescuers are generally lethal, but prompt and effective CPR may obviate the need for any other interventions. This was illustrated by a large prospective study in Houston where Sirbaugh and colleagues demonstrated that 41 children who had received bystander CPR following a drowning incident were not in cardiac arrest by the time of EMS arrival and all survived with good neurological outcomes [8]. Most were quite ill when they arrived at a hospital emergency department. In contrast, none of the other 24 children during the same period with drowning-related events who were still in cardiac arrest when the EMS personnel arrived survived with a good neurological outcome. These data and similar data from Hickey [9] are consistent with animal data, and in-patient paediatric CPR data, namely basic CPR can be quite effective for asphyxial cardiac arrests, but the timing of the interventions is critically important.

Important tenets of paediatric basic life support are PUSH HARD, PUSH FAST and minimise interruptions. Traditional recommendations for basic life support in children include a 5:1 ratio of compressions-ventilation with a chest compression rate of 100 per minute. However, it is very likely, in the near future, that such guidelines will be modified to prevent frequent interruptions of compressions (see Chap. 6.4). Chest compressions should be performed at a compression depth of approximately 1/3 to 1/2 the depth of the chest (1.25–2.5 cm for infants, 2.5–3.75 cm for young children and 3.75–5 cm for older children). Compressions should be sufficient to produce a palpable pulse. Each rescue breath should be adequate enough to provide visible chest rise, but the actual rates and ratios are less important than taking action.

As with adults, use of the Heimlich manoeuvre in an attempt to express water from the lungs of drowning victims is contraindicated [10]. Under most circumstances, drowning victims initially have little excess water in their lungs, but may have substantial quantities of water in their stomach. Compression of the chest or upper abdomen is likely to push gas from the lungs more than water, thereby decreasing the functional residual capacity, the amount of gas in the lungs at the end of a breath and worsening hypoxemia. In addition, such compression of the torso can cause emesis and subsequent aspiration. Moreover, efforts to initially remove water from the lungs can result in life-threatening delays in the implementation of CPR.

Cervical spine injury can accompany drowning. This concern has likely been over-emphasised. A study in 2001 by Watson and colleagues [11] demonstrated a low prevalence of C-spine injury in drowning victims and all such injuries were associated with high-impact trauma. C-spine precautions are recommended in the setting of high-impact trauma prior to or accompanying the submersion event. In this setting, airway opening should be accomplished with a combined jaw-thrust and spinal immobilisation manoeuvre.

Ventricular tachycardia or ventricular fibrillation (VF/VT) does occur in paediatric drowning victims, though uncommonly [8]. The incidence of VF/VT is not well known, but generally VF/VT seems to be a late finding except in icy-water drowning. The diagnosis of long QT syndrome should be considered in such cases. Piglet data indicate that VF/VT rarely occurs prior to cardiac arrest (loss of aortic pulsations) but occurs in nearly 30% of the piglets after prolonged cardiac arrest and resuscitation [12]. Clearly, the definitive therapy for VF is defibrillation. Therefore, rapid determination of electrocardiographic rhythm and prompt defibrillation, if indicated, are also important for successful resuscitation.

A unique paediatric aspect of drowning resuscitation is the paucity of paediatric-specific CPR training. Citizens are not adequately trained to perform CPR on young children. Adequate training includes the technical aspects of CPR as well as the psychological aspects, both of which are quite different for toddlers than for adults. Adequate training for rare occurrences is difficult. Health care providers are often inexperienced and lack expertise in the BLS and ALS of small children. Emergency rooms, particularly in rural settings, may have difficulty maintaining adequate equipment for paediatric resuscitation.

The post-resuscitation phase must include meticulous cardiopulmonary care to avoid exacerbation of existing hypoxic-ischemic damage. Ventilation should also be directed toward avoiding hypoxemia or hypercapnia. Also ventilator induced lung injury and compromised cardiac output from positive pressure breaths should be avoided, particularly in patients already predisposed to the development of ARDS. It is increasingly clear that excessive hyperventilation can lead to increased intrathoracic pressure, diminished venous return and reduced cardiac output. The associated hypocapnia can also cause cerebral ischemia and worsen neurological outcome. Fluid and inotropic support should be provided as needed to improve haemodynamics, maximise tissue perfusion, and maintain adequate arterial pressure for adequate cerebral perfusion. Preliminary reports favour dobutamine in children as the preferred inotrope.

Measures directed specifically toward neurological resuscitation have not to date been demonstrated to improve outcome from drowning events [13]. To some extent, this lack of positive findings may be linked to the difficulty in obtaining adequate sample sizes in studies of paediatric drowning. Certainly further study is warranted to clarify whether neurologic resuscitation measures can benefit paediatric drowning victims. Nevertheless, as noted in the section on neuro-protection, there is great interest in the use of therapeutic mild-to-moderate hypothermia to improve outcome from various neurological insults, including drowning-associated cardiac arrests [14, 15]. This modality may be especially beneficial for children. For many years, deep hypothermia has been effectively utilised during cardiac surgery for children because the surface area is relatively large in small children and therefore rapid control of core temperature is easier. In the prehospital setting there are difficulties in terms of monitoring and titrating core temperature. This is an area ripe for further clinical investigation.

6.10.4
Outcome

Epidemiological studies indicate that submersion for longer than 25 min, continued need for cardiopulmonary resuscitation for greater than 25 min, pulselessness on arrival to the emergency department of a hospital, and continued neurologic dysfunction post-resuscitation predict death or severe neurologic sequelae for the few survivors in these categories [4, 7, 16]. Unfortunately, most of the paediatric epidemiologic studies are retrospective and all are relatively small. Virtually every apparently certain predictor of poor outcome from one of these epidemiologic studies has been undermined by a case report or rare occurrence in another series. Study of all predictors is complicated by the difficulty in quantifying neurologic outcome in children, particularly younger children. Exciting case reports of children surviving neurologically intact after prolonged ice water drownings [5] have suggested that more aggressive intervention is indicated. Conversely, several retrospective studies have suggested that discontinuation of resuscitative efforts is appropriate when various indicators of poor outcome are present [16].

With such conflicting reports, it is difficult to establish standard recommendations for the length or aggressiveness of resuscitation that will be of use for individual cases. No one factor or combination of factors has been found that has reliably predicted who will have a good versus a poor outcome after resuscitation from drowning. The use of coma or fixed, dilated pupils to predict lack of response to resuscitation, although proposed by some studies, has been shown in other studies to be unreliable as predictors [13, 16, 17]. Similarly, the use of Glasgow Coma Scores to predict outcome has not been supported by ongoing studies. Despite reports in the media of survival following prolonged submersion in icy water and despite the potential benefit of induced hypothermia following initial resuscitation, hypothermia on arrival generally portends a poor prognosis [18], as it is strongly associated with the duration of submersion. Due to the lack of specific predictors, it is generally believed that resuscitation should be attempted in all drowning victims unless they are clearly dead (for example, presence of rigour mortis or documented to be submerged in non-icy water for prolonged periods). On the other hand, it should be realised that in some studies all survivors with eventual favourable neurologic outcome showed spontaneous, purposeful movement within 24 hours of admission to a hospital [19]. At present, repeated clinical examinations provide the most valuable information in predicting the eventual degree of functional outcome following drowning injury.

6.10.5
Psychosocial Aspects

Coping with a sudden unexpected death is always difficult. When the victim is a child, the loss is generally even more devastating. In modern, developed countries, childhood death is unusual and many people have a strong belief that children are not supposed to die. Consequently, childhood death is often difficult to accept. Children are an integral part of a family unit with their death causing deep and lasting impact for those close to them. The death of their children is frequently inconceivable to parents. In addition to immediate family, the profound and long-lasting impact often affects large numbers of people who have relationships with the child and family.

Childhood death is also stressful for health care providers. They may feel an additional burden in caring for the family as well as for the victim while concurrently attempting to deal with their own emotions regarding childhood death. Many prehospital and emergency personnel are inexperienced in caring for children and feelings of inadequacy may provoke additional stress after an unsuccessful paediatric resuscitation. Decision-making is different when the victim is a child and some health care providers are uncomfortable with a process that involves an extended family unit. Others may appreciate the support system that families typically provide for their children. Support for families of childhood drowning victims and for health care providers involved in the unsuccessful resuscitation deserves greater emphasis.

6.10.6
Future Research

Determination of standards for the care of paediatric drowning victims has been hampered by the lack of data. Studies of paediatric drowning have primarily been small, retrospective reviews of epidemiology. Standardised trials of resuscitation and post-resuscitation care are lacking. The research that has been done has used varying definitions and assessments of outcome which limits comparison between studies. Lack of uniform definitions and consistent reporting to a centralised registry of paediatric CPR impedes comparison of outcomes. A uniform style (Utstein) has been recommended for reporting outcomes from CPR, with emphasis on four standards of outcome: (a) return of spontaneous circulation, (b) survival of event, (c) survival to hospital discharge, and (d) intact neurologic survival [20].

Goals for future paediatric resuscitation research in drowning should include further epidemiologic investigations, studies of preventative interventions, and therapeutic interventional trials to increase survival from cardiac arrest and to maximise the probability that these survivors remain neurologically intact. There is a need for prospective and multi-centre studies, in order to attain adequate numbers to further delineate pathophysiology and appropriate treatment in drowning victims. Such studies can be targeted toward providing both predictors of poor outcome and predictors of successful resuscitation and good functional outcome. In addition, long-term follow-up with measures of neuro-psychological outcome of victims and psychological outcome of families and health care providers would improve our understanding and lead to better care. We must also find innovative ways to encourage bystander CPR for drowned children after drowning. Animal studies can target the pathophysiology and optimal treatment of asphyxial cardiac arrest at various times in the asphyxial process. Both animal studies and multi-centre investigational trials are needed to investigate moderate hypothermia and other innovative techniques for cerebral protection. Finally, educational and programmatic research is warranted to find more ways to teach and motivate bystanders to provide CPR for paediatric drowning victims.

References

1. Kuisma M, Suominen P, Korpela R (1995) Pediatric out-of-hospital cardiac arrest – epidemiology and outcome. Resuscitation 30:141–150
2. Orlowski JP, Szpilman D (2001) Rescue, resuscitation, and reanimation. Pediatr Clin North Am 48:627–645
3. Orlowski JP (1988) Adolescent drowning: swimming, boating, diving, and scuba accidents. Pediatr Ann 17:125–128, 131–132

4. Quan L, Wentz KR, Gore EJ, Copass MK (1990) Outcome and predictors of outcome in pediatric submersion victims receiving prehospital care in King County, Washington. Pediatrics 86:586–593
5. Orlowski JP (1987) Drowning, near-drowning, and ice-water submersions. Pediatr Clin North Am 34:75–92.
6. Berg RA (2002) Cardiac arrest in children. In: Vincent JL (ed) 2002 Yearbook of intensive care and emergency medicine. Springer-Verlag, Berlin, pp 877-888
7. Quan L, Kinder D (1992) Pediatric submersions: prehospital predictors of outcome. Pediatrics 90:909–913
8. Sirbaugh PE, Pepe PE, Shook JE, et al. (1999) A prospective, population-based study of the demographics, epidemiology, management and outcome of out-of-hospital pediatric cardiopulmonary arrest. Ann Emerg Med 33:174–184
9. Hickey RW, Cohen DM, Strausbaugh S, Detrich AM (1995) Pediatric patients requiring CPR in the prehospital setting. Ann Emerg Med 25:495–501
10. Ruben A, Ruben H (1962) Artificial respiration. Flow of water from the lung and the stomach. Lancet 1:780–781
11. Watson RS, Cummings P, Quan L, et al. (2001) Cervical spine injuries among submersion victims. J Trauma 51:658–662
12. Berg RA, Kern KB, Otto CW, et al. (2002) Ventricular fibrillation in a swine model of acute pediatric asphyxial cardiac arrest. Resuscitation 33:147–153
13. Allman FD, Nelson WB, Pacentine GA, McComb G (1986) Outcome following cardiopulmonary resuscitation in severe pediatric near-drowning. Am J Dis Child 140:571–575
14. Bernard SA, Gray TW, Buist MD, et al. (2002) Treatment of comatose survivors of out-of-hospital cardiac arrest with induced hypothermia. NEJM 346:557–563
15. The Hypothermia after Cardiac Arrest Study Group (2002) Mild therapeutic hypothermia to improve the neurologic outcome after cardiac arrest. NEJM 346:549–556
16. Peterson B (1977) Morbidity of childhood near-drowning. Pediatrics 59:364–370
17. Orlowski JP (1979) Prognostic factors in pediatric cases of drowning and near-drowning. J Am Coll Emerg Physicians 8:176–179
18. Kyriacou D, Arcinue E, Peek C, Kraus J (1994) Effect of immediate resuscitation on children with submersion injury. Pediatrics 94:137–142
19. Bratton SL, Jardine DS, Morray JP (1994) Serial neurologic examinations after near drowning and outcome. Arch Pediatr Adolesc Med 148:167-170
20. Idris AH, Berg RA, Bierens J, et al. (2003) ILCOR advisory statement. Recommended guidelines for uniform reporting of data from drowning: the Utstein style. Resuscitation 59:45-57

6.11
Termination of Resuscitation Efforts in Drowning

MARTIN NEMIROFF and PAUL PEPE

Resuscitation following submersion events is most often guided by the history of the incident itself. Certain variables such as age of the patient, underwater time, water temperature, associated injuries, quality and timelines of cardiopulmonary resuscitation (CPR), cleanliness of the water or other liquid, amount of struggle, and whether or not there was suicidal intent, all help in determining prognosis as well as magnitude of resuscitative efforts needed [1–5]. As would be expected, the younger the patient, the better the prognosis. Reports of survivors in large series are heavily weighted towards the youngest age groups, particularly in water with temperatures below 21°C. Medical literature is replete with examples of unwanted newborns surviving attempts at drowning. A three-year-old child and a 75-year-old adult have markedly different tolerances to hypoxia. But while all of these factors determine risk, they are not necessarily absolutes in terms of determining outcomes for individuals. The following chapter will provide a more detailed discussion of these factors and areas for further research.

6.11.1
Should Resuscitations Not Be Attempted if Submersion Has Been Lengthy?

The underwater time is a key fact in any decision-making in both the initiation and termination of resuscitation of drowned victims. It is generally accepted that, with current resuscitative techniques and in a typical cardiac arrest situations, most persons without oxygenation to the brain would have permanent brain damage within 5–10 min. However, drowning may be a different story in that pulses and brain perfusion may continue for a period of time, even without optimal oxygenation. In fact, in the US, the general practice is to attempt resuscitation if the victim was underwater for 1 hour or less, particularly in cold water. A frequent analogy has been to refer to the golden hour discussed in the trauma literature because successful resuscitation (that is, a return to former level of functioning) has been reported most often during this time parameter.

Citing 60 min is not to say that there are no deaths within the 1 hour time frame, as well as rare survivals following submersions longer than 1 hour. However, this factor is relatively so important in decision-making that it is worth extra effort and time to question bystanders, family members and emergency personnel to arrive at a best estimate. One question that arises is one of whether the underwater time is accurate. Should longer submersions preclude resuscitation or should we alter the magnitude of resuscitative efforts beyond 1 hour submersions?

6.11.2
Terminating Resuscitation Efforts

Also, the decisions to attempt resuscitation do not preclude the concept of on-scene termination of efforts. In recent studies, it has been demonstrated that in all cardiac arrests, including drowning incidents, patients not regaining pulses within 25 min after initiation of advanced life support (ALS) interventions will not survive neurologically intact, regardless of the previous arrest interval or the extent to which basic life support (BLS) was performed [6–8]. Exceptions to these findings are those with persistent ventricular fibrillation in applicable cases and the usual caveats about suspected hypothermia [6–8]. As a result, water temperature is an important factor in determining the length of resuscitation efforts.

6.11.2
Water Temperature as a Factor

The colder the water, the better the survival characteristics for drowning victims, and, in turn, the longer one would persist in resuscitating. More specifically, there appears to be a markedly improved prognosis with drowning in waters below 21°C. Treating the associated hypothermia often facilitates cardiac resuscitation and ensures a full cerebral resuscitation. In the meantime, hypothermic resuscitation also entails a difference in ventilatory rates and even the threshold for chest compressions if any pulses are present. The question remains, should cold water drowning always be considered a special case and have different parameters for termination of resuscitation delineated from warm water cases?

6.11.3
Trauma as a Factor

Some submersion incidents are associated with trauma such as car submersions, air crashes in the water, and jumping from bridges in suicide attempts. Closed head injuries, thoracic acceleration injuries, burns and blast injuries, all markedly reduce the survivability previously ascribed to cold water submersion. A study of jumpers from San Francisco's Golden Gate Bridge showed these were primarily trauma cases rather than cold water submersion victims, although the latter was necessarily part of the whole spectrum of injuries. Asystolic victims were treated as per trauma protocols, but not resuscitated. In contrast, when there was so-called relatively clean water entry (after an 80-meter fall), little or no trauma resulted. In such cases 7% survived (n=1020) and were successfully treated for submersion and hypothermia.

6.11.4
Bystander CPR as a Factor

In these days of ubiquitous video camera coverage of accidents, one sees many varied attempts at cardiopulmonary resuscitation (CPR) at the scene. When there are major lapses in technique, such as a delay in initiating CPR, ventilation without circulation (or vice versa), poor outcomes result. The quality of BLS is considered an important determinant of what the eventual outcome will be, though not an absolute determinant. But based on what we know about the relative futility of ALS without bystander CPR in drowning [9–11], this still begs the question, that if CPR is improper or not performed at all, should resuscitations be terminated rapidly?

6.11.5
Dirty Water

Immersion and submersion incidents occurring in fluids other than clear clean water lead to a poorer prognosis. Sewerage, swamp water, industrial chemicals and even liquid fertiliser submersions have been reported. These scenarios have a grave prognosis and pulmonary bacterial loads have proven fatal despite heroic attempts at antibiotic and antifungal coverage. When relatively clear water is the agent, the prognosis is much better, especially if the samples are transparent or translucent and have less suspended particulate matter. This then raises the question as to whether or not there are better techniques available to manage massive bacterial and fungal exposure in contaminated drowning events.

6.11.6
The Degree of Struggle Involved

Interestingly, if the submersion occurred after a mammoth struggle to stay afloat, the eventual prognosis is poor. If the history suggests that the person disappeared suddenly or fell or was pushed into the water, then quickly recovered, survival rates are much better depending on the underwater time. Of particular interest is the finding in drug or alcohol intoxicated individuals. Presumably, they tend to struggle less and appear to be easier to resuscitate.

In contrast, if one is attempting suicide by drowning, the resuscitations are often ineffectual. Along with the factors above, there appears to be some ill-defined factor of the will to live which enters into the prognosis.

6.11.7
Physical and Laboratory Findings

Physical findings have been considered in early termination of resuscitation. For example, the presence of fixed and dilated pupils on admission has been considered a universally grave sign. However, this can be confusing because hypothermia alone can lead to this finding and there have been full survivors despite this initial appearance. The Glasgow Coma Scale (GCS) has been used with success to quantify the severity of the neurologic injury associated with submersion accidents, but even initial presentations with decerebration and decorticate posturing do not exclude normal neurological recovery. An excellent area for research would be to find some physical finding that correlates with survivability or non-survivability so as to dictate termination of resuscitation.

Likewise, when available in the prehospital setting, laboratory findings such as the level of hypoxemia are not good determinants of outcome. Drowning patients have some of the lowest partial pressures of oxygen measured and yet can be successfully ventilated, supported and taken to cardiopulmonary bypass (CPB) if available, for circulation, oxygenation and re-warming. Markedly elevated serum potassium and lactate levels, and pH levels below 7.0 do correlate with poor resuscitation results, but should not be used exclusively to terminate resuscitation. A persistent end-tidal carbon dioxide level less than 10 mm Hg for more than 20 min uniformly predicts non-survival in typical cardiac arrests [7]. However, this same concept may not be applicable in drowning cases, particularly with accompanying hypothermia. An excellent area for research would be to isolate some laboratory finding that correlates with survivability or non-survivability so as to dictate termination of resuscitation.

6.11.7
Facility and Resources

Termination of resuscitation also depends on many other factors, including the access and capabilities of medical facilities, its staffing, the involvement of multiple other victims and resources in general. Each submersion victim can paralyse an emergency department of a community hospital for hours. If there is more than one victim, resources are stressed and some resuscitation efforts may need to be shortened.

6.11.8
Summary

Given a young patient, with a short submersion, in cold water, with no injuries, and an unintentional clear water entry, the prognosis should be very good, and resuscitative efforts should be maximal. Current data about futility of resuscitation efforts in drowning are limited, not absolute and the prognosis is multi-factorial. However, almost all normothermic adult patients are resuscitated within 25 min of the initiation of advanced life support techniques and although there are rare exceptions, almost all neurologically-intact survivors, including cold water victims, are resuscitated within 1 hour of the initiating event.

6.11.9
Recommendations

Future research efforts should attempt to delineate the circumstances and applicable stratifications for the futility of continued resuscitation efforts following drowning incidents.

In addition to demographic, historical, physical examination and laboratory information and water temperature considerations, future research efforts should determine maximum time intervals for resuscitation efforts under these various circumstances and stratifications, particularly with any proposed neuroprotective or resuscitative interventions.

References

1. Allman FD, Nelson WB, Pacentine GA, McComb G (1986) Outcome following cardiopulmonary resuscitation in severe pediatric near-drowning. Am J Dis Child 140:571–575
2. Modell JH, Graves SA, Ketover A (1976) Clinical course of 91 consecutive near drowning victims. Chest 70:231–238
3. Nemiroff MJ (1992) Near-drowning. Respir Care 37:600–608
4. Orlowski JP (1979) Prognostic factors in pediatric cases of drowning and near-drowning. J Am Coll Emerg Physicians 8:176–179
5. Peterson B (1977) Morbidity of childhood near-drowning. Pediatrics 59:364–370
6. Bonnin MJ, Pepe PE, Kimball KT, Clark PS (1993) Distinct criteria for termination of resuscitation in the out-of-hospital setting. JAMA 270:1457-1462
7. Pepe PE, Swor RA, Ornato JP, et al. (2001) Resuscitation in the out-of-hospital setting: Medical futility criteria for on-scene pronouncement of death. Prehosp Emerg Care 5:79–87
8. Pepe PE, Brown CG, Bonnin MJ, et al. (1993) Prospective validation of criteria for on-scene termination of resuscitation efforts after out-of-hospital cardiac arrest. Ann Emerg Med 22:884–885
9. Pepe PE, Wigginton JG, Mann DM, et al. (2002) Prospective, decade-long, population-based study of pediatric drowning-related incidents. Acad Emerg Med 9:516–517
10. Kyriacou D, Arcinue E, Peek C, Kraus J (1994) Effect of immediate resuscitation on children with submersion injury. Pediatrics 94:137–142
11. Goh SH, Low B (1999) Drowning and near-drowning – some lesions learned. Acad Med Singapore 28:183–188

6.12
Unusual Circumstances of Drowning

PETER MORLEY

The circumstances surrounding submersion injuries are often far more complex than initially apparent, and are often more complex than those associated with the usual resuscitation of heart or trauma patients. Many factors influence this complexity including: the fluid involved, the environment, the characteristics of the victim themselves, the aetiology of the incident, the resuscitation itself and the potential ramifications after the event. The unusual circumstances are classified by three case reports.

6.12.1
The Fluid

The amount of fluid required to result in a serious drowning injury to the victim may be much less than expected. The type of fluid encountered may be of various degrees of salinity, from fresh water all the way through to the hypertonic Dead Seawater and may be significantly contaminated, even with kerosene [1]. Occasionally, the fluid is not even water but for example mineral oil [2].

6.12.2
The Environment

The environment may add challenges of its own. Submersion has been reported in buckets, toilets, washing machines, showers, bathtubs, jacuzzis and of course rivers, lakes and the sea. Interestingly, the design of toilet bowls may have a significant impact on the incidence of submersion in them. Extremes of temperature may also be encountered, with the hypothermia induced by icy water offering some potential benefits with regard to organ preservation, but adding complex management issues with regard to the appropriate timing, amount and techniques for rewarming. The weather and sea conditions may not only contribute to the likelihood of incidents but also may hamper the rescue and resuscitation. Vertical removal of the victim from water may be necessary, but results in the sudden withdrawal of the hydrostatic squeeze and may be associated with significant and even fatal hemodynamic compromise.

6.12.3
The Victim

Victims of submersion injuries come from a variety of sources. To many, the picture conjured up is that of a young child drowning in a backyard swimming pool [3]. Yet the victims encompass the extremes of age, the complete spectrum of health and disease, and include recreational and workplace incidents. Indeed, for many professions, drowning becomes an occupational health and safety issue, especially in the ocean-going fishing industry [4]. Seamen are a particularly interesting group, as they seem to be at an increased risk of dying from a number of causes other than submersion including accidental poisoning, suicide and homicide [5]. Healthy adult males may be at particular risk because of hazardous behaviour, and heavy alcohol and/or drug use [5, 6]. The male:female ratio for drowning victims increases to a peak of 10 in the 20–24 age group and then declines slowly toward 1 when over 80 years.

Cervical spine injuries are only approximately 1% in drowning victims. In certain situations, these and other associated injuries may be much more likely, such as in bridge jumpers, where they are really victims of trauma and not of submersion, and in crashes associated with the increasingly popular personal water craft [7].

The possibility of spinal injury complicates the management of the drowning victim by raising a conflicting priority between optimal resuscitation and optimal spine immobilisation. Appropriate strategies and techniques for the rescue of victims with suspected spinal injuries should continue to be evaluated. Multiple medical complications can also occur as a result of the submersion ranging from the induction of otherwise asymptomatic conditions [8], to various acute stresses on the respiratory and cardiovascular systems including aspiration, myocardial infarction and stroke. Finally, a significant number of submersion incidents occur in victims foreign to the area where language difficulties may cause problems. An example are the overseas tourists at Australian surfing beaches [9].

6.12.4
The Aetiology

Lack of supervision is a common theme, particularly in children less than 5 years of age. However, in older children and adults, associated conditions may also result in submersion. Children up to the age of 19 years with epilepsy are far more likely to have a submersion or to actually drown [10], and this may be related, in turn, to suboptimal medical treatment prior to the incident [11]. Other medical conditions are also commonly encountered, including myocardial infarction and cerebrovascular accidents [12]. They must be considered when managing the victim. Unfortunately, a large number of fatal and near-fatal submersion incidents are as a result of suicide attempts [12]. Psychiatric conditions may be present in those who are resuscitated.

6.12.5
The Resuscitation

The victim is often exhausted or suffering from a complication of a medical condition by the time they are reached. As a result of asphyxia and aspiration hypoxemia may well be present long before a cardiac arrhythmia ensues. In direct opposition to some of the recent trends, the initial basic life support (BLS) should be directed to maintenance of airway patency, and the commencement of rescue breathing. Ventricular fibrillation (VF) is rare in submersion victims, so the urgency of defibrillation is replaced by an emphasis on good cardiopulmonary resuscitation (CPR). The ability to perform the components of CPR may be delayed or limited by an unstable or unsafe environment [13].

Hypothermia may in itself prolong the window of opportunity for successful resuscitation, and whether due to this or the predominantly respiratory aetiology, the victims of a cardiac arrest secondary to submersion have a much better outcome than would be otherwise expected [14]. Submersion in icy water is occasionally associated with miraculous outcomes possibly due to the rapid cooling of the victim, resulting in some cerebral preservation. Some prediction of the likelihood of successful resuscitation can be made, in the field, based on clinical criteria [15]. However, many authors recommend that resuscitation attempts should always be continued in the pre-hospital setting because of the difficulty of predicting outcome with sufficient accuracy at the scene [16]. This area is still controversial, and requires further investigation.

6.12.6
The Psycho-Social Aftermath

The submersion may well have been as a result of inadequate supervision or lack of simple safety precautions. Grieving bystanders themselves, especially when family, may have significant guilt and may well need careful supportive management and counselling in the short and the long term. The victim themselves may go on to have significant psychological sequelae as a result of the incident, or require careful medical and/or psychiatric evaluation because of the high prevalence of associated conditions

References

1. Segev D, Szold O, Fireman E, et al. (1999) Kerosene-induced severe acute respiratory failure in near drowning: reports on four cases and review of the literature. Crit Care Med 27:1437–1440
2. Hussain IR, Edenborough FP, Wilson RS, Stableforth DE (1996) Severe lipoid pneumonia following attempted suicide by mineral oil immersion. Thorax 51:652–653, discussion 656–657
3. Ellis AA, Trent RB (1995) Hospitalizations for near drowning in California: incidence and costs. Am J Public Health 85:1115–1118
4. Lincoln JM, Conway GA (1999) Preventing commercial fishing deaths in Alaska. Occup Environ Med 56:691–695
5. Rafnsson V, Gunnarsdottir H (1993) Risk of fatal accidents occurring other than at sea among Icelandic seamen. BMJ 22:1379–1381
6. Howland J, Hingson R, Mangione TW, et al. (1996) Why are most drowning victims men? Sex differences in aquatic skills and behaviors. Am J Public Health 86:93–96
7. Shatz DV, Kirton OC, McKenney MG, et al. (1998) Personal watercraft crash injuries: an emerging problem. J Trauma Injury Infect Crit Care 44:198–201
8. Yoshinaga M, Kamimura J, Fukushige T, et al. (1999) Face immersion in cold water induces prolongation of the QT interval and T-wave changes in children with nonfamilial long QT syndrome. Am J Cardiol 83:1494–1497
9. Leahy SJ, Fenner PJ, Harrison SL, Tebb N (1999) Olympic visitors need to be told about the dangers of the Australian surf. Aust N Z J Public Health 4:442
10. Diekema DS, Quan L, Holt V (1993) Epilepsy as a risk factor for submersion injury in children. Pediatrics 91:612–616
11. Ryan CA, Dowling G (1993) Drowning deaths in people with epilepsy. CMAJ 148:781–784
12. Bierens JJLM (1996) Drowning in the Netherlands. Pathophysiology, epidemiology and clinical studies. University Utrecht PhD-thesis
13. Anonymous (2000) Advanced challenges in resuscitation. Section 3: special challenges in emergency cardiovascular care 3B: submersion or near-drowning. Resuscitation 23:1–3, 273–277
14. Kuisma M, Jaara K (1997) Unwitnessed out-of-hospital cardiac arrest: is resuscitation worthwhile? Ann Emerg Med 30:69–75
15. Szpilman D (1997) Near-drowning and drowning classification: a proposal to stratify mortality based on the analysis of 1,831 cases. Chest 112:660–665
16. Christensen DW, Jansen P, Perkin RM (1997) Outcome and acute care hospital costs after warm water near drowning in children. Pediatrics 99:715–721

6.13
A Case Report of an Extreme Situation

MARTIN STOTZ and WOLFGANG UMMENHOFER

For medical teams involved in rescuing victims after near drowning, especially children, it would be helpful to have predictors of survival and neurologic outcome. Attempts to define these predictors have been made [1–4], but, unfortunately, individual outcome generally cannot be predicted on-scene. We present a paediatric case non-fotal drowning in cold water with a subsequent cardiopulmonary arrest of at least 15 min without attempts of CPR that resulted in an outcome with no neurologic impairment.

6.13.1
The Case Report

A 25-month-old boy was found lifeless in a swimming pool by his parents. The estimated drowning time was 10 min with a presumed water temperature of 4°C. He remained unconscious and apneic while his parents transferred him to the hospital in their private car (5 min) without attempting cardiopulmonary resuscitation. In the emergency department he was in cardiorespiratory arrest with asystole, exhibited flaccid paralysis, had a Glasgow Coma Score (GCS) of 3, dilated pupils without reaction to light, and a body core temperature of 29°C. Cardiopulmonary resuscitation was started immediately, his trachea was intubated and he was ventilated with 100% oxygen. Chest compressions were performed successfully with a palpable carotid pulse. Before gaining venous access, 1 mg epinephrine was administered intratracheally. Spontaneous circulation returned after 5 min and chest compressions were stopped. Blood gas analysis showed acidosis (◻ **Table 6.4**) and a low potassium concentration. After a further 10 min of ventilation and external rewarming, the boy moved spontaneously all four extremities and improved neurologically to a GCS score of 6. He was then transferred to the intensive care unit where he showed stable hemodynamic parameters with supraventricular tachycardia and pupils that were reactive to light. Chest radiography showed no evidence of aspiration. The following night, the patient remained hemodynamically stable. The next morning he was extubated normothermic and he improved neurologically to a GCS of 15 after extubation. Blood glucose levels were within normal range during the whole course. He was discharged to the ward the next day and left hospital 1 day later without neurologic deficit.

6.13.2
Applicable Discussion

Water temperature seems to be the major determinant for outcome of victims following drowning. Hypothermia, resulting from cold water drowning may

◘ **Table 6.4.** pH-values, blood potassium and body core temperature after cold-water near-drowning

Time after accident	30 min	40 min	4 hours	10 hours
pH	7.03	7.19	7.28	7.34
Blood potassium (mmol/L)	2.1	2.4	3.8	4.3
Temperature (°C)	29	32	34	38

offer some degree of brain protection to hypoxia that warm water does not. Neurologically intact survival even after 45 min of drowning in cold water has been reported [5, 6]. On the other hand, hypothermia cannot render its cerebral protective effect if it is preceded by hypoxemia. The time to resuscitation of cardiac arrest may be less important for victims drowned in cold water, as seen in our case. In warm water drowning, this protective effect is not present, and CPR should start immediately to be successful. A stay-and-play approach is always indicated for warm water drowning victims with cardiopulmonary resuscitation on scene, whereas in cold water drowning victims, scoop-and-run approaches may be a valuable alternative with respect to outcome.

Hypothermia is known to cause blood acidosis and a potassium shift [7]. There is clear evidence that an elevated serum potassium level above 10 mmol/l is a poor prognostic sign [8, 9]. The hypothermia induced acidosis seems to have minor predictive value and survival after extreme acidosis (pH 6.33) has been reported without neurologic deficit [10]. An initial arterial pH of 7.03 and serum potassium of 2.1 mmol/l were associated with a favourable outcome in our case. Re-warming of hypothermic drowning victims has traditionally been of major concern. It seems to be reasonable to start re-warming as soon as possible if return of spontaneous circulation can be achieved. When the victim is hemodynamically stable, external re-warming techniques can be used. The use of convective warm air devices (Bair-Hugger®) is widespread and they are also available in smaller hospitals. A re-warming rate of 3.9°C to 4.4°C per hour in children has been reported and has been successfully used in profound hypothermia (less than 20°C) [11]. Rewarming techniques, such as peritoneal and pleural lavage, have inherent risk and offer no obvious advantage to drowning victims. In the absence of a rhythm associated with spontaneous circulation, extracorporeal life support remains the golden standard and it has been used successfully in children [12, 13].

In conclusion, our case report demonstrates that, as there is no definite proof of survival rate and predictable neurologic outcome after cold water submersion, aggressive management and resuscitation of the paediatric victim should be performed even after prolonged periods of submersion and cardiac arrest [14]. The decision to subsequently withdraw life support generally should not be made in the field for cases of cold water drowning and the decision to continue or terminate resuscitative efforts should be made by a team of specialists with experience with drowning patients.

References

1. Christensen DW, Jansen P, Perkin RM (1997) Outcome and acute care hospital costs after warm water near drowning in children. Pediatrics 99:715–721
2. Gonzalez-Luis G, Pons M, Cambra FJ, et al. (2001) A use of the Pediatric Risk of Mortality Score as predictor of death and serious neurologic damage in children after submersion. Pediatr Emerg Care 17:405–409
3. Graf WD, Cummings P, Quan L, Brutocao D (1995) Predicting outcome in pediatric submersion victims. Ann Emerg Med 26:312–319
4. Suominen P, Baillie C, Korpela R, et al. (2002) Impact of age, submersion time and water temperature on outcome in near-drowning. Resuscitation 52:247–254
5. Chochinov AH, Baydock BM, Bristow GK, Giesbrecht GG (1998) Recovery of a 62-year-old man from prolonged cold water submersion. Ann Emerg Med 31:127–131
6. Perk L, Borger van de Burg F, Berendsen HH, Wout JW van't (2002) Full recovery after 45 min accidental submersion (letter). Intensive Care Med 28:524
7. Koht A, Cane, R, Cerullo LJ (1983) Serum potassium levels during prolonged hypothermia. Intensive Care Med 9:275–277
8. Mair P, Kornberger E, Furtwaengler W, et al. (1994) Prognostic markers in patients with severe accidental hypothermia and cardiocirculatory arrest. Resuscitation 27:47–54
9. Schaller MD, Fischer AP, Perret CH (1990) Hyperkalemia. A prognostic factor during acute severe hypothermia. JAMA 264:1842–1845
10. Opdahl H (1997) Survival put to the acid test: extreme arterial blood acidosis (pH 6.33) after near drowning. Crit Care Med 25:1431–1436
11. Caen A de (2002) Management of profound hypothermia in children without the use of extracorporeal life support therapy. Lancet 360:1394–1395
12. Walpoth BH, Walpoth-Aslan BN, Mattle HP, et al. (1997) Outcome of survivors of accidental deep hypothermia and circulatory arrest treated with extracorporeal blood warming. N Engl J Med 337:1500–1505
13. Wollenek G, Honarwar N, Golej J, Marx M (2002) Cold water submersion and cardiac arrest in treatment of severe hypothermia with cardiopulmonary bypass. Resuscitation 52:255–263
14. Jacinto SJ, Gieron-Korthals M, Ferreira JA (2001) Predicting outcome in hypoxic-ischemic brain injury. Pediatr Clin North Am 48:647–660

6.14
A Case Report of a Successful Resuscitation from Accidental Hypothermia of 22°C and Submersion with Circulatory Arrest

GERT-JAN SCHEFFER

On April 2, 2002, at 6:11 (am), a security officer on his way to work noticed a car upside down in a canal and called the local alarm number. At 6.18 a rescue team arrived at the scene of the accident and, at 6.23, divers managed to enter the car and removed a 41-year-old man from the water. Paramedics immediately evaluated the man who was in deep coma with fixed and dilated pupils, had no spontaneous breathing but still had a palpable pulse. Once connected to the monitor, he had a spontaneous rhythm. Intubation was not immediately possible. The patient was artificially ventilated by bag-mask and he was transported to a nearby hospital. At 6.33, during transport to the hospital, the patient developed ventricular fibrillation (VF) and external chest compressions were started. Upon arrival at the hospital, the patient was still in deep coma and the ECG still showed VF. The measured rectal temperature was 22°C. There were no signs of a major injury. The patient was intubated and several attempts to defibrillate failed. It was decided to transfer the patient to our centre for cardiac surgery with the aim of starting extracorporeal circulation. The patient arrived at 7.45 and was immediately taken to the operating room. A team of cardiac surgeons, anaesthesiologists, perfusionists and specialised nurses continued CPR, while the patient was prepared for cardiopulmonary bypass by mid-sternal access. At 8.05 the patient was on bypass and full flow was reached after a total period of 92 min of CPR. At 28°C, defibrillation was performed, and the patient was further re-warmed until 35.4°C. He was successfully weaned from cardiopulmonary bypass after 121 min. The post-operative course was uneventful and after 7 hours the patient woke up and could be extubated. The patient had good neurological recovery and could be discharged in excellent condition from the hospital after 7 days.

6.14.1
Applicable Discussion

While traditional advanced life support (ALS) techniques applied in the out-of-hospital context cannot be definitively identified as life-saving, extraordinary ALS techniques can change the apparent outcome in drowning, even after more than 90 min of CPR, especially when hypothermia is present. Decisions regarding termination of resuscitation efforts following a drowning incident should take cases like this one into account.

6.15
A Care Report of 22-Minute Submersion in Warm Water Without Sequelae

DAVID SZPILMAN

On a sunny day, with air temperature of 30°C and water temperature of 21°C, the submersion of a healthy black 33-year-old male, in brackish dark water of a canal with slow current, was noticed by bystanders. Later it was reported that the man had used a small amount of alcohol. At 7 min after the submersion, the first lifeguard arrived and after another 15 min of search by lifeguards and a helicopter, the victim was found and brought to shore.

No in-water resuscitation was performed. The victim was taken out of the water with his head up, positioned parallel to the shore and cardiorespiratory arrest was confirmed. Basic life support (BLS) was started by two lifeguards. After 2 min, bag-mask ventilation with 15 litres of oxygen was started and after another 2 min the victim was orotracheally intubated. A total of 1 mg of epinephrine

IV was given immediately after the intubation. At this moment clinical signs of acute pulmonary oedema were identified; 3 mg epinephrine IV every 3–5 min were then given (total of 22 mg). After 33 min of BLS and advanced life support (ALS) supraventricular tachycardia was notice and spontaneous ventilation started 4 min later. Soon after, the cardiac rhythm changed into a sinus tachycardia. At 20 min after restoration of spontaneous circulation the victim was transferred to a hospital with a Glasgow Coma Scale of 6 (1; 1; 4). In the hospital, the Glasgow Coma Scale raised to 9 (3; 1; 5). The patient was sedated because of acute pulmonary oedema and mechanical ventilation was maintained After a period with pneumonia, the patient was extubated after 7 days, discharged from the ICU after 9 days and went home 16 days after the drowning event. At discharge there was no motor or psychological damage and he started to work again 24 days after drowning.

6.15.1
Applicable Discussion

In general, it is believed that resuscitation has to start within 4–6 min to avoid cerebral damage but those victims who drown in cold water can be resuscitated after this time frame without neurological sequelae [1, 2]. In 1993, a resuscitation of a young girl with 41 min submersion in cold water was successful after 80 min of CPR (personal observation) The longest submersion time registered in cold water with complete recovery is 66 min [3]. Several authors have stated that at the rescue site and in the hospital, no one indicator appeared to be absolutely reliable. Therefore, resuscitation should be started without delay in each victim without palpable pulse who has been submerged for less than 1 hour.

For these reasons, the Rio de Janeiro Drowning Resuscitation Centre proceeds according to the following guidelines for drowning resuscitation:

- CPR should always be started when time of submersion is under 1 hour or when there is no obvious physical evidence of death
- Resuscitation efforts should be maintained until the victim is warm and an asystole is still diagnosed
- Both BLS and ALS are performed at the accident site
- High doses of IV epinephrine are allowed in these cases

Of the 114 resuscitations undertaken in our Drowning Resuscitation Center between 1998 and 2002, 18 victims were resuscitated with submersion time of over 10 min. Of these:

- Two were without sequelae (11%)
- Five survived with severe neurological sequelae (28%)
- 11 Died within 24 hours (61%)

In this case report the water was not cold, so maybe water should always be considered to be relatively cold in relation to body temperature.

The use of alcohol may have increased the loss of body heat allowing the temperature to drop faster.

The diving reflex in combination with hypothermia may be an explanation. This case report shows again that there is no reliable indicator for the outcome of CPR in drowning.

References

1. Peterson B (1977) Morbidity of childhood near-drowning. Pediatrics 59:364–370
2. Orlowski JP (1988) Drowning, near-drowning and ice-water drowning. JAMA 260:390–391
3. Bolte RG, Block PG, Bowers RS, et al. (1988) The use of extracorporal rewarming in a child submerged for 66 minutes. JAMA 260:377–379

Further Reading

Allman FD, Nelson WB, Gregory AP, et al. (1986) Outcome following cardiopulmonary resuscitation in severe near-drowning. Am J Dis Child 140:571–575
Orlowski JP(1987) Drowning, near-drowning, and ice water submersion. Pediatr Clin North Am 34:92–93
Southwick FS, Dalglish PH (1980) Recovery after prolonged asystolic cardiac arrest in profound hypothermia. JAMA 243:1250–1253
Szpilman D (1997) Near-drowning and drowning classification: a proposal to stratify mortality based on the analysis of 1,831 cases. Chest 112:660–665

6.16
Recommended Guidelines for Uniform Reporting of Data from Drowning: The Utstein Style

AHAMED IDRIS, ROBERT BERG, JOOST BIERENS, LEO BOSSAERT, CHRISTINE BRANCHE, ANDREA GABRIELLI, SHIRLEY GRAVES, ANTHONY HANDLEY, ROBYN HOELLE, PETER MORLEY, LINDA PAPA, PAUL PEPE, LINDA QUAN, DAVID SZPILMAN, JANE WIGGINTON and JEROME MODELL

This chapter presents the consensus of a group of international investigators (■ Fig. 6.8) who met to establish guidelines for the uniform reporting of data from studies of drowning incidents. Similar consensus guidelines for reporting surveillance and resuscitation research have been developed for both adult and paediatric cardiac arrest [1, 2].

The principal purpose of the recommendations in this publication is to establish consistency in the reporting of drowning-related studies, both in terms of nomenclature and guidelines for reporting data. The following section highlights the overall concepts published in detail in [6] and [7].

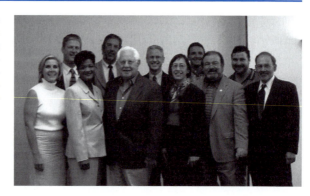

◘ Fig. 6.8. Some of the participants of the Utstein drowning group: Wigginton, Bierens, Branche, Bossaert, Modell, Berg, Quan, Szpilman, Pepe, Morley, and Idris

6.16.1
History of the Utstein-Style Approach

Both laboratory and clinical investigators from many different specialities contribute to the multidisciplinary knowledge base of both injury prevention and resuscitation science. While diversity can be a strength, it can also be an obstacle due to the lack of a common language and communication between investigators from different backgrounds.

In response to these problems, an international group of scientists concerned with out-of-hospital cardiac arrest research met at the Utstein Abbey in Norway in June 1990. Participants recognised the lack of standardised nomenclature and definitions as key problems in research reports. They developed definitions and recommended data that should be reported in studies of out-of-hospital cardiac arrest and resuscitation [3]. Drowning is another important problem within resuscitation research that also shares many of the same nomenclature and reporting problems. Drowning research is based on clinical events, time intervals and points, pathophysiological changes, autopsy findings, and other observations common to cardiac arrest and cardiopulmonary resuscitation research.

6.16.2
The Need for Standardised Nomenclature
and Reporting in Drowning

Drowning accounts for at least half a million deaths annually worldwide. This number is probably a gross underestimate due to under-reporting [4]. Physicians and other healthcare workers across the world deal frequently with the consequences of drowning, yet there are few population-based surveillance studies on drowning incidents or prospective clinical studies of prognostic factors and outcomes of drowning. A review of existing studies reveals a lack of standardised definitions [5]. Something as fundamental as the definition of drowning itself varies among reports, as do the clinical characteristics of outcome measures. This lack of consistency makes assessment and analysis of studies, both individually and as a whole, difficult.

◻ Table 6.5. Participating organisations for the Utstein-style process for drowning

Maatschappij tot Redding van Drenkelingen

International Liaison Committee on Resuscitation

American Heart Association

Australian Resuscitation Council

Comitê Latino-America de Ressuscitação

European Resuscitation Council

Heart and Stroke Foundation of Canada

Resuscitation Councils of Southern Africa

Centers for Disease Control and Prevention

In an attempt to solve these problems, an international Utstein-style consensus conference convened in Amsterdam in June 2002 to develop guidelines for definitions and the reporting of data related to drowning. The Utstein Task Force on Drowning consisted of representatives from major organisations concerned with resuscitation and epidemiology (◻ **Table 6.5**), as well as other recognised experts from around the world. In the following discussion, we report the results of this consensus project including a definition of drowning and recommended core and supplemental data (◻ **Tables 6.6–6.10**). As in previous Utstein-style reports, the primary language for the consensus process was English.

Data in the tables have been categorised as core data (Core) – which are pieces of information that could be expected to be collected at almost any venue, and supplemental data (Supplemental) – which are pieces of information that are very much advantageous to have and are encouraged to be collected by all investigators.

6.16.3
Definitions

Drowning is defined as:

The process of experiencing respiratory impairment from submersion/immersion in liquid.

Implicit in this definition is that a liquid/air interface is present at the entrance of the victim's airway, thus preventing the victim breathing air. A person may live or die after this process has occurred, but all who experience this process have had a drowning incident. The drowning process is a continuum beginning

■ **Table 6.6.** Drowning victim information

Victim identifier	Core
Gender	Core
Age (estimate, if necessary)	Core
Race or ethnic category	Supplemental
Incident date and time of day	Core
Resident of city, county, state, country?	Supplemental
Precipitating event: known/unknown	Core
If precipitating event is known, then specify	
Pre-existing illness: yes/no	Supplemental
If yes, then specify	

when the airway of the victim is below the surface of the liquid, usually water, at which time the victim voluntarily holds his breath. During this period of breath holding and laryngospasm, the victim does not have the ability to breathe gas. Therefore, oxygen is depleted and carbon dioxide is not eliminated. This results in the victim becoming hypercarbic, hypoxemic and acidotic [8–12].

A victim can be rescued at any time during the drowning process and may not require any intervention at all or may receive appropriate resuscitative measures, in which case the drowning process is interrupted. If the victim is not ventilated soon enough, then circulatory arrest will ensue and, in the absence of effective resuscitative efforts, multiple organ dysfunction and death will result, primarily due to tissue hypoxia.

Most resuscitations begin at the scene of the drowning and not in a hospital and, therefore, on-scene data are extremely important. Furthermore, many, possibly most, drowning victims have mild symptoms, recover at the scene, and may or may not be transported to a hospital [13]. Thus, to have a complete understanding of drowning and to capture the full scope of this problem, it is crucial that data at the scene be included in drowning reports.

The task force also decided to abandon the miscellaneous terms:

— Dry versus wet drowning
— Active versus passive versus silent drowning
— Secondary drowning
— Near-drowned and near-drowning

▣ Table 6.7. Drowning scene information

Witnessed (seeing submersion into water)	
Yes/No	Core
Body of water	
Bathtub, swimming pool, ocean, lake, river, bucket, or other bodies of water or containers	Core
Water/liquid type	
Fresh, salt, chemical, other	Supplemental
Approximate water temperature	
Non-icy, icy	Supplemental
Time of submersion, if known	Supplemental
Time of removal, if known	Supplemental
Unconscious when removed from the water	
Yes/No	Core
Cyanosis	Supplemental
Resuscitation before EMS arrived:	
Yes/No	Core
If yes, who gave CPR: lay, lifeguard	Supplemental
Method of CPR	
Mouth-to-mouth (MTM) ventilation alone, MTM+chest compression (CC), CC only, automatic external defibrillation	Supplemental
EMS called:	
Yes/No	Core
EMS vehicle dispatched	
Yes/No	Supplemental
Time of First EMS assessment	Supplemental
Initial Vital signs	
Spontaneous breathing, palpable pulse	Core
Oxygen saturation, temperature, blood pressure, pupillary reaction	Supplemental
Time of First EMS resuscitation attempts	Core
Neurological status: awake, blunted, coma (ABC), or other neurological assessment (AVPU, GCS)	Core

AVPU, alert/verbal/painful/unresponsive scale; GCS, Glasgow Coma Score.

◨ Table 6.8. Emergency department evaluation and treatment of the drowning patient

A. Vital signs: Temperature, heart rate, respiratory rate, blood pressure	Core
B. Oxygen haemoglobin saturation	Core
C. Arterial blood gas analysis, if unconscious or when SaO_2 <95% on room air	Core
D. Initial neurological status (GCS, AVPU, or ABC)	Core
E. Pupillary reaction	Supplemental
F. Airway and ventilation requirements	Core
G. Toxicology testing: Blood alcohol level and other drugs	Supplemental

GCS, Glasgow Coma Score; AVPU, alert/verbal/painful/unresponsive scale; ABC, awake, blunted, coma.

◨ Table 6.9. Hospital course of drowning patients

A. Airway and ventilation requirements	Core
B. Serial neurological function (Admission, 6 h, 24 h, 72 h, Discharge)	Supplemental
C. Complicated illness	Supplemental

◨ Table 6.10. Disposition of drowning outcomes

A. Alive or dead	Core
If dead, report date, place and time of death	
B. Date of hospital discharge	Core
C. Neurological outcome at hospital discharge	Core
D. Quality of life (OPC, CPC, other)	Supplemental
E. Cause of death:	Supplemental
1. How was cause decided	
2. Autopsy: Yes/No	
3. Forensic information (suicide, homicide)	
F. Other injuries and morbidities	Supplemental

6.16.4
Outcome

The primary outcome of a drowning episode should be categorised as either death or survival [14–24]. Survival indicates that the drowning victim remained alive after the acute event and following any acute or subacute sequelae. Drownings in which the victims are successfully resuscitated at the scene, but succumb to any condition that is causally related to the drowning should be categorised as deaths due to drowning.

Multiple outcome scales exist and have been validated. Commonly used assessment tools for adults are the ABC score (awake, blunted, comatose) [18, 19], the Glasgow Coma Score (GCS) [20, 21], Glasgow-Pittsburgh Cerebral Performance Categories (CPC) and Overall Performance Categories (OPC) [22], and for children, the Pediatric Cerebral Performance Category Scale and Pediatric Overall Performance Category Scale [23]. However, there have been other important schemas for measuring non-fatal health outcomes that are applicable to drowning survivors that expand the range of possible outcomes and better describe how survivors and families really function after injury.

◘ **Figure 6.9** one possible scheme that can be used to chart outcome. The outcome categories are derived, in part, from the Cerebral and Overall Performance Categories (CPC, OPC).

6.16.5
Summary

In summary, these are recommendations for unified drowning-related definitions and guidelines for reporting data contributed by a group of international experts. They are intended to improve the clarity of scientific communication and the comparability of scientific investigations. Improved validity, clarity and data compatibility of future scientific investigations of drowning will improve our knowledge base, improve epidemiological stratification, improve appropriate treatment of victims of drowning, and, ultimately, save lives.

References

1. American Heart Association ACLS and BLS subcommittees (1992) Standards and guidelines for cardiopulmonary resuscitation and emergency cardiac care. JAMA 268:2171–2302
2. Anonymous (2000) Guidelines 2000 for cardiopulmonary resuscitation and emergency cardiovascular care. International Consensus on Science. Circulation 102:I-1–I-384; Resuscitation 46:1–448
3. Cummins RO, Chamberlain DA, Abramson NS, et al. (1991) Recommended guidelines for uniform reporting of data from out-of-hospital cardiac arrest: the Utstein style. A statement for health professionals from a task force of the American Heart Association, the European Resuscitation Council, the Heart and Stroke Foundation of Canada, and the Australian Resuscitation Council. Circulation 84:960–975

Patient ID

_____

Gender = M ❑ F ❑ U* ❑
Age = _____ or
Date of birth __/__/__
            DDMMYY

Date of event:
    __/__/__
    DDMMYY

Times:

Call received _____
EMS rescue _____

Location of Drowning:

bucket	❑	toilet	❑
bathtub	❑	lake	❑
ocean	❑	pool	❑
river/flowing water ❑		Other	❑

Event witnessed?   Yes ❑   No ❑
If yes: time of event = _____
witnessed/monitored by
layperson ❑   healthcare personnel ❑

At scene:

Loss of consciourness	Yes ❑	No ❑
CPR before EMS	Yes ❑	No ❑
by layperson ❑	healthcare personnel ❑	
techniques used:	rescue breathing	❑
	chest compression	❑

Precipitating event knows?

No	❑	If yes:	Intoxication	❑	Pre-existing medical
Yes	❑		Trauma	❑	List _____
					Drugs ❑
					Other _____

ED assessment/management:

Spont. breathing	Yes ❑ No ❑ U* ❑	Initial neuro state: GCS: E___ V___ M___
Palpable pulse	Yes ❑ No ❑ U* ❑	or A ❑ V ❑ P ❑ U ❑
Airway interventions	Yes ❑ No ❑ U* ❑	or A ❑ B ❑ C ❑

ED assessment/management:

Spont. breathing	Yes ❑ No ❑ U* ❑	Initial neuro state: GCS: E___ V___ M___
Palpable pulse	Yes ❑ No ❑ U* ❑	or A ❑ V ❑ P ❑ U ❑
Trachsal Tube/ventilation		or A ❑ B ❑ C ❑

Yes ❑ No ❑ U* ❑
Initial temp_____ BP_____ RR_____ SpO$_2$_____ FIO$_2$_____

Outcome:

ROSC: Survived to:

Any	Yes ❑ No ❑ U* ❑	ICU/ED	Yes ❑ No ❑ U* ❑
>20 min	Yes ❑ No ❑ U* ❑	hosp. admission	Yes ❑ No ❑ U* ❑
		hosp. discharge	Yes ❑ No ❑ U* ❑
DNAR order	Yes ❑ No ❑ U* ❑	If discharged alive, CPC _____	U* ❑

Date of discharge or death: __/__/__
                            DDMMYY

Fig. 6.9. Example of an Utstein drowning data form

4. DeNicola LK, Falk JL, Swanson ME, et al. (1997) Submersion injuries in children and adults. Crit Care Clin 13:477–502
5. Idris AH, Hoelle R, Papa L (2002) Lack of uniform definitions and reporting in drowning. Proceedings, Resuscitation 2002, Florence, Italy
6. Idris A, Berg R, Bierens J, et al. (2003) ILCOR advisory statement. Recommended guidelines for uniform reporting of data from drowning: the Utstein style. Resuscitation 59:45–57; and
7. Idris AH, Berg RA, Bierens J, et al. (2003) Recommended guidelines for uniform reporting of data from drowning: the Utstein style. Circulation 108:2565–2574
8. Modell JH, Gaub M, Moya F, et al. (1966) Physiologic effects of near drowning with chlorinated fresh water, distilled water, and isotonic saline. Anesthesiology 27:33–41
9. Modell JH (1971) Pathophysiology and treatment of drowning and near-drowning. Charles C Thomas, Springfield, Ill.
10. Modell JH, Graves SA, Ketover A (1976) Clinical course of 91 consecutive near-drowning victims. Chest 70:231–238
11. Modell JH, Moya F (1966) Effects of volume of aspirated fluid during chlorinated fresh water drowning. Anesthesiology 27:662–672
12. Modell JH, Moya F, Newby EJ, et al. (1967) The effects of fluid volume in sea water drowning. Ann Intern Med 67:68–80
13. Szpilman D (1997) Near-drowning and drowning classification: a proposal to stratify mortality based on the analysis of 1,831 cases. Chest 112:660–665
14. Modell JH, Graves SA, Kuck EJ (1980) Near-drowning: correlation of level of consciousness and survival. Can Anaesth Soc J 27:211–215
15. Graf WD, Cummings P, Quan L, Brutocao DL (1995) Predicting outcome in pediatric submersion victims. Ann Emerg Med 26:312–319
16. Causey AL, Tilelli JA, Swanson ME (2000) Predicting discharge in uncomplicated near-drowning. Am J Emerg Med 18:9–11
17. Kyriacou DN, Arcinue EL, Peek C, Kraus JF (1994) Effect of immediate resuscitation on children with submersion injury. Pediatrics 94:137–142
18. Conn AW, Montes JE, Barker GA, Edmonds JF (1980) Cerebral salvage in near-drowning following neurological classification by triage. Can Anaesth Soc J 27:201–210
19. Conn AW, Edmonds JF, Barker GA (1979) Cerebral resuscitation in near-drowning. Pediatr Clin North Am 26:691–701
20. Jennett B, Bond M (1975). Assessment of outcome after severe brain damage. Lancet 1:480–484
21. Teasdale G, Jennett B (1974) Assessment of coma and impaired consciousness. A practical scale. Lancet 2:81–84
22. Brain Resuscitation Clinical Trial I Study Group (1986) A randomized clinical study of cardiopulmonary-cerebral resuscitation: design, methods, and patient characteristics. Brain Resuscitation Clinical Trial I Study Group. Am J Emerg Med 4:72–86
23. Fiser DH (1992) Assessing the outcome of pediatric intensive care. J Pediatr 121:68–74
24. Pepe PE, Wigginton JG, Mann DM, et al. (2002) Prospective, decade-long, population-based study of pediatric drowning-related incidents. Acad Emerg Med 9:516–517

Hospital Treatment

TASK FORCE ON HOSPITAL TREATMENT
Section editors: HARRY GELISSEN, JEAN-LOUIS VINCENT and LAMBERT THIJS

Task Force Chairs

- Lambert Thijs
- Jean-Louis Vincent

Task Force Members

- Jean Carlet
- Luciano Gattinoni
- Jordi Mancebo
- Antony Simcock
- Hans van Vught
- Volker Wenzel
- Max Harry Weil

Other contributors

- Giel van Berkel
- E. Carlesso
- Davide Chiumello
- Harry Gelissen
- Sjef van Gestel
- Shirley Graves
- Jack Haitsma
- Walter Hasibeder
- Koos Jansen
- Burt Lachmann
- Jerome Modell
- Tomasso Pellis
- David Szpilman
- Nigel Turner

7.1
Overview

HARRY GELISSEN, JEAN-LOUIS VINCENT and LAMBERT THIJS

Hospital treatment of drowning victims includes in-hospital resuscitation as well as treatment of drowning related disorders of the pulmonary system, the neurological system and the temperature regulating systems. Resuscitation, brain and spinal cord injuries and problems of temperature regulation due to immersion hypothermia are addressed by other task forces of the project World Congress on Drowning. The hospital treatment task force had its focus on the hospital treatment of the pulmonary problems in drowned patients and during the World Congress on Drowning in Amsterdam in 2002 several aspects of the treatment of drowning victims were discussed.

This section of the handbook focuses on the diagnosis and treatment of respiratory complications of drowning in adults and children and on the clinical classification and stratification of drowning victims in the emergency room and intensive care unit (ICU). Members of the World Congress on Drowning Task Force on Hospital Treatment and other experts give their opinions on these topics. The authors of this chapter include many of the task force members. All are clinicians, some of whom have build up large expertise during a life-time of interest in the clinical treatment of drowning, and others who are outstanding experts in related subjects and were prepared to extrapolate their knowledge to the area of drowning. The recommendations of the task force are summarised in ▶ Chapter 7.2 and have also been published [1].

Few clinicians have build up sufficient clinical experience to publish data on the results of treatment after drowning. In ▶ Chapter 7.3, Antony Simcock describes his guidelines for the treatment of drowning victims in the emergency room, while in ▶ Chapter 7.4, Walter Hasibeder, Volker Wenzel and Antony Simcock focus on treatment in the ICU. All of these guidelines and protocols specifically aim at restoration and optimisation of oxygen delivery by treating both the pulmonary and cardiovascular system.

In ▶ Chapter 7.5, Hans Van Vught, Niger Turner, Koos Jansen and Sjet van Gestel overview the most important aspects of drowning in children. Epidemiology, pathophysiology, emergency treatment and clinical complications are discussed. As in adults, the ultimate outcome in children is largely determined by the severity of the neurological injury.

The key problems in most hospital admitted drowning victims are caused by aspiration. An overview of the effects of aspiration of water is given by Jerome Modell in ▶ Chapter 7.6. Until recently it was thought that 80−90% of drowning victims aspirated while drowning. In most of these patients, the amount of aspirated water is rather small, in which case there is no difference between the pathophysiological consequences of fresh- and salt-water drowning. In animal models the development of pulmonary oedema may be delayed by up to 48 hours after aspiration. However, clinical studies show that patients who present to the emergency room without respiratory symptoms can be safely discharged after an observation period of 8 hours. The management of the most prominent clinical problems in an ICU, the acute respiratory distress syndrome (ARDS) and drowning related pneumonia, are discussed by Davide Chiumello, E. Carlesso and Luciano Gattinoni in ▶ Chapter 7.7. Although there is a lack of randomised controlled clinical trials of the treatment of ARDS in drowning victims, early phase ARDS after drowning resembles ARDS after lung lavage. Lung lavage is often used in laboratory models for ARDS and relevant data for drowning can be extrapolated from these data. The late proliferative stage of ARDS is considered a final stage of unresolving ARDS regardless of the cause. Mechanical ventilatory support for early stage ARDS should be based on opening the lung and keeping the lung open with the right PEEP level, prevention of ventilator-induced lung injury and maybe ventilation in the prone position, although this has not been shown to be definitely beneficial.

Another pulmonary problem after drowning is pneumonia. Aspiration of water can cause early onset infections with water-borne micro-organisms. Also the aspiration of stomach contents may cause pneumonia. Late onset nosocomial pneumonias may be caused by secondary aspiration from the oropharynx. Nosocomial pneumonia is quite common in patients supported with mechanical ventilation. In ▶ **Chapter 7.8**, Giel van Berkel discusses the risk factors for pneumonia during and after drowning and describes the micro-organisms involved and the specific treatment required for such infections.

Water aspiration during drowning causes washout of surfactant. Furthermore, inactivation of functional alveolar surfactant takes place due to increased alveolocapillary permeability. In ▶ **Chapter 7.9**, Jack Haitsma and Burt Lachmann report the potential role of exogenous surfactant in acute respiratory failure related to drowning. Promising results from animal studies and case reports of surfactant use in humans after submersion have led to the first trials which are currently taking place.

Jerome Modell, Tomasso Pellis and Max Weil describe current insights into the cardiovascular alterations during submersion in ▶ **Chapter 7.10**. After sea-water aspiration, alveoli become fluid filled which causes intrapulmonary shunts. Artificial ventilation further compromises the cardiovascular system. The authors explain that treatment of decreased cardiac output by fluid replacement is more effective than by inotropic drugs. Also the effects of hypothermia on heart rhythm are discussed.

David Szpilman, Antony Simcock and Shirley Graves present several classification systems in ▶ **Chapter 7.11**. All classifications are based on the severity of neurological and cardiopulmonary symptoms upon presentation of the drowning victim. Classification of the severity of drowning facilitates the comparison of different treatment protocols and of the clinical results between centres where drowning patients are treated. The use of classification systems is also essential for the collection of data, the evaluation of treatment and for comparison of outcome in drowning.

Reference

1.   Bierens JJLM, Knape JTA, Gelissen HPMM (2002) Drowning. Curr Opin Crit Care 8:578–586

7.2
Recommendations

HARRY GELISSEN, JEAN-LOUIS VINCENT and LAMBERT THIJS

The following recommendations were made during the World Congress on Drowning by the Task Force on Hospital Treatment:
- *Registration of drowning victims and collection of clinical data on in-hospital resuscitation and treatment of complications of drowning are recommended.*

▬ *A uniform reporting system to register and collect these data should be developed.*

▬ *Hospital treatment of severe drowning victims should be concentrated in specialised centres.*

7.3
Treatment Protocols – Emergency Room

ANTHONY SIMCOCK

The relief of hypoxia and restoration of cardiorespiratory stability is a primary consideration in drowning. Where possible this should already occur at the accident site as soon as the victim has been removed from the water and treatment should be continued during transfer to hospital. Transfer should always be to a well-equipped hospital with an emergency department, ICU and advanced facilities for rewarming. A severe case of drowning is a medical emergency and if treatment can be instituted before cardiac arrest occurs, then full recovery without cerebral damage can be expected in the vast majority of cases [1–3].

7.3.1
Initial Assessment

The most important aspect of the initial assessment is speed. The objective is to reduce hypoxia to a minimum and decrease the hypoxic gap [4]. The basic questions to ask at this stage are: Is this patient breathing and is the breathing adequate?

Any patient who has inhaled water but is conscious and breathing with a reasonable depth and rate of respiration should be given oxygen until it can be confirmed that arterial oxygenation is indeed satisfactory. Any patient with suspected respiration problems should attend the emergency room. Patients who are apneic but not in cardiac arrest should be ventilated with 100% oxygen as soon as the apnoea is recognised.

7.3.2
Pathophysiology

There may be many ways in which a patient can drown. The final common pathway is always the same, no matter what the cause is. There is ventilation-perfusion mismatch with right to left shunt due to the inhalation of water. The resulting hypoxaemia is often accompanied by metabolic acidosis. Both hypoxaemia and acidosis can be severe. The cardiovascular response is very similar to response during hypovolaemia: tachycardia, narrow pulse pressure, low blood pressure and poor peripheral circulation. This is most likely due to fluid shifts and occurs in both fresh- and seawater drowning. In patients who die from drowning, aspiration of vomit is commonly found on post-mortem, and must be the terminal event.

7.3.3
Classification of Drowning Incidents

In general, the treatment of drowning can be based on four patient groups (◘ Table 7.1).

7.3.3.1
Group 1: Patients with No Apparent Inhalation

The treatment protocol is shown in ◘ Table 7.2. A significant number of victims who had to be rescued and received immediate care at the accident site have not inhaled at all. By the time they reach the emergency room they appear to have fully recovered. In general they are at low risk. Anyone who has to be rescued and has received immediate care at the site should however be admitted for close observation. These patients may not require oxygen. Nevertheless ventilation should be continuously monitored with a pulse oximeter (SaO_2) wherever possible. Arterial gas analysis may only be necessary if the peripheral circulation is shut down, for example due to stress, hypotension or hypothermia. Further observation consists of checking lung sounds, central temperature, basic biochemical screening and a chest X-ray. Criteria for discharge were set out for the first time in the European Resuscitation Council ALS Manual in 1994 and are shown in modified form as ◘ Table 7.3.

7.3.3.2
Group 2: Patients with Adequate Ventilation

This group of patients has inhaled water but on initial assessment appear to have adequate ventilation. These patients should be assumed to be hypoxaemic until proven otherwise and should be treated with high flow oxygen through a non-rebreathing mask with reservoir bag as soon as they are admitted to the emergency room. Wherever possible they should be admitted to the ICU for close cardiorespiratory monitoring. Any respiratory deterioration should be treated aggressively with either a continuous positive airway pressure circuit (CPAP) or, when this fails, intubation and ventilation. The aim is not to become hypoxic under any circumstances. Treatment is summarised in ◘ Table 7.4.

7.3.3.3
Group 3: Patients with Inadequate Ventilation

These patients are usually unconscious and have gasping respiration with a low respiratory rate. They are hypoxaemic and it is of paramount importance that the hypoxaemia is relieved as soon as possible. Endotracheal intubation can normally take place without depressant or muscle-relaxant drugs as reflexes are

Table 7.1. Classification of immersion incidents

Group 1	No evidence of inhalation
Group 2	Clinical evidence of inhalation, but with adequate ventilation
Group 3	Patients with inadequate ventilation
Group 4	Patients with absent ventilation and heart-beat

Table 7.2. Group 1: patients with no apparent inhalation

Admit for close observation

Blood gas analysis, monitor SaO_2

Assess hypothermia

Check electrolytes, blood film, glucose

Chest X-ray

Table 7.3. Criteria for 6-hour discharge

No fever, no cough, no respiratory symptoms

No crepitations in lungs

Normal PaO_2 on 21% oxygen

Normal chest X-ray

markedly depressed. Continuous positive pressure ventilation should begin with 100% oxygen. Blood pressure is invariably low and an intravenous infusion with warmed crystalloid is the second priority. It is only when the patient is being ventilated, that a transfer to the ICU for the cardiorespiratory assessment and treatment can take place. This is summarised in **Table 7.5**.

◻ Table 7.4. Group 2: patients with adequate ventilation

Oxygen by mask or CPAP circuit

Monitor SaO_2 and PaO_2

IV infusion of warmed fluid

Assess hypothermia and metabolic acidosis

Check chest X-ray, full blood count, urea, electrolytes, glucose

Admit to ICU wherever possible

◻ Table 7.5. Group 3: patients with inadequate ventilation

Intubate and ventilate with 100% oxygen

Continue IPPV. Maintain PaO_2 >8 kPa

Intravenous infusion

Use PEEP if necessary

Transfer to ICU

7.3.4
The Apparently Dead

There have been regular reports of cerebrally normal survival after prolonged submersion in cold water [5, 6]. These reports usually, but not invariably, involve children and extremely cold water. However, even more remarkable survival has occurred after prolonged partial submersion in snow or ice and has been reported in this handbook. It is probable that no acute immersion victim should be declared dead without some knowledge of the period of submersion, the temperature of the water, an ECG and central temperature recording. If there is any doubt, then resuscitation should be commenced and continued until the patient is rewarmed to at least 32°C.

■ **Table 7.6.** Treatment of cardiac arrest

Airway clearance

Immediate IPPV

External thoracic compressions

ECG as soon as possible

Intravenous cannulation

Assess hypothermia

7.3.5
Treatment of Hypothermic Cardiac Arrest

Resuscitation should follow the most recent Advanced Life Support Guidelines. It should be remembered, however, that there may be increased chest wall stiffness if hypothermia is severe. Both ventilation and external cardiac massage may not be as easy as in a conventional normothermic person. Treatment is summarised in ■ **Table 7.6**. It is important that once a decision to resuscitate is made, resuscitation should continue until the heart is restarted or the patient is rewarmed to at least 32°C before a decision on death can be made. The question of defibrillation in presence of hypothermia is controversial but most experts would accept that, without regard to the temperature and if ventricular fibrillation is diagnosed, a single three-shock cycle may restore sinus rhythm, but repeated cycles of defibrillation should be avoided due to the risk of myocardial damage.

7.3.6
Summary

The most essential rule for hospital treatment of drowning can be quoted from Haldane: "A lack of oxygen does not simply involve stoppage of the engine, but total ruin of what we took to be the machinery" [7]. This is also true for drowning victims.

References

1. Kemp A, Sibert J (1991) Outcome in children who drown, a British Isle study. Br Med J 302:931–933
2. Simcock AD (1999) Near drowning. In: Grieves I, Porter K (eds) Pre-hospital medicine. Arnold, London

3. Conn A, Barker G (1984) Fresh-water drowning and near drowning – an update. Can Anaesth Soc J 31:538–544
4. Simcock AD (1997) Drowning, near-drowning and immersion hypothermia. In: Garrard C, Foex P, Westaby S (eds) Principles and practice of intensive care. Blackwell, London
5. Botte RG, Black PG, Bowers RS, Kent-Thorne J, Correlli HM (1988) The use of extracorporeal rewarming in a child submerged for 66 minutes. JAMA 260:377–379
6. Theilade D (1977) The danger of fatal misjudgement in hypothermia after immersion. Anaesthesia 32:889–892
7. Haldane JS (1922) In respiration. York University Press, New Haven

7.4
Treatment Protocols: Intensive Care Department

WALTER HASIBEDER, VOLKER WENZEL and ANTONY SIMCOCK

Drowning is a frequent, preventable accident with a significant morbidity and mortality in a mostly healthy population. Prompt resuscitation and aggressive respiratory and cardiovascular treatment are crucial for optimal survival. In most patients the primary injury is pulmonary, resulting in severe arterial hypoxaemia and secondary damage to other organs. Damage to the central nervous system is most critical in terms of survival and subsequent quality of life. Immediate reversal of hypoxia, aggressive treatment of hypothermia and cardiovascular failure are the cornerstones of correct medical treatment. Accurate neurologic prognosis cannot be predicted from initial clinical presentation and laboratory, radiological or electrophysiological examinations. Therefore, aggressive initial therapeutic efforts are indicated in most drowning victims.

Epidemiological data [1–17] demonstrate a large variety in patient characteristics and concomitant clinical problems in patients who are admitted to the emergency room and ICU. In spite of this variety, the pathophysiological problem is basically the same. In most patients the primary injury is pulmonary due to fluid aspiration, resulting in severe arterial hypoxaemia and secondary damage to other organs. Immediate reversal of tissue hypoxia is the mainstay of emergency and hospital therapy.

7.4.1
Emergency Treatment

Hypoxia is the major cause of death in non-fatal patients. Therefore, the primary goal of treatment is to restore adequate oxygen delivery to tissues. Immediate rescue from the water is of utmost importance. After successful resuscitation, continuing heat loss must be prevented by adequate insulation against the environment [18]. Co-existing trauma to the cervical spine has to be anticipated in approximately 0.5% of submersion victims and is commonly associated with other clinical signs of severe injury [19]. A simple protocol for the initial treatment is shown in ◘ Fig. 7.1.

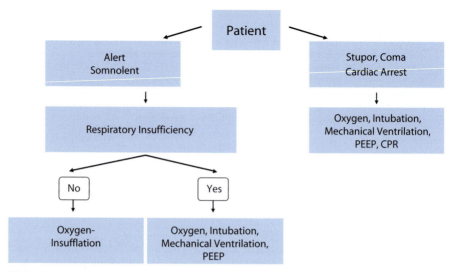

■ **Fig. 7.1.** Simple protocol for the initial treatment of drowning victims in the intensive care unit

Alert patients without clinical signs of pulmonary insufficiency should receive supplemental oxygen by mask or a nasal catheter. In these patients pulmonary function should be observed in a hospital for further 8 hours. A recent study reported that patients with a Glasgow Coma Scale ≥13, normal chest X-ray, lack of clinical signs of respiratory distress and normal room air oxygen saturation can be safely discharged home 8 hours after emergency room presentation [20]. Patients presenting awake or somnolent but with clinical signs of respiratory distress receive oxygen at high inspiratory concentrations. In the emergency situation this can only be accomplished by a tight fitting mask combined with reservoir bag and an oxygen source. In non-comatose patients with progressive deterioration of respiratory function, emergency intubation with cricoid pressure and muscle relaxation has to be performed and mechanical ventilation with positive end-expiratory pressure (PEEP) and 100% oxygen has to be initiated without delay. Ventilation with PEEP of 8–12 mm H_2O may be expected to prevent or attenuate the development of atelectasis after fluid aspiration and therefore significantly improve arterial oxygenation. A nasogastric tube will decompress a full stomach. After decompression of the stomach, the ventilation in these patients often becomes more effective.

All comatose patients need immediate tracheal intubation and mechanical ventilation with PEEP and 100% oxygen. Asystole and ventricular fibrillation warrant aggressive cardiopulmonary resuscitation as the prognosis still is not hopeless. Numerous case reports have been published demonstrating that especially submersion in cold water is compatible with long-term survival, even when the period of submersion is relatively long [21–23]. Unfortunately cardiopulmonary resuscitation is still under-utilised for victims of submersion accidents [24]. In a recent investigation on prognosis of unwitnessed out-of-hospital cardiac arrest drowning appeared to be an independent factor related to survival [25]. These findings strongly suggest that aggressive resuscitative measures, including reversal of hypoxia and cardiovascular stabilisation, should be instituted urgently in drowning victims regardless of clinical presentation.

Patients of submersion accidents usually are hypovolaemic and need adequate volume resuscitation. In adults, rapid infusion of 1500 cc crystalloid can be performed without delay.

There is no systematic evidence to support the usefulness of prophylactic antibiotics or steroid therapy in the emergency setting in order to decrease or attenuate the incidence and severity of ARDS or infectious complications.

7.4.2
Hypothermia

Victims of drowning accidents will present with varying degrees of hypothermia. In haemodynamically stable patients rewarming should be performed using warmed humidified inspiratory gases, warmed intravenous fluids, heating blankets or forced air surface rewarming. With these methods body temperature may be increased by approximately 1–2°C per hour [18, 26]. When the patient is haemodynamically unstable, more aggressive rewarming strategies have proven successful including bladder irrigation, gastric or pleural lavage, peritoneal dialysis using warmed fluids, or extracorporal rewarming using haemofiltration [4, 18]. In severely hypothermic patients with cardiocirculatory arrest rewarming on cardiopulmonary bypass (CPB) is the method of choice [18, 27]. CPB immediately restores tissue perfusion regardless of myocardial performance. Body temperature can be increased most effectively at a rate of approximately 10°C per hour. Additional ultrafiltration can treat severe pulmonary oedema. CPB has been performed as partial bypass from the femoral artery to the femoral vein or as full bypass using the median sternotomy access to the heart [18, 28, 29]. The latter procedure allows higher blood flow rates, successful decompression of a cold and dilated ventricle, and access to the myocardium for defibrillation and massage. However, if the body temperature is above 33°C and stable cardiovascular function cannot be achieved, resuscitation efforts should be terminated.

7.4.3
Pulmonary Problems

Recent studies suggest that the clinical course of ARDS may be significantly influenced by the mode of mechanical ventilation [30–32]. Application of PEEP to patients with ARDS results in improved arterial oxygenation. This has been attributed to recruitment of previously atelectatic alveoli, reopening of peripheral airways in units with trapped gas and reduction of regional inequality of intrinsic PEEP [33–35]. Artificial ventilation with PEEP above the lower inflection point of the compliance curve of the respiratory system and selection of tidal volumes preventing overexpansion of lung areas probably attenuate the pulmonary inflammatory response and systemic inflammatory response after injury [36, 37]. This "lung protective strategy" of mechanical ventilation may also reduce secondary infection of the respiratory system [38].

Lung failure resistant to mechanical ventilation after drowning has been successfully treated with extracorporal membrane oxygenation, intrapulmonary application of surfactant and inhalation therapy with nitric oxide and prostacyclin derivatives in single patients [39–42].

7.4.4
Circulation Problems

Correct management of cardiovascular failure after severe submersion accidents requires invasive haemodynamic monitoring. In some patients a pulmonary artery catheter or PiCCO-system is used [43]. Patients commonly present volume depleted and with a transient myocardial dysfunction. Rapid restoration of normovolaemia and pharmacological treatment of persistent hypotension and myocardial failure in order to restore adequate oxygen supply to tissues are of utmost importance to reduce secondary organ damage. There is no evidence demonstrating that complex cerebral salvage techniques, such as induction of barbiturate coma, mild to moderate hypothermia, intracerebral pressure monitoring, the use of corticosteroids and osmotic diuretics will significantly impact neurological outcome [44–46]. Neurologic prognosis cannot definitively be predicted from initial evaluations. Therefore, prompt resuscitation and aggressive respiratory and cardiovascular treatment are crucial for optimal survival.

References

1. Fields AI (1992) Near drowning in the paediatric population. Critical Care Clin 8:113–129
2. Olshaker JS (1992) Near drowning. Environ Emerg 10:339–350
3. Hasibeder W, Schobersberger W (2001) Near drowning. In: Søreide E, Grande CM (eds) Prehospital trauma care. Marcel Dekker, New York, Basel, pp 603–614
4. Golden FC, Tipton MJ, Scott RC (1997) Immersion, near-drowning and drowning. Br J Anaesth 79:214–225
5. Sibert JR, Lyons RA, Smith BA, et al. (2002) Preventing deaths by drowning in children in the United Kingdom: have we made progress in 10 years? Population based incidence study. Brit Med J 324:1070–1071
6. Brenner RA, Smith GS, Overbeck MD (1994) Divergent trends in childhood drowning rates, 1971 through 1988. JAMA 271:1606–1608
7. Mitic W, Greschner J (2002) Alcohol's role in the deaths of BC children and youth. Can J Public Health 93:173–175
8. Rimsza ME, Schackner RA, Bowen KA, Marshall W (2002) Can child deaths be prevented? The Arizona Child Fatality Review Program experience. Pediatrics 110:e11
9. Crume TL, Diguiseppi C, Beyers T, et al. (2002) Underascertainment of child maltreatment fatalities by death certificates, 1990–1998. Pedriatics 110:e18
10. McGraw EP, Pless JE, Pennington DJ, White SJ (2002) Postmortem radiography after unexpected death in neonates, infants, and children: should imaging be routine? Am J Röntgenol 178:1517–1521

11. Kemp AM, Sibert JR (1993) Epilepsy in children and the risk of drowning. Arch Dis Child 68:684–685
12. Ackerman MJ, Tester DJ, Porter CJ (1999) Swimming, a gene-specific arrhythmogenic trigger for inherited long QT syndrome. Mayo Clin Proc 11:1088–1094
13. Yoshinaga M, Kamimura J, Fukushige T, et al. (1999) Face immersion in cold water induces prolongation of the QT interval and T-wave changes in children with nonfamilial long QT syndrome. Am J Cardiol 83:1494–1497
14. Ishmael HA, Begleiter ML, Butler MG (2002) Drowning as a cause of death in Angelman syndrome. Am J Ment Retard 107:69–70
15. Shavelle RM, Strauss DJ, Pickett J (2001) Causes of death in autism. J Autism Dev Disord 6:569–576
16. Nguyen S, Kuschel C, Teele R (2002) Water birth – a near-drowning experience. Pedriatics 110:411–413
17. Spira A (1999) Diving and marine medicine review part II: diving diseases. J Travel Med 6:180–198
18. Giesbrecht GG (2000) Cold stress, near drowning and accidental hypothermia: a review. Aviat Space Environ Med 71:733–752
19. Watson RS, Cummings P, Quan L, et al. (2001) Cervical spine injuries among submersion victims. J Trauma 51:658–662
20. Causey AL, Tilelli JA, Swanson ME (2000) Predicting discharge in uncomplicated near-drowning. Am J Emerg Med 18:9–11
21. Edwards ND, Timmins AC, Randalls B, et al. (1990) Survival in adults after cardiac arrest due to drowning. Int Care Med 16:336–337
22. Lopez-Pison J, Pineda-Ortiz I, Oteiza C, et al. (1999) Survival with no sequelae after near-drowning with very poor signs for prognosis including persistent bilateral non-reactive mydriasis. Rev Neurol 28:388–390
23. Perk L, Borger van de Burg F, Berendsen HH, van't Wout JW (2002) Full recovery after 45 min accidental submersion. Intensive Care Med 28:524
24. Wyatt JP, Tomlinson GS, Busuttil A (1999) Resuscitation of drowning victims in south-east Scotland. Resuscitation 41:101–104
25. Kuisma M, Jaara K (1997) Unwitnessed out-of-hospital cardiac arrest:Is resuscitation worthwhile ? Ann Emerg Med 30:69–75
26. Kornberger E, Schwarz B, Lindner KH, Mair P (1999) Forced air surface rewarming in patients with severe accidental hypothermia. Resuscitation 41:105–111
27. Vretenar DF, Urschel JD, Parrott JC, Unruh HW (1994) Cardiopulmonary bypass resuscitation for accidental hypothermia. Ann Thorac Surg 58:895–898
28. Gilbert M, Busund R, Skagseth A, et al. (2000) Resuscitation from accidental hypothermia of 13.7°C with circulatory arrest. Lancet 355:375–376
29. Wollenek G, Honarwar N, Golej J, Marx M (2002) Cold water submersion and cardiac arrest in treatment of severe hypothemia with cardiopulmonary bypass. Resuscitation 52:255–263
30. Amato M, Barbas C, Bigelow DB, et al. (1998) Effect of a protective-ventilation strategy on mortality in acute respiratory distress syndrome. N Engl J Med 338:347–354
31. The ARDS Network (2000) Ventilation with lower tidal volumes as compared with traditional tidal volumes for acute lung injury and the acute respiratory distress syndrome. N Engl J Med 18:1301–1308
32. Gillette MA, Hess DR (2001) Ventilator-induced lung injury and the evolution of lung-protective strategies in acute respiratory distress syndrome. Respir Care 46:826–828
33. Falke KJ, Pontoppidan H, Kumar A, et al. (1972) Ventilation with end-expiratory pressure in acute lung disease. J Clin Invest 51:2315–2323
34. Ranieri VM, Eissa NT, Corbeil C, et al. (1991) Effects of positive end-expiratory pressure on alveolar recruitment and gas exchange in patients with the adult respiratory distress syndrome. Am Rev Respir Dis 145:355–360
35. Koutsoukou A, Bekos B, Sotiropoulou Ch, et al. (2002) Effects of positive end-expiratory pressure on gas exchange and expiratory flow limitation in adult respiratory distress syndrome. Crit Care Med 30:1941–1949

36. Ranieri VM, Suter PM, Tortorella C, et al. (1999) Effects of mechanical ventilation on inflammatory mediators in patients with acute respiratory distress syndrome: a randomized controlled trial. JAMA 282:54–61
37. Stuber F, Wrigge H, Schroeder S, et al. (2002) Kinetic and reversibility of mechanical ventilation-associated pulmonary and systemic inflammatory response in patients with acute lung injury. Intensive Care Med 28:834–841
38. Meduri GU, Kanangat S, Stefan J, et al. (1999) Cytokines IL-1beta, IL-6, and TNF-alpha enhance in vitro growth of bacteria. Am J Respir Crit Care Med 160:961–967
39. Staudinger T, Bankier A, Strohmaier W, et al. (1997) Exogenous surfactant therapy in a patient with adult respiratory distress syndrome after near drowning. Resuscitation 35:179–182
40. Moller JC, Schaible TF, Reiss I, et al. (1995) Treatment of severe non-neonatal ARDS in children with surfactant and nitric oxide in a "pre-ECMO"-situation. Int J Artif Organs 18:598–602
41. Thalmann M, Rampitsch E, Haberfellner N, et al. (2001) Resuscitation in near drowning with extracorporal membrane oxygenation. Ann Thorac Surg 72:607–608
42. Lowson SM (2002) Inhaled alternatives to nitric oxide. Anesthesiology 96:1504–1513
43. Della Rocca G, Costa MG, Pompei L, et al. (2002) Continuous and intermitted cardiac output measurements: pulmonary artery versus aortic transpulmonary technique. Br J Anesth 88:350–356
44. Gonzales-Rothi RJ (1987) Near drowning: consensus and controversies in pulmonary and cerebral resuscitation. Heart Lung 16:474–482
45. Bohn DJ, Biggar WD, Smith CR, et al. (1986) Influence of hypothermia, barbiturate therapy, and intracranial pressure monitoring on morbidity and mortality after near-drowning. Crit Care Med 14:529–534
46. Sarnaik AP, Preston G, Lieh-Lai M, Eisenbrey AB (1985) Intracranial pressure and cerebral perfusion pressure in near drowning. Crit Care Med 13:224–227

7.5
Paediatric Considerations

HANS VAN VUGHT, NIGEL TURNER, KOOS JANSEN and SJEF VAN GESTEL

Submersions are frequently encountered events in the paediatric age group. Therefore, all first-line medical personnel and all hospital staff must be familiar with the basic principles of treating children after a submersion incident. This chapter presents an overview of the problems to be anticipated following such an accident. For details the reader is referred to the specific literature mentioned in the text and the reference list.

7.5.1
Epidemiology

The incidence of drowning in the Netherlands is 0.8 per 100.000 inhabitants. One third of all drowning victims are under 15 years old, the majority being under 5 years old. Between 1 and 4 years of age 10% of death is caused by drowning, as compared with 0.1% for the whole Dutch population [1]. The number of paediatric hospital admissions following immersion injury is many times higher. Hence, fatal drowning and non-fatal drowning are typical paediatric topics. Prevention is a major issue in all discussions of submersion accidents: fencing public pools and ponds, professional supervision in swimming pools and swimming instruction for children as young as 4 years old (see also ▶ **Sect. 3**).

7.5.2
Pathophysiology

The most important factors in the pathogenesis of submersion accidents are asphyxia and hypothermia, with primary or secondary aspiration as an additional factor.

Submersion is immediately followed by reflex apnoea. Subsequent asphyxia with combined hypoxia, hypercapnia and acidosis provokes breathing movements. Aspiration of small amounts of fluid elicits laryngospasm. If laryngospasm relaxes before breathing movements have ceased, aspiration of fluid will occur. In general only small amounts of water are aspirated and sometimes no water at all. Attempts to remove this water are futile. There are no clinically relevant differences between submersion in salt- or in freshwater [2]. However, submersion in water contaminated with petrol products as in harbours or after boating accidents, may result in very severe ARDS [3]. Asphyxia is the first step in a process which eventually leads to ARDS, infection and neurological damage. Following submersion hypothermia generally develops during and after asphyxia. This situation differs from those in which hypothermia precedes asphyxia or ischaemia.

7.5.3
Hypothermia

Hypothermia may contribute to morbidity and mortality by inducing cardiorespiratory depression, coagulation disorders and by increasing susceptibility to infections [4]. On the other hand hypothermia is said to protect submersion victims against hypoxic-ischaemic injury by decreasing the metabolic demands of the tissues. However, this is only true if hypothermia leads to a decrease in metabolic demand to the same degree as the decrease in oxygen supply. Although children cool faster than adults following submersion the protective effect of hypothermia is often disappointing. In temperate climates hypothermia correlates with longer submersion times and consequently goes along with a bad neurological prognosis [5, 6].

The diving reflex is a vagally mediated apnoea, bradycardia and redistribution of blood to the brain triggered by cold in the trigeminal region. Observations in animals and isolated paediatric cases have suggested a protective effect for this reflex in children. However, its practical contribution is questionable.

The afterdrop during rewarming, the continued drop in core temperature while the outer surface rewarms, is mainly a physical phenomenon, only marginally influenced by physiological factors.

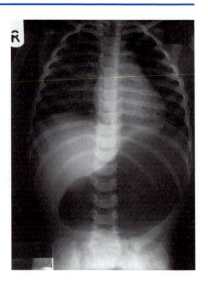

◘ **Fig. 7.2.** Gastric overdistension due to swallowing of water or inflating during emergency treatment of a paediatric drowning victim

7.5.4
Emergency Treatment

Standard ABC stabilisation according to the Advanced Paediatric Life Support (APLS) guidelines remains the mainstay of the emergency treatment [7]. A high degree of suspicion for additional pathological conditions (cervical spine lesions, intoxication, pre-existing diseases) is necessary [8, 9]. Establishing a patent airway at the site may be impeded by laryngospasm. Gastric overdistension due to swallowing of water or inflating during CPR may lead to vomiting and aspiration of gastric contents (◘ **Fig. 7.2**).

A central temperature below 28°C can induce ventricular fibrillation, which may be refractory to defibrillation until the temperature has been raised. It remains controversial whether mild hypothermia (32–35°C) should be treated or not, and if so how it should be treated and how fast the central temperature should be allowed to rise. The general rule to rewarm not faster than 1°C per hour may be overcautious; however, the limiting factor is often haemodynamic instability during rewarming. Therefore, close haemodynamic monitoring, including continuous central venous and arterial pressure monitoring, is mandatory. Children cool down faster than adults, but they can also be rewarmed more quickly. In the presence of circulation children can most easily, and thus best, be rewarmed with external means such as overhead heating devices and warm blankets. The use of peritoneal dialysis, gastric lavage or bladder lavage to rewarm a child remains controversial [10]. Hyperthermia, which is probably the result of a systemic inflammatory response (SIRS), may follow even mild hypothermia and must be anticipated. During cardiac arrest children, like adults, are difficult to rewarm. Cardiopulmonary bypass (CPB) is a highly efficacious tool for rewarming and has the advantage of restoring circulation and oxygenation virtually instantaneously [11]. However, CPB is only available in a limited number of specialised centres and even there it takes time to establish. No comparative studies have demonstrated a superior outcome of rewarming with CPB compared with external heating in children. Currently, institution of advanced life support measures as soon as possible takes priority over distant transfer of an unstable child to a CPB facility. In any case, resuscitation in children should be continued until death is unequivocally ascertained at a central temperature of at least 32°C.

7.5.5
Respiratory Complications

Respiratory complications in submersion victims are typical secondary events and may be due to aspiration of water during submersion, aspiration of gastric contents after rescue or due to ARDS caused by hypoxaemia or hypercapnia induced activation of inflammatory mediators in the blood and the lung. Characteristic for submersion victims is the development of respiratory distress in the first 6 hours after submersion, even in a child who has initially apparently recovered from the submersion injury. Chest X-ray abnormalities appear somewhat later than the clinical signs of respiratory distress.

Treatment is supportive and intubation and mechanical ventilation should be considered early. As in adults, the ventilatory strategy in a child with ARDS is a low-stretch lung protective strategy with adequate levels of PEEP (to improve oxygenation and to prevent shear stress) and low tidal volumes, 5–8 ml/kg, to prevent barotrauma and volutrauma. Permissive hypercapnia is not appropriate in submersion victims. If ventilatory goals (SaO_2 100% with F_iO_2 <0.6 and normocapnia) are not met with conventional mechanical ventilation, high-frequency oscillatory ventilation (HFOV) is indicated. Treatment of ARDS in paediatric submersion victims is usually uncomplicated with a good outcome in most cases.

7.5.6
Infectious Complications

Infectious complications in submersion victims with ARDS are frequent and often difficult to diagnose. Mild ARDS and a systemic inflammatory response may mimic infection. Up till now there is no evidence that prophylactic antibiotic therapy prevents these complications. Therefore, antibiotic therapy should be instituted early but only when signs of infection emerge. The choice of antibiotics should preferably be based on cultures from the suspected infected sites, predominantly the airways [12, 13]. As in other patients in the paediatric ICU, submersion victims are sensitive to nosocomial infections. Leucopenia, which can occur in association with developing ARDS, carries an increased risk of common commensal micro-organisms becoming invasive leading to bacteraemia and sepsis.

7.5.7
Neurological Complications

Neurological damage remains the main threat to complete recovery after non-fatal drowning. The damage is the result of asphyxia and subsequent circulatory failure (see ▶ **Section 8**). Cerebral oedema appears to be the result of post-hypoxic cerebral damage rather than its cause. Strategies for preventing or treating cerebral oedema have not been shown to improve outcome [14, 15].

7.5.8
Prognosis

Outcome after an initially successful resuscitation of a submersion victim is an almost exclusively neurological issue. Indicators for a poor outcome are prolonged submersion time, circulatory arrest on arrival in the emergency room, persistent coma, arterial blood pH less than 7.0 despite adequate resuscitation and a rectal temperature less than 33°C on arrival in the emergency room. There are several scoring systems for quantifying the severity of submersion injury [16]. Although these are indispensable for comparative multi-centre intervention studies, most of these systems have not been validated properly. As with all scoring systems they will not help to establish the individual prognosis in a particular patient. For the moment the ultimate prognosis and the decision to continue or forgo further treatment, must be based on the clinical course and neurophysiological observations.

7.5.9
Concluding Remarks

Instant restoration of ventilation and circulation are the mainstays for the successful treatment of submersion victims. Resuscitation efforts may only be finished if death has unequivocally been ascertained at a core temperature of at least 32°C, or when it is evident from the submersion time of more than 1 hour that further efforts are futile. Further treatment of submersion victims requires skilled and experienced paediatric intensive care and children must be transferred as soon as possible to a paediatric ICU with full facilities. Conscious submersion victims must be kept under close medical supervision during the first 8 hours for signs of respiratory distress.

References

1. CBS (2002) Statistics Netherlands. Visited at: www.CBS.nl. 1-6-2002. Electronic Citation
2. Orlowski JP, Szpilman D (2001) Drowning. Rescue, resuscitation, and reanimation. Pediatr Clin North Am 48:627–646

3. Segev D, Szold O, Fireman E, et al. (1999) Kerosene-induced severe acute respiratory failure in near drowning: reports on four cases and review of the literature. Crit Care Med 27:1437–1440
4. Bernardo LM, Henker R, O'Connor J (2000) Treatment of trauma-associated hypothermia in children: evidence-based practice. Am J Crit Care 9:227–234
5. Suominen P, Baillie C, Korpela R, et al. (2002) Impact of age, submersion time and water temperature on outcome in near-drowning. Resuscitation 52:247–254
6. Veenhuizen L, Haasnoot K, van Vught AJ, et al. (1994) [Submersion in children; the role of hypothermia and development of adult respiratory distress syndrome]. Ned Tijdschr Geneeskd 138:906–910
7. Advanced Life Support Group (2001) Advanced paediatric life support, the practical approach, 3rd edn. BMJ Books, London
8. Watson RS, Cummings P, Quan L, et al. (2001) Cervical spine injuries among submersion victims. J Trauma 51:658–662
9. Ackerman MJ, Tester DJ, Porter CJ (1999) Swimming, a gene-specific arrhythmogenic trigger for inherited long QT syndrome. Mayo Clin Proc 74:1099–1094
10. Bernardo LM, Gardner MJ, Lucke J, Ford H (2001) The effects of core and peripheral warming methods on temperature and physiologic variables in injured children. Pediatr Emerg Care 17:138–142
11. Wollenek G, Honarwar N, Golej J, Marx M (2002) Cold water submersion and cardiac arrest in treatment of severe hypothermia with cardiopulmonary bypass. Resuscitation 52:255–263
12. Ender PT, Dolan MJ (1997) Pneumonia associated with near-drowning. Clin Infect Dis 25:896–907
13. Berkel M van, Bierens JJ, Lie RL, et al. (1996) Pulmonary oedema, pneumonia and mortality in submersion victims; a retrospective study in 125 patients. Intensive Care Med 22:101–107
14. Biggart MJ, Bohn DJ (1990) Effect of hypothermia and cardiac arrest on outcome of near-drowning accidents in children. J Pediatr 117:179–183
15. Bohn DJ, Biggar WD, Smith CR, et al. (1986) Influence of hypothermia, barbiturate therapy, and intracranial pressure monitoring on morbidity and mortality after near-drowning. Crit Care Med 14:529–534
16. Graf WD, Cummings P, Quan L, Brutocao D (1995) Predicting outcome in pediatric submersion victims. Ann Emerg Med 26:312–319

7.6
Aspiration

JEROME MODELL

The drowning process begins when the entrance of the respiratory track has been immersed or submersed under water. Initially, a victim may struggle to remove himself from the aqueous environment. However, during the time that he is submerged he will first voluntarily hold his breath to avoid aspirating water. This usually is followed by a period of involuntary laryngospasm during which time substantial respiratory movement may occur but aspiration does not take place. Once the degree of hypoxia is sufficient so that the victim loses consciousness and no longer has his protective reflexes intact, the laryngospasm will abate, and the victim will actively breathe water into his lungs. During the period of breath-holding and laryngospasm, it is not uncommon for victims to swallow significant quantities of water as well. The aspiration of water, obviously, compounds the degree of hypoxaemia, and this then is followed by circulatory arrest.

A recent publication suggests that drowning to the point of death may not actually occur without evidence of aspiration in the lungs and in that situation, other causes of death should be considered as well [1]. In persons who are rescued from the drowning process, if rescue takes place before active breathing of water occurs, then it is possible for them to have experienced drowning without aspiration. It frequently is very difficult to tell at the scene of the accident whether victims have aspirated water or not, particularly when the quantity is small. One study relied upon the arterial oxygen tension upon admission to the hospital as a presumptive indicator of whether aspiration occurred. In that study, the authors assumed that if the arterial oxygen tension while breathing room air was at least 80 mm Hg, that either no aspiration occurred or the quantity was insignificant. In this situation they found that 12% of their patients fit into the category of non-aspiration [2].

In any event, what prevents aspiration while submerged? First of all, breath-holding and airway obstruction such as occurs in laryngospasm will prevent water from entering the trachea. For water to be aspirated and dispersed throughout the lungs, active respiration must be present [3]. In other words, if the victim were dead when placed in the water or if sudden death and immediate cessation of circulation occurred from another cause, then active respiratory effort would not be present and water would not be aspirated. It is possible for one who has had an acute circulatory arrest to take a few gasps as cell death is occurring. However, these breaths are few in number and not very effective in movement of air to the alveolar level of the lung.

An intrapulmonary shunt and hypoxaemia is produced if water is aspirated. Because seawater is hypertonic, it will pull fluid from the circulation, thereby, expanding the amount of liquid in those alveoli that are affected, resulting in fluid-filled but perfused alveoli [4]. Freshwater, being hypotonic, is absorbed very rapidly from the alveoli into the circulation. However, it alters the surface tension characteristics of pulmonary surfactant, thereby, causing instability of the alveoli and collapse [5]. In addition, if sufficient quantities are absorbed into the circulation, transient hypervolaemia occurs, resulting in pulmonary oedema [6].

The treatment of water aspiration is intensive pulmonary support. Key to this is positive pressure ventilation to expand the alveoli and some method of continuous positive airway pressure to maintain expansion [7]. A variety of ventilatory techniques are now available to accomplish this. Also, increasing the percentage of oxygen breathed will be helpful. It should be pointed out that an effective circulating blood volume of adequate proportion must be maintained to preserve the cardiac output so that the improvement in oxygenation of the blood that occurs in the lungs will be reflected in the tissues [8]. To increase the arterial oxygen tension but to decrease the oxygen delivery to the tissues is not of benefit.

It is known that drowning victims frequently regurgitate stomach contents either as part of the drowning process or during the resuscitation attempts. The factors leading to regurgitation are distension of the stomach with water secondary to swallowing movements of the victim, distension of the stomach with air, particularly when the rescuer is not able to maintain an effective patent airway, and cerebral hypoxia. If the aspiration of stomach contents occurs, this leads to aspiration pneumonitis. The pathophysiology of aspiration pneumonitis has been described as obstruction with foreign material, a chemical burn and secondary infection. It is uncommon to have a foreign body of sufficient size to produce blockage of the airway. The aspirate is more than likely partially digested food or liquid in nature. It is doubtful that a chemical burn of the lung will occur in a drowning victim who regurgitates and aspirates stomach contents because the water swallowed during the drowning process will dilute the pH of the acid in the stomach and a pH of less then 2.5 is thought to be necessary to produce a chemical burn of the lung [9]. Whether secondary infection occurs will depend upon the degree to which the water was contaminated and the efficiency of the body in combating that situation. Aspiration of the regurgitated liquid will increase intrapulmonary shunting and hypoxia.

At one time, treatment of victims recovering from drowning with prophylactic antibiotics and corticosteroids was recommended [10]. Corticosteroids have been shown experimentally to decrease the inflammatory response that may occur with aspiration of acidic foodstuff [11]. However, they also interfere with the normal healing process and in those experiments when animals were studied long term, there was evidence of granulomata in their lungs due to the breakdown of the normal response of the body to infection [11]. Likewise, animal studies that used prophylactic corticosteroids as treatment of freshwater aspiration did not show any improvement in parameters measured over those animals that did not receive corticosteroids [12]. As far as prophylactic antibiotics are concerned, reports in humans have not demonstrated a beneficial effect in regard to the percent of drowning survivors with and without prophylactic antibiotic therapy [2]. Obviously, if signs of infection are present or if the water that was aspirated is grossly contaminated, then treatment with antibiotics specific for those organisms is indicated.

In summary, if one has died in the water and evidence of having aspirated water is not present at autopsy, causes of death other than drowning should strongly be considered [1]. It is doubtful that one would die in a state of laryngospasm prior to its abating and respiratory movement taking place. In persons who are rescued from the drowning process, it appears that approximately 12% of them, at least from one study, may have been rescued before aspiration occurred [2]. If water or stomach contents have been aspirated, intensive pulmonary support, which includes methods of increasing functional residual capacity, decreasing intrapulmonary shunting and maintaining effective circulating blood volume, must be implemented. Utilising these types of techniques has resulted in an excellent normal survival rate in multiple reported series [2, 13, 14]. If the period of time from submersion to rescue and effective CPR is prolonged, it is far more likely that permanent cerebral damage will occur and results will be far less rewarding.

References

1. Modell JH, Bellefleur M, Davis JH (1999) Drowning without aspiration: is this an appropriate diagnosis? J Forensic Sci 44:1119–1123
2. Modell JH, Graves SA, Ketover A (1976) Clinical course of 91 consecutive near-drowning victims. Chest 70:231–238
3. Cot C (1931) Les asphyxies accidentecelles (submersion, electrocution, intoxication oxycarbonique) etude clinique, therapeutique et preventive. Editions medicales N. Maloine, Paris
4. Modell JH, Moya F, Newby EJ, et al. (1967) The effects of fluid volume in sea water drowning. Ann Intern Med 67:68–80
5. Giammona ST, Modell JH (1967) Drowning by total immersion: effects on pulmonary surfactant of distilled water, isotonic saline and sea water. Am J Dis Child 114:612–616
6. Modell JH (1971) The pathophysiology and treatment of drowning and near-drowning, Chap. IV and V. Charles C Thomas, Springfield, Illinois, pp 26–40
7. Bergquist RE, Vogelhut MM, Modell JH, et al. (1980) Comparison of ventilatory patterns in the treatment of freshwater near-drowning in dogs. Anesthesiology 52:142–148
8. Tabeling BB, Modell JH (1983) Fluid administration increases oxygen delivery during continuous positive pressure ventilation after freshwater near-drowning. Crit Care Med 11:693–696
9. James CF, Modell JH, Gibbs CP, et al. (1984) Pulmonary aspiration: effects of volume and pH in the rat. Anesth Analg 63:665–668
10. Modell JH, Davis JH, Giammona ST, et al. (1968) Blood gas and electrolyte changes in human near-drowning victims. JAMA 203:337–343
11. Wynne JW, Modell JH (1977) Respiratory aspiration of stomach contents. Ann Intern Med 87:466–474
12. Calderwood HW, Modell JH, Ruiz BC (1975) The ineffectiveness of steroid therapy for treatment of fresh water near-drowning. Anesthesiology 43:642–650
13. Conn AW, Montes JE, Barker GA, Edmonds JF (1980) Cerebral salvage in near-drowning following neurological classification by triage. Can Anaesth Soc J 27:201–210
14. Modell JH, Graves, SA, Kuck EJ (1980) Near-drowning: correlation of level of consciousness and survival. Can Anaesth Soc J 27:211–215

7.7
Management of ARDS

Davide Chiumello, E. Carlesso and Luciano Gattinoni

By June 2002, only 49 papers dealing with ARDS in drowning have appeared in the literature and most of them are anecdotal. Moreover, to our knowledge no study has been performed specifically on mechanically ventilated drowning patients. Consequently, our discussion will be based on the pathophysiological characteristics of ARDS in drowning which may dictate a physiological approach for mechanical ventilation.

7.7.1
Incidence

In a series of 91 consecutive drowning patients, 53% presented with severe hypoxaemia (defined as the ratio of arterial oxygenation and oxygen fraction below 300 mm Hg) and 36% of them received mechanical ventilation [8]. ARDS may develop in up to 40% of drowning patients and is mainly due to a direct toxic effect of freshwater on lung epithelium [12]. Although the degree of hypoxaemia 24 and 48 hours after the onset of ARDS is predictive of outcome, the development of secondary complications (sepsis, acute myocardial infarction, multiple organ failure) can further worsen this outcome [2].

7.7.2
Pathophysiology

Every drowning patient is characterised by arterial hypoxaemia. However, both the pathophysiology and the severity of arterial hypoxaemia depend on the stage of drowning. Three stages of drowning have been recognised [5]. In stage 1 (in less than 10% of patients) there is no water aspiration but only a severe laryngospasm which blocks the passage of air and lung ventilation. Consequently the inspiratory effort, creating a negative alveolar pressure may cause pulmonary oedema. Recently, however, this interpretation has been challenged [10]. In stage 2 and 3, in which there is water aspiration (fresh- or seawater), there is an alteration of the pulmonary surfactant, damage to the alveolar-capillary endothelium and alveolar flooding. The combination of these factors favour the increase in lung mass, the formation of lung compressive atelectasis, decrease in lung compliance, with an increase of pulmonary shunt and dead space. Lung damage may be worsened if the aspirate is contaminated by gastric content or water contaminants. In this case lung infection may develop.

The classical physiopathological view of early ARDS after drowning strictly resembles the ARDS lung lavage model which is characterised by a great potential for lung recruitment while in the late stage of ARDS there is a low potential for lung recruitment.

7.7.3
Computed Tomography Imaging

At computed tomography in stage 1, the pulmonary oedema is characterised by Kerley lines, peribronchial cuffing and patchy perihilar alveolar areas of airspace consolidation [4]. At stages 2 and 3 the lung CT scan shows a non specific image from tiny, ill-defined lesions to large lobar airspace consolidation [4].

7.7.4
Artificial Mechanical Support

The aim of mechanical ventilation is to support an adequate gas exchange while the patient recovers. Since mechanical ventilation per se may be harmful and may further damage the lung, the key principle is to select the less harmful form of mechanical ventilation in any given patient.

7.7.5
Non-invasive Positive Pressure Ventilation

The primary goal in every drowning victim is to ensure an adequate oxygen delivery. The level of arterial hypoxaemia should be evaluated by performing an arterial blood gas analysis during breathing pure oxygen through a non-rebreathing facial mask.

If the PaO_2/F_iO_2 ratio is lower than 200 mm Hg or the respiratory rate is higher than 24 beats per minute with severe dyspnea and use of accessory muscles, non-invasive positive pressure ventilation (NPPV) should be started. However, NPPV can be applied only in conscious patients, with good airway reflexes and in whom gas exchange impairment is mild [7]. NPPV is defined as any form of ventilatory support delivered without the use of an endotracheal tube. CPAP is the most common and easy way to deliver NPPV. CPAP, by ensuring a continuous positive pressure during the whole respiratory cycle, is able to increase the functional residual capacity and to counteract the effects of pulmonary oedema and consequently improve arterial oxygenation. During CPAP the PEEP level should be increased to reach at least an arterial saturation above 90% with the lowest possible level of the inspired oxygen fraction. If the patients remain severely dyspneic or if there is an increase in arterial carbon dioxide, volume-cycled or pressure support ventilation should be started. Compared to CPAP, volume-cycled or pressure support ventilation are more able to reduce the work of breathing to ameliorate alveolar ventilation and assure a set tidal volume or a set inspiratory ventilation. Using volume-cycled or pressure support ventilation an expired tidal volume between 6 and 9 ml per kg should be reached.

7.7.6
Invasive Mechanical Ventilation

When NPPV fails to correct gas exchange within the first hours, invasive mechanical ventilation should be started [7]. Invasive mechanical ventilation should be promptly applied in comatose patients or in case of severe gas exchange impairment. At the beginning of invasive mechanical ventilation adequate levels of sedation with or without paralysis are necessary to rest the patient, to ameliorate patient synchrony or when the patient is treated in the prone position. Because sedation and paralysis may impair neurologic evaluation, these measures should be limited to patients in whom it is strictly necessary.

In the early phase of ARDS, when using invasive mechanical ventilation, the following five objectives should be applied: recruit the lung, keep the lung open, select the right PEEP level, ventilate with a non-injurious tidal volume and consider using the prone position.

Recruit the Lung

As previously stated the ARDS lung in drowning is in part similar to the ARDS lung in the lavage model with a great potential for recruitment. Consequently, we should try to reopen the atelectatic lung regions. Different types of recruitment manoeuvres have been proposed such as the application of CPAP at 40 cmH_2O for 40 seconds, or the use of intermittent big breaths or pressure controlled ventilation set to reach 40–45 cmH_2O [6]. However, independent of the proposed recruitment manoeuvres, in order to obtain maximal lung recruitment, an adequate transpulmonary pressure (TP) must be applied to overcome the critical opening pressure. In supine position the transpulmonary pressure required may be high, up to 30–35 cmH_2O. The TP depends on the airway pressure applied and the lung and chest wall elastance: $TP=Paw*[E_L/(E_L+E_W)]$, in which Paw is the airway pressure, EL is the lung elastance and EW is the chest wall elastance. For the same amount of Paw the resulting TP will be higher if the EL is increased or lower if the EL is reduced. Because ARDS patients may present huge differences in lung and chest wall elastance it is not possible to predict the resulting TP. Although it is cumbersome and time-consuming we suggest calculating the lung and chest wall elastance.

Keep the Lung Open

After recruitment of the lung an adequate level of PEEP must be applied to oppose the critical closing pressure. Because the critical closing pressures are lower in the not-dependent regions and higher in the dependent regions, the PEEP to maintain open dependent regions may simultaneously overdistend the not-dependent regions. PEEP could also translocate oedema fluid from airways and alveoli to the interstitial perivascular space.

Select the Right PEEP Level

The optimal PEEP is defined as: "the level of PEEP required to minimise the intrapulmonary shunt with minimal negative effects on cardiac output" [3]. The most common method to select PEEP is the gas exchange trial. Different PEEP levels from 5 to 15 cmH_2O are randomly applied and gas exchange is measured. Both changes in oxygenation (PaO_2) and in carbon dioxide ($PaCO_2$) are evaluated. An increase in oxygenation likely reflects the amount of aerated tissue present at end expiration, or on the other hand, the amount of collapsed non-aerated tissue which has been maintained open at end expiration. We usually consider as a positive response to the gas exchange trial an improvement in oxygenation of at least 10–15 mm Hg (whatever inspired oxygen fraction is used). On the other hand, we have to consider the changes in $PaCO_2$. Our hypothesis is that when $PaCO_2$ decreases during the PEEP test this likely means prevalent alveolar recruitment, whereas no change in $PaCO_2$ indicates a balance between recruitment and overdistension, and finally even small increases in $PaCO_2$ likely indicate prevalent overdistension compared to the amount of recruitment. Thus we believe that when a gas exchange trial is performed both oxygenation and carbon dioxide changes have to be taken into account to optimise the selection of PEEP.

Similarly during the PEEP trial the arterial to end tidal carbon dioxide gradient should be evaluated. In the presence of maximal lung recruitment and no change in cardiac output this gradient is minimal, in the presence of alveolar overdistension this gradient increases [11]. However, PEEP by increasing the airway pressure could reduce venous return and cardiac output, although mean blood pressure may remain within normal values if the systemic vascular resistance increases. Consequently PEEP could increase arterial oxygenation due to a shunt reduction whilst at the same time the oxygen delivery could be decreased. In order to better understand the real PEEP effects we suggest in every PEEP trial to evaluate all haemodynamic parameters by a pulmonary artery catheter or by transesophageal echocardiography. If not available, a venous sample from a central venous catheter placed in the superior vena cava could roughly give an idea of the overall effect.

Ventilate with a Non-injurious Tidal Volume

At the present time there is convincing evidence that ARDS patients should be ventilated with moderate to low levels of tidal volume. As stated above, the really dangerous force is the transpulmonary pressure that depends in part on airway pressure. However, the effect of tidal volume (V_T) on the airway pressure depends on the elastance of the respiratory system.

Since $Paw=ETOT*V_T$, it is not possible for every ARDS patient to assess what the safe tidal volume is. A safe solution could be to maintain the plateau airway pressure below $30-40$ cmH_2O or better to measure the transpulmonary pressure and maintain it below $25-30$ cmH_2O [1].

Use the Prone Position

Although the use of the prone position was not specifically evaluated in drowning patients, this manoeuvre should always be considered. The prone position may induce lung recruitment, reduce the harmful effects of mechanical ventilation and ameliorate gas exchange. The prone position should be used with caution in drowning patients with increased intracranial pressure, because the prone position could further increase intracranial pressure by impairing venous return.

7.7.7
Adjuvant Therapy

Different methods such as surfactant replacement, high frequency ventilation or nitric oxide can be applied in these patients [9], although the definitive role of these therapies is still unclear.

As soon as the patient reaches a relative stability the physician should stop the use of paralysis, decrease the level of sedation and begin to wean the patient from mechanical ventilation.

Water aspiration can also cause severe bronchospasms with an increase in airway resistance, which can induce air trapping, barotrauma and haemodynamic impairment. In the presence of bronchospasms, bronchodilator therapy is beneficial. However, an increase of airway resistance can also be due to the aspiration of particulate matter which may obstruct the smaller bronchi and bronchioles. In such situations a fiberoptic bronchoscopy should be performed.

7.7.8
Late ARDS Stage

During the late ARDS stage the potential for recruitment is very low as the lung structure has been remodelled due to the presence of lung infection. In this case the above rules for mechanical ventilation should be applied, keeping in mind the possible contraindications of permissive hypercapnia in patients with elevated intracranial pressure.

7.7.9
Conclusions

ARDS in non-fatal drowning may develop in up to 40% of patients and part of these victims may need invasive mechanical ventilation. The final outcome depends on the level of arterial hypoxaemia and secondary complications. Although the outcome in these patients is better compared to ARDS of other aetiologies, mechanical ventilation with as few harmful effects as possible should be aimed for.

References

1. Artigas A, Bernard GR, Carlet J, et al. (1988) The American European Consensus conference on ARDS, Part 2. Intensive Care Med 24:378–398
2. Bernard G, Artigas A, Brigham KL, et al. (1994) Report of the American European consensus conference on ARDS: definitions, mechanism, relevant outcomes and clinical trial coordination. Intensive Care Med 20:225–232
3. Downs JB, Klein EF, Modell JH (1973) The effect of incremental PEEP on PaO_2 in patients with respiratory failure. Anesth Analg 52:210–214

4. Gluecker T, Capasso P, Schnyder P, et al. (1999) Clinical and radiologic features of pulmonary edema. RadioGraphics 19:1507–1531
5. Golden FS, Tipton MJ, Scott RC (1997) Immersion, near drowning and drowning. Br J Anaesth 79:214–225
6. Kacmarek RM (2002) Strategies to optimize alveolar recruitment. Curr Opin Crit Care 7:15–21
7. Mehta S, Hill NS (2001) Noninvasive ventilation. Am J Respir Crit Care Med 163:540–577
8. Modell JH, Graves SA, Ketover A (1975) Clinical course of 91 consecutive near drowning victims. Chest 70:231–238
9. Modell JH (1993) Drowning. New Engl J Med 328:253–256
10. Modell JH, Bellefleur M, Davis JH (1999) Drowning without aspiration: is this an appropriate diagnosis? J Forensic Sci 44:1119–1123
11. Murray IP, Modell JH, Gallagher TJ, Banner MJ (1984) Titration of PEEP by the arterial minus end tidal carbon dioxide gradient. Chest 85:100–104
12. Oakes DD, Sherck JP, Maloney JR (1982) Prognosis and management of victims of near drowning. J Trauma 22:544–564

7.8
Risk Factors and Treatment of Pneumonia

GIEL VAN BERKEL

Survivors of drowning present with features related to three aspects of submersion: asphyxia, hypothermia and aspiration. The relative contributions of each depends on the specifics of the incident, such as temperature of the water, length of submersion, seawater or freshwater, and the specifics of the individual, such as age and previous health status. Submersion is immediately followed by reflex apnoea. Subsequent asphyxia (the combination of hypoxia, hypercapnia and acidosis) provokes breathing movements, which results in aspiration. In general only small amounts of water are aspirated and attempts to remove the water are useless.

Initial treatment consists of emergency resuscitation based on standard Airway, Breathing, Circulation principles, patient re-warming, and assessment of additional associated injuries, such as intoxication and cervical spine injuries. Thereafter, hospital treatment focuses on the management of respiratory complications.

Respiratory complications in submersion victims are typically secondary events and may be due to the effects of asphyxia, due to the aspiration of water during submersion, or to the aspiration of gastric contents after rescue. Many non-fatal drowning patients will develop acute respiratory distress syndrome (ARDS) caused by activation of inflammatory mediators in blood and lung due to hypoxaemia and hypercapnia. Aspirated water alters the surface tension of the natural surfactant, making the alveoli unstable and promoting collapse and atelectasis, thus resembling the experimental model of bronchoalveolar lavage-induced lung injury.

Characteristically, ARDS will develop some 4–8 hours after submersion in an initially apparently recovered individual. Treatment of ARDS is by intubation and mechanical ventilation. Administration of continuous positive pressure ventilation and high FiO_2 are the most efficient way to reverse hypoxaemia.

Several experimental techniques, including recruitment manoeuvres, nitric oxide inhalation and the intratracheal administration of surfactant or perfluorochemicals, may be beneficial. Prone positioning of the patients with ARDS may also be of benefit. Further studies are needed in all these fields.

Diagnosis of pneumonia in these patients can be difficult as it is often superimposed on ARDS. The diagnosis of pneumonia can be based on four criteria. A new and persistent pulmonary infiltrate must be visible on the chest X-ray. Signs and symptoms of infection have to be present (fever, leucocytosis, purulence of sputum, pathogenic micro-organisms from sputum culture). The problem with these signs is that they are not specific. Protected brush specimens or bronchoalveolar lavage for microbiological culture can also be helpful for the diagnosis. Also the concomitant finding of positive cultures of pleural fluid or blood are considered as a diagnostic parameter.

The common denominator of pneumonia associated with drowning is hypoxaemia and ischaemic organ damage. Severe and prolonged hypoxaemia can cause lung damage through the activation of inflammatory mediators. In addition most drowning victims aspirate some of the water they are in. This water can contain particulate matter and both human and animal infectious material. Especially in the comatose victims and in those who need resuscitation there is a great risk of aspiration of gastric contents as well. The risk of vomiting and aspiration of gastric contents is increased because drowning victims often swallow significant amounts of water. Also the circumstances which led to drowning are important factors which influence the risk of pneumonia such as seizures, thoracic trauma and drug overdose. Finally, when mechanical ventilation is needed, there is a prolonged risk of aspirating oropharyngeal contents and developing nosocomial pneumonia.

It seems common sense that the type of water you submerge in makes a difference. The risk seems lower for submersion in a bath tub with clean water than in a flamingo pond, as one of our patients did. In the Netherlands, river deltas consist of wide, shallow sluggish rivers, and also brooks, lakes and coastal waters which are heavily polluted and harbour lots of aquatic birds, who add to the pollution by their excreta. The situation may be somewhat better in public swimming pools, lakes or on beaches.

The incidence of pneumonia might be quite different between patient populations from countries where most drowning incidents occur in clean ocean water or countries where most drownings occur in private swimming pools. One study diagnosed 15 cases of pneumonia in 125 victims (◘ Table 7.7) [1].

Some of these bacteria are obviously exogenous, for example the *Aeromonas* species, others are most likely endogenous such as *Streptococcus pneumoniae* and *Haemophilus influenzae*.

In other studies and case reports the occurrence of pneumonia by less common micro-organisms are mentioned (◘ Table 7.8) [2].

Burkholderia pseudomallei is reported from the Philippines and South Vietnam. *Chromobacterium violaceum* occurs in tropical and subtropical areas, including Florida. Fungi typically cause systemic infection. *Pseudoallescheria boydii* is known for brain abscesses, meningitis and pulmonary infection and is difficult to treat.

◼ **Table 7.7.** Bacteriology (results of cultures in 15 submersion victims with pneumonia)
[1]

	Sputum	Blood	Pleural fluid
Escherichia coli	7	1	2
Aeromonas spp.	4	1	1
Klebsiella spp.	3	1	1
Pseudomonas spp.	4	1	1
Haemophilus influenzae	3		
Staphylococcus aureus	3		1
Streptococcus pneumoniae	1		
Branhamella spp.	1		
Candida spp.	1		
Bacteroides spp.	1		
Streptococcus spp.	1	1	1
Clostridium spp.			1
Peptostreptococcus			1
Propionibacterium spp.			1

◼ **Table 7.8.** Less common micro-organisms that have complicated treatment of drowning patients [2]

Aerobic gram-negative
Burkholderia pseudomallei
Chromobacterium violaceum
Francisella philoniragia
Legionella species
Fungi
Aspergillus species
Pseudoallescheria boydii

Early onset pneumonia can be due to aspiration of polluted water, can be a complication of aspirations of gastric contents, and can be caused be endogenous flora such as *Streptococcus pneumoniae* in a submersion victim with chronic obstructive pulmonary disease. All patients with severe ARDS in whom prolonged mechanical ventilation is necessary are at risk for ordinary nosocomial pneumonia. However, in the differential diagnosis fungal and anaerobic infections should be considered.

In a series of 125 submersion victims there was a 17 times greater risk for pneumonia in patients who needed mechanical ventilation. Of patients requiring mechanical ventilation 52% developed pneumonia in contrast to 3% in patients not requiring mechanical ventilation. This finding underscores that severe lung damage due to aspiration of sufficient quantities of water and gastric contents is necessary for the development of pneumonia. In the study, pneumonia was not related to water type, body temperature at admission, neurological state at rescue or at admission, use of corticosteroids or the prophylactic use of antibiotics.

Most experts agree that pneumonia in submersion victims should be treated with a broad spectrum beta-lactam penicillin or cephalosporin with or without the addition of an aminoglycoside. Specific choices will depend on local experience.

There are no studies favouring the prophylactic use of antibiotics. No reduction in the incidence or the mortality of pneumonia has been proven. When pneumonia develops in patients on prophylactic antibiotics, it will probably be due to selected resistant bacteria.

However, those who advocate selective decontamination will start antibiotics in these patients on admission. The recognition and treatment of fungal and other exotic organisms requires a high index of suspicion and a high standard of clinical skills. Corticosteroids or not of any use.

References

1. Berkel M van, Bierens JJLM, Lie RL, et al. (1996) Pulmonary oedema, pneumonia and mortality in submersion victims; a retrospective study in 125 patients. Intensive Care Med 22:101–107
2. Ender PT, Dolan MJ (1997) Pneumonia associated with drowning. Clin Infect Dis 25:896–907

7.9
Surfactant Therapy

Jack Haitsma and Burt Lachmann

Fluid aspiration during submersion impairs normal lung function [1]. Aspiration of both freshwater (hypotonic) and seawater (hypertonic) impairs the pulmonary surfactant system by increasing the surface tension at the air-liquid interface [1]. The rise in surface tension will result in end-expiratory collapse, atelectasis, increase in right-to-left shunt and a decrease in PaO_2, leading finally to acute respiratory failure (ARF). ARF is characterised by increased capillary permeability, often associated with damage to the alveolar epithelium, leading to high permeability oedema. The capillary leakage combined with damage to the alveolar epithelium leads to an immediate, or moderately slow, loss of active surfactant by inactivation due to plasma components (mainly fibrinogen and fibrin monomers) or depletion from the alveoli and the small airways. In principle, the loss of active surfactant will be compensated by release of stored surfactant from type II cells. When the balance between compensation or production and loss or inactivation of surfactant favours the latter, the surface tension will rise. Because submersion patients lack active surfactant at the alveolar level, it would be logical to replenish the surfactant at the alveolar level by giving exogenous surfactant or, if not available, to compensate the high retractive forces by sufficient PEEP levels.

7.9.1
Exogenous Surfactant Therapy: Lessons from Animal Models

The use of different animal models has led to increased understanding of delivery techniques, timing of administration and type of exogenous surfactant to be used.

Bolus administration is the most frequently used method of instillation with its ability to rapidly deliver large quantities of surfactant that are necessary to overcome the inhibitory effects of serum proteins present in the alveoli. Because of the presence of strong surfactant inhibitors in the alveoli, the dosage of exogenous surfactant needs to be sufficiently high, up to 800 mg/kg bodyweight. Approximately 1 mg of surfactant is needed to overcome the inhibitory effect of 1 mg plasma proteins [2]. In ARF there is an accumulation of proteins in the lungs over time, again resulting in the need for higher doses [3]. Another important aspect of optimal surfactant therapy is the time elapsed between initial damage and start of the therapy. Respiratory failure can be prevented with exogenous surfactant given before deterioration of lung function (this is within 10 min after acid aspiration), whereas after development of respiratory failure exogenous surfactant only prevents further decline of lung function but does not restore gas exchange [3]. When treatment starts in a later stage of lung injury the amount of inhibitory proteins that have accumulated in the lung require larger amounts of surfactant, or several consecutive administrations, to improve lung function.

Various surfactant preparations are available on the market and are being used in the treatment of RDS in neonates. Studies performed in animal models under standardised conditions showed marked differences in efficacy in improving lung function between the various preparations [4]. Natural surfactants containing the hydrophobic proteins SP-B and SP-C, which are able to withstand to a certain extent the inactivation by plasma proteins, are more effective in improving lung function than artificial surfactants [4].

7.9.2
First Clinical Results

Although less than 1% of adult ARF patients develop ARF due to submersion [5], the risk to develop ARF after drowning is much greater. Because there have been only a couple of case reports on surfactant treatment in submerged ARF patients [6, 7], data available from surfactant treatment in ARF patients in general have to be translated to this patient population.

In 1987, Lachmann treated a 4-year-old patient suffering from ARF and bacterial pneumonia with exogenous surfactant. The successful treatment has shown the great potential of surfactant as the lifesaver for ARF patients [8]. Since 1987 there have been about 25 case reports of exogenous surfactant therapy in ARF patients [9]. The results of the first multi-patient studies have been published. Walmrath, studying 27 patients with established severe ARF and sepsis, showed that bronchoscopic application of a natural surfactant (300 mg/kg) resulted in an immediate, impressive, and highly significant improvement of arterial oxygenation in all patients, due to a marked reduction of shunt flow. In seven patients a second dose of 200 mg per kilogram was required. A total of 15 patients survived the 28-day observation period. The mortality rate was 44.4%, compared to a calculated risk of death for the given APACHE II scores of $74.0\pm3.5\%$. All causes of death were of non-respiratory origin [10, 11].

Gregory studied four different dosing strategies in 48 adults with ARF and showed that maximum improvement in oxygenation, minimum ventilatory requirements, and the lowest mortality rate were obtained by using four doses of 100 mg/kg of a natural surfactant (total amount of 400 mg/kg) [12]. The instillation of up to 2200 ml surfactant suspension over a 48-hour period was generally well tolerated.

In a phase II study of aerosolised artificial surfactant, Weg observed no differences in any physiological parameters between the treatment groups, but there was a dose-dependent trend in reduction of mortality from 47% in the combined placebo group to 41% and 35% in the groups treated with 12 hours and 24 hours of surfactant per day, respectively [13]. Anzueto demonstrated that administration of aerosolised artificial surfactant had no effect on mortality and lung function in a multicenter, randomised placebo-controlled trial in 725 patients with sepsis-induced ARF [14]. The authors speculated that one of the reasons for the lack of response could be that less than 5 mg surfactant per kg body weight was actually delivered into the lungs due to the method of administration. This is only one-sixteenth of the dosage used by Gregory et al. [12].

Recently, Kesecioglu used a natural porcine surfactant in patients with acute lung injury (ALI) or ARF in a prospective, randomised, multi-centre phase II study. Patients were randomised to receive standard therapy plus surfactant (mortality 9%) or only standard therapy (mortality 43%). He also demonstrated a significant reduction in 28-day mortality [15].

Two case reports of patients with drowning in which exogenous surfactant was administered confirmed the benefits from these multi-patient studies [6, 7]. Suzuki administered natural surfactant in a 3-year-old drowning victim, in which surfactant administration lead to a significant improvement of arterial oxygenation (141 mm Hg up to 294 mm Hg) and a concomitant reduction in peak inspiratory pressures (51 cmH$_2$O to 36 cmH$_2$O) [7]. The child was successfully weaned from the ventilator over the next days without any further complications [7]. Staudinger applied natural surfactant in a 24-year-old female drowning victim who did not respond to conventional ventilation, prone positioning and inhaled nitric oxide [6]. After repeated surfactant administration (total dose 300 mg per kg; 18,000 mg surfactant) PaO$_2$ rose from 43 mm Hg to 362 mm Hg and allowed conventional ventilation again [6]. Unfortunately this patient developed septic shock and died, but this was not related to a pulmonary origin [6].

7.9.3
Conclusion and Future Considerations

In drowning patients with ARF, increased alveolocapillary permeability is known to inactivate the functional alveolar surfactant, resulting in the failure of the lung as a gas exchange organ. The value of surfactant therapy is that the functional impairment of active surfactant can be reversed by the instillation of an excess of exogenous surfactant. Data from animal studies and preliminary clinical studies increase the insight into how to optimise exogenous surfactant therapy. Furthermore, the role of surfactant in controlling pulmonary infections [16], emphasises the potential of surfactant therapy in patients who submerge in contaminated water.

The first randomised clinical trials with surfactant are currently taking place. However, before surfactant becomes a routine therapy, these clinical trials have to confirm all the benefits expected from exogenous surfactant instillation.

References

1. Modell JH (1993) Drowning. N Engl J Med 328:253–256
2. Lachmann B, Eijking EP, So KL, Gommers D (1994) In vivo evaluation of the inhibitory capacity of human plasma on exogenous surfactant function. Intensive Care Med 20:6–11
3. Eijking EP, Gommers D, So KL, et al. (1993) Prevention of respiratory failure after hydrochloric acid aspiration by intratracheal surfactant instillation in rats. Anesth Analg 76:472–477
4. Gommers D (1998) Comparison of eight different surfactant preparations on improvement of blood gases in lung-lavaged rats. Appl Cardiopulm Pathophysiol 7:95–102
5. Luhr OR, Antonson K, Karlsson M, et al. (1999) Incidence and mortality after acute respiratory failure and acute respiratory distress syndrome in Sweden, Denmark, and Iceland. The ARF Study Group. Am J Respir Crit Care Med 159:1849–1861
6. Staudinger T, Bankier A, Strohmaier W, et al. (1997) Exogenous surfactant therapy in a patient with adult respiratory distress syndrome after near drowning. Resuscitation 35:179–182
7. Suzuki H, Ohta T, Iwata K, Sato T (1996) Surfactant therapy for respiratory failure due to near-drowning. Eur J Pediatr 155:383–384
8. Lachmann B (1987) The role of pulmonary surfactant in the pathogenesis and therapy of ARDS. In: Vincent JL (ed.) Update in intensive care and emergency medicine. Springer, Berlin Heidelberg, pp 123–134

9. Gommers D, Lachmann B (1993) Surfactant therapy: does it have a role in adults? Clin Intensive Care 4:284–295
10. Walmrath D, Gunther A, Ghofrani HA, et al. (1996) Bronchoscopic surfactant administration in patients with severe adult respiratory distress syndrome and sepsis. Am J Respir Crit Care Med 154:57–62
11. Walmrath D, Grimminger F, Pappert D, et al. (2002) Bronchoscopic administration of bovine natural surfactant in ARDS and septic shock: impact on gas exchange and haemodynamics. Eur Respir J 19:805–810
12. Gregory TJ, Steinberg KP, Spragg R, et al. (1997) Bovine surfactant therapy for patients with acute respiratory distress syndrome. Am J Respir Crit Care Med 155:1309–1315
13. Weg JG, Balk RA, Tharratt RS, et al. (1994) Safety and potential efficacy of an aerosolized surfactant in human sepsis-induced adult respiratory distress syndrome. JAMA 272:1433–1438
14. Anzueto A, Baughman RP, Guntupalli KK, et al. (1996) Aerosolized Surfactant in adults with sepsis-induced acute respiratory distress syndrome. N Engl J Med 334:1417–1421
15. Kesecioglu J (2002) Treatment of acute lung injury (ALI/ARDS) with surfactant. Am J Respir Crit Care Med 163:A819
16. Haitsma JJ, Lachmann U, Lachmann B (2001) Exogenous surfactant as a drug delivery agent. Adv Drug Deliv Rev 47:197–207

7.10
Cardiovascular Changes

JEROME MODELL, TOMASSO PELLIS and MAX HARRY WEIL

The studies of Swann in the 1940s and 1950s called attention to the cardiovascular effects of the drowning process [1]. These experiments subjected awake dogs to total submersion until death and resulted in the conclusion that seawater victims died a respiratory death, secondary to pulmonary oedema, but freshwater victims died a cardiac death, secondary to ventricular fibrillation. Subsequent studies revealed that only approximately 15% of human victims who died in the water [2] and, virtually, none of those who were rescued, revived and admitted to hospital [3], aspirated sufficient quantities of water to produce the severe serum electrolyte changes seen in Swann's dogs. Swann assumed that it was hyponatraemia that provoked ventricular fibrillation in conjunction with profound hypoxia. Yet, ventricular fibrillation has been rarely documented in human victims of drowning.

In the early 1960s, Redding demonstrated fluid shifts following seawater aspiration produced life-threatening hypovolaemia and, prompted early management with intravenous fluids for repletion of intravascular volume [4]. Yet it was only after Modell [5–7] investigated the physiological effects of aspirating variable quantities of water, that it was appreciated that the cardiovascular changes after drowning are extremely variable.

Both experiments in animals and observations in human victims demonstrated a wide variety of arrhythmias after a drowning episode. These included bradycardia, tachycardia, absent P waves, decreased amplitude of the P waves, widening of the PR interval, decreased amplitude of the R wave, widening of the QRS interval, both ST segment elevation and depression, inverted T or peaked T waves, atrioventricular dissociation, atrial fibrillation, premature ventricular contractions and ventricular fibrillation [8]. The aetiology of these arrhythmias together with their haemodynamic effects on arterial pressure, central venous pressure, pulmonary artery pressure, and cardiac output, were all highly variable. The contributory role of hypoxia, hypercarbia, acidosis, increased catecholamine release, increases or decreases in blood volume, increases in serum potassium concentration, decreases in serum sodium concentration, and increases in mean intrathoracic pressure produced by mechanical ventilation together with the possible presence of unrelated diseases provide a complex clinical state.

The aetiology of the hypoxia that occurs in the drowning process is both apnoea and intrapulmonary shunting. When seawater is aspirated, it is hypertonic. Because the alveolar capillary interface acts as a semipermeable membrane, there is movement of fluid from the capillaries into the alveoli displacing alveolar gas. After seawater aspiration, fluid-filled but perfused alveoli explain intrapulmonary shunts [6]. When freshwater is aspirated, hypotonic water is rapidly absorbed into the alveolar capillaries [5]. This produces a two-fold effect. First, it alters the surface tension properties of pulmonary surfactant, accounting for collapsed alveoli [9]. Secondly, the hypervolaemia produced by absorption of water from alveoli is followed by impaired capillary permeability and subsequent fluid flow from the alveolar capillaries into the alveoli, and accounts for permeability pulmonary oedema. Both mechanisms account for intrapulmonary shunting and arterial hypoxia [10]. Arterial hypoxia and decreases in intravascular volume and cardiac output are the major causes of cerebral hypoxia and ischaemic brain injury.

Treatment includes two priorities. The first is ventilatory support, including mechanical ventilation and increase in the inspired oxygen concentration. The goal is to restore more normal functional residual capacity (FRC) and more normal ventilation-perfusion ratios [10]. This usually requires use of positive end expiratory pressure (PEEP) or continuous positive airway pressure (CPAP), which increases the FRC [11]. The second priority is circulatory support to assure adequacy of oxygen delivery to tissues [4, 12]. After significant quantities of seawater are aspirated, hypovolaemia threatens survival. After freshwater aspiration, hypervolaemia is typically transient but secondary pulmonary oedema subsequently decreases the effective circulating blood volume. The use of inotropes and vasopressor agents may transiently augment cardiac output and arterial blood pressure but their ultimate benefit with respect to outcome are unproven. They cannot substitute for adequate oxygenation and fluid replacement to support cardiac output, which should be considered definitive therapy.

It is important that oxygen delivery be optimised. Increases in the arterial oxygen saturation and oxygen tension of blood are of questionable benefit unless the oxygen is delivered to vital tissues [12]. Although monitoring of arterial oxygen tension, carbon dioxide tension, and pH define pulmonary gas exchange and the acid-base status of the victim, these measurements do not necessarily reflect the adequacy of oxygen delivery to the tissues. Mechanical ventilation as presently used increases the airway pressure and therefore the mean intrathoracic pressure. Increases in intrathoracic pressure act to decrease venous return and therefore compromises cardiac output and oxygen delivery.

After significant fluid shifts due to water aspiration, the effective circulating blood volume may be profoundly altered. Although pulmonary management may restore arterial oxygen saturation and tension to normal, oxygen delivery to the tissues is dependent on maintaining adequate threshold levels of cardiac output. Administration of generous volumes of intravenous fluids may be required to sustain cardiac output and forward blood flow, as recognised by Redding [4]. These investigators showed that mechanical ventilation alone fails to resuscitate dogs after seawater drowning, whereas adding fluid replacement was lifesaving. This also applied to experimental animal models of freshwater drowning in which increases in oxygen delivery after fluid repletion was essential in conjunction with mechanical ventilation [12]. Inotropes alone failed to produce a significant increase in oxygen delivery. Oxygen delivery did not increase adequately until intravascular volume was expanded by administration of intravenous fluids [12]. Because precision in fluid repletion is facilitated by monitoring the patient with a pulmonary artery catheter or transesophageal echocardiography, such measurements are recommended in the severely compromised patient.

Many drowning accidents occur in cold water, in which case the body cools quite rapidly. A distinction must be made with respect to the temperature of the water and especially the reflex response to cold water. A 10°C cold stimulus applied to the face, causes bradycardia and peripheral vasoconstriction and is generally identified as the diving reflex. It is characterised by a negative chronotropic effect in which the heart rate is typically reduced by approximately one fifth within 10 seconds [13]. Although stroke volume is increased, peripheral blood flow is reduced quite strikingly [14]. Two temporal autonomic responses follow face immersion in cold water, including an initial parasympathetic response characterised by bradycardia, due to baroreceptor stimulation, and a late efferent peripheral sympathetic response. Similar but less profound responses are observed following immersion of the face in water in which temperature approximates 33°C [14].

The most important haemodynamic effect of cold is on myocardial irritability and conduction. This can also occur during the afterdrop of core temperature after removal of chronic cold stress. Some authors attributed the afterdrop to peripheral vasodilation associated with external rewarming and, therefore, paradoxical central cooling by shunting of stagnant cold blood to the central circulation. In other theories this is a thermophysical phenomenon (▶ Section 9). In any case, when the myocardium is chilled, the vulnerability to ventricular fibrillation (VF) is increased [15–19].

Homogenous cooling of the entire heart causes an increase in T wave duration without a change in polarity [20]. Hypothermia is frequently associated with the appearance of a J wave or Osborne wave, which is a slow upright deflection between the end of the QRS complex and the early portion of the ST segment [21]. When the body temperature is reduced to below 32°C and especially below 30°C, there is widening of the QRS complex, and the J wave appears. When the temperature continues to decrease after the J wave has appeared, there is high likelihood of imminent onset of VF [22]. Unfortunately, the hypothermic heart is relatively unresponsive to both electrical and pharmacological interventions for control of arrhythmias [23, 24].

Under conditions of severe hypothermia, there is a high risk of ventricular arrhythmias and VF during rewarming with fatal outcome [25–28]. There is, as yet, no clear consensus on the optimal rate of rewarming. In some experimental studies, core temperature was allowed to increase at a rate of 7°C per hour or from 23°C to 37°C in 2 hours [29]. Rewarming techniques, however, should recognise that the capability of the heart to deliver adequate amounts of oxygenated blood must be restored before there is an increased temperature of other tissues, with its concurrent increase in metabolic rate and therefore its increased oxygen requirements.

In summary, it is now clear that the cardiovascular changes that follow drowning predominately result from decreases in oxygenation, abnormalities in acid-base balance and decreases in effective circulating blood volume. Although sufficient aspiration to produce severe serum electrolyte changes seldom occurs, aspiration of large volumes of water can significantly effect blood components and especially serum electrolyte concentrations. Mechanical ventilation may compromise the adequacy of the circulating blood volume and therefore prompt fluid repletion. Fluid repletion is indicated for minimising decreases in oxygen delivery to the tissues, especially to the heart and to the brain. Thus, if therapy is aimed at restoring normal respiratory function, adequate circulating blood volume and vascular stability, success may be anticipated, provided the period of cerebral hypoxia was not sufficient to cause permanent neurologic damage. Significant hypothermia complicates the physiologic responses and must be given special consideration when present.

References

1. Swann HG (1956) Mechanism of circulatory failure in fresh and sea water drowning, editorial. Circ Res 4:241–244
2. Modell JH, Davis JH (1969) Electrolyte changes in human drowning victims. Anesthesiology 30:414–420
3. Modell JH, Graves SA, Ketover A (1976) Clinical course of 91 consecutive near-drowning victims. Chest 70:231–238
4. Redding JS, Voigt GC, Safar P (1997) Treatment of sea water aspiration. J Appl Physiol 15:1113–1116
5. Modell JH, Moya F (1966) Effects of volume of aspirated fluid during chlorinated fresh water drowning. Anesthesiology 27:662–672
6. Modell JH, Moya F, Newby EJ, et al. (1967) The effects of fluid volume in seawater drowning. Ann Intern Med 67:68–80
7. Modell JH, Gaub M, Moya F, et al. (1966) Physiologic effects of near-drowning with chlorinated fresh water, distilled water and isotonic saline. Anesthesiology 27:33–41
8. Modell JH (1971) The pathophysiology and treatment of drowning and near-drowning, Chap. VIII. Charles C Thomas, Springfield, Illinois, pp 61–68
9. Giammona ST, Modell JH (1967) Drowning by total immersion. Effects on pulmonary surfactant of distilled water, isotonic saline and sea water. Am J Dis Child 114:612–616
10. Modell JH, Moya F, Williams HD, Weibley TC (1968) Changes in blood gases and A-aDO$_2$ during near-drowning. Anesthesiology 29:456–465
11. Bergquist RE, Vogelhut MM, Modell JH, et al. (1980) Comparison of ventilatory patterns in the treatment of freshwater near-drowning in dogs. Anesthesiology 52:142–148

12. Tabeling BB, Modell JH (1983) Fluid administration increases oxygen delivery during continuous positive pressure ventilation after freshwater near-drowning. Crit Care Med 11:693–696
13. Paulev PE, Pokorski M, Honda Y, et al. (1990) Facial cold receptors and the survival reflex „diving bradycardia" in man. Jpn J Physiol 40:701–712
14. Heath ME, Downey JA (1990) The cold face test (diving reflex) in clinical autonomic assessment: methodological considerations and repeatability of responses. Clin Sci (Lond) 78:139–147
15. Berne RM (1954) Myocardial function in severe hypothermia. Circ Res 2:90–95
16. Mouritzen CV, Andersen MN (1965) Myocardial temperature gradients and ventricular fibrillation during hypothermia. J Thorac Cariovasc Surg 49:937–944
17. Duguid H, Simpson RG, Stowers JM (1961) Accidental hypothermia. Lancet 2:1213–1219
18. Pickering BG, Bristow GK, Craig DB (1977) Core rewarming by peritoneal irrigation in accidental hypothermia with cardiac arrest. Anesth Analg 56:574–577
19. Althaus U, Aerberhard P, Shupbach P, et al. (1982) Management of profound accidental hypothermia with cardiorespiratory arrest. Ann Surg 195:492–495
20. Paparella N, Ouyang F, Fuca G, et al. (2000) Significance of newly acquired negative T waves after interruption of paroxysmal reentrant supraventricular tachycardia with narrow QRS complex. Am J Cardiol 85:261
21. Surawicz B, Knilans TK (eds) (2001) Chou's electrocardiography in clinical practice. WB Saunders, Philadelphia
22. Schwab RH, Lewis DW, Killough JH, Templeton JY (1964) Electrocardiographic changes occurring in rapidly induced deep hypothermia. Am J Med Sci 284:290
23. Towne WD, Geiss WP, Yanes HO, Rahimtoola SH (1972) Intractable ventricular fibrillation associated with profound accidental hypothermia – successful treatment with partial cardiopulmonary bypass. N Engl J Med 287:1135–1136
24. Truscott DG, Firor WB, Clein LJ (1973) Accidental profound hypothermia: successful resuscitation by core rewarming and assisted circulation. Arch Surg 106:216–218
25. Laub GW, Banaszak D, Kupferschmid J, et al. (1989) Percutaneous cardiopulmonary bypass for the treatment of hypothermic circulatory collapse. Ann Thorac Surg 47:608–611
26. Splittgerber FH, Talbert JG, Seezer WP, Wilson RF (1986) Partial cardiopulmonary bypass for core rewarming in profound accidental hypothermia. Am Surg 52:407–412
27. Vretnar DF, Urschel JD, Parrot JCW, Unruh HW (1994) Cardiopulmonary bypass resuscitation for accidental hypothermia. Ann Thorac Surg 58:895–898
28. Wollenek G, Honarwar N, Golej J, Marx M (2000) Cold water submersion and cardiac arrest in treatement of severe hypothermia with cardiopulmonary bypass. Resuscitation 52:255–263
29. Rekand T, Sug IA, Bjaernes L, Jolin A (1991) Neuromonitoring in hypothermia and in hypothermic hypoxia. Arch Med Res 50 (Suppl. 6):32–36

7.11
Classification Systems

Dᴀᴠɪᴅ Sᴢᴘɪʟᴍᴀɴ, Aɴᴛᴏɴʏ Sɪᴍᴄᴏᴄᴋ and Sʜɪʀʟᴇʏ Gʀᴀᴠᴇs

Drowning is a public health problem that affects the population of all nations. Standard definitions for drowning [1, 2] and classification of drowning incidents [3, 4] have evolved in an attempt to develop treatment protocols and analyse data for outcome purposes. One of the earlier classifications was by type of water – seawater or freshwater. Treatment in these early days was frequently aimed first at electrolyte evaluation. While these changes do occur when massive quantities of freshwater are aspirated, those surviving the drowning episode rarely aspirate that amount of water and, therefore, do not develop serum electrolyte changes requiring specific therapy [5, 6]. In later studies it was demonstrated that pathophysiology created by aspiration of either seawater or freshwater is hypoxia secondary to an intrapulmonary shunt [7]. In many of the subsequently developed classification systems for drowning the pulmonary lesion has been emphasised [3, 4]. In addition, classification by the central nervous system changes secondary to lack of cerebral oxygenation and adequate cardiac output has been proposed [8].

In 1979, Simcock [3] reported a classification that resulted from a 5-year study of drowning incidents in Cornwall, UK. Classification of the victims into groups was assigned once they arrived at the hospital. Victims were divided into four groups: Group 1, those with no apparent inhalation; Group 2, those with evidence of inhalation of water but adequate ventilation; Group 3, those with inadequate ventilation; Group 4, those with no ventilation or cardiac output. Emphasis was placed on the importance of immediate care and timely relief of hypoxia. There was little evidence that drowning in freshwater or seawater made a difference to resuscitation or prognosis. Intact survival was excellent in those who did not suffer cardiac arrest. Even those in the cardiac arrest group who were given rapid, aggressive intensive therapy produced encouraging results. Water temperature, however, was important in determining outcome. These studies have continued since 1974. There have been 407 drowning incidents analysed from 1974–2000 [9], and findings are consistent with those reported in 1979 [3]. All survivors in Groups 1, 2, and 3 were cerebrally normal. Those suffering cardiac arrest, Group 4, had a 25% survival rate but 3 of the 14 survivors were neurologically impaired. The use of the above groups has provided a useful framework for immediate and intensive care.

Szpilman [4] has developed a severity of drowning classification with treatment recommendations. This classification is extremely valuable to the pre-hospital attendant. One of the most difficult medical decisions a lifeguard or an emergency medical technician (EMT) must make is how to treat a drowning victim appropriately. It is evident that cardiopulmonary or isolated respiratory arrest indicates that resuscitation should begin immediately. These cases compose approximately 0.5% of all rescues done by lifeguards. The questions that arise in the other 99.5% of cases rescued at the beach are: should the rescuer administer oxygen, call an ambulance, transport the person to a hospital, or observe for a time at the site. Even hospital emergency physicians may be in doubt as to the most appropriate immediate and continued support, as the drowning victims vary in the severity of injury.

Based on these questions, a classification system was developed in Rio de Janeiro (Brazil) in 1972 and updated in 1997 [4] to assist lifeguards, ambulance personnel and doctors. It was based on analysis of 41,279 rescues of which 2304 (5.5%) needed medical attention. It was revalidated in 2001 by a 10-year study with 46,080 rescues [10]. This classification encompasses all the support from the site of the accident to the hospital, recommends treatment and shows the likelihood of death based on the severity of injury. This classification (Table 7.9) allows lifeguards and medical staff to speak the same language.

The classifications of Simcock [3] and Szpilman [4] are aimed at cardiopulmonary evaluation and resuscitation, the primary concern to prevent or decrease the hypoxia common to the drowning victim. Modell and Conn [8] in 1980 developed a classification based on the degree of neurological deficit

■ **Table 7.9.** Severity of drowning classification and treatment [4, 10, 15]

Grade	Mortality (%)	Signs and symptoms (lifeguards' terms)	Treatment (first aid)
Rescue	0%	Alive with normal pulmonary auscultation (No coughing, foam, difficulty breathing, or cardiac arrest)	Evaluate and release from the accident site without further medical care
1	0%	Cough, without foam in mouth or nose	Rest, warm and calm the victim Advanced medical attention or oxygen should not be required
2	0.6%	Rales in some pulmonary fields (Small amount of foam in mouth/nose)	5 Litres/min of oxygen by nasal cannula Warm and calm the victim Recovery position if unconscious Hospitalisation required for 6–48 hours Request chest X-ray and arterial blood gas
3	5.2%	Acute pulmonary oedema without hypotension or shock (Large amount of foam in mouth or nose with palpable radial pulse)	Oxygen 15 litres/min by face mask or tracheal tube at accident site Recovery position if unconscious Hospitalisation required (ICU) for 48–96 hours. 1. Mechanical ventilation with PEEP, F_IO_2 1.0 until arterial blood gas available 2. Sedation as necessary for 48 hours 3. Restore pH to normal 4. Request chest X-ray, arterial blood gas, electrolytes, urea, creatinine, glucose, urinalysis and if any abnormal level of consciousness, axial cranial tomography

Table 7.9. *Cont.*

Grade	Mortality (%)	Signs and symptoms (lifeguards' terms)	Treatment (first aid)
4	19.4%	Acute pulmonary oedema with hypotension/shock (Large amount of foam in mouth or nose, without palpable radial pulse, but carotid pulse present)	Carefully monitor breathing (respiratory arrest can still occur) Follow the treatment for grade 3 and start crystalloid intravenously via peripheral vein (independent of type of water) until restoration of normal blood pressure Inotropic or vasopressor drugs rarely needed
5	44%	Isolated respiratory arrest	Artificial ventilation (mouth-to-mouth) immediately at the scene at 12–20 breath/min, with 15 litres of oxygen if possible, until restoration of normal breathing Then treat as grade 4
6	93%	Cardiopulmonary arrest	Start CPR – monitor ECG and defibrillate if necessary Insert a tracheal tube as early as possible and obtain venous access to give epinephrine each 3 min After CPR follow grade 4
Dead body	100%	Submersion time over 1 hour or obvious physical evidence of death (rigor mortis, putrefaction or dependent lividity)	Do not start resuscitation – follow to the morgue

on arrival at a tertiary referral centre. The drowning victims were classified into three categories, category A (awake), category B (blunted), and category C (comatose). Modell [11] used these categories in a retrospective review of 121 cases of drowning. Those in category A survived with normal brain function, in category B 89% of adults and 92% of children survived normally, in category C 73% of adults survived with normal brain function and 44% of children recovered neurologically intact. Treatment of all these patients was aimed at the cardiopulmonary systems. Conn [12], reported similar results using this classification. The patients in category C in the study by Conn received special therapy aimed at brain preservation. Their normal survival rate was identical to those in the series reported by Modell [11].

There is value in classification systems not only in developing standardised treatment protocols but also in comparing outcomes with different levels of severity of injury. Classifications and studies [13, 14] that are based on geographic site of injury, developmental age of the victim, and other factors are valuable for epidemiological studies that can lead to development of preventive strategies. Classifications are helpful as guides to appropriate therapy and standardised reporting of drowning incidents.

References

1. Christoffel KK, Scheidt PC, Agran PF, et al. (1994) Standard definitions for childhood injury research: excerpts of a conference report. Pediatrics 89:1027–1034
2. Modell JH (1971) Pathophysiology and treatment of drowning and near drowning. Charles C. Thomas, Springfield, IL
3. Simcock AD (1979) Sequelae of near drowning. Practitioner 22:202–206
4. Szpilman D (1997) Near-drowning and drowning classification: A proposal to stratify mortality based on the analysis of 1,831 cases. Chest 112:660–5
5. Modell JH, Gaub M, Moya F, et al. (1966) Physiologic effects of near drowning with chlorinated fresh water, distilled water, and isotonic saline. Anesthesiology 27:33–41
6. Modell JH, Graves SA, Ketover A (1976) Clinical course of 91 consecutive near drowning victims. Chest 70:231–238
7. Modell JH, Moya F, Williams H, Weibley TC (1968) Changes in blood gases and A-aDO$_2$ during near-drowning. Anesthesiology 29:456–465
8. Modell JH, Conn AW (1980) Current neurological considerations in near-drowning, editorial. Can Anaesth Soc J 27:197
9. Simcock AD (2002) The value of a classification system. Book of Abstracts, World Congress on Drowning, Amsterdam 2002, p 65
10. Szpilman D, Elmann J, Cruz-Filho RES (2002) Drowning classification: a revalidation study based on the analysis of 930 cases over 10 years. World Congress on Drowning, Amsterdam 2002, Book of Abstracts, p 66
11. Modell JH, Graves SA, Kuck EJ (1980) Near-drowning: correlation of level of consciousness and survival. Can Anaesth Soc J 27:211–218
12. Conn AW, Montes JE, Barker GA, Edmonds JF (1980) Cerebral salvage in near drowning following neurological classification by triage. Can Anaesth Soc J 27:201–209
13. Sibert JA, Lyons BA, Smith BA, et al. (2002) Classifying drowning deaths in children by developmental stages rather than sites. Book of Abstracts, World Congress on Drowning, Amsterdam 2002, p 64

14. Sibert JA, Lyons BA, Smith BA, et al. (2002) Preventing deaths by drowning in children in the United Kingdom: have we made progress in 10 years? Population based incidence study. Br Med J 324:1070–1071

15. Orlowski JP, Szpilman D (2001) Drowning. Rescue, resuscitation, and reanimation. Pediatr Clin North Am 48:627–646

Brain Resuscitation in the Drowning Victim

TASK FORCE ON BRAIN RESUSCITATION
Section editors: DAVID WARNER and JOHANNES KNAPE

This chapter is dedicated to the memory of Peter Safar, MD. Peter Safar combined genius, incredible purpose, elegance, and humanism to move the collective fields of acute medicine to a new level. His work in resuscitation medicine, critical care, anaesthesiology, emergency medicine, and disaster medicine saved countless lives. As a mentor he taught us a great deal. Peter left us with an important message – in both clinical care and research: namely, to always ask "What is your intervention or research doing for the patient?". Whether physician or scientist, it is a critical message never to forget.

Task Force Chairs

- David Warner
- Johannes Knape

Task Force Members

- Udo Illievich
- Cor Kalkman
- Laurence Katz
- Patrick Kochanek
- Bengt Nellgård
- Peter Safar
- Takefumi Sakabe

8.1
Overview

DAVID WARNER and JOHANNES KNAPE

Although drowning is a common cause of death, little medical research has been specifically devoted to improving management of this disease. All organ systems are affected by an asphyxial insult, but the brain is the most sensitive and its function is most likely to define quality of life following a drowning accident. In the 1950s and 1960s major advances were made in understanding the pathophysiology of drowning, with particular emphasis on the pulmonary system. In parallel, major advances were made in basic methods of cardiopulmonary resuscitation (CPR), most of which remain employed to this day.

From the 1970s to the present, intense investigation has been made into how the brain responds to acute injury. Knowledge gained from stroke, traumatic brain injury (TBI), and circulatory arrest has only begun to show us how complex brain biology becomes when it is deprived of adequate oxygen delivery. Because all forms of brain injury involve the same tissue, it is no surprise that many commonalities of the response of the brain to injury exist, regardless of the nature of the insult. Paralleling this advance has been a cornucopia of pharmacologic and physiologic therapies which have been tested in both laboratory animals and humans. To date, no pharmacologic therapies have been shown to alter outcome in a sufficient magnitude to allow adoption in clinical medicine. The search for such therapies remains intense and it is likely that future pharmacologic therapy for the injured brain will include multiple different drugs, each having a specific mechanism of action known to be important at different stages of recovery from the initial insult.

Fortunately, despite the lack of meaningful pharmacologic intervention, major advance has occurred in our understanding of how physiologic factors affect outcome from acute brain injury. Most prominent are the roles of temperature and glucose. We have solid human data demonstrating a beneficial effect of sustained mild to moderate induced hypothermia on outcome from acute brain injury. We also have overwhelming laboratory and clinical evidence that outcome from acute brain injury is dependent on the glycaemic state. However, none of this work has been specifically validated in either human drowning studies or in laboratory models of drowning. Similarly, there has been little or no study of neuromonitoring techniques or neurochemical markers of anoxic injury in drowning patients for use in either prognostication or guiding treatment.

It is clear that further research is required to improve neuroresuscitation in the drowning victim. However, drowning events are not predictable, presentation is typically to community hospitals as opposed to research centres and there is a lack of an organised constituency to advocate for research resources. It seems unlikely, therefore, that randomised double-blind trials of neuroresuscitative interventions for the drowning patient will occur in the foreseeable future. As a result, current discussion of cerebral resuscitation in the drowning victim borrows heavily from knowledge gained from the study of different forms of brain injury. This is not optimal, particularly because there are unique factors associated with drowning including feasibility of CPR in the water, ingestion or aspiration of fresh, sea and contaminated water with associated electrolyte and osmotic effects, effects of water temperature on body temperature and the fact that drowning asphyxia usually precedes cardiac arrest. Nevertheless, in the absence of direct evidence from studies in the drowning victim, medical care is still required. Because of the similar response of brain to a variety of forms of acute insult, it is likely that meaningful improvement in neuroresuscitation can be made for the drowning patient by adopting knowledge from other domains of neuroresuscitation. This section provides a systematic review of these findings. This review has provided a basis for a consensus statement by the authors with respect to recommendations that can now be applied to the care of drowning victims with central nervous system injury.

8.2
Consensus and Recommendations

David S. Warner and Johannes Knape

The Brain Resuscitation Task Force met at the World Congress on Drowning from June 26–28, 2002. This meeting consisted of a series of plenary sessions, pro-con debates, and open public working sessions devoted to review of all available scholarly and clinical material relevant to resuscitation of the brain in humans suffering a drowning accident. Based on this Congress and extensive review of the literature, the following consensus statement and recommendations were generated and have been approved in full by all authors of this chapter.

Consensus: In the prehospital phase, the first priority is to achieve restoration of spontaneous circulation in the drowning patient. In normothermic dogs, cardiac arrest (no flow) due to asphyxia causes more post-ischaemic encephalopathy than does the same duration of ventricular fibrillation induced no-flow [242].

Consensus: Continuous monitoring of core and/or brain (tympanic) temperature is mandatory in drowning patients in the emergency department and intensive care unit and in the prehospital setting to the extent that it is possible.

Consensus: In hypothermic patients, rewarming to about 32°C can be important to achieve restoration of spontaneous circulation. Temperature should be monitored after restoration of spontaneous circulation. Drowning victims with restoration of adequate spontaneous circulation who remain comatose should not be actively rewarmed to temperature values >32–34°C (see below).

Consensus: Numerous clinical trials have shown that hyperthermia is prevalent in adults and children resuscitated from cardiac arrest [3, 92]. There is extensive evidence from laboratory animal studies and correlative data in human brain injury that hyperthermia (as little as 1°C above normal), even if delayed, exacerbates neurologic damage. Hyperthermia in the drowning-induced asphyxial encephalopathy victim should be prevented at all times in the acute recovery period.

Consensus: Randomised clinical trials that define ideal temperature management in drowning victims are not possible. However, a large body of multi-species laboratory animal evidence and two human trials in adults resuscitated from ventricular fibrillation cardiac arrest convincingly demonstrate a beneficial effect of induced hypothermia (32–34°C) on neurologic outcome [26, 201, 204, 232]. Therefore, the Brain Resuscitation Task Force recommends drowning victims remaining comatose after restoration of spontaneous circulation be treated with deliberate mild hypothermia (32–34°C) initiated as soon as possible and sustained for 12–24 hours. Patients treated with mild hypothermia should be endotracheally intubated and mechanically ventilated. Shivering must be prevented. Hypnotics, analgesics, and neuromuscular blockade may be used as required to maintain hypothermia. Electroencephalographic monitoring is recommended to detect seizures. Vigilance should be maintained for pneumonia. At completion of induced hypothermia, passive rewarming is recommended at a rate no greater than 0.5–1.0°C per hour.

Consensus: There is insufficient evidence to support use of any specific brain oriented neuroresuscitative pharmacologic therapy in drowning victims. Seizures should be appropriately treated.

Consensus: Numerous laboratory animal studies and numerous clinical correlative studies convincingly demonstrate that hyperglycaemia present during arrest worsens outcome from acute brain injury. There are no clinical randomised trials of glucose management in patients after drowning. There is one randomised prospective trial in critically ill patients that demonstrated improved outcome when blood glucose was controlled between 80–110 mg/dl

(4.4–6.1 mM) while carefully avoiding hypoglycaemia [243]. Based on this evidence, blood glucose concentration in the drowning patient should be frequently monitored and normoglycaemic values should be maintained.

Consensus: There is insufficient evidence that routine intracranial pressure (ICP) monitoring and ICP management will alter outcome from drowning induced asphyxial encephalopathy. Increased ICP as a result of cerebral hyperaemia may be a concern if permissive hypercapnia is deemed necessary in patients with acute respiratory distress syndrome.

Consensus: After initial resuscitation is completed, there is insufficient evidence to support either hyperventilation or hypoventilation during intensive care management. Until further evidence to the contrary is provided, maintenance of normocapnia is recommended. There is insufficient evidence to make a recommendation on management of arterial pH. Although there is insufficient evidence to support a specific target PaO_2 or oxygen saturation during and after resuscitation, hypoxaemia should be avoided.

Consensus: Studies in experimental models suggest benefit of hypertension early after cardiac arrest. Similarly, in a large clinical database, hypertension after restoration of spontaneous circulation was associated with a favourable outcome. However, a direct comparison of therapies targeting specific blood pressure levels has not been carried out after drowning-induced cardiac arrest. Hypotension, however, should be avoided.

Consensus: A central registry for drowning victims with asphyxial encephalopathy should be established in conjunction with other task forces at the World Congress on Drowning. Members of the Brain Resuscitation Task Force should be consulted so that key parameters associated with use of induced hypothermia and neurologic outcome can be tracked.

Consensus: There are no investigations of use of neurochemical markers for outcome prediction in drowning patients. In cardiac arrest studies, repeated assessment of S-100B and neuron specific enolase have been shown to have value in predicting neurologic outcome [190, 206]. Although promising, there is insufficient evidence at this time to recommend routine use of these neurochemical markers in guiding management of drowning encephalopathy.

8.2.1
Summary of Consensus

Treatment of the patient with brain injury resulting from cardiopulmonary arrest attributable to drowning must be based on scientific evidence. Due to the absence of interventional outcome studies in human drowning victims, current therapeutic strategies must be extrapolated from studies of humans or animals having similar forms of acute brain injury.

The following recommendations for care of drowning victims who remain unresponsive due to anoxic encephalopathy are made on the basis of best available scientific evidence.

The highest priority is restoration of spontaneous circulation. Subsequent to this, continuous monitoring of core and/or brain (tympanic) temperature is mandatory in the emergency department and intensive care unit and to the extent possible in the prehospital setting. Drowning victims with restoration of adequate spontaneous circulation who remain comatose should not be actively rewarmed to temperature values above 32–34°C. If core temperature exceeds 34°C, hypothermia (32–34°C) should be achieved as soon as possible and sustained for 12–24 hours. Hyperthermia should be prevented at all times in the acute recovery period. There is insufficient evidence to support the use of any neuroresuscitative pharmacologic therapy. Seizures should be appropriately treated. Blood glucose concentration should be frequently monitored and normoglycaemic values maintained. Although there is insufficient evidence to support a specific target $PaCO_2$ or oxygen saturation during and after resuscitation, hypoxaemia should be avoided. Hypotension should also be avoided. Research is needed to evaluate specific efficacy of neuroresuscitative therapies in drowning victims.

8.3
Prehospital and Emergency Department Management of the Drowning Victim

Laurence Katz

8.3.1
Prehospital Management

Recognition of asphyxia from submersion in water is straightforward if the patient is unconscious, apneic, cyanotic or pulseless. However, many patients rescued from the water have a spontaneous pulse, respirations, and a relatively normal mental status. Therefore, unless there are physicians or experienced paramedics with close physician supervision on the scene with advanced diagnostic capabilities, all drowning victims should be treated presumptively for persistent brain hypoxia resulting from submersion asphyxia and transported to hospital for further evaluation and care. Initial therapy should focus on opening the airway and providing mouth-to-mouth ventilation to apneic patients while they are still in the water, if possible. Restoration of ventilation in an apneic patient before cardiac arrest develops can dramatically improve neurological outcome, especially in children [115]. Opening the airway with the backward tilt of the head or jaw thrust manoeuvre is required to provide adequate ventilation [196]. Adjuncts such as a snorkel or a SCUBA regulator may also assist with ventilations in the water [128]. Hyperextension of the neck to open the airway is discouraged because it can exacerbate a cervical injury that may be present in drowning victims who have sustained trauma during a diving accident [215]. Removal of the patient from the water should be the next priority because performance of chest compressions in the water without a floatation device and back support is relatively ineffective [128]. Once the patient is removed from the water, the need for CPR should be determined [107]. Help from emergency medical services should be requested as early as possible upon discovery of a drowning victim. Use of the Heimlich (abdominal thrust) manoeuvre has been discouraged before initiating CPR because it does not convincingly empty water from the lungs and may cause abdominal trauma or aspiration of stomach contents [191]. However, if there is a solid foreign body in the airway that prevents ventilation, the Heimlich manoeuvre may be beneficial.

Drowning patients may aspirate 3–4 ml/kg of water [86]. This volume is usually not sufficient to cause alterations in volume or electrolyte status, regardless of whether the aspiration is fresh or saltwater [147, 148]. In drowning to pulselessness, electrolyte changes can be considerable but do not usually obviate resuscitation. Aspirated fluid can cause ventilation-perfusion mismatches by either surfactant washout or transudation of fluid into the alveoli [146]. Therapy needs to be directed at reducing hypoxaemia from shunting caused by the ventilation-perfusion mismatch. Oxygen needs to be administered as soon as possible. For unconscious patients, the trachea should be intubated and the lungs mechanically ventilated. Positive end expiratory pressure (PEEP) should be utilised if available [193]. The severity of respiratory distress will help guide management of the conscious patient. Conscious patients with severe respiratory distress should be intubated and ventilated with 100% oxygen and PEEP. The patient presenting with an increased respiratory rate, rales on lung examination, or mild hypoxaemia demonstrated by a pulse oximeter reading of less than 93% may benefit from oxygen delivered by a non-rebreathing mask, continuous positive airway pressure ventilation (CPAP) or bi-level positive airway pressure (BiPAP) support delivered by a sealed nasal mask if available [65, 174]. Patients with wheezing may also benefit from a beta-agonist aerosolised therapy such as albuterol [149]. Many patients become volume depleted or may require cardiotonic medications after drowning. Therefore, intravenous access and fluids may be beneficial, especially if ventilation with PEEP is required. En route to the hospital, the patient should be monitored for cardiac arrhythmias, temperature should be obtained, and wet clothing should be removed to protect the rescuer from electrocution during defibrillation attempts if ventricular fibrillation should occur. However, unless the patient is haemodynamically unstable, no efforts at active rewarming should be made because hyperthermia has been consistently associated with worse neurologic outcome after cerebral ischaemia in laboratory animal models [77, 145]. Patients with altered mental status should have blood glucose levels measured and hypoglycaemia or hyperglycaemia treated. Radio communication with the hospital emergency department can be critical for efficient transfer of care in the emergency department, especially if the victim has sustained hypothermic submersion requiring cardiopulmonary bypass (CPB) support.

8.3.2
Emergency Department Management

On arrival at the emergency department, the prehospital care provider should give a concise report of the circumstances surrounding the drowning event, initial patient condition (Glasgow Coma Scale score and vital signs), estimated submersion time, approximate water temperature, resuscitative efforts and response to resuscitative efforts. Treatment of the drowning victim in the emergency department should maintain the same priorities as prehospital, including detecting and treating hypoxia and hypoperfusion and treating blood glucose abnormalities. A pulse oximeter should be connected to the patient and in line capnometry should be used when available in intubated patients to avoid hyperventilation which may decrease perfusion to the brain. Intubated patients should have PEEP adjusted to maximise oxygen delivery while minimising hypotension due to compromised venous return. A tidal volume of 6 ml/kg instead of the standard 12 ml/kg during mechanical ventilation may decrease lung injury and improve outcome [231]. Intubated patients should also have a nasogastric tube and Foley catheter placed for decompression of the stomach and monitoring of urinary output, respectively. A low temperature rectal or bladder thermometer is helpful to detect significant hypothermia and direct therapy. Patients with temperatures below 32°C may need passive or active warming to prevent cardiac arrhythmias or haemodynamic instability [59]. Deep hypothermia (<28°C) with cardiovascular instability or arrest may warrant flow promotion such as CPB or extra corporal membrane oxygenation (ECMO). These interventions have been shown to have a dramatic improvement in outcome in patients with hypothermic submersion (<10°C), even after prolonged periods of cardiac arrest [32, 76, 134, 253]. CPAP or BiPAP may be beneficial in spontaneously breathing patients who present evidence of respiratory insufficiency or hypoxaemia. Arterial blood gases (ABG) can help determine acid-base status and confirm response to respiratory interventions. Sodium bicarbonate may be helpful for the treatment of severe acidosis and cardiovascular instability, although its use during cardiac arrest is less clear [70, 194]. A chest X-ray, electrolytes, blood urea nitrogen, creatinine, glucose, complete blood count, prothrombin time, partial thromboplastin time, alcohol level, toxin screens, cardiac enzymes, electrocardiogram and levels of anti-seizure medications (in patients with history of seizures) are helpful to detect and guide therapy of complications that may arise after drowning. The physical examination should also be directed towards finding occult injuries and a cervical spine X-ray and computed tomography (CT) of the head may be warranted, especially in patients with a history of trauma and head injury or neurological deficits. Finally, patients stabilised in the emergency department of hospitals without critical care services should be considered for transfer to a tertiary care facility [256].

8.3.3
Brain Directed Therapy

Restoration of spontaneous circulation with delivery of oxygenated blood at an adequate perfusion pressure is the foundation of cerebral resuscitation. Beyond this, neuroresuscitative therapies other than management of temperature, blood glucose and seizures have little or no documented value. Steroids and prophylactic antibiotics are not recommended for reduction of brain damage and infection after drowning [46, 164]. HYPER therapy (diuretics, hyperventilation, hypothermia, barbiturates and chemical paralysis) has also been shown to be ineffective in reducing brain damage after drowning [31]. The effects of most of the individual components of HYPER therapy on cerebral outcome have not been adequately evaluated. However, mild hypothermia (32–34°C) has clearly been demonstrated to have benefit in improving outcome from cardiogenic cardiac arrest and is recommended in patients remaining comatose after restoration of spontaneous circulation (see below) [26, 232]. In contrast, hyperthermia occurs frequently in patients with acute brain injury and there is sufficient direct laboratory and circumstantial human evidence to dictate that hyperthermia be corrected [3, 92]. Since hyperglycaemia frequently occurs in association with an hypoxic-ischaemic event and worsens neurological outcome, administration of insulin to normalise blood glucose should be considered [141, 243, 246, 249]. Seizures after drowning can worsen neurological outcome and should be treated aggressively. Institution of these therapies in the emergency department or even in transport may save critical time.

8.3.4
Discharge from the Emergency Department

Patients who arrive in the emergency department and have no symptoms, a normal respiratory rate, peak expiratory flow, chest X-ray and arterial blood gasses should be observed for 6 hours. If the patient remains normal after this interval and has access to good follow-up, he or she can safely be discharged from the emergency department.

8.3.5
Prognosis and Family Counselling

There is currently no accurate method for determining outcome early after resuscitation from drowning. Patients with submersion times greater than 10 min or no return of spontaneous circulation within 25 min of initiating advanced cardiac life support usually have a poor prognosis [178]. However, there have been multiple reports of patients who arrive in the emergency department with non-reactive pupils, no pulse and asystole, yet following resuscitation have good neurological outcomes, especially after hypothermic submersion [119]. The paediatric mortality score (PRIMS), which has been modified for adults, can provide some basis for a discussion with the family about prognosis, but even this extensive physiological assessment can not sufficiently predict outcome and should be used with caution [173]. Patients who sustain an ice water submersion may have a better prognosis, but unfortunately there currently are no methods available for deciding which patients may benefit from heroic measures. Therefore, the decision to proceed with such measures must be based on clinical experience, availability of resources, and the patient's premorbid state.

8.4
Intensive Care Management of the Drowning Victim

Udo Illievich

The main indications for admitting a drowning victim to the intensive care unit are respiratory failure, cardiac arrest or arrhythmias, and coma. In addition, there are patients in whom submersion injury is associated with initially unsuspected conditions (epilepsy, traumatic cervical spine injury, intoxication from alcohol or drugs). An active search for pre-existing diseases or occult traumatic injuries should be made in addition to treatment of the obvious immediate threats of hypoxic-ischaemic encephalopathy, pulmonary injury, hypothermia related complications, disseminated intravascular coagulation, and rhabdomyolysis [80]. Finally, autosomal dominant long QT syndrome (LQTS; Romano Ward syndrome) must be considered in the investigation of children who present with unexplained drowning accidents [37] (▶ Chapter 6.9).

8.4.1
Hypervolaemia or Hypovolaemia

Systemic fluid overload may occur secondary to fluid absorbed through the pulmonary and gastric circulation. The pulmonary volume load varies between patients but usually does not exceed 5 ml/kg. A further problem is that 80%−90% of drowning victims swallow large amounts of water. This leads to gastric distension resulting in an increased risk of vomiting and aspiration during resuscitation.

Paradoxically, drowning victims tend to develop hypovolaemic shock. This is due to hypoxic endothelial cell damage leading to increased capillary permeability that results in loss of proteins with resultant displacement of water into tissues causing intravascular hypovolaemia. Central venous pressure monitoring may be necessary to manage intravascular volume status to optimise cerebral perfusion and reduce pulmonary complications.

8.4.2
Pulmonary Considerations

Aspiration of either fresh or salt water may result in reduced pulmonary compliance and pulmonary oedema. Oedema augments the intrapulmonary shunt and causes difficulty in ventilating and oxygenating the patient. Fresh water is hypotonic and therefore is readily absorbed whereas seawater is hypertonic, drawing water into the alveoli. The result is intrapulmonary shunt due to ventilation-perfusion mismatch. Large amounts of water in the lungs will also wash away surfactant leading to atelectasis. In animal drowning models, use of artificial surfactant did not prove to be of greater benefit than simple mechanical ventilation [8]. However, anecdotal clinical reports have indicated that application of artificial surfactant may be beneficial depending on the application technique [137]. Aspirated water often contains bacteria and foreign objects such as sand, chemicals and oil. Fortunately, unlikely bacteria are to be initially resistant to antibiotics, perhaps facilitating treatment of aspiration pneumonia, although empiric use of antibiotics is not recommended. More problems are to be expected from acute respiratory distress syndrome (ARDS).

Aspiration of water can also increase ICP by causing a neurogenic intrapulmonary shunt. Currently the mechanism of neurogenic pulmonary shunt is not fully understood.

In patients with cerebral oedema requiring mechanical ventilation, high PEEP is problematic because it inhibits cerebral venous outflow. High-frequency low volume ventilation is helpful but only to a certain degree. Permissive hypercapnia is not a solution in patients with cerebral oedema and intracranial hypertension. Alternative ventilation techniques including superimposed high frequency ventilation are an option [207]. Extracorporeal CO_2 removal is a further possibility [239]. Prone positioning of the patient can recruit atelectatic lung areas and improve pulmonary shunt [75]. The hesitance to move the patient to a prone position lies in the expected reduction of venous return from the brain and the limited possibility to monitor the patient's pupils as a diagnostic tool. Optimal positioning of the patient's head can minimise cerebral venous congestion. ICP monitoring may be helpful. However, there is insufficient evidence that routine ICP monitoring and management will alter outcome from drowning asphyxial encephalopathy [31].

8.4.3
Hyperglycaemia and Hypoglycaemia

Stress of drowning is believed to cause hyperglycaemia secondary to excessive endogenous catecholamine release. Pre-existing hyperglycaemia exacerbates neurologic injury following episodes of global ischaemia in a variety of species [117, 176]. Although an elevated initial blood glucose is highly predictive for poor outcome or death [10], hyperglycaemia may also be an epiphenomenon reflecting the severity of global cerebral ischaemia in humans [223]. Regardless, there is now sufficient evidence to recommend prompt correction of hyperglycaemia to normoglycaemic values with insulin, if required, to reduce neurologic morbidity.

Severe hypoglycaemia, due to the administration of excess insulin, should also be avoided because severe hypoglycaemia alone can cause brain damage. Cessation of spontaneous electroencephalographic (EEG) activity often occurs in association with energy failure and loss of ion homeostasis, with cellular efflux of potassium and cellular calcium uptake [87] with eventual tissue destruction [13]. Thus, hypoglycaemia should be rapidly corrected.

Maintenance of normoglycemia (blood glucose concentration between 80 and 110 mg/dl; 4.4 and 6.1 mmol/l) dramatically reduces mortality and morbidity during intensive care treatment of critically ill patients [243]. Although the mechanism for this effect remains undefined, this evidence, and that indicated above, is sufficient to recommend that blood glucose concentrations be frequently monitored with appropriate treatment to maintain normoglycaemia in all patients requiring intensive care treatment.

8.4.4
Temperature

Cerebral hypothermia may be accidental or deliberate. Either case may afford some degree of permanent cerebral protection.

Evidence for the neuroprotective effect of accidental hypothermia is based on a large body of case reports where victims, who despite prolonged submersion in cold water, had good neurologic recovery [9, 96, 159, 161, 251]. Accidental hypothermia is unlikely to be caused by surface cooling alone. Brain cooling might be achieved through pulmonary heat exchange with the cold aspirated water before cardiac arrest occurs. Children tend to loose heat faster because they have a greater body surface area and less fat than adults. Drugs or alcohol are often involved in adult drowning and may cause additional heat loss due to vasodilation. Brain death cannot be assessed until rewarming has occurred and in some cases use of CPB may be required to achieve rewarming sufficient to allow recovery of cardiac function.

Deliberate hypothermia has been used as a therapeutic adjunct for a variety of medical procedures. Two human trials have definitively demonstrated that deliberate hypothermia (lasting 12–24 hours at 32–34°C body core temperature), induced shortly after the restoration of spontaneous circulation in humans who had out-of-hospital cardiac arrest, improves overall neurologic outcome and reduces mortality [26, 232]. There have been no such studies in drowning patients. Further, because of the sporadic nature of drowning events, such studies seem unlikely in the foreseeable future. There are differences between cardiogenic cardiac arrest and cardiac arrest resulting from drowning. The primary difference is the progressive total body hypoxia and acidosis that precedes cardiac arrest with drowning. In contrast, with cardiogenic cardiac arrest, delivery of oxygen is abruptly halted. From the perspective of the brain, the duration of hypoxia prior to asphyxial circulatory arrest is longer than with cardiogenic cardiac arrest. Therefore, it may prove more difficult to provide effective improvement in outcome from asphyxial arrest. Nevertheless, the two insults bear sufficient pathophysiologic similarity, that use of deliberate hypothermia can be recommended in the drowning victim who remains comatose after restoration of cardiopulmonary function.

Use of hypothermia has implications for intensive care management of these patients. Animal studies have shown two important factors that determine the value of neuroresuscitation derived from post-ischaemic induced hypothermia. The earlier hypothermia is initiated, the more likely it will be effective. Second, the effectiveness of deliberate hypothermia is dependent on its duration. Brief intervals of post-ischaemic hypothermia (several hours) do not provide protection. For hypothermia to be effective, when initiated after the insult has occurred, it must be sustained for at least 12 hours. As a result, institution of deliberate hypothermia should occur as soon as possible and it is likely that this will already be in process prior to intensive care admission. Because the duration of hypothermia is critical in defining efficacy, induction of hypothermia in the field or emergency department that is not sustained in the intensive care unit will likely be of little of no benefit. It is therefore incumbent on the intensivist to obtain information regarding when hypothermia was initiated relative to the time of the drowning accident so that it can be determined how long it should be continued in the intensive care unit.

Should deliberate hypothermia be employed there are other implications for intensive care management. Sustained maintenance of core temperature at 32–34°C will likely require endotracheal intubation, mechanical ventilation and pharmacologic adjuncts for sedation and to prevent shivering. This will interfere with neurologic evaluation and definition of prognosis. Possible side-effects of hypothermia should be considered. Hypothermic vasoconstriction and impaired neutrophil oxidative function may contribute to reduced resistance to infection [255], which may be particularly relevant if there is aspiration of contaminated water. Should deliberate hypothermia be employed, after 12–24 hours of hypothermic therapy, haemodynamically stable patients may be rewarmed actively at a slow rate (maximum of 0.5–1°C per hour) considering possible increases in ICP. Core temperature should not exceed normothermia to prevent aggravation of neuronal injury by hyperthermia.

Two human studies have shown that acute CNS injury results in spontaneous hyperthermia [3, 92]. Considering the growing number of publications linking temperature modulation to the extent of neurological injury, the importance of temperature control in patients at risk for cerebral injury is still underestimated. Because hyperthermia has been consistently associated with worsened outcome from a variety of acute brain insults in both laboratory animals and humans, monitoring of body core temperature is highly recommended in the drowning victim, but is useless if documented fever is not treated.

8.4.5
Seizures

Patients with primary neurologic disorders and hypoxic-ischaemic encephalopathy have a high incidence of seizures that may be of special concern in drowning victims. Moreover, hypoxia and anoxia is a common aetiology for nonconvulsive status epilepticus in comatose patients [236]. Therefore, EEG monitoring is recommended for seizure detection. The EEG should be recorded in the raw form, which is considered the most reliable standard for documentation of seizures.

8.5
Paediatric Considerations

PATRICK KOCHANEK

8.5.1
Background

Classic paediatric studies on cerebral resuscitation of the drowning victim involved the use of aggressive cerebral resuscitation and monitoring strategies [52, 53, 122, 142, 162, 170, 184–186, 188]. However, reports in the late 1980s suggested that initial optimism for application of brain-targeted therapies, including the use of hypothermia and barbiturates, was overstated [28, 31, 163]. These reports almost completely halted the investigation of brain-specific resuscitative therapies in both paediatric laboratory models of drowning and the clinical arena. Unfortunately, these reports included small numbers of children and thus may not have provided definitive answers.

During the past 10 years, investigation into paediatric drowning has focused on epidemiological, diagnostic, and prognostic issues. Laboratory and clinical investigation of cerebral resuscitation in the developing organism has been restricted to perinatal asphyxia. This compounds the difficulties in translating results to the clinical setting of drowning, because the model used by investigators studying perinatal asphyxia [187] shares few features with asphyxial cardiopulmonary arrest. The lack of investigation in the last decade on cerebral resuscitation of the drowning victim limits our ability to recommend, with any confidence, specific paediatric brain oriented therapies with the exception of temperature management.

8.5.2
Induced Hypothermia

Beneficial effects of mild-to-moderate induced hypothermia (32–34°C), whether instituted during or after an hypoxic or ischaemic insult, are established. Two trials of induced hypothermia after ventricular fibrillation (VF) cardiopulmonary arrest in adults [26, 232], a recent study of rapid post-resuscitation cooling after VF in adults [25], and extensive studies in experimental models of global cerebral ischaemia, cardiopulmonary arrest, and asphyxial arrest in adult animals support this statement. This is also the case for studies in experimental models of brain ischaemia in the developing organism [82–84, 195, 216, 247, 259] and is similarly suggested in reports of favourable outcome despite prolonged submersion in cold-water drowning [9, 27, 96, 125, 159, 161, 167, 251]. Regarding clinical application, most of these reports suggest that hypothermia should be initiated as soon as possible after the insult or even during CPR if technically feasible [160]. In canine VF arrest, mild hypothermia (34°C) is effective, however a delay of 15 min in application reduced its efficacy [112]. In experimental perinatal asphyxia, delayed application of moderate hypothermia was still efficacious [82]. Details of the optimal application of hypothermia remain to be clarified, but application of mild hypothermia should not be delayed.

Reports have been published concerning risks of hypothermia-induced stress in the normal neonate [102, 140]. However, there is no compelling experimental or clinical evidence to suggest that hypothermia should be less efficacious in the treatment of hypoxic-ischaemic brain injury in developing versus mature organisms. The use of resuscitative hypothermia in perinatal asphyxia has been suggested since the mid 1960s [55, 58, 67].

One aspect of hypothermia-mediated cerebral protection, selective head cooling, may have unique importance and application to infants and young children [82, 84]. A number of studies, including those in large animal models of cardiopulmonary arrest and adult victims of severe traumatic brain injury (TBI) and cardiopulmonary arrest have reported that adequate brain cooling cannot be achieved by isolated head cooling [156, 157, 258, 263]. However, in infants, this does not seem to be the case [83]. Foetal head cooling to an extradural temperature of 30–33°C was effective and improved EEG and histological outcome, even when initiated as late as 5.5 hours after a 30 min hypoxic-ischaemic insult [83]. Isolated head cooling may have unique cerebrovascular and metabolic effects [113]. Cooling of the human newborn can be achieved through isolated cooling of head and neck. In newborn infants with moderate to severe hypoxic-ischaemic encephalopathy, selective brain cooling was able to rapidly achieve a nasopharyngeal temperature of 34°C, which was 1.2°C lower than rectal temperature. A multi-centre study of hypothermia in perinatal asphyxia is ongoing. Study of infants and children randomised to moderate hypothermia after severe head injury suggests a powerful reduction in oxidative stress by this therapy [17]. Other beneficial mechanistic effects may also be operating.

8.5.3
Rewarming from Accidental Hypothermia

A wealth of experimental data, across literally every category of brain injury model, has demonstrated that even mild hyperthermia, applied during or after the insult, exacerbates neuronal death and worsens outcome [63]. Often, victims of submersion episodes present with spontaneous hypothermia. It has been demonstrated that hyperthermia often inadvertently results after cardiopulmonary arrest in infants or children, even when rewarming is carefully performed [92]. Although the optimal rate of rewarming remains to be determined, based on the most successful trial of the application of resuscitative hypothermia in haemodynamically stable brain-injured patients to date, rewarming should probably not exceed a rate of 1°C per hour [129]. The optimal temperature to which rewarming should be targeted has not been defined. However, because we know that core temperatures of 32–33°C are neuroprotective in humans in the acute post-resuscitation interval [26, 232], this may be an appropriate target range if haemodynamic stability is not threatened.

8.5.4
100% Oxygen

Controversy exists regarding the optimal fraction of inspired oxygen (F_iO_2) for resuscitation after cardiopulmonary arrest. Studies in adult experimental models of cardiopulmonary arrest suggest that resuscitation with 100% oxygen is less efficacious than resuscitation with room air [124, 269]. In perinatal asphyxia, this question has been subjected to both feasibility and multi-centre clinical trials in over 600 infants. No difference in either acute or long-term outcome was reported between resuscitation with a F_iO_2 of 0.21 and 1.0. However, in the drowning victim, pulmonary aspiration of water and gastric contents are an important concomitant finding. Thus, the use of room air would introduce potential risk of a deleterious hypoxaemic resuscitation [270]. An F_iO_2 of 1.0 should be used in the initial resuscitation, even in infants. Studies with brain-penetrating antioxidant agents are also warranted.

8.5.5
Pharmacological Agents

No pharmacological agent has been proven to be neuroprotective (either alone or in combination with hypothermia) in cerebral resuscitation of either children or adults after cardiopulmonary arrest (▶ **Chapter 8.7**). In light of this, it is difficult to recommend any specific drug regimen for the paediatric drowning victim.

8.6
Neuromonitoring in the Intensive Care Unit for the Drowning Victim

Cor Kalkman

It has become clear that rapid and successful initial resuscitation can improve outcome from drowning. However, there is far less consensus, let alone evidence, regarding optimal cerebral monitoring and treatment strategies in patients who demonstrate asphyxial encephalopathy. Secondary brain ischaemia remains a common pathway to irreversible brain damage following an anoxic primary insult in critically ill patients, including the drowning victim. It would therefore seem logical to monitor the brain for the occurrence of secondary cerebral ischaemia and attempt corrective intervention.

Neuromonitoring techniques in the intensive care unit can be applied to estimate prognosis. The same techniques can also be used in an attempt to improve outcome by allowing early detection of cerebral ischaemia or seizures and early institution of aggressive treatment. Neuromonitors can be divided into those that measure or estimate:

- Cerebral perfusion pressure (CPP) by ICP monitoring
- Cerebral blood flow (CBF) or derivatives such as red blood cell velocity by transcranial Doppler
- Balance between oxygen supply and demand by cerebral oximetry, jugular bulb oximetry, near infrared spectroscopy (NIRS), brain tissue pO_2
- Neuronal function such as spontaneous and evoked electrical activity by EEG or evoked potentials

8.6.1
Intracranial Pressure Monitoring

To reliably calculate CPP (mean arterial pressure – ICP) in the presence of acute brain swelling, it is necessary to measure ICP using either an intraventricular, intraparenchymal, subdural, or epidural pressure transducer. The value of ICP monitoring following resuscitation from a hypoxic-ischaemic insult is unknown. Theoretically, maintaining CPP above 60 mmHg reduces the probability of secondary cerebral ischaemia. However, there is insufficient evidence that routine ICP monitoring and management will alter outcome from drowning induced asphyxial encephalopathy. Increased ICP as a result of cerebral hyperaemia may be a concern if permissive hypercapnia is deemed necessary in patients with ARDS.

8.6.2
Transcranial Doppler Ultrasonography

Little is known about the value of transcranial Doppler ultrasonography (TCD) monitoring following resuscitation from cardiac arrest. Iida et al. [98] suggested that delayed hyperaemia can occur in humans after resuscitation from cardiac arrest. They argued that this delayed hyperaemia can lead to intracranial hypertension and acute brain swelling, resulting in poor outcome. Although TCD may detect this change, the therapeutic implications are unknown.

8.6.3
Mixed Jugular Venous Oxygen Content (SjvO₂)

Jugular venous oxygenation provides information about global brain oxygenation and is used in several centres to provide early detection of cerebral ischaemia that might otherwise go unrecognised, such as in patients with TBI, especially those being hyperventilated. $S_{jv}O_2$ can be measured intermittently with a co-oximeter or continuously using a fibre optic catheter. A $S_{jv}O_2$ of less then 50% suggests cerebral ischaemia that may be reversible by increasing CPP. Takasu et al. [228] monitored $S_{jv}O_2$ in a small group of patients resuscitated after cardiac arrest, and found that high $S_{jv}O_2$ values were associated with poor outcome, suggesting an inability of damaged neurons to use oxygen. Limitations of $S_{jv}O_2$ monitoring include inability to provide information about regional cerebral ischaemia, contamination with extracranial venous blood, and catheter related technical problems.

8.6.4
Near Infrared Spectroscopy

Near infrared spectroscopy (NIRS) can be used to non-invasively measure the oxygen status of intracranial mixed arterial-venous blood using a sensor on the forehead. Although the technique is steadily improving, there are at present many unsolved issues including the problems of extracranial contamination, and variations in optical path length, making reliable calibration difficult [45]. If these problems can be solved, NIRS has the potential to become a non-invasive method of assessing regional cerebral oxygenation, that might be of use both for prognosis and treatment of patients following asphyxial cerebral insults.

8.6.5
Electroencephalogram

The availability of electroencephalogram (EEG) equipment specially designed for use in the intensive care unit or operating room has become more widespread. The value of EEG for the diagnosis and management of convulsive and nonconvulsive status epilepticus is established [100, 101], but the value of EEG for early detection of cerebral ischaemia in the intensive care setting is much less clear. One reason is that hypnotic and sedative medication and ischaemia can produce very similar EEG patterns, which hampers reliable diagnosis of cerebral ischaemia.

8.6.6
Somatosensory Evoked Potentials

Somatosensory evoked potentials (SSEPs) reflect conduction in neural pathways from the site of stimulation to the recording electrodes. An intact conducting pathway is a prerequisite for a normal SSEP waveform. These signals are robust, even in the presence of high concentrations of barbiturate [66]. Cortical SSEPs can provide prognostic information in TBI patients [217]. Of 51 TBI patients with normal bilateral central conduction times, 57% had a good outcome. Any delay in central conduction time was associated with a decreased incidence of good outcome (30%). Unilateral absence of the cortical SSEP component was usually associated with a poor outcome (death or severe disability) and bilateral absence was always associated with a poor outcome. Berek et al. [24] found that brain lactate measured by proton magnetic resonance and absent N2 waves in short-latency SSEPs were significant predictors of a poor prognosis in patients recovering from CPR. Poor neurological outcome was correlated both with the duration of anoxia and CPR. Zandbergen et al. [267] recently performed a meta-analysis of 33 studies and assessed the overall prognostic accuracy of variables that had a specificity of 100% for poor outcome. Absence of pupillary light reflexes on day 3, absent motor response to pain on day 3 and bilateral absence of early cortical SSEPs within the first week were all strong predictors of poor outcome. SSEPs had the smallest confidence interval of its pooled positive-likelihood ratio and its pooled false-positive test rate. Thus, SSEPs may have a role in the care of the drowning victim but there is absence of specific evidence to support this conclusion.

8.6.7
Conclusions

It is clear that neuromonitoring techniques, in particular the SSEPs, can contribute to estimating prognosis following a severe hypoxic ischaemic cerebral insult. Do clinical decisions guided by the results of multimodality neuromonitoring affect patient outcome? There are no data to support the claim that the use of these monitors will increase the proportion of survivors with good neurological function. Evidence to support or refute the use of neuromonitoring techniques during the care for drowning victims will have to come from carefully designed prospective studies in properly defined patient groups. Considering the relatively low annual frequency of drowning patients per centre, it seems logical to study these issues first in all patients following cardiopulmonary resuscitation who enter the intensive care unit after return of spontaneous circulation.

8.7
Neurochemical Markers of Brain Injury

BENGT NELLGÅRD

In some neurodegenerative conditions such as Alzheimer's disease (AD), measurement of neurochemical markers in blood and cerebrospinal fluid (CSF) is now routine. These markers may detect axonal and synaptic degeneration or regeneration, as well as structural changes like plaques. In contrast, for brain asphyxia, caused by cardiac arrest or drowning, only a few investigations have examined the prognostic value of biochemical markers. Drowning is an asphyxia condition. Because no specific studies have been done on neurochemical markers in this patient population, information must be extrapolated from studies of both humans and laboratory animals that have been subjected to hypoxaemia, ischaemia, or traumatic brain injury (TBI). Hopefully, ongoing investigations of neurochemical markers in these conditions may give us new prognostic tools of relevance to the drowning victim.

8.7.1
Immunology

TBI in animals and humans elicits an acute inflammatory response with production of both pro- and anti-inflammatory cytokines. In children, interleukin-8 (IL-8) is increased in CSF after TBI and correlates strongly with outcome and mortality [257]. In adults with TBI, IL-6 correlated with severity of brain damage [261]. In stroke patients, increased concentrations of IL-1, IL-8 and IL-17 correlated with Scandinavian Stroke Scale scores [110]. In stroke patients, C-reactive protein induced by IL-6, correlated with outcome [62]. The anti-inflammatory IL-10, increased in CSF and modestly in plasma in TBI patients. The IL-10 increase also correlated with concomitant increases in IL-6 and the anti-inflammatory mediator transforming growth factor-beta (TGF-β), whereas increases in tumour necrosis factor (TNF-α) corresponded to decreased IL-10 concentrations [57]. In another investigation in TBI patients, TGF-β increased in CSF with a maximum the first day, then decreased paralleling blood–brain barrier function [152]. In CSF, alternative pathway proteins C3 and factor B were increased following TBI in patients speculatively contributing to secondary brain injury [109]. Coagulopathy after TBI has been demonstrated both in experimental animals and humans. Fibrin degradation products increased after TBI in children and this predicted poor outcome [244]. In adults with TBI, local micro-thrombi are found [222]. Thus, major immunologic changes are evident after TBI and may have prognostic significance but the implications of these findings for the drowning patient are undefined.

8.7.2
Apolipoprotein E

Apolipoprotein E (apoE) plays a role in lipid transport, but is also important in mechanisms of neural injury. There are three human apoE alleles (E2, E3, E4). ApoE3 is far more prevalent than apoE2 and apoE4. Individuals who carry the apoE4 allele have a higher risk of developing Alzheimer's disease [226]. Recently, studies demonstrate that the presence of the apoE4 allele increases risk of poor outcome after TBI [230], stroke [136, 211], and CPB [229] potentially because of altered calcium homeostasis or immunomodulatory properties [118, 245]. Its effect on outcome from drowning has not been studied. Although promising, genotyping of patients for apoE has not yet become routine practice in prognosticating outcome from acute brain injury.

8.7.3
S-100B

S-100B is a small cytosolic protein highly specific for brain tissue. S-100B, derived from astroglial or Schwann cells, is measurable in blood and CSF. It is the most extensively investigated biochemical marker of brain injury in humans. After severe TBI, S-100B concentrations peak by 24 hours post-injury and have been correlated with neurological outcome [139, 179]. In moderate TBI, a weak correlation between serum S-100B and neurological outcome and lesion size has also been shown [99]. Cerebral contusion size, as defined by CT has been shown to correlate with S-100B concentrations [90]. It has been suggested that persistent elevation of S-100B for 2–6 days indicates ongoing secondary damage. In patients undergoing cardiac surgery a correlation between S-100B, within 5 hours after onset of by-pass, and neuropsychological performance has been reported [106]. After cardiac arrest, S-100B was found to increase the first day after resuscitation and a correlation was shown between S-100B levels on day 2 and 3 and degree of coma and time of anoxia. A high level of S-100B on days 1 and 2 was associated with mortality [190]. In a study where patients were unconscious after acute global cerebral ischaemia, S-100B levels in serum at 24 hours were predictive of regaining consciousness [133]. These findings indicate potential for S-100B to be of value in the drowning victim but this has not been investigated.

8.7.4
Neuron-Specific Enolase

Neuron-specific enolase (NSE) is another widely used biochemical marker of brain injury specific to neurons measurable in both blood and CSF. NSE concentrations at admission after TBI have been correlated with neurologic outcome [139]. Others have demonstrated a correlation between NSE and CT scan documented lesion size [90]. In patients resuscitated from cardiac arrest,

NSE correlated with outcome at 12, 24 and 72 hours after anoxia, with the 72-hour values being the best predictor [206]. Finally, NSE has also been shown to predict the recovery of consciousness after global cerebral ischaemia [133]. Therefore, like S-100B, investigation of NSE as an outcome prognosticator in patients with drowning encephalopathy is warranted.

8.7.5
Heat Shock Proteins

Ubiquitin is a heat-shock protein associated with the degradation of abnormal cellular proteins. In humans resuscitated from cardiopulmonary arrest, a strong correlation between presence of this protein in the CSF and Glasgow Outcome Scale score has been reported [114].

8.7.6
Conclusions

The only clinically available biochemical markers of anoxia or cerebral ischaemia are S-100B and NSE. Measurement of these markers in blood may be considered at admission and daily for the first week. If possible, CSF values may also be analysed. A secondary ischaemic event could thus be detected. Within a few years new biochemical markers will be available with more sensitivity and specificity than S-100B and NSE.

8.8
Post-hypoxic Treatment with Pharmacologic Agents

Takefumi Sakabe

Energy depletion is the central mechanism for brain damage following an hypoxic or ischaemic insult. Thus, there is no substitute for restoration of cerebral circulation. However, accumulating data show that various secondary events initiated by the hypoxic insult also contribute to irreversible brain damage [214]. These secondary events may allow a sufficient therapeutic window for pharmacologic intervention to, at least in part, reduce damage. Because prophylactic pharmacologic therapy is not applicable to drowning victims, evidence derived from pre-treatment studies has little relevance to this patient population. Attention must be focused on post-insult treatment investigations and on whether favourable laboratory results can be extended to clinical situations.

8.8.1
Barbiturates and Propofol

There is much evidence to support the notion that barbiturates have beneficial effect, which is mainly attributed to the suppression of metabolic demand. However, the benefit has been questioned in the situation of complete global cerebral ischaemia such as cardiac arrest and administration of barbiturates following cardiac arrest is no longer advocated [38]. The attitude is the same for drowning. No beneficial effects of pentobarbital could be demonstrated in non-fatal drowning in children [163]. The neuroprotective effect of propofol in experimental brain ischaemia has been claimed by some [108, 266] but not all. No data is available whether propofol has beneficial effects following cardiac arrest in humans.

8.8.2
Corticosteroids

Corticosteroids have long been used to reduce brain oedema in various forms of brain pathology. However, routine use has been broadly questioned with the exception of peritumoral brain oedema. Recent guidelines from the Brain Trauma Foundation on the Management of Severe Head Injury state that glucocorticoids are not recommended [42]. Nevertheless, a recent meta-analysis could not exclude a beneficial effect of corticosteroids [4]. The second National Acute Spinal Cord Injury Study revealed a small improvement in neurologic outcome in patients who suffered spinal cord injury and received large doses of methylprednisolone beginning within 8 hours of injury [35]. The beneficial effect was attributed to inhibition of lipid peroxidation. However, routine use of methylprednisolone, even in this patient population has been questioned [97, 151].

In post-cardiac arrest patients, the use of corticosteroid has been questioned. Corticosteroid increases plasma glucose concentrations in the setting of ischaemia [250]. It is known that hyperglycaemia during ischaemia leads to lactic acidosis which exacerbates ischaemic brain damage. A recent randomised prospective trial in critically ill patients demonstrated improved outcome when blood glucose was controlled between 80–110 mg/dl with intensive insulin therapy [243]. Furthermore, it has been demonstrated in animals that metyrapone, an inhibitor of glucocorticoid production, reduces brain injury induced by ischaemia and seizures [219]. Corticosteroids have no beneficial effects on pulmonary injury caused by aspiration of water, and may actually cause harm by impairing the immune response [150, 164]. Therefore, corticosteroids are not recommended for routine use in drowning victims.

8.8.3
Excitatory Amino Acid (EAA) Antagonists

Excessive accumulation of extracellular excitatory amino acid (EAA) during energy failure and the subsequent increase in intracellular calcium cause serial events leading to neuronal necrosis and apoptosis [192]. High glutamate concentrations in CSF have been reported in patients with severe TBI [41].

Glutamate receptor antagonists have been shown to protect against brain damage in various experimental ischaemic and traumatic conditions. Selective NMDA (N-methyl-D-aspartate) and AMPA (α-amino-3-hydroxy-5-methyl-4-isoxazole propionic acid) receptor antagonists may have beneficial effects when given immediately after laboratory insults, although this remains controversial. With the exception of ketamine [93, 210], glutamate antagonists are not clinically available. Furthermore, most glutamate receptor antagonists themselves have neurotoxic properties [153, 166] and adverse effects such as hypertension, hallucination and catatonia. Although use of EAA antagonists is attractive based on the excitotoxicity hypothesis, clinical outcome studies in stroke and acute traumatic brain injury (TBI) patients failed to demonstrate a beneficial effect [60, 61, 120]. No data are available for use of these drugs in humans following CPR. Use of EAA antagonists for brain resuscitation in the drowning victim is, therefore, not recommended.

8.8.4
Calcium-Entry Blockers

Pharmacologic blockade of calcium influx through voltage sensitive calcium channels has been shown to protect against experimental focal and global ischaemic damage in some patients. Clinical trials on acute stroke patients suggest that nimodipine improves neurologic function if ischaemia is mild but not if ischaemia is severe [74]. In cardiac arrest patients the effects of calcium entry blockers have been inconsistent. A trial of nimodipine in patients showed no overall improvement in 1-year survival rate, but showed encouraging effects in a subset of patients in whom advanced life support was delayed for more than 10 min [189]. A trial of lidoflazine in patients remaining comatose after resuscitation found no beneficial effect [39].

At present, despite the suggested favourable effect of some of those compounds for post-arrest treatment, clinical application of calcium-entry blockers has only been approved for the treatment of vasospasm after subarachnoid haemorrhage [171].

8.8.5
Magnesium

Magnesium blocks both ligand and voltage dependent calcium entry. Beneficial effects of magnesium have been shown in various experimental ischaemia models including spinal cord ischaemia, mostly with pretreatment. The results from a preliminary trial of magnesium treatment in stroke patients are encouraging [154]. The use of magnesium in cardiac arrest patients showed a suggested favourable effect in pilot studies [144, 209]. However, a randomised trial of magnesium for in-hospital cardiac arrest failed to demonstrate benefit [233]. Although magnesium may have a potential role in resuscitation, more information is needed before this drug is accepted as a routine therapy for drowning encephalopathy.

8.8.6
Sodium-Channel Blockers and Related Drugs

Sodium channel blockers confer protection in some, but not all, models of brain ischaemia probably by preventing presynaptic sodium influx thereby attenuating glutamate release.

Protective effects of lubeluzole have been shown in animal ischaemia models [88]. The protective effect may be attributable to prevention of glutamate release and inhibition of glutamate-induced nitric oxide-related neurotoxicity [127]. A clinical multi-centre study in stroke patients failed to demonstrate an improvement in mortality but did show a trend towards better functional recovery [81].

Lamotrigine and riluzole have been shown to have anti-ischaemic properties by blocking glutamatergic neurotransmission [15, 56]. No data are available for the use of these drugs in post-CPR patients. However, riluzole is currently in clinical use in patients with amyotrophic lateral sclerosis [116]. Thus, these drugs may be of use in variable brain disorders including post-hypoxic conditions. However, again, more information is needed before this class of drug is accepted as a routine therapy for drowning encephalopathy.

8.8.7
Diphenylhydantoin

Diphenylhydantoin is an anticonvulsant and has been shown to have neuroprotective effects in various forms of experimental brain pathology [34, 252]. Human investigation is limited but one study showed that 90% of patients given diphenylhydantoin shortly after cardiac arrest exhibited complete recovery [5]. The situations in this report were special, i.e., cardiac arrest during anaesthesia, and no control group was studied. Therefore, these results are inconclusive. Diphenylhydantoin has been shown to reduce pulmonary oedema associated cerebral hypoxia in animals [260]. Diphenylhydantoin is relatively free of side effects when given slowly. Because seizures are a common sequel to cardiac arrest [220], it may be justified to consider the use of diphenylhydantoin in patients with drowning encephalopathy.

8.8.8
Local Anaesthetics

Whether local anaesthetics, serving as sodium channel blockers, possess a cerebral protective effect is controversial. Lidocaine, given intravenously, reduced K^+ efflux during complete ischaemia [12]. Lidocaine also ameliorated cerebral damage induced by air embolism [71]. Recent animal studies showed that intracerebroventricular administration of lidocaine or procaine attenuated glutamate increases induced by ischaemia and dose-dependently decreased neuronal damage in hippocampal CA_1 [2, 72]. However, possible toxic effects of lidocaine on oxidative phosphorylation have also been reported [143]. Tetracaine, given intrathecally prior to ischaemia, failed to improve neurologic and histologic outcome and did not prevent CSF glutamate increase following transient spinal cord ischaemia [248]. There have been no data showing beneficial effects of local anaesthetics given after CPR in humans. Lidocaine is often given systemically to prevent cardiac irritability following resuscitation. It would be interesting to define whether the dose used for this purpose also ameliorates hypoxic brain injury.

8.8.9
Antioxidants and Free Radical Scavengers

The resumption of oxygen supply following ischaemia may generate reactive oxygen species that are toxic to neural tissue. Furthermore, inflammatory responses to acute brain injury may induce sustained formation of reactive oxygen species. As a result, antioxidants and free radical scavengers have potential to ameliorate brain damage.

Tirilazad mesylate reduces neuronal damage in a variety of experimental models. However, clinical trials have been disappointing. Tirilazad, used in stroke or subarachnoid haemorrhage patients, failed to show consistent efficacy [85]. Only an early co-operative study showed a significant decrease in 3-month mortality [103]. Failures with tirilazad may have been, in part, attributable to co-administration of anticonvulsant medications which can influence the metabolism of tirilazad. However, a clinical trial in acute spinal cord injury showed no advantage of tirilazad over methylprednisolone [36].

Superoxide dismutase (SOD) is an enzyme that provides natural defence against oxidative stress. In humans with TBI, polyethylene glycol-conjugated SOD given 4 hours after injury was effective but a subsequent study failed to show any benefit [155]. The hydroxyl radical scavenger, nicaraven, ameliorated ischaemic brain and traumatic spinal cord damage in animal experiments [237, 265]. The beneficial effects on brain injury were observed even with post-ischaemic treatment. Post-treatment with the (spin) trapping agents α-phenyl-N-tert-butyl-nitrone (PBN) [268] and s-PBN [208] substantially reduced damage from focal ischaemia and damage induced by an intrastriatal injection of malonate, a mitochondrial toxin. A derivative of PBN, NXY-059, has shown the most promise providing reduction in neurologic deficits and lesion size for up to

10 weeks in primates subjected to focal ischaemic insults given as late as 4 hours after onset of ischaemia [132]. Clinical trials are underway in stroke studies but little information is available regarding cardiac arrest. Nitric oxide synthase (NOS) inhibitors have been reported to be either beneficial or detrimental [11, 135]. More information is needed to establish a therapeutic strategy using antioxidants following cardiac arrest.

8.8.10
Other Drugs

It is known that post-ischaemic circulatory disturbances (no-reflow or hypoperfusion), at least in part, may be responsible for the final outcome after cerebral ischaemia. Increased blood viscosity, intravascular coagulation, vasospasm, free radical formation, neutrophil adhesion, and oedema, all contributing to hypoperfusion, have been postulated as mechanisms for reperfusion disturbances. Measures to improve microcirculation such as haemodilution and anticoagulation may be of value. A recent clinical trial of tissue type plasminogen activator (t-PA) for stroke showed a reduction of focal ischaemic brain damage in humans [131]. Presumably, however, the mechanism was stenotic clot lysis which would not be applicable to hypoxic encephalopathy. Moreover, other research has shown that t-PA exacerbated neuronal damage induced by excitotoxins or ischaemia [238]. Plasminogen activator inhibitor also protects against brain damage. Thus, it is not justified to use t-PA following cardiac arrest.

Induced hypertension and intracarotid haemodilution with dextran 40 and heparinisation have been shown to improve outcome in an animal cardiac arrest model [197]. Furthermore, a recent report showed that intra-aortic saline flush with the antioxidant agent Tempol enhanced mild or moderate hypothermic cerebral preservation [21]. With this type of therapeutic strategy, it may be possible to buy time for delayed resuscitation.

Inflammatory cytokines are believed to contribute to ischaemic and TBI [16]. Cytokines stimulate the production of free radicals, arachidonic acids, and up-regulate the activity of adhesion molecules, all of which contribute to secondary injury. IL-6 and TNF-α are known to be released following TBI [138]. An increase in adhesion molecules has been observed which can produce disturbances of microcirculation. However, a trial of anti-intracellular adhesion molecule (ICAM-1) antibody in stroke patients showed increased morbidity and mortality rather than improvement [212]. There have been no data available for the use of this drug after CPR. Further study is necessary before these drugs can be recommended for use in drowning victims.

Calpain is a protease implicated in several downstream events in the neuronal injury cascade. Calpain inhibitor has been shown to protect against or ameliorate ischaemic damage [14, 73]. The potent and rapidly brain penetrating calpain inhibitor MDL 28, 170 ameliorated damage even when therapy was initiated up to 6 hours after the onset of ischaemia [130]. Clinical data for these substances have not been reported.

As a result, despite major efforts to define mechanisms of ischaemic-anoxic brain injury and pharmacologic therapy, current recommendations for pharmacologic neuroprotective intervention in the drowning victim is limited to consideration use of prophylactic anticonvulsants.

8.9
Animal Experimentation
on Cardiopulmonary Cerebral Resuscitation
Relevant for Drowning

PETER SAFAR

Drowning to cardiac arrest is a challenge for cerebral resuscitation [169, 177]. Asphyxia is a combination of decrease in blood oxygen, increase in blood CO_2, and acidaemia caused by airway obstruction, alveolar blockage, hypoventilation, or apnoea. Protection is treatment initiated before the insult (which is not an issue in drowning). Preservation is treatment initiated during the insult (which would apply to cold-water drowning). Resuscitation is treatment to reverse the insult and support recovery. Normothermic submersion is drowning in tepid or warm water with cardiac arrest occurring at near-normal body and cerebral temperatures. Hypothermic submersion is drowning in cold water resulting in brain cooling during asphyxiation to cardiac arrest, with preservative cerebral hypothermia reached at the moment of cardiac arrest [6, 234].

Cardiopulmonary cerebral resuscitation (CPCR) consists of three phases: basic life support (BLS) to be initiated as rapidly as possible by a bystander (co-swimmer, lifesaver); advanced life support (ALS) predominantly designed for restoration of spontaneous circulation (ROSC), to be most commonly initiated by EMS; and prolonged life support (PLS), usually to be carried out en route to and in the hospital. BLS consists of step A [airway control], step B [breathing control, to be initiated by mouth-to-mouth or mouth-to-nose ventilation (MMV)], and step C [circulation support, usually initiated by external cardiac massage, also called external chest (cardiac, sternal) compressions]. ALS is meant primarily to achieve ROSC as rapidly as possible. It includes reversal of ventricular fibrillation (VF) by electric countershocks; vigorous continuance of steps A–C with tracheal intubation, tracheobronchial clearing, and increased inhaled oxygen concentration; epinephrine or other vasoconstrictor and other drugs and fluids. PLS should be brain-oriented intensive care life support until recovery of consciousness. That includes therapeutic hypothermia. For cerebral resuscitation in the drowning victim, all steps of CPCR are important with steps A–C being started in the water if possible.

In these animal experiments, the temperature levels were defined as follows: mild hypothermia is 33–36°C, moderate 28–32°C, deep 16–27°C, profound 5–15°C, and ultra-profound below 5°C. Spontaneous circulation ceases below about 25°C. There are differences between sites of temperature measurements. Tympanic and nasopharyngeal temperatures reflect brain temperature; which under normal circulation equilibrate quite well with core temperatures such as oesophageal, vena cava, and pulmonary artery. Temperatures in the urinary bladder or rectum, or on the skin, do not reflect brain or heart temperatures.

8.9.1
Animal Models

The most important factors which determine cerebral outcome after drowning are arrest time (no flow), CPCR time (BLS-ALS) (low flow or trickle flow), and temperature. What to teach for CPCR delivery should be based on pathophysiologic facts, best obtained from experiments with clinically realistic models in large animals high on the phylogenetic scale, such as dogs and pigs. [198]. Whom to teach should be based on local circumstances and priorities. To be prepared for resuscitation of drowning victims, all fit human beings, starting from about 10 years of age, should acquire life supporting first aid skills, which include CPCR-BLS. How to teach should be based on the results of education research [69]. Observations on human drowning victims are not suitable for pathophysiologic studies, not even for randomised clinical treatment trials. Few variables can be controlled in clinical trials of CPCR. Almost everything can be controlled in well-conducted models of large animals. In order for results in animal models to be meaningful for cerebral resuscitation and recovery, there must be controlled life support of extracerebral organs throughout the 3–7 day duration of the 'maturing' of the post-ischaemic-anoxic encephalopathy. Some neurons can die even later. Outcome evaluation should be in terms of function and morphology, including histopathologic damage scoring throughout the brain [158, 180, 181]. Cerebral resuscitation innovations are aiming for histologically normal brains, but more important is normal neurologic function. Cerebral resuscitation from cardiac arrest has been studied mostly without water in the lungs – after global brain ischaemia by neck tourniquet in monkeys [30, 78, 79, 158], after VF cardiac arrest in dogs [112, 121, 197, 198, 200, 201, 240], and after forebrain ischaemia in rats [44, 175, 218]. Few cardiac arrest outcome studies have been reported on asphyxial cardiac arrest in dogs and rats. There are no published reproducible cerebral outcome data on pigs after any kind of cardiac arrest and long-term life support. Seemingly beneficial outcome results in studies of cerebral resuscitation potentials with the clinically less relevant incomplete forebrain ischaemia rat models (or even the clinically somewhat more relevant rat models of asphyxial cardiac arrest) may not be reproducible in large animal outcome models or clinical trials. Emergency portable CPB is valuable as an experimental tool for control of reperfusion blood pressure, flow, composition and temperature [200]; and is essential for some patients with cold-water drowning. CPB has been proven superior to standard ALS in cardiac arrest dog models [7, 9, 200, 251] and recently found also feasible in rat models [126]. Clinical emergency CPB is limited by time and skills required for vessel access and initiation of CPB.

8.9.2
Pathophysiology

Accidental human drowning has been studied mostly from anecdotal case reports, which, of course, are uncontrollable in terms of the many factors that influence cerebral damage and recovery. In the 1950s, Swann and Brucer documented patterns of dying from submersion [227]; and Redding et al. [186] documented cardiovascular resuscitation from obstructive asphyxia without water in the lungs [184]; asphyxia with seawater aspiration to cardiac arrest (mostly in asystole) [183]; and asphyxia with freshwater aspiration to cardiac arrest (mostly in VF) [185]. These studies did not evaluate cerebral recovery. In dogs, the brain can fully recover after normothermic VF cardiac arrest (no-flow) of up to 5 min (loss of energy) [180, 199]; and VF cardiac arrest of 10 min if treated promptly with prolonged resuscitative (post-cardiac arrest) mild hypothermia (see later).

Complete airway obstruction after air breathing in dogs results in cardiac arrest within 5–10 min [111, 184]. When acute asphyxia is reversed before pulselessness, using CPCR steps A-B-C (zero arrest time), complete cerebral recovery can occur. The effects on the brain of prolonged asphyxia to hypotension but without cardiac arrest, which causes maximal cerebral vasodilation plus tissue hypoxia and acidosis, need study. When asphyxia leads to cardiac arrest at normothermia, after resuscitation the brain suffers more permanent damage than after the same arrest time with VF [241, 242]. Vaagenes et al. [242] have shown some ischaemically damaged cerebral neurons in histologic pictures after only 2 min normothermic asphyxial cardiac arrest (no-flow) time and normothermic reperfusion, similar to a VF-cardiac arrest time of 5 min.

8.9.3
Cerebral Resuscitation Potentials

Cerebral resuscitation from submersion starts with steps A and B. Results of studies of novel cerebral resuscitation potentials in the clinically less relevant incomplete forebrain ischaemia rat models [175, 218], or even the clinically more relevant rat model of asphyxial cardiac arrest [104] may not be reproducible in large animal outcome models or clinical trials. Pharmacologic and hypothermic resuscitation potentials have been identified in non-drowning cardiac arrest models and should be evaluated in drowning models with water aspiration; and then introduced via clinical feasibility trials to clinical use.

Pharmacologic cerebral resuscitation potentials have been disappointing and have been reviewed above. After normothermic global brain ischaemia or cardiac arrest, barbiturate loading gave mixed results [30, 78]. In the only randomised clinical trial of barbiturate loading after cardiac arrest (BRCT I) [38], there was only a suggestion of benefit in a subgroup with long cardiac arrest. Subsequent pharmacologic combination treatments, in dogs, including barbiturate, also have given only suggestive benefit, but no breakthrough effect [68]. Calcium entry blockers after cardiac arrest have given promising results in dogs [240] and monkeys [221], but again, in the only randomised clinical trial (BRCT II) [39], there was significant benefit only in a subgroup [1]. Antioxidants deserve further evaluation [21, 48, 49]. A recent dog study shows suggestive outcome benefit from an antioxidant given during cardiac arrest but not during reperfusion [21]. Optimal blood glucose levels [105] and PaO_2 levels [124, 269] after cardiac arrest and ROSC are still unclear.

The only normothermic reperfusion treatment that clearly improves cerebral outcome has been hypertensive reperfusion in animals models [94, 197, 202, 224] and patients [205]. This is to combat both immediate no-reflow and the delayed cerebral hypoperfusion. Treatments for the latter, by CBF-promoting measures over the long-term, need outcome studies.

In contrast to the disappointing results with drugs [38–40], therapeutic hypothermia has documented breakthrough effects. Moderate hypothermia (28–32°C) has been in use, for protection and preservation of heart and brain in thoracic surgery and neurosurgery, since the 1950s. Trials after cardiac arrest in patients were recommended around 1960, and found seemingly effective in a few patients [23, 51, 54, 182], but then abandoned for 25 years because of management difficulties and because moderate hypothermia can produce arrhythmias and coagulopathy. Therapeutic hypothermia received renewed research interest when in the 1980s mild protective and resuscitative hypothermia (33–36°C), which is simple and safe, was discovered to reduce post-cardiac arrest brain damage in dogs [112, 121, 199, 201, 225, 254] and in rats [43, 262]. The best cerebral outcome after prolonged normothermic VF cardiac arrest in dogs has been with mild hypothermia combined with CBF promotion [201]. The beneficial effect of mild hypothermia in coma after normothermic cardiac arrest has also recently been documented in two randomised clinical outcome studies [26, 204, 232]. Fortunately, patients often spontaneously develop mild hypothermia during prolonged cardiac arrest and CPR [26, 92, 232]. Ideally, induction of mild hypothermia should begin during prolonged CPCR BLS-ALS (steps A–C) [29] even before ROSC [160]. Fever (up to 42°C) is tolerated by the normal brain but even mild hyperthermia can add damage to the already injured brain.

Controlled therapeutic hypothermia (without shivering, vasoconstriction, catecholamine release, thermogenesis) helps preserve and resuscitate vital organs by synergism of many mechanisms [121], more than by simple reduction in oxygen demand, which may not occur with mild hypothermia [165]. ROSC and spontaneous circulation do not seem to be hampered by mild hypothermia, but may be hampered by moderate hypothermia. This remains to be examined in patients with diseased hearts. Profound hypothermia preserves viability of the heart, although it produces cardiac arrest. Many cooling methods have been tried since the 1950s. Many are now under re-investigation. In general, blood cooling [22] has advantages over attempts at external head and brain cooling or whole body surface cooling [22, 26, 83, 232, 258].

Cerebral resuscitation data in dog outcome studies were mostly for VF cardiac arrest. Mechanism-oriented data were mostly from forebrain ischaemia rat models. Mild resuscitative hypothermia for asphyxial cardiac arrest has been documented only in rats [262]. It has been shown that once complete cerebral recovery on days 3–7 is achieved, one has to have such "normal" animals also survive for several months to make sure that the damage has not merely been postponed [64]. Permanent benefit, however, can be achieved with long-term mild resuscitative hypothermia (12–24 hours) after prolonged cardiac arrest, even with delayed cooling [50, 91]. On levels of hypothermia after normothermic cardiac arrest, mild hypothermia seems more effective than moderate or deep hypothermia [254].

Preservative hypothermia during cardiac arrest is of course more effective than resuscitative hypothermia after cardiac arrest [262]. Cooling before or during cardiac arrest is more beneficial the lower the temperature [19, 20]. This has been shown clearly in the dramatic recoveries of humans after cold-water submersion: after up to 1 hour of submersion, with lowest core temperatures recorded close to 10°C [28, 32, 51, 76, 89, 95, 159, 213]. Animal studies without asphyxia, mostly in dogs, with exsanguination cardiac arrest [203], have documented complete cerebral functional recovery after cardiac arrest (no-flow) of up to 20 min at 30°C [20], 30 min at 20°C [19], and 60–120 min at 10°C. While standard CPCR will usually be adequate for achieving ROSC from cardiac arrest at 30–37°C, this is not the case with lower temperatures. After cold-water submersion to pulselessness at ≤20°C, either very prolonged and vigorous external CPR or, better, CPB is needed. Open-chest CPR with direct heart warming should also be evaluated.

8.10
Future Research Questions

David Warner

It is evident from extensive review of medical literature that little specific effort has been made to define either the pathobiology or treatment of brain injury resulting from drowning. Almost all data pertaining to medical management of this condition is derived from studies performed more than 30 years ago or data borrowed from study of other forms of acute brain injury which may have some generalisable but not specific reference to the condition of drowning. Further, there is no active organised constituency dedicated to fostering research concerning brain resuscitation after drowning, despite the fact that drowning induced encephalopathy is a relatively common problem. Dedication of the biomedical research community to specific study of this disorder, along with commitment of research funding agencies, is required for meaningful advances to be made. Listed below are suggestions for future research offered by the Brain Resuscitation Task Force that are believed to have potential to improve medical care.

- Research should be focused towards optimal timing and speed of induction of hypothermia, the optimal magnitude of hypothermia, the optimal duration of hypothermia, and the optimal rate of rewarming.
- Methods of rapid brain cooling should be developed and evaluated for safety and efficacy.
- Research into the mechanistic basis of mild resuscitative hypothermia will allow optimisation of therapy and/or development of adjunctive and/or mimetic pharmacologic therapy.

- Age-related aspects of the application of mild hypothermia in non-fatal drowning induced encephalopathy should be investigated. Drowning represents a leading cause of death in children. Most questions relevant to the development and implementation of novel cerebral resuscitation strategies in paediatric drowning victims are relevant in adults. It is likely that if a breakthrough therapy were to be developed, it would be efficacious in both paediatric and adult drowning victims. However, application of these approaches in infants and young children will warrant specific separate investigation. Certain mechanisms, particularly apoptosis [172], inflammation [123], or blood brain-barrier injury [33], may play more important and/or different roles in infants and young children. Investigation in both animal models specifically relevant to drowning and in patients are needed in the paediatric arena.
- Novel pharmacologic therapies are being advanced for other forms of acute brain injury. Specific examination of breakthrough therapies should be performed in the context of drowning in both the laboratory and the clinical setting.
- Clinically relevant contemporary laboratory models of drowning encephalopathy are almost non-existent. Development of laboratory in vivo models of drowning, with standardised physiologic conditions and long-term neurologic and histologic outcome, is needed to allow study of mechanisms and treatment of drowning related anoxic encephalopathy. Verification of any breakthrough therapies should be made in multiple species which includes study in large animals with prolonged post-arrest intensive care life support.
- It is desirable to develop and evaluate contemporary neuromonitors (such as biochemical, molecular, physiological, neurophysiological and imaging technologies) to guide therapy of drowning encephalopathy. Effectiveness of interventions guided by the use of these monitors on long-term outcome should be established. In addition, these tools should also be evaluated for their usefulness to provide an accurate early prognosis.
- Additional information is needed on the development and treatment of intracranial hypertension in patients with drowning encephalopathy.
- Investigation into the rehabilitation of patients with asphyxial brain injury is insufficient and deserves emphasis (pharmacologic intervention, stem cell transplantation, electrical stimulation, enriched environment, among others).
- Study of unclear pathophysiologic factors [169]. Examples include: (a) effects of different electrolyte fluxes, with seawater versus freshwater inhalation, on cerebral recovery and determine if asphyxial encephalopathy is altered by the presence or absence of aspirated water; (b) functional and morphologic outcome differences between prolonged VF cardiac arrest and asphyxial cardiac arrest of the same no-flow time (for example, does asphyxial cardiac arrest more likely lead to intracranial hypertension and cerebral microinfarcts?); and (c) are cerebral oedema and osmolality factors in post-drowning encephalopathy [162, 168, 264]?
- Optimise initiation of CPCR, starting with water rescue. Simulate realistic field scenarios in animal models. Evaluate in human volunteers the feasibility of applying head-tilt, jaw thrust, and MMV (or MNV) in deep water, and to add external cardiac massage in shallow water.

■ Ultra-advanced CPCR. Would 'suspended animation (preservation) for delayed resuscitation', using hypothermic aortic cold flush and CPB, have something to offer in pulseless victims rescued from water at normothermia? This approach has been introduced and investigated primarily for use in exsanguination cardiac arrest of trauma casualties [18, 22, 47, 203, 235].

References

1. Abramson NS, Kelsey SF, Safar P, Sutton-Tyrrell K (1992) Simpson's paradox and clinical trials: what you find is not necessarily what you prove. Ann Emerg Med 21:1480–1482
2. Adachi N, Chen J, Nakanishi K, Arai T (1999) Pre-ischaemic administration of procaine suppresses ischaemic glutamate release and reduces neuronal damage in the gerbil hippocampus. Br J Anaesth 83:472–474
3. Albrecht RF 2nd, Wass CT, Lanier WL (1998) Occurrence of potentially detrimental temperature alterations in hospitalized patients at risk for brain injury. Mayo Clin Proc 73:629–635
4. Alderson P, Roberts I (1997) Corticosteroids in acute traumatic brain injury: systematic review of randomised controlled trials. BMJ 314:1855–1859
5. Aldrete JA, Romo-Salas F, Mazzia VD, Tan SL (1981) Phenytoin for brain resuscitation after cardiac arrest: an uncontrolled clinical trial. Crit Care Med 9:474–477
6. Alfonsi G, Gilberston L, Safar P, Stezoski W, Bircher N (1982) Cold water drowning and resuscitation in dogs. Anesthesiology 57:A80
7. Angelos M, Safar P, Reich H (1991) External cardiopulmonary resuscitation preserves brain viability after prolonged cardiac arrest in dogs. Am J Emerg Med 9:436–443
8. Anker AL, Santora T, Spivey W (1995) Artificial surfactant administration in an animal model of near drowning. Acad Emerg Med 2:204–210
9. Antretter H, Dapunt OE, Mueller LC (1994) Portable cardiopulmonary bypass: resuscitation from prolonged ice-water submersion and asystole. Ann Thorac Surg 58:1786–1787
10. Ashwal S, Schneider S, Tomasi L, Thompson J (1990) Prognostic implications of hyperglycemia and reduced cerebral blood flow in childhood near-drowning. Neurology 40:820–823
11. Ashwal S, Cole DJ, Osborne TN, Pearce WJ (1994) Dual effects of L-NAME during transient focal cerebral ischemia in spontaneously hypertensive rats. Am J Physiol 267:H276–284
12. Astrup J, Skovsted P, Gjerris F, Sorensen HR (1981) Increase in extracellular potassium in the brain during circulatory arrest: effects of hypothermia, lidocaine, and thiopental. Anesthesiology 55:256–2562
13. Auer RN, Wieloch T, Olsson Y, Siesjö BK (1984) The distribution of hypoglycemic brain damage. Acta Neuropathol 64:177–191
14. Banik NL, Matzelle D, Gantt-Wilford G, Hogan EL (1997) Role of calpain and its inhibitors in tissue degeneration and neuroprotection in spinal cord injury. Ann NY Acad Sci 825:120–127
15. Bareyre F, Wahl F, McIntosh TK, Stutzmann JM (1997) Time course of cerebral edema after traumatic brain injury in rats: effects of riluzole and mannitol. J Neurotrauma 14:839–849
16. Barone FC, Feuerstein GZ (1999) Inflammatory mediators and stroke: new opportunities for novel therapeutics. J Cereb Blood Flow Metab 19:819–834
17. Bayir H, Kagan VE, Tyurina YY, Tyurin VA, Ruppel RA, Adelson PD, Graham SH, Janesko K, Clark RSB, Kochanek PM (2002) Therapeutic hypothermia preserves antioxidant defenses after traumatic brain injury in infants and children. J Neurotrauma 19:1343
18. Behringer W, Prueckner S, Kentner R, Safar P, Radovsky A, Stezoski W, Wu X, Henchir J, Tisherman SA (1999) Exploration of pharmacologic aortic arch flush strategies for rapid induction of suspended animation (SA) (cerebral preservation) during exsanguination cardiac arrest (ExCA) of 20 min in dogs. Crit Care Med 27:A65
19. Behringer W, Prueckner S, Kentner R, Tisherman SA, Radovsky A, Clark R, Stezoski SW, Henchir J, Klein E, Safar P (2000) Rapid hypothermic aortic flush can achieve survival without brain damage after 30 minutes cardiac arrest in dogs. Anesthesiology 93:1491–1499

20. Behringer W, Prueckner S, Safar P, Radovsky A, Kentner R, Stezoski SW, Henchir J, Tisherman SA (2000) Rapid induction of mild cerebral hypothermia by cold aortic flush achieves normal recovery in a dog outcome model with 20-minute exsanguination cardiac arrest. Acad Emerg Med 7:1341–1348

21. Behringer W, Safar P, Kentner R, Wu X, Kagan VE, Radovsky A, Clark RS, Kochanek PM, Subramanian M, Tyurin VA, Tyurina YY, Tisherman SA (2002) Antioxidant Tempol enhances hypothermic cerebral preservation during prolonged cardiac arrest in dogs. J Cereb Blood Flow Metab 22:105–117

22. Behringer W, Safar P, Wu X, Nozari A, Abdullah A, Stezoski SW, Tisherman SA (2002) Veno-venous extracorporeal blood shunt cooling to induce mild hypothermia in dog experiments and review of cooling methods. Resuscitation 54:89–98

23. Benson DW, Williams GR, Spencer FC, et al. (1959) The use of hypothermia after cardiac arrest. Anesth Analg 38:423–428

24. Berek K, Lechleitner P, Luef G, Felber S, Saltuari L, Schinnerl A, Traweger C, Dienstl F, Aichner F (1995) Early determination of neurological outcome after prehospital cardiopulmonary resuscitation. Stroke 26:543–549

25. Bernard S, Buist M, Monteiro O, Smith K (2003) Induced hypothermia using large volume, ice-cold intravenous fluid in comatose survivors of out-of-hospital cardiac arrest: a preliminary report. Resuscitation 56:9–13

26. Bernard SA, Gray TW, Buist MD, Jones BM, Silvester W, Gutteridge G, Smith K (2002) Treatment of comatose survivors of out-of-hospital cardiac arrest with induced hypothermia. N Engl J Med 346(8):557–563

27. Bierens JJ, van der Velde EA, van Berkel M, van Zanten JJ (1990) Submersion in The Netherlands: prognostic indicators and results of resuscitation. Ann Emerg Med 19:1390–1395

28. Biggart MJ, Bohn DJ (1990) Effect of hypothermia and cardiac arrest on outcome of near-drowning accidents in children. J Pediatr 117:179–183

29. Bircher N, Safar P (1985) Cerebral preservation during cardiopulmonary resuscitation. Crit Care Med 13:185–190

30. Bleyaert AL, Nemoto EM, Safar P, Stezoski SM, Mickell JJ, Moossy J, Rao GR (1978) Thiopental amelioration of brain damage after global ischemia in monkeys. Anesthesiology 49:390–398

31. Bohn DJ, Biggar WD, Smith CR, Conn AW, Barker GA (1986) Influence of hypothermia, barbiturate therapy, and intracranial pressure monitoring on morbidity and mortality after near-drowning. Crit Care Med 14:529–534

32. Bolte R, Black P, Bowers R, Thorne K, Corneli H (1988) The use of extracorporeal rewarming in a child submerged for 66 minutes. JAMA 260:377–379

33. Bolton SJ, Perry VH (1998) Differential blood-brain barrier breakdown and leucocyte recruitment following excitotoxic lesions in juvenile and adult rats. Exp Neurol 154:231–240

34. Boxer PA, Cordon JJ, Mann ME, Rodolosi LC, Vartanian MG, Rock DM, Taylor CP, Marcoux FW (1990) Comparison of phenytoin with noncompetitive N-methyl-D-aspartate antagonists in a model of focal brain ischemia in rat. Stroke 21:III47–51

35. Bracken MB, Shepard MJ, Collins WF, Holford TR, Young W, Baskin DS, Eisenberg HM, Flamm E, Leo-Summers L, Maroon J, et al. (1990) A randomized, controlled trial of methylprednisolone or naloxone in the treatment of acute spinal-cord injury. Results of the Second National Acute Spinal Cord Injury Study. N Engl J Med 322:1405–1411

36. Bracken MB, Holford TR, Leo-Summers L, Aldrich EF, Fazl M (1997) Administration of methylpredonisolone for 24 or 48 h or trilazad mesylate for 48 h in the treatment of acute spinal cord injury. 277:1597-1-604

37. Bradley T, Dixon J, Easthope R (1999) Unexplained fainting, near drowning and unusual seizures in childhood: screening for long QT syndrome in New Zealand families. N Z Med J 112:299–302

38. Brain Resuscitation Clinical Trial I Study Group (1986) Randomized clinical study of thiopental loading in comatose survivors of cardiac arrest. N Engl J Med 314:397–403

39. Brain Resuscitation Clinical Trial II Study Group (1991) A randomized clinical study of a calcium-entry blocker (lidoflazine) in the treatment of comatose survivors of cardiac arrest. N Engl J Med 324:1225–1231

40. Brambrink AM, Martin LJ, Hanley DF, Becker KJ, Koehler RC, Traystman RJ (1999) Effects of the AMPA receptor antagonist NBQX on outcome of newborn pigs after asphyxic cardiac arrest. J Cereb Blood Flow Metab 19:927–938
41. Brown JI, Baker AJ, Konasiewicz SJ, Moulton RJ (1998) Clinical significance of CSF glutamate concentrations following severe traumatic brain injury in humans. J Neurotrauma 15:253–263
42. Bullock R, Chesnut RM, Clifton G, Ghajar J, Marion DW, Narayan RK, Newell DW, Pitts LH, Rosner MJ, Wilberger JW (1996) Guidelines for the management of severe head injury. Brain Trauma Foundation. Eur J Emerg Med 3:109–127
43. Busto R, Dietrich WD, Globus MYT, Valdés I, Scheinberg P, Ginsberg MD (1987) Small differences in intraischemic brain temperature critically determine the extent of neuronal injury. J Cereb Blood Flow Metab 7:729–738
44. Busto R, Globus MY, Dietrich WD, Martinez E, Valdes I, Ginsberg MD (1989) Effect of mild hypothermia on ischemia-induced release of neurotransmitters and free fatty acids in rat brain. Stroke 20:904–910
45. Buunk G, van der Hoeven JG, Meinders AE (1998) A comparison of near-infrared spectroscopy and jugular bulb oximetry in comatose patients resuscitated from a cardiac arrest. Anaesthesia 53:13–19
46. Calderwood H, Modell J, Ruiz B (1975) The ineffectiveness of steroid therapy for treatment of fresh water near-drowning. Anesthesiology 43:642–650
47. Capone A, Safar P, Radovsky A, Wang YF, Peitzman A, Tisherman SA (1996) Complete recovery after normothermic hemorrhagic shock and profound hypothermic circulatory arrest of 60 minutes in dogs. J Trauma 40:388–395
48. Cerchiari EL, Hoel TM, Safar P, Sclabassi RJ (1987) Protective effects of combined superoxide dismutase and deferoxamine on recovery of cerebral blood flow and function after cardiac arrest in dogs. Stroke 18:869–878
49. Cerchiari EL, Sclabassi RJ, Safar P, Hoel TM (1990) Effects of combined superoxide dismutase and deferoxamine on recovery of brainstem auditory evoked potentials and EEG after asphyxial cardiac arrest in dogs. Resuscitation 19:25–40
50. Colbourne F, Corbett D (1995) Delayed postischemic hypothermia: A six month survival study using behavioral and histologic assessments of neuroprotection. J Neurosci 15:7250–7260
51. Conn AW, Edmonds JF, Barker GA (1978) Near-drowning in cold fresh water: current treatment regimen. Can Anaesth Soc J 25:259–265
52. Conn AW (1979) Near-drowning and hypothermia. Can Med Assoc J 120:397–400
53. Conn AW, Edmonds JE, Barker GA (1979) Cerebral resuscitation in near drowning. Pediatr Clin North Am 26:691
54. Conn AW, Edmonds JF, Barker GA (1979) Cerebral resuscitation in near-drowning. Pediatr Clin North Am 26:691–701
55. Cordey R, Chiolero R, Miller JA (1973) Resuscitation of neonates by hypothermia: report on 20 cases with acid-base determination on 10 cases and the long-term development of 33 cases. Resuscitation 2:169–181
56. Crumrine RC, Bergstrand K, Cooper AT, Faison WL, Cooper BR (1997) Lamotrigine protects hippocampal CA1 neurons from ischemic damage after cardiac arrest. Stroke 28:2230–2236; discussion 37
57. Csuka E, Morganti-Kossmann MC, Lenzlinger PM, Joller H, Trentz O, Kossman T (1999) IL-10 levles in cerebrospinal fluid and serum of patients with severe traumatic brain injury: relationship to IL-6, TNF-alpha, TGF-beta1 and blood-brain barrier function. J Neuroimmunol 101:211–221
58. Daniel SS, Dawes GS, James LS, Ross BB, Windle WF (1966) Hypothermia and the resuscitation of asphyxiated fetal rhesus monkeys. J Pediatr 68:45–53
59. Danzl D, Pozos R (1994) Accidental hypothermia. N Engl J Med 1756–1760
60. Davis SM, Albers GW, Diener HC, Lees KR, Norris J (1997) Termination of Acute Stroke Studies Involving Selfotel Treatment. ASSIST Steering Committee. Lancet 349:32
61. Davis SM, Lees KR, Albers GW, Diener HC, Markabi S, Karlsson G, Norris J (2000) Selfotel in acute ischemic stroke : possible neurotoxic effects of an NMDA antagonist. Stroke 31:347–354
62. Di Napoli M (2002) C-reactive protein in ischemic stroke. An independent prognostic factor. Stroke 32:917–924

63. Dietrich WD, Busto R, Valdes I, Loor Y (1990) Effects of normothermic versus mild hyperthermic forebrain ischemia in rats. Stroke 21:1318–1325
64. Dietrich WD, Busto R, Alonso O, Globus MY, Ginsberg MD (1993) Intraischemic but not postischemic brain hypothermia protects chronically following global forebrain ischemia in rats. J Cereb Blood Flow Metab 13:541–549
65. Dottorini M, Eslami A, Baglioni S, Fiorenzano G, Todisco T (1996) Nasal-continuous positive pressure in the treatment of near-drowning in freshwater. Chest 110:1122–1124
66. Drummond JC, Todd MM, Schubert A, Sang H (1987) Effect of the acute administration of high dose pentobarbital on human brain stem auditory and median nerve somatosensory evoked responses. Neurosurgery 20:830–835
67. Dunn JM, Miller JA (1969) Hypothermia combined with positive pressure ventilation in resuscitation of the asphyxiated neonate. Clinical observations in 28 infants. Am J Obstet Gynecol 104:58–67
68. Ebmeyer U, Safar P, Radovsky A, Xiao F, Capone A, Tanigawa K, Stezoski SW (2000) Thiopental combination treatments for cerebral resuscitation after prolonged cardiac arrest in dogs. Exploratory outcome study. Resuscitation 45:119–131
69. Eisenburger P, Safar P (1999) Life supporting first aid training of the public–review and recommendations. Resuscitation 41:3–18
70. Emergency Cardiac Care Committee and Subcommittees (1992) American Heart Association: Guidelines for cardiopulmonary resuscitation and emergency cardiac care. JAMA 268:2172–2180
71. Evans DE, Kobrine AI, LeGrys DC, Bradley ME (1984) Protective effect of lidocaine in acute cerebral ischemia induced by air embolism. J Neurosurg 60:257–263
72. Fujitani T, Adachi N, Miyazaki H, Liu K, Nakamura Y, Kataoka K, Arai T (1994) Lidocaine protects hippocampal neurons against ischemic damage by preventing increase of extracellular excitatory amino acids: a microdialysis study in Mongolian gerbils. Neurosci Lett 179:91–94
73. Fukuda S, Harada K, Kunimatsu M, Sakabe T, Yoshida K (1998) Postischemic reperfusion induces alpha-fodrin proteolysis by m-calpain in the synaptosome and nucleus in rat brain. J Neurochem 70:2526–2532
74. Gelmers HJ, Gorter K, Weerdt CJ de, Wiezer HJ (1988) A controlled trial of nimodipine in acute ischemic stroke. N Engl J Med 318:203–207
75. Germann P, Poschl G, Leitner C, Urak G, Ullrich R, Faryniak B, Roder G, Kaider A, Sladen R (1998) Additive effect of nitric oxide inhalation on the oxygenation benefit of the prone position in the adult respiratory distress syndrome. Anesthesiology 89:1401–1406
76. Gilbert M, Busund R, Skagseth A, Nilsen PA, Solbo JP (2000) Resuscitation from accidental hypothermia of 13.7 degrees C with circulatory arrest [letter]. Lancet 355:375–376
77. Ginsberg MD, Sternau LL, Globus MT, Dietrich WD, Busto R (1992) Therapeutic modulation of brain temperature – relevance to ischemic brain injury. Cerebrovasc Brain Metab Rev 4:189–225
78. Gisvold SE, Safar P, Hendrickx HH, Rao G, Moossy J, Alexander H (1984) Thiopental treatment after global brain ischemia in pigtailed monkeys. Anesthesiology 60:88–96
79. Gisvold SE, Safar P, Rao G, Moossy J, Kelsey S, Alexander H (1984) Multifaceted therapy after global brain ischemia in monkeys. Stroke 15:803–812
80. Goh SH, Low BY (1999) Drowning and near-drowning – some lessons learnt. Ann Acad Med Singapore 28:183–188
81. Grotta J (1997) Lubeluzole treatment of acute ischemic stroke. The US and Canadian Lubeluzole Ischemic Stroke Study Group. Stroke 28:2338–2346
82. Gunn AJ, Gunn TR, Haan HH de, Williams CE, Gluckman PD (1997) Dramatic neuronal rescue with prolonged selective head cooling after ischemia in fetal lambs. J Clin Invest 99:248–256
83. Gunn AJ, Gunn TR, Ginning MJ, Williams CE, Gluckman PD (1998) Neuroprotection with prolonged head cooling started before postichemic seizures in fetal sheep. Pediatrics 102:1098–1106
84. Gunn AJ (2000) Cerebral hypothermia for prevention of brain injury following perinatal asphyxia. Curr Opin Pediatr 12:111–115
85. Haley EC Jr, Kassell NF, Apperson-Hansen C, Maile MH, Alves WM (1997) A randomized, double-blind, vehicle-controlled trial of tirilazad mesylate in patients with aneurysmal subarachnoid hemorrhage: a cooperative study in North America. J Neurosurg 86:467–474

86. Harries M (1981) Drowning in man. Crit Care Med 9:407–408
87. Harris RJ, Wieloch T, Symon L, Siesjo BK (1984) Cerebral extracellular calcium activity in severe hypoglycemia: relation to extracellular potassium and energy state. J Cereb Blood Flow Metab 4:187–193
88. Haseldonckx M, Van Reempts J, Van de Ven M, Wouters L, Borgers M (1997) Protection with lubeluzole against delayed ischemic brain damage in rats. A quantitative histopathologic study. Stroke 28:428–432
89. Hayward JS, Hay C, Matthews BR, Overweel CH, Radford DD (1984) Temperature effect on the human dive response in relation to cold water near-drowning. J Appl Physiol 56:202–206
90. Hermann DM, Mies G, Hossmann KA (1999) Expression of C-fos, JUNB, C-JUN, MKP-1 and HSP72 following traumatic neocortical lesions in rats – relation to spreading depression. Neuroscience 88:599–608
91. Hickey RW, Ferimer H, Alexander HL, Garman RH, Callaway CW, Hicks S, Safar P, Graham SH, Kochanek PM (2000) Delayed, spontaneous hypothermia reduces neuronal damage after asphyxial cardiac arrest in rats. Crit Care Med 28:3511–3516
92. Hickey RW, Kochanek PM, Ferimer H, Graham SH, Safar P (2000) Hypothermia and hyperthermia in children after resuscitation from cardiac arrest. Pediatrics 106:118–122
93. Hoffman WE, Pelligrino D, Werner C, Kochs E, Albrecht RF, Schulte am Esch J (1992) Ketamine decreases plasma catecholamines and improves outcome from incomplete cerebral ischemia in rats. Anesthesiology 76:755–762
94. Hossmann KA (1988) Resuscitation potentials after prolonged global cerebral ischemia in cats. Crit Care Med 16:964–971
95. Huckabee HC, Craig PL, Williams JM (1996) Near drowning in frigid water: a case study of a 31-year-old woman. J Int Neuropsychol Soc 2:256–260
96. Hudome S, Palmer C, Roberts RL, Mauger D, Housman C, Towfighi J (1997) The role of neutrophils in the production of hypoxic-ischemic brain injury in the neonatal rat. Pediatr Res 41:607–616
97. Hugenholtz H (2003) Methylprednisolone for acute spinal cord injury: not a standard of care. CMAJ 168:1145–1146
98. Iida K, Satoh H, Arita K, Nakahara T, Kurisu K, Ohtani M (1997) Delayed hyperemia causing intracranial hypertension after cardiopulmonary resuscitation. Crit Care Med 25:971–976
99. Ingebrigtsen T, et al. (1999) Traumatic brain damage in minor head injury: relation of serum S-100 protein measurements to magnetic resonance imaging and neurobehavioral outcome. Neurosurgery 45:468–475
100. Jordan KG (1999) Nonconvulsive status epilepticus in acute brain injury. J Clin Neurophysiol 16:332–340; discussion 53
101. Jordan KG (1999) Continuous EEG monitoring in the neuroscience intensive care unit and emergency department. J Clin Neurophysiol 16:14–39
102. Kaplan M, Eidelman AI (1984) Improved prognosis in severely hypothermic newborn infants treated by rapid rewarming. J Pediatr 105:470–474
103. Kassell NF, Haley EC Jr, Apperson-Hansen C, Alves WM (1996) Randomized, double-blind, vehicle-controlled trial of tirilazad mesylate in patients with aneurysmal subarachnoid hemorrhage: a cooperative study in Europe, Australia, and New Zealand. J Neurosurg 84:221–228
104. Katz L, Ebmeyer U, Safar P, Radovsky A, Neumar R (1995) Outcome model of asphyxial cardiac arrest in rats. J Cereb Blood Flow Metab 15:1032–1039
105. Katz LM, Wang Y, Ebmeyer U, Radovsky A, Safar P (1998) Glucose plus insulin infusion improves cerebral outcome after asphyxial cardiac arrest. Neuroreport 9:3363–3367
106. Kilminster S, et al. (1999) Neuropsychological change and S-100 protein release in 130 unselected patients undergoing cardiac surgery. Stroke 30:1869–1874
107. Kloeck W, Cummins R, Chamberlain D, Bossaert Lea (1997) Special resuscitation situations. An advisory statement from the International Liaison Committee on Resuscitation. Circulation 95:2196–2210
108. Kochs E, Hoffman WE, Werner C, Thomas C, Albrecht RF, Schulte am Esch J (1992) The effects of propofol on brain electrical activity, neurologic outcome, and neuronal damage following incomplete ischemia in rats. Anesthesiology 76:245–252

109. Kossman T, Stahel PF, Morganti-Kossmann MC, Jones JL, Barnum SR (1997) Elevated levels of the complement components C# and factor B in ventricular cerebrospinal fluid of patients with traumatic brain injury. J Neuroimmunol 73:63–69
110. Kostulas N, et al. (1999) Increased IL-1beta, IL-8 and IL17 mRNA expression in blood mononuclear cells observed in a prospective ischemic stroke study. Stroke 30:2174–2179
111. Kristoffersen MB, Rattenborg CC, Holaday DA (1967) Asphyxial death: the roles of acute anoxia, hypercarbia and acidosis. Anesthesiology 28:488–497
112. Kuboyama K, Safar P, Radovsky A, Tisherman SA, Stezoski SW, Alexander H (1993) Delay in cooling negates the beneficial effect of mild resuscitative cerebral hypothermia after cardiac arrest in dogs: a prospective, randomized study. Crit Care Med 21:1348–1358
113. Kuluz JW, Prado R, Chang J, Ginsberg MD, Schleien CL, Busto R (1993) Selective brain cooling increases cortical cerebral blood flow in rats. Am J Physiol 265:H824–827
114. Kurimura M, Shirai H, Takada K, Manaka H, Kato T (1997) An increase in cerebrospinal fluid ubiquitin in human global brain ischemia – a prognostic marker for anoxic-ischemic encephalopathy. Rinsho Shinkeigaku 37:963–968
115. Kyriacou D, Arcinue E, Peek C, Kraus J (1994) Effect of immediate resuscitation on children with submersion injury. Pediatrics 94:137–142
116. Lacomblez L, Bensimon G, Leigh PN, Guillet P, Meininger V (1996) Dose-ranging study of riluzole in amyotrophic lateral sclerosis. Amyotrophic Lateral Sclerosis/Riluzole Study Group II. Lancet 347:1425–1431
117. Lanier WL, Stangland KJ, Scheithauer BW, Milde JH, Michenfelder JD (1987) The effects of dextrose infusion and head position on neurologic outcome after complete cerebral ischemia in primates: examination of a model. Anesthesiology 66:39–48
118. Laskowitz DT, Goel S, Bennet ER, Matthew WD (1997) Apolipoprotein E suppresses glial secretion of TNFα. J Neuroimmunol 76:70–74
119. Lavelle J, Shaw K (1993) Near-drowning: Is emergency department cardiopulmonary resuscitation or intensive care unit cerebral resuscitation indicated? Crit Care Med 21:368–373
120. Lees KR (1997) Cerestat and other NMDA antagonists in ischemic stroke. Neurology 49: S66–69
121. Leonov Y, Sterz F, Safar P, Radovsky A, Oku K, Tisherman S, Stezoski SW (1990) Mild cerebral hypothermia during and after cardiac arrest improves neurologic outcome in dogs. J Cereb Blood Flow Metab 10:57–70
122. Levin DL (1980) Near-drowning. Crit Care Med 8:590–595
123. Liu X-H, Kwon D, Schielke GP, Yang G-Y, Silverstein FS, Barks JDE (1999) Mice deficient in interleukin-1 converting enzyme are resistant to neonatal hypoxic-ischemic brain damage. J Cereb Blood Flow Metab 19:1099–1108
124. Liu Y, Rosenthal RE, Haywood Y, Miljkovic-Lolic M, Vanderhoek JY, Fiskum G (1998) Normoxic ventilation after cardiac arrest reduces oxidation of brain lipids and improves neurological outcome. Stroke 29:1679–1686
125. Lopez-Pison J, Pineda-Ortiz I, Oteiza C, Loureiro B, Abenia P, Melendo J (1999) Survival with no sequelae after near-drowning with very poor signs for prognosis including persistent bilateral non-reactive mydriasis. Rev Neurol 28:388–390
126. Mackensen GB, Sato Y, Nellgard B, Pineda J, Newman MF, Warner DS, Grocott HP (2001) Cardiopulmonary bypass induces neurologic and neurocognitive dysfunction in the rat. Anesthesiology 95:1485–1491
127. Maiese K, TenBroeke M, Kue I (1997) Neuroprotection of lubeluzole is mediated through the signal transduction pathways of nitric oxide. J Neurochem 68:710–714
128. March N, Matthews R (1980) Feasibility study of CPR in the water. Undersea Biomed Res 7:141–148
129. Marion DW, Penrod LE, Kelsey SF, Obrist WD, Kochanek PM, Palmer AM, Wisniewski SR, DeKosky ST (1997) Treatment of traumatic brain injury with moderate hypothermia. N Engl J Med 336:540–546
130. Markgraf CG, Velayo NL, Johnson MP, McCarty DR, Medhi S, Koehl JR, Chmielewski PA, Linnik MD (1998) Six-hour window of opportunity for calpain inhibition in focal cerebral ischemia in rats. Stroke 29:152–158

131. Marler JR, Brott T, Broderick J, Kothari R, ODonoghue M, Barsan W, Tomsick T, Spilker J, Miller R, Sauerbeck L, et al. (1995) Tissue plasminogen activator for acute ischemic stroke. N Engl J Med 333:1581–1587
132. Marshall JWB, Duffin KJ, Green R, Ridley RM (2003) NXY-059, a free radical-trapping agent, substantially lessens the functional disability resulting from cerebral ischemia in a primate species. Stroke 32:190–198
133. Martens P, et al. (1998) Serum S-10 and neuron-specific enolase for prediction of regaining consciousness after global cerebral ischemia. Stroke 29:2363–2366
134. Martin T (1984) Near-drowning and cold water immersion. Ann Emerg Med 13:263–273
135. Matsumoto M, Iida Y, Wakamatsu H, Ohtake K, Nakakimura K, Xiong L, Sakabe T (1999) The effects of N(G)-nitro-L-arginine-methyl ester on neurologic and histopathologic outcome after transient spinal cord ischemia in rabbits. Anesth Analg 89:696–702
136. McArron MO, Muir KW, Weir CJ, Dyker AG, Bone I, Nicoll JA, Lees KR (1998) The apolipoprotein E epsilon-4 allele and outcome in cerebrovascular disease. Stroke 29:1882–1887
137. McBrien M, Katumba JJ, Mukhtar AI (1993) Artificial surfactant in the treatment of near drowning. Lancet 342:1485–1486
138. McClain C, Cohen D, Phillips R, Ott L, Young B (1991) Increased plasma and ventricular fluid interleukin-6 levels in patients with head injury. J Lab Clin Med 118:225–231
139. McKeating EG, et al. (1998) Relationship of neuron specific enolase and protein S-1000 concentrations in systemic and jugular venous serum to injury severity and outcome after traumatic brain injury. Acta Neurochir Suppl (Wien) 71:117–119
140. Melini CB, Kusakcioglu A, Kendall N (1969) Acute accidental hypothermia in a newborn infant: Case report. J Pediatr 74:960–962
141. Michaud L, Rivara F, Longstreth W, Grady M (1991) Elevated initial blood glucose levels and poor outcome following severe brain injuries in children. J Trauma 31:1356–1362
142. Mickell JJ, Reigel DH, Cook DR, Binda RE, Safar P (1977) Intracranial pressure: monitoring and normalization therapy in children. Pediatrics 59:606–613
143. Milde LN, Milde JH (1987) The detrimental effect of lidocaine on cerebral metabolism measured in dogs anesthetized with isoflurane. Anesthesiology 67:180–184
144. Miller B, Craddock L, Hoffenberg S, Heinz S, Lefkowitz D, Callender ML, Battaglia C, Maines C, Masick D (1995) Pilot study of intravenous magnesium sulfate in refractory cardiac arrest: safety data and recommendations for future studies. Resuscitation 30:3–14
145. Minamisawa H, Smith ML, Siesjö BK (1990) The effect of mild hyperthermia and hypothermia on brain damage following 5, 10, and 15 minutes of forebrain ischemia. Ann Neurol 28:26–33
146. Modell J, Moya F (1966) Effects of volume of aspirated fluid during chlorinated fresh water drowning. Anesthesiology 27:662–672
147. Modell J, Moya F, Newby E, Ruiz B, Showers A (1967) The effects of fluid volume in seawater drowning. Ann Int Med 67:68–80
148. Modell J, Davis J (1969) Electrolyte changes in human drowning victims. Anesthesiology 30:414–420
149. Modell J (1980) Drowning and near-drowning. Soc Crit Care Med-State of the Art F:10–38
150. Modell JH, Graves SA, Ketover A (1976) Clinical course of 91 consecutive near-drowning victims. Chest 70:231–238
151. Molano Mdel R, Broton JG, Bean JA, Calancie B (2002) Complications associated with the prophylactic use of methylprednisolone during surgical stabilization after spinal cord injury. J Neurosurg 96:267–272
152. Morganti-Kossmann MC, Hans VH, Lenzlinger PM, Dubs R, Ludwig E, Trentz O, Kossmann T (1999) TGF-beta is elevated in the CSF of patients with severe traumatic brain injuries and parallels blood-brain barrier function. Journal of Neurotrauma 16:617–628
153. Muir KW, Lees KR (1995) Clinical experience with excitatory amino acid antagonist drugs. Stroke 26:503–513
154. Muir KW, Lees KR (1995) A randomized, double-blind, placebo-controlled pilot trial of intravenous magnesium sulfate in acute stroke. Stroke 26:1183–1188

155. Muizelaar JP (1994) Clinical trials with Dismutec (pegorgotein; polyethylene glycol- conjugated superoxide dismutase; PEG-SOD) in the treatment of severe closed head injury. Adv Exp Med Biol 366:389–400
156. Natale JE, D'Alecy LG (1989) Protection from cerebral ischemia by brain cooling without reduced lactate accumulation in dogs. Stroke 20:770–777
157. Nelson DA, Nunneley SA (1998) Brain temperature and limits on transcranial cooling in humans: quantitative modeling results. Eur J Appl Physiol 78:353–359
158. Nemoto EM, Bleyaert AL, Stezoski SW, Moossy J, Rao GR, Safar P (1977) Global brain ischemia: a reproducible monkey model. Stroke 8:558–564
159. Norberg WJ, Agnew RF, Brunsvold R, Sivanna P, Browdie DA, Fisher D (1992) Successful resuscitation of a cold water submersion victim with the use of cardiopulmonary bypass. Crit Care Med 20:1355–1357
160. Nozari A, Safar P, Wu X, Stezoski SW, Tisherman S (2003) Intact survival in dogs after cardiac arrest (CA) of 40 min with mild hypothermia (34°C) during closed chest CPR: Myocardial and cerebral preservation. Crit Care Med Suppl 30:A121
161. Nugent SK, Rogers MC (1980) Resuscitation and intensive care monitoring following immersion hypothermia. J Trauma 20:814–815
162. Nussbaum E, Galant SP (1983) Intracranial pressure monitoring as a guide to prognosis in the nearly drowned, severely comatose child. J Pediatr 102:215–218
163. Nussbaum E, Maggi JC (1988) Pentobarbital therapy does not improve neurologic outcome in nearly drowned, flaccid-comatose children. Pediatrics 81:630–634
164. Oakes D, Sherck J, Maloney J (1982) Prognosis and management of victims of near-drowning. J Trauma 22:544–549
165. Oku K, Sterz F, Safar P, Johnson D, Obrist W, Leonov Y, Kuboyama K, Tisherman SA, Stezoski SW (1993) Mild hypothermia after cardiac arrest in dogs does not affect postarrest multifocal cerebral hypoperfusion. Stroke 24:1590–1597; discussion 98
166. Olney JW, Labruyere J, Price MT (1989) Pathological changes induced in cerebrocortical neurons by phencyclidine and related drugs. Science 244:1360–1362
167. Orlowski JP (1987) Drowning, near-drowning, and ice-water submersions. Pediatr Clin North Am 34:75–92
168. Orlowski JP, Abulleil MM, Phillips JM (1989) The hemodynamic and cardiovascular effects of near-drowning in hypotonic, isotonic, or hypertonic solutions. Ann Emerg Med 18:1044–1049
169. Ornato JP (1986) The resuscitation of near-drowning victims. JAMA 256:75–77
170. Pfenninger J, Sutter M (1982) Intensive care after fresh water immersion accidents in children. Anaesthesia 37:1157–1162
171. Pickard J, Murray G, Illingworth R, Shaw M, Teasdale G, Foy P, Humphrey P, Lang D, Nelson R, Richards P, Sinar J, Bailey S, Skene A (1989) Effect of oral nimodipine on cerebral infarction and outcome after subarachnoid haemorrhage: British aneurysm nimodipine trial. Br Med J 298:636–642
172. Pohl D, Bittigau P, Ishimaru MJ, Stadthaus D, Hubner C, Olney JW, Turski L, Ikonomidou C (1999) N-Methyl-D-aspartate antagonists and apoptotic cell death triggered by head trauma in developing rat brain. Proc Natl Acad Sci USA 96:2508–2513
173. Pollack M, Ruttimann U, Getson P (1988) Pediatric risk of mortality (PRISM) score. Crit Care Med 16:1110–1116
174. Poponick J, Renston J, Bennett R, Emerman C (1999) Use of ventilatory support system (BiPAP) for acute respiratory failure in the emergency department. Chest 116:166–171
175. Pulsinelli WA, Brierley JB, Plum F (1982) Temporal profile of neuronal damage in model of transient forebrain ischemia. Ann Neurol 11:491–498
176. Pulsinelli WA, Waldman S, Rawlinson D, Plum F (1982) Moderate hyperglycemia augments ischemic brain damage: a neuropathologic study in the rat. Neurology 32:1239–1246
177. Quan L, Gore EJ, Wentz K, Allen J, Novack AH (1989) Ten-year study of pediatric drownings and near-drownings in King County, Washington: lessons in injury prevention. Pediatrics 83:1035–1040
178. Quan L (1993) Drowning issues in resuscitation. Ann Emerg Med 22:366–369

179. Raabe A, Seifert V (1999) Fatal secondary increase in serum S-100B protein after severe head injury. Report of three cases. J Neurosurg 91:875–877
180. Radovsky A, Safar P, Sterz F, Leonov Y, Reich H, Kuboyama K (1995) Regional prevalence and distribution of ischemic neurons in dog brains 96 hours after cardiac arrest of 0 to 20 minutes. Stroke 26:2127–2133; discussion 33–34
181. Radovsky A, Katz L, Ebmeyer U, Safar P (1997) Ischemic neurons in rat brains after 6, 8, or 10 minutes of transient hypoxic ischemia. Toxicol Pathol 25:500–505
182. Ravitch M, Lane R, Safar P, Steichen F, Knowles P (1961) Lightning stroke. Report of case with recovery after cardiac massage and prolonged artificial respiration. N Engl J Med 264:36–38
183. Redding J, Voigt C, Safar P (1960) Treatment of seawater aspiration. J Appl Physiol 15:1113–1116
184. Redding J, Voigt GC, Safar P (1960) Drowning treated with intermittent positive pressure breathing. J Appl Physiol 15:849–854
185. Redding JS, Cozine RA (1961) Restoration of circulation after fresh water drowning. J Appl Physiol 16:1071–1074
186. Redding JS, Cozine RA, Voigt GC, Safar P (1961) Resuscitation from drowning. JAMA 178:1136–1139
187. Rice JE, Vannucci RC, Brierley JB (1981) The influence of immaturity on hypoxic-ischemic brain damage in the rat. Ann Neurol 9:131–141
188. Rockoff MA, Marshall LF, Shapiro HM (1979) High-dose barbiturate therapy in humans: a clinical review of 60 patients. Ann Neurol 6:194–199
189. Roine RO, Kaste M, Kinnunen A, Nikki P, Sarna S, Kajaste S (1990) Nimodipine after resuscitation from out-of-hospital ventricular fibrillation. A placebo-controlled, double-blind, randomized trial. JAMA 264:3171–3177
190. Rosen H, Rosengren L, Herlitz J, Blomstrand C (1998) Increased serum levels of the S-100 protein are associated with hypoxic brain damage after cardiac arrest. Stroke 29:473–427
191. Rosen P, Stoto M, Harley J (1995) The use of the Heimlich maneuver in near-drowning: Institute of Medicine Report. J Emerg Med 13:397–405
192. Rothman SM, Olney JW (1987) Excitotoxicity and the NMDA receptor. Trends Neurosci 10:299–302
193. Rutledge R, Flor J (1973) The use of mechanical ventilation with positive end-expiratory pressure in the treatment of near-drowning. Anesthesiology 38:194–196
194. Sachdeva R (1999) Near-drowning. Crit Care Med 15:281–296
195. Saeed D, Goetzman BW, Gospe SM (1993) Brain injury and protective effects of hypothermia using triphenyltetrazolium chloride in neonatal rat. Pediatr Neurol 9:263–267
196. Safar P, Escarraga L, Elam J (1958) A comparison of the mouth-to-mouth and mouth-to-airway methods of artificial respiration with the chest-pressure arm-lift methods. N Engl J Med 258:671–677
197. Safar P, Stezoski W, Nemoto EM (1976) Amelioration of brain damage after 12 minutes' cardiac arrest in dogs. Arch Neurol 33:91–95
198. Safar P (1985) Long-term animal outcome models for cardiopulmonary-cerebral resuscitation research. Crit Care Med 13:936–940
199 Safar P (1988) Resuscitation from clinical death: pathophysiologic limits and therapeutic potentials. Crit Care Med 16:923–941
200. Safar P, Abramson NS, Angelos M, Cantadore R, Leonov Y, Levine R, Pretto E, Reich H, Sterz F, Stezoski SW, et al. (1990) Emergency cardiopulmonary bypass for resuscitation from prolonged cardiac arrest. Am J Emerg Med 8:55–67
201. Safar P, Xiao F, Radovsky A, Tanigawa K, Ebmeyer U, Bircher N, Alexander H, Stezoski SW (1996) Improved cerebral resuscitation from cardiac arrest in dogs with mild hypothermia plus blood flow promotion. Stroke 27:105–113
202. Safar P, Kochanek P (2000) Cerebral blood flow promotion after prolonged cardiac arrest. Crit Care Med 28:3104–3106
203. Safar P, Tisherman SA (2002) Suspended animation for delayed resuscitation. Curr Opin Anesthesiol 203–210

204. Safar PJ, Kochanek PM (2002) Therapeutic hypothermia after cardiac arrest. N Engl J Med 346:612–613
205. Sasser HC, Safar P, Kelsey SF, Ricci EM, Sutton-Tyrrell KC, Wisniewski SR (1999) Arterial hypertension after cardiac arrest is associated with good cerebral outcome in patients. Crit Care Med 27: A29 (abstract)
206. Schoerkhuber W, Kittler H, Sterz F, Behringer W, Holzer M, Frossard M, Spitzauer S, Laggner AN (1999) Time course of serum neuron-specific enolase. A predictor of neurological outcome in patients resuscitated from cardiac arrest. Stroke 30:1598–1603
207. Schragl E, Pfisterer W, Reinprecht A, Donner A, Aloy A (1995) Behavior of cerebral blood flow velocity in conventional ventilation and superimposed high frequency jet ventilation. Anasthesiol Intensivmed Notfallmed Schmerzther 30:283–289
208. Schulz JB, Matthews RT, Jenkins BG, Brar P, Beal MF (1995) Improved therapeutic window for treatment of histotoxic hypoxia with a free radical spin trap. J Cereb Blood Flow Metab 15:948–952
209. Schwartz AC (1985) Neurological recovery after cardiac arrest: clinical feasibility trial of calcium blockers. Am J Emerg Med 3:1–10
210. Shapira Y, Lam AM, Eng CC, Laohaprasit V, Michel M (1994) Therapeutic time window and dose response of the beneficial effects of ketamine in experimental head injury. Stroke 25:1637–1643
211. Sheng H, Laskowitz DT, Bennett E, Schmechel DE, Bart RD, Saunders AM, Pearlstein RD, Roses AD, Warner DS (1998) Apolipoprotein E isoform-specific differences in outcome from focal ischemia in transgenic mice. J Cereb Blood Flow Metab 18:361–366
212. Sherman DG (1997) The enlimomab acute stroke trial: final results. Neurology 48:A270
213. Siebke H, Rod T, Breivik H, Link B (1975) Survival after 40 minutes; submersion without cerebral sequeae. Lancet 1:1275–1277
214. Siesjo BK, Katsura K, Zhao Q, Folbergrova J, Pahlmark K, Siesjo P, Smith ML (1995) Mechanisms of secondary brain damage in global and focal ischemia: a speculative synthesis. J Neurotrauma 12:943–956
215. Simonsen J (1983) Injuries sustained from high-velocity impact with water after jumps from high bridges. Am J For Med Path 4:139–142
216. Sirimanne ES, Blumberg RM, Bossano D, Gunning M, Edwards AD, Gluckman PD, Williams CE (1996) The effect of prolonged modification of cerebral temperature on outcome after hypoxic-ischemic brain injury in the infant rat. Pediatr Res 39:591–597
217. Sleigh JW, Havill JH, Frith R, Kersel D, Marsh N, Ulyatt D (1999) Somatosensory evoked potentials in severe traumatic brain injury: a blinded study. J Neurosurg 91:577–580
218. Smith ML, Bendek G, Dahlgren N, Rosen I, Wieloch T, Siesjo BK (1984) Models for studying long-term recovery following forebrain ischemia in the rat. 2. A 2-vessel occlusion model. Acta Neurol Scand 69:385–401
219. Smith-Swintosky VL, Pettigrew LC, Sapolsky RM, Phares C, Craddock SD, Brooke SM, Mattson MP (1996) Metyrapone, an inhibitor of glucocorticoid production, reduces brain injury induced by focal and global ischemia and seizures. J Cereb Blood Flow Metab 16:585–598
220. Snyder BD, Hauser WA, Loewenson RB, Leppik IE, Ramirez-Lassepas M, Gumnit RJ (1980) Neurologic prognosis after cardiopulmonary arrest: III. Seizure activity. Neurology 30:1292–1297
221. Steen PA, Gisvold SE, Milde JH, Newberg LA, Scheithauer BW, Lanier WL, Michenfelder JD (1985) Nimodipine improves outcome when given after complete cerebral ischemia in primates. Anesthesiology 62:406–414
222. Stein SC, et al. (2002) Intravascular coagulation: a major secondary insult in nonfatal traumatic brain injury. 97:1372–1377
223. Steingrub JS, Mundt DJ (1996) Blood glucose and neurologic outcome with global brain ischemia. Crit Care Med 24:802–806
224. Sterz F, Leonov Y, Safar P, Radovsky A, Tisherman SA, Oku K (1990) Hypertension with or without hemodilution after cardiac arrest in dogs. Stroke 21:1178–1184
225. Sterz F, Safar P, Tisherman S, Radovsky A, Kuboyama K, Oku K (1991) Mild hypothermic cardiopulmonary resuscitation improves outcome after prolonged cardiac arrest in dogs. Crit Care Med 19:379–389

226. Strittmatter W, Saunders A, Goedert M, Weisgraber K, Dong L-M, Jakes R, Hunag D, Pericak-Vance M, Schmechel D, Roses A (1994) Isoform-specific interactions of apolipoprotein E with microtubule-associated protein tau: implications for Alzheimer disease. Proc Natl Acad Sci 91:11183–11186

227. Swann H, Brucer M (1949) The cardiorespiratory and biochemical events during rapid anoxic death. Crit Care Med 169

228. Takasu A, Yagi K, Ishihara S, Okada Y (1995) Combined continuous monitoring of systemic and cerebral oxygen metabolism after cardiac arrest. Resuscitation 29:189–194

229. Tardiff BE, Newman MF, Saunders AM, Strittmatter WJ, White W, Blumenthal JA, Croughwell ND, Smith LR, Davis RD, Roses AD, Reves JG (1997) Preliminary report of a genetic basis for cognitive decline after cardiac operations. Ann Thorac Surg 64:715–720

230. Teasdale GM, Nicoll JAR, Murray G, Fiddes M (1997) Association of apolipoprotein E polymorphism with outcome after head injury. Lancet 350:1069–1071

231. The Acute Respiratory Distress Syndrome Network (2000) Ventilation with lower tidal volumes as compared with traditional tidal volumes for acute lung injury and the acute respiratory distress syndrome. N Engl J Med 342:1301–1308

232. The Hypothermia After Cardiac Arrest Study Group (2002) Mild therapeutic hypothermia to improve the neurologic outcome after cardiac arrest. N Engl J Med 346:549–556

233. Thel MC, Armstrong AL, McNulty SE, Califf RM, O'Connor CM (1997) Randomised trial of magnesium in in-hospital cardiac arrest. Duke Internal Medicine Housestaff. Lancet 350:1272–1276

234. Tisherman S, Chabal C, Safar P, Stezoski W (1985) Resuscitation of dogs from cold-water submersion using cardiopulmonary bypass. Ann Emerg Med 14:389–396

235. Tisherman SA, Safar P, Radovsky A, Peitzman A, Marrone G, Kuboyama K, Weinrauch V (1991) Profound hypothermia (less than 10 degrees C) compared with deep hypothermia (15 degrees C) improves neurologic outcome in dogs after two hours' circulatory arrest induced to enable resuscitative surgery. J Trauma 31:1051–1061; discussion 61–62

236. Towne AR, Waterhouse EJ, Boggs JG, Garnett LK, Brown AJ, Smith JR Jr, DeLorenzo RJ (2000) Prevalence of nonconvulsive status epilepticus in comatose patients. Neurology 54:340–345

237. Toyoda T, Kassell NF, Lee KS (1997) Attenuation of ischemia-reperfusion injury in the rat neocortex by the hydroxyl radical scavenger nicaraven. Neurosurgery 40:372–377; discussion 77–78

238. Tsirka SE, Gualandris A, Amaral DG, Strickland S (1995) Excitotoxin-induced neuronal degeneration and seizure are mediated by tissue plasminogen activator. Nature 377:340–344

239. Ullrich R, Lorber C, Roder G, Urak G, Faryniak B, Sladen RN, Germann P (1999) Controlled airway pressure therapy, nitric oxide inhalation, prone position, and extracorporeal membrane oxygenation (ECMO) as components of an integrated approach to ARDS. Anesthesiology 91:1577–1586

240. Vaagenes P, Cantadore R, Safar P, Moossy J, Rao G, Diven W, Alexander H, Stezoski W (1984) Amelioration of brain damage by lidoflazine after prolonged ventricular fibrillation cardiac arrest in dogs. Crit Care Med 12:846–855

241. Vaagenes P, Safar P, Moossy J, Rao G, Diven W, Cantadore R (1988) Differences in the effects of CNS treatments after ventricular fibrillation (VF) vs. asphyxiation (A) cardiac arrest (CA) in dog models. Crit Care Med 16:447

242. Vaagenes P, Safar P, Moossy J, Rao G, Diven W, Ravi C, Arfors K (1997) Asphyxiation versus ventricular fibrillation cardiac arrest in dogs. Differences in cerebral resuscitation effects – a preliminary study. Resuscitation 35:41–52

243. van den Berghe G, Wouters P, Weekers F, Verwaest C, Bruyninckx F, Schetz M, Vlasselaers D, Ferdinande P, Lauwers P, Bouillon R (2001) Intensive insulin therapy in the critically ill patients. N Engl J Med 345:1359–1367

244. Vavilala MS, et al. (2001) Coagulopathy predicts poor outcome following head injury in children less than 16 years of age. J Neurosurg Anesthesiol 13:13–18

245. Veinbergs I, Everson A, Sagara Y, Masliah E (2002) Neurotoxic effects of apolipoprotein E4 are mediated via dysregulation of calcium homeostasis. J Neurosci Res 67:379–387

246. Voll C, Auer R (1991) Insulin attenuates ischemic brain damage independent of its hypoglycemic effect. J Cereb Blood Flow Metabol 11:1006–1014

247. Wagner CL, Eicher DJ, Katikaneni LD, Barbosa E, Holden KR (1999) The use of hypothermia: a role in the treatment of neonatal asphyxia? Pediatr Neurol 21:429–443

248. Wakamatsu H, Matsumoto M, Nakakimura K, Sakabe T (1999) The effects of moderate hypothermia and intrathecal tetracaine on glutamate concentrations of intrathecal dialysate and neurologic and histopathologic outcome in transient spinal cord ischemia in rabbits. Anesth Analg 88:56–62
249. Warner DS, Gionet TX, Todd MM, McAllister A (1992) Insulin-induced normoglycemia improves ischemic outcome in hyperglycemic rats. Stroke 23:1775–1781
250. Wass CT, Scheithauer BW, Bronk JT, Wilson RM, Lanier WL (1996) Insulin treatment of corticosteroid-associated hyperglycemia and its effect on outcome after forebrain ischemia in rats. Anesthesiology 84:644–651
251. Waters DJ, Belz M, Lawse D, Ulstad D (1994) Portable cardiopulmonary bypass: resuscitation from prolonged ice-water submersion and asystole. Ann Thorac Surg 57:1018–1019
252. Weber ML, Taylor CP (1994) Damage from oxygen and glucose deprivation in hippocampal slices is prevented by tetrodotoxin, lidocaine and phenytoin without blockade of action potentials. Brain Res 664:167–177
253. Weber R, Kountzman B (1998) Extracorporeal membrane oxygenation for nonneonatal pulmonary and multiorgan failure. J Ped Surg 11:1605–1609
254. Weinrauch V, Safar P, Tisherman S, Kuboyama K, Radovsky A (1992) Beneficial effect of mild hypothermia and detrimental effect of deep hypothermia after cardiac arrest in dogs. Stroke 23:1454–1462
255. Wenisch C, Narzt E, Sessler DI, Parschalk B, Lenhardt R, Kurz A, Graninger W (1996) Mild intraoperative hypothermia reduces production of reactive oxygen intermediates by polymorphonuclear leukocytes. Anesth Analg 82:810–816
256. Werman H, Falcone R, Shaner S, Herron H, Johnson R ea (1999) Helicopter transport of patients to tertiary care centers after cardiac arrest. Am J Emerg Med 17:130–134
257. Whalen MJ, et al. (2000) Interleukin-8 is increased in cerebrospinal fluid of children with severe head injury. Crit Care Med 28:929–934
258. White RJ, Brown HW, Albin MS, Verdura J (1983) Rapid selective brain-cooling using head immersion and naso-oral perfusion in dogs. Resuscitation 10:189–191
259. Williams GD, Dardzinski bJ, Buckalew AR, Smith MB (1997) Modest hypothermia preserves cerebral energy metabolism during hypoxia-ischemia and correlates with brain damage: a ^{31}P Nuclear magnetic resonance study in unanesthetized neonatal rats. Pediatr Res 42:700–708
260. Wohns RN, Kerstein MD (1982) The role of dilantin in the prevention of pulmonary edema associated with cerebral hypoxia. Crit Care Med 10:436–443
261. Woiciechosky C, et al. (2002) Early IL-6 plasma concentrations correlate with severity of brain injury and pneumonia in brain-injured patients. J Trauma 52:339–345
262. Xiao F, Safar P, Radovsky A (1998) Mild protective and resuscitative hypothermia for asphyxial cardiac arrest in rats. Am J Emerg Med 16:17–25
263. Xu X, Tikuisis P, Giesbrecht G (1999) A mathematical model for human brain cooling during cold-water near-drowning. J Appl Physiol 86:265–272
264. Yagil Y, Stalnikowicz R, Michaeli J, Mogle P (1985) Near drowning in the dead sea. Electrolyte imbalances and therapeutic implications. Arch Intern Med 145:50–53
265. Yamamoto K, Ishikawa T, Sakabe T, Taguchi T, Kawai S, Marsala M (1998) The hydroxyl radical scavenger Nicaraven inhibits glutamate release after spinal injury in rats. Neuroreport 9:1655–1659
266. Yamasaki T, Nakakimura K, Matsumoto M, Xiong L, Ishikawa T, Sakabe T (1999) Effects of graded suppression of the EEG with propofol on the neurological outcome following incomplete cerebral ischaemia in rats. Eur J Anaesthesiol 16:320–329
267. Zandbergen EG, de Haan RJ, Stoutenbeek CP, Koelman JH, Hijdra A (1998) Systematic review of early prediction of poor outcome in anoxic-ischaemic coma. Lancet 352:1808–1812
268. Zhao Q, Pahlmark K, Smith ML, Siesjo BK (1994) Delayed treatment with the spin trap alphaphenyl-N-tert-butyl nitrone (PBN) reduces infarct size following transient middle cerebral artery occlusion in rats. Acta Physiol Scand 152:349–350
269. Zwemer CF, Whitesall SE, D'Alecy LG (1994) Cardiopulmonary-cerebral resuscitation with 100% oxygen exacerbates neurological dysfunction following nine minutes of normothermic cardiac arrest in dogs. Resuscitation 27:159–170
270. Zwemer CF, Whitesall SE, D'Alecy LG (1995) Hypoxic cardiopulmonary-cerebral resuscitation fails to improve neurologic outcome following cardiac arrest in dogs. Resuscitation 29:225–236

Immersion Hypothermia

Task Force on Immersion Hypothermia
Section editors: Beat Walpoth and Hein Daanen

Task Force Chairs

- Beat Walpoth
- Hein Daanen

Task Force Members

- Michel Ducharme
- Anton Fischer
- Gordon Giesbrecht
- Paul Husby
- Peter Tikuisis
- Michael Tipton
- Durk Zandstra

Other Contributors

- Wolfgang Baumeier
- Joost Bierens
- Marit Farstad
- Frank Golden
- Alan Steinman

9.1
Overview

Beat Walpoth and Hein Daanen

Humans are homeotherms. This implies that the temperature in the essential organs has to be maintained at a constant temperature. Therefore, heat production and heat loss have to be in equilibrium over a prolonged period. When heat loss exceeds heat production, the temperature in the body will drop below the normal value of 37°C and hypothermia occurs when the temperature falls below 35°C. Mild hypothermia is defined as core temperatures as low as 32°C, moderate hypothermia as core temperatures between 32 and 28°C and severe hypothermia as core temperatures below 28°C.

The occurrence of hypothermia is often related to the immersion in water. People can be immersed or submersed in water. Immersion means that a part of the body is exposed to water (head out, no asphyxia), as opposed to submersion (full body under water, asphyxia). Water has 25 times the thermal conductivity of air but only cools the body 4–5 times faster than the rate seen in air of the same temperature. Heat loss will exceed metabolic heat production in cold water below 25°C. Therefore, victims rescued from the water are often in a hypothermic condition. Severe hypothermia is life threatening and even mild hypothermia may be a complicating factor in drowning victims.

This section on immersion hypothermia includes several aspects of immersion hypothermia: from rescue to treatment and from cooling to rewarming strategies.

▶ **Chapter 9.2** summarises the consensus and recommendations of the task force on immersion hypothermia that were formulated during the World Congress on Drowning in short and easy to understand sentences.

Tipton and Golden address the physiology of cooling in ▶ **Chapter 9.3**. The responses observed on immersion in cold water and the hazards to be faced are directly related to the body tissues that are cooled. The skin, nerves, muscles, deep tissues and body core are cooled respectively.

In ▶ **Chapter 9.4** Tikuisis and Daanen proceed with body cooling and present a model to assess the core temperature after immersion in cold water. The Cold Exposure Survival Model (CESM) includes weather information such as water and air temperature, clothing information and individual information like body weight. The model is validated and a useful tool for instruction and assessment of the severity of an emergency situation.

In ▶ **Chapter 9.5** Michael Tipton and Michel Ducharme argue that rescue collapse is primarily due to cardiovascular rather than thermal problems. Victims who have been immersed or have stayed in a life raft for a long time, should be treated as potentially critical ill and removed from the water carefully and horizontally, but only as long as their airway is not under threat. They should be kept horizontal if possible and not have to assist in their own rescue. If the airway is under threat, the victim should be removed from the water as soon as possible.

Ducharme, Steinman and Giesbrecht compare current guidelines on pre-hospital rewarming with recent scientific insights on these topics in ▶ **Chapter 9.6**. Based on this information they compile a comprehensive list of guidelines for conscious and shivering casualties, unconscious and non-shivering casualties and casualties with cardiorespiratory arrest. One additional list with guidelines applies to all casualties.

Durk Zandstra gives an overview of rewarming methods in ▶ **Chapter 9.7**, focussing on methods that are available in hospital. He concludes that the treatment of accidental hypothermia in the hospital should preferably be realised via a hospital protocol. There are however no randomised controlled trials that definitively establish the most optimal rewarming strategy. Based on sound theoretical considerations, he advises active rewarming in any case where thermogenesis fails to increase central temperature at more than 0.5°C per hour. In patients with spontaneous circulation a combination of non-invasive rewarming methods may be used. The choice for the optimal rewarming strategy depends on clinical presentation.

Walpoth and Fisher discuss the treatment of patients with cardiorespiratory arrest in ▶ **Chapter 9.8**. They give the following topics for consideration:

- Submersion hypothermia is accompanied by various levels of asphyxia and thus shows many similarities with asphyxiated avalanche victims. Therefore, some of the reported data and clinical and laboratory indicators of avalanche victims can be applied to drowning victims.

- Clinical signs on rescue have been reported in mountain and drowning accidents and are a positive survival predictor in most cases. Some of these can go into secondary cardiac arrest called sheltering or rescue death, but if rescue and prehospital treatment are rapid and professional such patients have a good chance of recovery after cardiopulmonary bypass rewarming. In contrast, patients without vital signs on rescue can be fatally asphyxiated, especially when the measured temperature is above 30°C, indicating that some patients can be warm and dead
- Laboratory parameters may represent a help for the hospital clinician. Mainly potassium levels in excess of 10 mmol/l for adults and possibly higher for children have been associated with fatal outcomes.
- The reported extraordinary survival cases of prolonged, sub-ice immersion of children have seldom been duplicated for adult victims. Some possible explanations are the diving reflex in small children, the extremely fast cooling rate in cold water accentuated by the large body surface area of the head of children and the aspiration of cold water into the large surface area of the lungs. This can selectively cool the lungs, heart and brain by as much as 7°C in 2 minutes, giving immediate brain protection to the anoxic state (▶ Chapter 9.3).
- There is no doubt that the state-of-the-art method for rewarming deep hypothermic victims in cardiac arrest is cardiopulmonary bypass. Recently, debate on the speed of rewarming has occurred since most rapidly rewarmed patients during cardiopulmonary bypass (8–10°C) have shown severe pulmonary and probably severe brain oedema as compared to non-invasive warm air rewarming with rewarming rates of 2–3°C per hour. Prolongation of bypass rewarming will bring other disadvantages such as bleeding disorders, mediator and cytokine activation which in turn has been found to increase neuropsychological disorders and multi-organ failure. Thus, some experts feels that rewarming by cardiopulmonary bypass should be stopped at 34–35°C. This is supported by two recent reports published in the *New England Journal of Medicine* of positive effects of mild hypothermia in out-of hospital cardiac arrest patients.

Farstad and Husby address the issue of fluid management in ▶ Chapter 9.9. They include a recent review of the literature on the topic. Based on the current, still incomplete, knowledge they come with the following recommendations:

- Fluid supplementation should in general be administered rapidly enough in sufficient quantity to maintain adequate tissue perfusion without overloading the cardiovascular system. The underlying cardiac and renal functions determine how well fluid replacement will be tolerated. The rate of fluid administration must be based on the severity of hypovolaemia and the haemodynamic response to volume replacement.
- Haemodynamic parameters should be assessed regularly together with vital signs, diuresis and clinical data such as breath sounds, skin colour and temperature. Absolute values must be related to actual temperature. Definite limits are still undefined. Thermodilution catheters should be used with care as their introduction can precipitate cardiac arrhythmias. Central haemodynamics can alternatively be assessed by use of a PICCO system.

Durk Zandstra briefly addresses acid base management during hypothermia in ▶ **Chapter 9.10**. He argues that blood pH should not be the focus of control, but the combination of blood pH and $PaCO_2$, called alfa-stat control.

In ▶ **Chapter 9.11** several authors present their data on hypothermia or express the need for an international data registry. Large series of drowning victims do exist but very few prognostic factors on deep hypothermia from immersion or submersion have been reported. Thus, an international register to gather more information may be helpful.

9.2
Consensus and Recommendations

BEAT WALPOTH and HEIN DAANEN

The task force on immersion hypothermia met several times during the drowning conference and compiled a list of practical recommendations, based on research and experience. The recommendations are related to prevention, rescue and treatment.

9.2.1
Prevention

Prevention of hypothermia can be achieved by the awareness that water can cool the body rapidly. Rescuers should also be aware of this and have the means to prevent themselves from cooling. Insulation garments such as wet suits, dry suits and life jackets with a splash guard, should be worn during water activities. Without flotation aids, a victim generally drowns within minutes due to swimming failure in cold water. On immersion, any unnecessary movements should be avoided until breathing is under control and recovery from cold shock has occurred.

Manual tasks should be performed as soon as possible before self help capability is impaired. The victim should make efforts to get out of the water, even partially.

It should be realised that swimming in cold water is severely impaired and may increase heat loss. However, swimming should be considered if no other rescue options are available.

9.2.2
Rescue

When possible, the subject should be removed from the water in a horizontal position and remain supine, unless the airway is under threat, in which case speed is more important. Handling should be done with care to avoid rescue death and the victim should not be required to exercise. Anticipate that vomiting is common and try to prevent aspiration

If a casualty is rescued from ice water, attempts at resuscitation should be made even if the victim has been totally submerged for up to 1 hour. Particularly in children, death should not be assumed. The diagnosis of death should only be made in hospital.

For water rescued victims without life signs, the primary attention should go to restoration of vital signs by CPR. Temperature is a secondary issue. This means that when vital signs are stable, further heat loss should be minimised and the subject should be insulated using available means.

After checking vital signs, the following measures have to be taken:

- Cardiorespiratory arrest: immediate start of continuous CPR, including intubation, arrange medical assistance and transport to a hospital immediately
- Unconscious and non-shivering victims: provision of external rewarming, oxygen, warm IV fluids and medical assistance as soon as possible. Be careful of rescue death (minimise motion)
- Fully consciousness victims, shivering: this is a favourable situation, that nevertheless requires observation

9.2.3
Treatment

Rescuers have to take care that the patient is admitted to a hospital. Patients in deep hypothermia or cardiac arrest should be admitted to a hospital with cardiopulmonary bypass facilities, when possible.

Patients should be treated under intensive care conditions and core temperature should be measured properly. In cardio-respiratory arrest, when body temperature exceeds 32°C, reasons other than hypothermia should be looked for.

When brain damage is suspected, subjects should not be actively rewarmed to temperature values exceeding 32–34°C. If core temperature exceeds 34°C, hypothermia should be induced as soon as possible and maintained for 12–24 hours.

Cardiopulmonary bypass is the recommended rewarming method for severe hypothermia in patients with cardiac arrest or haemodynamic instability. Other active rewarming methods can be used in hypothermic victims with a stable cardiovascular system.

9.3
The Physiology of Cooling in Cold Water

MIKE TIPTON and FRANK GOLDEN

During immersion in cold water there is a very clear chronology with regard to cooling of the tissues of the body. Firstly, in head-out immersion, the skin is cooled, followed by cooling of the superficial nerves and musculature and finally of the deep tissues. The stages of immersion in cold water associated with particular risk, and first outlined by Golden [50], are directly related to the cooling of these tissues:

- Stage 1. Initial responses to immersion: skin cooling
- Stage 2. Short-term immersion: cooling of superficial nerves and muscle
- Stage 3. Long-term immersion: cooling of deep tissues
- Stage 4. Post-immersion: delayed effects of drowning, cooling of deep tissues, and haemodynamic changes during rescue

9.3.1
Skin and Lung Cooling

Due to its physical characteristics, cold water reduces the temperature of the skin much more quickly than exposure to air at the same temperature. The peripheral cold receptors have a superficial subepidermal location, 0.18–0.22 mm below the surface of the skin. Sudden falls in skin temperature on immersion in cold water produce a dynamic response in these receptors which, in turn, evokes the initial cardiovascular and respiratory responses seen on immersion, given the generic title of the cold shock response. The loss of control of respiration, increased blood pressure, increased work demand placed upon the heart and raised plasma catecholamine levels associated with the cold shock response are amongst the most hazardous of the responses associated with cold water immersion, and are often the precursors to drowning or cardiovascular problems.

Cooling of the face stimulates cold receptors around the nose, eyes, and mouth. These in turn can evoke the diving response comprising selective vasoconstriction, bradycardia and apnoea. This response, conserves oxygen and is the physiological means by which diving mammals extend their underwater time. The diving response is regarded to extend the underwater survival time in man. However, when evoked concurrently with the cold shock response during whole body immersion in humans, the consequent and concurrent sympathetic (cold shock) and parasympathetic (diving response) chronotropic inputs to the heart can, very frequently, produce both supraventricular and ventricular arrhythmias. In young, fit individuals these ECG abnormalities are asymptomatic, however in older and less fit individuals they may be the precursor to cardiac problems.

The diving response is weaker in man than in diving mammals, although it is generally stronger in children than adults. The response has been implicated in the survival of individuals, usually children, following prolonged submersion in cold water. However, a number of factors suggest that it may be rapid deep body cooling rather than the diving response that is responsible for the remarkable survival and recovery of these rare cases. These factors include: the length of the submersions (over 1 hour in one case); the majority are found to have aspirated water; the presence of cardiac arrest rather than bradycardia; and all have very low deep body temperatures. To extend the hypoxic survival time of the brain, its temperature must be reduced rapidly before it is irreversibly damaged. At normal body temperature (37°C), 10 min of acute cerebral hypoxia is associated with significant lasting cerebral damage. Brain cooling slows this process by reducing metabolism and thus the tissue oxygen requirements. A 7°C fall in brain temperature doubles hypoxic survival time, while below 22°C brain activity almost ceases and hypoxic survival time is extended considerably. The question is how are such rapid rates of cooling achieved before cerebral damage from hypoxia occurs?

Even in children with their high surface area to mass ratio, surface cooling alone during immersion in ice water, is not fast enough to reduce brain temperature sufficiently in 10 min to offer any significant cerebral protection from hypoxia. However, in submersion, there is the potential for a significant heat exchange via the airways and lungs as a result of water flushing in and out of them on initial submersion. This will be particularly so if there is an associated hyperventilation. The lung is the largest surface area a human has in contact with the environment, and cold water entering the lungs can selectively cool the heart and brain, as long as breathing and cardiac output continue. Authors have reported that respiratory movements continue for around 70 seconds following submersion. Others have reported 7.5–8.5°C falls in the temperature of blood flowing in the carotid artery during the first 2 min of submersion, with much smaller falls in temperature occurring subsequently. Mathematical modelling of the various routes of heat exchange, including respiratory heat loss, available following submersion, support the hypothesis that rapid falls in brain temperature can occur if cold water is taken into the lung and cools the cerebral circulation. The generalised vasoconstriction to the superficial tissues of the body, that occurs during immersion in cold water, can help in this regard by restricting the circulation to the lungs, heart and brain. Prolonged survival, and with it the potential for successful resuscitation, is therefore dependent on the brain temperature achieved by the time hypoxia becomes significant and when respiratory and cardiac functions cease. It is worth noting that, although these cases are fascinating, they represent a very small percentage of the overall immersion-related accidents, many of which have a much more depressing outcome.

9.3.2
Nerve and Muscle Cooling

In head-out immersion, cooling of the superficial nerves and muscles can result in rapid incapacitation, especially if water conditions are rough and no specialist protection, such as a lifejacket with a splash guard is worn. In nerve tissue below a local temperature of 20°C, the rate of conduction and amplitude of action potentials is slowed. For example the conduction velocity of the ulnar nerve falls by 15 meter/second/10°C fall in local temperature, and nerve block can occur at a temperature of 5–15°C for 1–15 min. The maximum power output of muscle falls by 3% per degree centigrade fall in muscle temperature, and below a muscle temperature of 27°C fatigue occurs earlier and force production is reduced. The reasons for this decreased muscle function include:
- Reduced enzyme activity
- Decreased acetylcholine and calcium release
- Slower rates of diffusion
- Decreased muscle perfusion

- Increased viscosity
- Rate of conduction and depolarisation of action potentials is slowed

The decrements in performance resulting from nerve and muscle cooling are observed first, and are most noticeable in the arms. The relatively small circumference, high surface area to mass ratio and exposure to the prevailing conditions make these particularly susceptible to cooling following immersion. Deep muscle in the forearm can cool to 27°C within about 20 min of immersion in water at 12°C.

As a result of these changes, the ability of an individual to undertake essential survival actions can be quickly impaired. Grip strength, manual dexterity, speed of movement, and swimming ability, all decline and may prevent rescue flares being fired, life rafts being boarded and lifejackets being properly deployed. The inability to swim or keep the back to the oncoming waves can result in drowning.

Survival may depend on the immersion casualty understanding that his or her physical abilities will quickly diminish following immersion in cold water, and undertaking essential survival actions as soon as possible. Legislators and designers of survival equipment should also recognise and understand these physiological limitations when considering their safety standards and design criteria.

9.3.3
Deep Tissue Cooling

In normal circumstances cooling of the deep tissues of the body and hypothermia will not represent a problem before about 30 min following immersion in cold water. Consistent with the vast majority of biological activity, cooling slows down and therefore impairs physiological function. Hypothermia affects cellular metabolism, blood flow and neural activation.

Progressive hypothermia can cause: confusion, disorientation, introversion, aggression (35°C), amnesia (34°C), cardiac arrhythmias (33°C), clouding of consciousness (33–30°C), loss of consciousness (30°C), ventricular fibrillation (28°C) and cardiac arrest (25°C). The figures in parenthesis represent deep body temperatures and should only be regarded as a very rough guide, as great variation exists between individuals. This variation is due to well-known factors such as level of internal and external insulation, fitness and gender, as well as a wide range of more subtle non-thermal factors, such as blood levels of sugar, oxygen and carbon dioxide. Drugs, including alcohol, can also influence the way the temperature regulation system functions and consequent cooling rates.

Below a deep body temperature of about 28°C the following may be observed:

- Decreased spontaneous depolarisation of pacemaker cells of the heart
- Fluid shifts out of the vascular space
- Renal function is depressed, decreased glomerular filtration, augmented osmotic diuresis; hypovolaemia and increased blood viscosity

- Hepatic metabolism is impaired
- Opening and closing of membrane channels is slowed
- Sodium channel conduction is decreased
- Potassium ion regulation is impaired
- Function of the brain stem is impaired
- Enzyme reaction times are reduced
- Gastrointestinal smooth muscle motility is decreased
- Cold-induced collapse of the microvasculature has occured
- Role of insulin-dependent glucose transport ceases

As can be seen from the foregoing, depending on conditions, consciousness can be lost some time before death. This emphasises the importance of wearing a good lifejacket that will support the airway clear of the water and prevent death by drowning at an early stage. Protection against hypothermia is provided primarily by immersion suits, liferafts and lifejackets. Additionally, because individuals cool 4–5 times faster in water compared to air at the same temperature, the buoyancy provided by upturned hulls, large pieces of driftwood and so on can offer the opportunity for the survivor to get partially, or completely, out of the water. Despite the fact that it often feels colder out of the water than in it, a survivor will always be better out of the water.

9.3.4
Conclusion

In conclusion, the responses observed on immersion in cold water and the hazards to be faced are directly related to the cooled body tissues. This is summa-

■ Table 9.1. Responses and hazards of immersion in cold water

Time period	Tissue cooled	Responses	Hazard
Initial	Skin	Initial cardiorespiratory responses	Drowning, cardiovascular problems
Short-term	Superficial nerves and muscles	Decreased: co-ordination, strength, dexterity, swimming ability	Physical incapacitation, drowning
Long-term	Deep body tissues	Hypothermia	Unconsciousness, drowning, cardiac problems. Collapse of arterial blood pressure

rised in ◘ **Table 9.1**, from which it becomes clear that the primary threat to be faced on immersion in cold water is drowning.

9.4
Body Cooling, Modelling and Risk Assessment

PETER TIKUISIS and HEIN DAANEN

This chapter describes a model that can be used to assess cooling times during cold water immersion.

As pointed out in the previous chapter, there are three phases of increasing incapacitation leading to lethality: initial, short-term and long-term. Upon immersion, a poorly insulated individual will first experience debilitating cold shock that can lead to involuntary inspiration of water and subsequent drowning [116]. This initial phase normally lasts a few minutes and subsides when the skin temperature plateaus just above water temperature. The individual that survives cold shock, or circumvents it because of adequate protection, is then at risk of failure of limb motor function due to the cooling of the joints and musculature [32, 64]. The rate of limb cooling is governed by the temperature difference between the water and the skin, and by any insulation between the two. This phase can last from 10–20 min for the average unprotected individual immersed in very cold water (0–10°C). If death occurs during the first two phases, the probable cause is drowning either through an involuntary excessive inspiration of water or due to a failure of the individual to initiate or maintain survival performance by swimming, grasping onto floating debris or climbing into a life-raft. The individual that survives these initial phases is then dependent on external devices such as personal flotation to maintain a head-out posture to avoid drowning. The risk to such individuals shifts to hypothermia.

◘ **Figure 9.1** shows the mean oesophageal and rectal temperatures of seven semi-naked individuals immersed in 15°C water for 2 hours [26]. The initial vasoconstriction creates a protective shell that causes a temporary rise in core temperature lasting several minutes, followed by a gradual decrease. This decrease can level off if the heat produced by shivering matches the rate of heat loss, in which case survival time depends on how long the elevated shivering rate can be sustained [115]. If the rate of heat loss can not be compensated, as will occur in very cold water, survival time is essentially determined by the time it takes to lethal hypothermia. The decrease in core temperature is the focus of the Cold Exposure Survival Model (CESM) developed at Defence Research and Development Canada (DRDC) [112, 113].

9.4.1
Model Description

CESM is based on steady state heat conduction in a cylindrical core-shell configuration. Heat is generated uniformly within the core region and the central

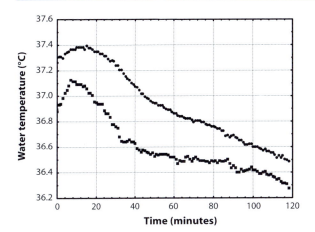

Fig. 9.1. Mean rectal (*circles*) and oesophageal (*squares*) temperatures of seven semi-nude individuals immersed in 15°C water for 2 hours

axis represents the deep body core temperature. Two outer concentric shells represent the fat plus skin and the clothing plus still boundary layer, respectively. The model is designed to predict body cooling for exposure to air only, water only, or a combination of the two. The water only condition assumes a head-out immersion, and this will be the assumed exposure in the present application of the model. A schematic of the model and the relevant heat transfer equations are outlined in two works by Tikuisis [112, 113].

The cold-exposed individual is also assumed to be sedentary (aside from any shivering activity) and therefore reliant on shivering as the only additional source of heat to resting values. Subject model inputs include gender, age, and basic anthropometric values of height, mass and body fatness. Environmental conditions include water temperature and sea state. Clothing options are listed under two separate menus. One menu involves a list of typical garments that can be selected in any combination, and the other list involves various ensembles having fixed insulation values based on the environmental conditions and level of wetness in the clothing. Greater detail on the availability and application of the model can be obtained from www.emssatcom.com/pdf/CESM.pdf.

9.4.2
Model Prediction

The primary model output is the predicted survival time based on deep body cooling to a temperature of 28°C, considered to represent the threshold of lethal hypothermia in most cases [113]. **Figure 9.2** shows the model prediction for an unprotected or essentially bare skinned individual immersed in rough water. In this example, predictions are shown for 35-year-old lean and fat males and females. Anthropometric values used for these predictions are based on the 25/75th percentiles of height and the 5/95th percentiles of mass of the general population. Corresponding body fatnesses based on regression are 14.3% (tall lean male), 19.0% (tall lean female), 28.1% (short fat male) and 32.3% (short fat female). Predictions

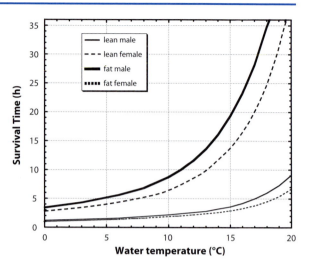

Fig. 9.2. Predicted times to lethal hypothermia for unprotected immersion in rough water for persons with different anthropometric values

beyond 36 hours of immersion are not provided because of increasing uncertainty of survival due to mitigating factors other than cold such as fluid balance.

▣ **Figure 9.3** shows the model prediction for unprotected 35-year-old anthropometrically-average males (19.3% body fatness) and females (23.4% body fatness) immersed in rough water. Predictions on the probability of being found alive are also superimposed on the figure. These probabilities are statistically derived from reported immersion incidents where the use of a buoyancy device was unknown and without specification on the cause of death in fatal cases [87]. The interpretation of these survival probabilities where they intersect the predicted survival times is the chance that the individual would not have died due to other causes such as drowning or an injury prior to lethal hypothermia.

9.4.3
Discussion

Drowning is likely responsible for most deaths in very cold water, as implied by the output of CESM. For example, while the average unprotected individual is predicted to survive lethal hypothermia from between 2.1 and 2.5 hours in 5°C rough water (▣ **Fig. 9.3**), the chance that they would still be alive at these times are 43% and 38%, respectively, suggesting that drowning precedes lethal hypothermia in more than 50% of cases under this condition. The survival probabilities are invariant to gender, unlike the predicted survival times. Despite having higher body fatness, females have lower predicted survival times due to hypothermia compared to males at similar anthropometric percentiles because of their higher surface area to body mass ratio, which enhances net heat loss. Increased body fatness, however, generally improves survival time, as demonstrated in ▣ **Fig. 9.2**.

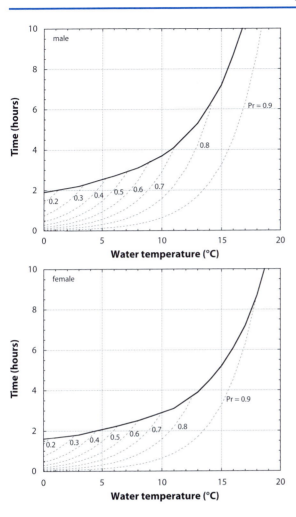

Fig. 9.3. Predicted times to lethal hypothermia (*solid line*) and probabilities (*Pr*) for being found alive during unprotected immersion in rough water for average males and females

9.4.4
Websites
— www.emssatcom.com/pdf/CESM.pdf

9.5
Rescue Collapse Following Cold Water Immersion

MICHAEL TIPTON and MICHEL DUCHARME

Approximately 20% of the immersion-related fatalities occur just before, during or shortly after rescue. The term circum rescue collapse has been applied to this phenomenon [52] (■ **Fig. 9.4**). Even survivors in lifeboats and life rafts, who have

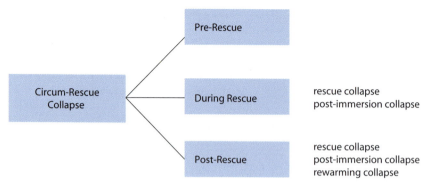

◘ Fig. 9.4. Circum-rescue collapse and associated terminology [52]

not been immersed, may collapse and die during rescue. A similar problem also appears to exist with those, such as avalanche victims, who are rescued after prolonged periods in cold environments.

9.5.1
Pre-Rescue Collapse

The mechanism causing pre-rescue collapse remains unclear, but the sudden deterioration in the condition of the survivors is suggestive of a cardiovascular mechanism. Catecholamines, particularly noradrenaline, have been shown to have a protective effect in hypothermia via the assistance they give to the maintenance of blood pressure. It is possible that the sense of relief engendered by imminent rescue results in a reduction in catecholamine secretion and the consequent withdrawal of their protective effect [51]. As a consequence, rescuers should encourage victims to continue to focus on their survival during and following rescue, and to be aware that the victims are still under threat. This mechanism can also play a significant role in rescue and post-rescue collapse.

9.5.2
Rescue Collapse

James Currie undertook the first reported cold water immersion experiments in 1798 [24]. Amongst other things, he noted a continued fall in deep body temperature following immersion, an afterdrop and the efficacy of hot bath rewarming. Following World War II the afterdrop was given as the mechanism for the deterioration in the condition of immersion victims during and following rescue. Originally, the term afterdrop was applied to the continued fall in rectal temperature observed when a cold casualty was transferred from cold to hot (40°C) water. The current accepted definition of afterdrop is a continued drop in core temperature following the cessation of a cold stress.

The cause of the afterdrop, still reported in some contemporary texts, was thought to be due to hot bath rewarming causing vasodilatation in the peripheral vasculature, and core blood perfusing cold tissue in the extremities, being cooled, and returning to cool the core (convective mechanism). This provided some of the rationale for leaving the limbs out of the water during bath rewarming. However, in 1981 Golden and Hervey proposed that the afterdrop during hot bath rewarming is mainly a conductive rather than convective phenomenon [50]. As a consequence, afterdrop is more pronounced at deep body temperature sites primarily dependent on conductive heat exchange (rectum) and not as much in sites where the temperature is primarily determined by blood flow (heart, brain). The fact that an afterdrop is not as pronounced in the heart suggests that the blood returning from the periphery during hot bath rewarming is unlikely to be a source of cold. Furthermore, it has been observed that perfusion of the extremities is re-established during rewarming only when the core temperature reaches a value above about 35°C. Consequently, the convective mass flow mechanism can hardly explain afterdrops observed below this value and is unlikely to be responsible for the rescue collapses observed in those with core temperatures below 35°C.

Another mechanism was therefore required to explain deaths during and immediately following rescue. The sudden deterioration in the condition of previously conscious subjects was too rapid and required too great a fall in deep body temperature to be caused by thermal changes. An alternative, cardiovascular mechanism, was proposed [50]. Head-out immersion can produce profound changes in cardiovascular, renal, and endocrine functions. These effects are a direct result of the high density of the water and the differential in hydrostatic pressure over the immersed body. A negative transthoracic pressure of about 14.7 mmHg is established which increases central blood volume by up to 700 ml very soon after immersion [75]. This is associated with enhanced diastolic filling, raised right atrial pressure and a 32%−66% increase in cardiac output, due entirely to an increase in stroke volume [93]. Most of the renal responses following immersion are due to the shift in blood volume, which the body senses as hypervolaemia. These responses include a significant diuresis within the first hour of cold water immersion [8]. A similar set of responses may also occur in those who have endured cold air environments with limited food and water supplies [51].

In these situations, circulatory collapse and cardiac arrest may occur during rescue as a result of a number of factors, including:
- Less venous return caused by loss of hydrostatic assistance and the re-imposition of the full effects of gravity on removal from the water
- Hypovolaemia caused by diuresis and inter-compartmental fluid shifts
- Increased blood viscosity as a result of cooling of blood
- Diminished work capacity of the hypothermic heart and reduced time for coronary filling
- Dulled baroreceptor reflexes
- Unattainable demands to perfuse skeletal muscle when asked to assist in the rescue
- Psychological stress
- Pre-existing coronary disease
- Possible reduction in catecholamine production

During rescue, assuming that the airway is not under threat, the greatest problems are likely to be encountered by those who are lifted vertically after prolonged immersion in a vertical position. The problems are likely to be potentiated by a requirement for activity by the casualty during rescue. Lifting casualties in a horizontal position is likely to be less traumatic and, with the inevitable proviso 'circumstances permitting', immersion victims should be handled with the utmost gentleness and as the potentially critically ill patients that they are. For the same reasons it is sensible to transport hypothermic casualties in a slightly head down attitude with the head towards the stern of a fast rescue craft and the front of a helicopter.

9.5.3
Post-Rescue Collapse

The most important cause of post-rescue collapse is hypoxia, secondary to the aspiration of water. Therefore, it is critical that, following rescue, a suitably qualified individual should check an immersion victim to determine whether water has been aspirated and if hospital screening is necessary. Anyone with extraneous sounds in the chest on auscultation, breathing difficulties or cyanosis should be admitted to hospital for X-ray and blood gas analysis to confirm or exclude aspiration.

A less common cause of post-rescue death is inappropriate rewarming, also referred to as rewarming collapse. Aggressive external rewarming of cold, hypovolaemic or dehydrated casualties can result in peripheral vasodilatation. An inability to compensate for the redistribution of blood flow in such casualties can result in the collapse of arterial blood pressure and poor coronary perfusion if no precaution is taken to maintain the systemic circulation. It is recommended that external rewarming as pre-hospital treatment of hypothermic victims should not be too aggressive and should be complemented by the injection of warm IV fluid and the provision of warm oxygen (see also the following chapter).

9.5.4
Conclusion

It is concluded that the rapid deterioration seen in cold casualties during rescue suggests mainly a cardiovascular rather than thermal problem. Therefore victims who are very cold or have been immersed or in a life raft for a long time, and whose airway is not under threat should be treated as potentially critically ill. If possible, they should be removed from the water carefully and horizontally, and kept horizontal. They should not have to assist in their rescue. However if the airway is under threat, the victim should be removed from the water as soon as possible.

9.6
Prehospital Management of Immersion Hypothermia

MICHEL DUCHARME, ALAN STEINMAN and GORDON GIESBRECHT

Establishing the proper prehospital treatment for hypothermic victims is a challenge because of two main factors: the value of field treatment is still open for debate and very few effective technologies are available. Lloyd [76] indicated that "hypothermia and its management are bedeviled by misunderstanding and dogmas...these dogmas may sometimes lead to inappropriate treatments". The main contributor to the misunderstanding and dogmas is the absence of randomised controlled trials to evaluate the efficacy, morbidity and mortality of various field or hospital rewarming methods [70], even though their value has been appreciated for some time. This can partially explain the large variability in the mortality rate of hypothermia casualties ranging between 12% and 100% depending on the treatment centre.

Valuable lessons can be learned, however, from successful cases of rewarming, particularly from a recent rewarming case of a young woman with a deep core temperature of 13.7°C and circulatory arrest [48]. Based on their experience with this case, the authors provided four key factors capable of improving the likelihood of survival from severe hypothermia: optimal mechanism of cooling (whole body cooling with subsequent circulatory arrest), rapid pre-hospital response, continuous CPR during transportation, and rapid extracorporeal blood rewarming during hospital treatment. Also a multi-year review of severe accidental hypothermia treatment, underlined short delay for rewarming after the accident and short rewarming time as key factors contributing to positive outcomes [124]. Proper early field management of hypothermia could significantly improve the likelihood of survival.

9.6.1
Current Guidelines on Prehospital Rewarming

For a long time, the classic approach to prehospital management of hypothermia victims has been summarised by four actions: rescue, examine, insulate, and transport [106]. Current guidelines remain ambiguous and non-uniform in their approach to prehospital management of hypothermia. The 2000 hypothermic guideline from the American Heart Association indicates that many experts believe that interventions to rewarm hypothermic victims should be limited to the hospital. The guidelines warn not to use external rewarming device for severe hypothermia in the field, although no specific reason is provided. The guidelines suggest the use of warm saline and warm oxygen instead, although those methods have very limited warming capabilities.

On the other hand, recently published guidelines in a textbook of wilderness emergency medicine [105] states that "After recovery of the victims from the water, and after management of immediate life threatening emergencies, the next objectives are prevention of further heat loss and efforts at moderate rewarming rates (1 to 2°C per hour)". The guidelines suggest the field use of active rewarming methods, applied primarily to the torso and neck, for moderate to severe hypothermia. Likewise, a recent review on emergency treatment of hypothermia in the wilderness suggests to warm hypothermic patients as soon as possible even in the case of severe hypothermia [45]. The practice of providing pre-hospital external warming to the torso has also recently been advocated in other medical standards including the State of Alaska Cold Injuries and Cold Water Near Drowning Guidelines [103], College of Physicians and Surgeons of Manitoba [22], and the Swedish military [20].

9.6.2
Rewarming Collapse

Early reports have linked external rewarming to rewarming collapse: an inability for a cold hypovolaemic and dehydrated casualty to compensate for the redistribution of blood flow during rewarming of the body. Application of external heat to moderate-to-severe hypothermic patient was considered hazardous because it could cause sudden peripheral vasodilatation and allow cold, acid-rich blood to return to the core and cause an afterdrop, a decrease in blood pressure and an increased likelihood of ventricular fibrillation. Although some afterdrop can be observed during rewarming, no clinical or experimental evidence can be found to support the peripheral vasodilatation theory during active warming of the skin [44] as long as deep core temperature does not increase above about 35°C (Ducharme, unpublished results) or unless arms and legs are placed in 45°C water [123]. Rescuers should thus be cognisant of potential core temperature afterdrop caused by conductive [50] and convective [46] components during field rewarming. An example of the convective component is the redistribution of blood to the limb muscles, without peripheral vasodilation, from voluntary or passive limb movements. However, rescuers should by no means withhold pre-hospital rewarming of hypothermic patients on this basis.

One of the most important aspects of resuscitation for moderate-to-severe hypothermia is the maintenance of an adequate systemic perfusion and blood pressure during the treatment. This is particularly important since myocardial depression caused by the direct effect of low tissue temperature on cardiac conduction velocity, and the loss of intravascular volume secondary to interstitial fluid shift to the third compartment and renal diuresis, would cause a progressive fall in systemic circulation. To minimise the risk of rewarming collapse, it is essential to maintain adequate systemic perfusion and oxygenation during the rewarming treatment. This approach will support the increase of cellular metabolic activity during the rewarming process parallel to the ability of the heart to distribute oxygen and metabolic substrates to the tissues, and will maintain an adequate blood pressure. This can be practically achieved by providing warm IV fluid (about 1 litre at about 43°C) and warm oxygen (42−46°C) as complementary treatments during active rewarming of the casualty.

9.6.3
Benefits of Early Hypothermia Management

Early effective prehospital treatment of hypothermia would ensure that the condition of the victim does not deteriorate and may even improve during the transportation to a hospital. It is often assumed that passive rewarming, which means the use of insulation, is sufficient to ensure the elimination of body heat loss to the environment. Laboratory testing simulating wilderness conditions showed that using only passive insulation, particularly on non-shivering casualties, could not prevent body heat loss, and consequently, body heat content could continued to decrease during passive rewarming [49]. This study demonstrates that in the absence of effective active heating, moderate to severe hypothermic victims with a suppressed metabolism due to the absence of shivering could see their condition deteriorate even in the presence of passive insulative protection. Effective active external heating of the vital organs in the head and torso regions complemented by the administration of warm intravenous fluid and oxygen, will minimise body heat loss, stabilise the condition of the patient, and eventually increase body heat content before admission to the hospital.

Improving the thermal and circulatory conditions of the hypothermic victim before admission to hospital could have several benefits during the hospital treatments. It could:

- Reduce the risks of ventricular fibrillation and cardiovascular collapse
- Minimise acidosis and hypoxia associated with hypothermia
- Facilitate the treatment of associated medical problems that appear to play a major role in hypothermia associated mortality
- Improve drug metabolism
- Decrease blood loss and risk of coagulopathy
- Increase resistance to wound infection and decrease the risk of sepsis syndrome
- Improve the effectiveness of defibrillation

9.6.4
Recommendations for Prehospital Treatment

The extent of the prehospital management of hypothermia would depend on a number of factors: the severity and complexity of the hypothermia condition, the availability of specialised equipment in the field, the experience of the rescue team, the remoteness of the site from a hospital, and the mode of transportation used. Therefore, the recommendations in ◘ Table 9.2 may not be possible or optimal for all conditions.

Some general care can be provided to all casualties while others will be aimed at specific categories of hypothermia.

◘ **Table 9.2.** Recommendations for prehospital treatment

All casualties:

Remove from water and maintain the casualty in a horizontal position

Avoid rough handling, excessive movement and activity

Practice first aid ABC

Stabilise serious injuries

Assess responsiveness of the victim and intensity of shivering: this will correlate with mild, moderate or severe hypothermia

Measure core temperature, if possible

Eliminate heat loss by conduction (by insulation from the ground), convection and evaporation (by the use of insulated vapour barrier which is preferable to removing wet clothing in exposed cold conditions). However, careful efforts should be made to gently remove or cut off wet clothing once shelter from the elements is achieved

Consider airway insulation with warm saturated air or oxygen. However, this will not provide significant heat to the body

Monitor symptoms and evacuate to a hospital

Conscious and shivering casualties:

Vigorously shivering victims will re-warm on their own if dry and adequately insulated

External heat source is optional depending on the resources and equipment available. The rescuer must be aware that cold, unperfused skin is easily burned

Any external heating could improve morale of victim and recovery time

Forced-air convective warming, heat packs (charcoal, chemical), body-to-body contact, heated blanket or sleeping bag, or hot sweet drink can be considered, although those methods are not all effective in rewarming body core

Table 9.2. *Cont.*

Unconscious and non-shivering casualties:

Victims will not rewarm by themselves because of their suppressed metabolism

Any effective external heat source applied to the torso and neck (forced-air convective warming, charcoal heat packs) will increase likelihood of survival and improve recovery as long as proper oxygenation and systemic circulation are maintained

Provide warm oxygen (42–46°C) and warm intravenous fluid (1 litre at about 43°C) as complementary treatments to any active external rewarming

Regard casualties as critical and avoid unnecessary movement: this can trigger ventricular fibrillation

Casualties with cardiorespiratory arrest:

More research is required for an optimal prehospital treatment

Some significant success with:

Leaving the victim cold but elimination of heat loss

Intubation and ventilation of victims with oxygen

Continuous cardiac massage during transportation

Before initiating CPR, a considerable effort must be made to confirm that the heart is in arrest or VF. First, 60 seconds should be taken to feel for a pulse. If no pulse can be detected, rescue breathing should be initiated for 3 min as this may improve heart function. If a pulse cannot be detected after a second 60-second attempt, chest compression should commence

In hospital, application of extracorporeal blood warming for fast warming

Limit the warming to a deep core temperature of 34°C to minimise risk of brain damage

Finally, rescue personnel are reminded of the following maxim: no one is dead until warm and dead

9.7
Hospital Rewarming of Hypothermic Victims

Durk Zandstra

The incidence of accidental hypothermia varies from 1.4–13.1 per million inhabitants in the registration area of the Centers of Disease Control (CDC news 1996). Half of these victims are older than 64 years of age. Underregistration is acknowledged and the magnitude of the hypothermia incidence is probably severely underestimated.

Hypothermia is associated with substantial morbidity and mortality. A multi-centre study reports that 85% of the non-survivors were admitted with a central temperature of below 32.2°C. Victims with a temperature above 32.2°C had a mortality of 7%, while victims with a temperature below 32.2°C had a mortality of 22.7%. Of these hypothermic victims 38% was resuscitated prior to hospital admission [28].

In 61 hypothermic patients with a temperature below 32°C admitted to one ICU, an increasing mortality with lower admission temperature was observed: No one died with a body temperature between 30 and 32°C, 10% when between 28–30°C, 12% when between 26–28°C and 29% when below 26°C. It is noteworthy to mention that none of the patients died during the rewarming phase [134].

Both Vassal and Suominen, in contrast, describe that the initial temperature is not associated with bad outcome [108, 124]. Hypothermic victims admitted to their ICUs did not seem to have an excess mortality.

A 14%–40% good outcome is reported of hypothermic victims who arrested prior to hospital admission [16, 108, 134]. A substantially higher survival rate is reported for hypothermic victims arresting in the hospital [16].

Usually most cases presenting with hypothermia are no immersion or submersion accidents. From the 47 hypothermic patients in the study by Vassal [124], none was reported to be a drowning victim although hypothermia was associated with outdoor exposure in approximately 50% of the cases. Immersion was present in 27% of the hypothermic victims who died in the multi-centre hypothermia study by Danzl [28]. Apart from hypothermia, many hypothermic immersion or submersion victims also suffer from co-morbidity like trauma, intoxication and post-anoxic neurological disease.

Submersion time appeared to be the only independent predictor of survival in a linear regression analysis. A cut-off temperature could not be indicated. Patient age (children versus adults), water temperature and rectal temperature in the emergency room were not significant predictors of survival [108].

Especially in drowning, post-anoxic brain injury after cardiac arrest with successful resuscitation contributes significantly to mortality and morbidity. In a series of 115 cases of submersion, only one victim with a palpable pulse at the site of drowning died, and 55 patients recovered. Of the resuscitated victims 50% had return of spontaneous circulation (ROSC), but only 25% of the victims after cardiopulmonary resuscitation (CPR) with return of spontaneous circulation (ROSC) survived with little or no neurological damage [40]. These results seem to be unaltered in time. Mortality from accidental hypothermia and drowning

▪ Table 9.3. Topics in the ICU in the treatment of accidental hypothermia

- Restoration of caloric deficit

- Optimisation of circulation to prevent circulatory shock

- Optimisation of gas-exchange to prevent ARDS and aspiration pneumonia

- Correction of acid-base balance

- Correction of electrolyte disorders

- Post-resuscitation therapy for brain protection

- Anticipation of complications such as systemic inflammatory response syndrome (SIRS), aspiration and ventilator associated pneumonia, renal failure and diffuse intravascular coagulation

- Treatment of co-morbidity as trauma, sepsis, intoxication, alcoholism, underlying disease

is about 10%–50%. Conn report an overall mortality in 96 cases of drowning of 13.5% [23]. In the 39 patients who were comatose on arrival at hospital, 33% died and 27% suffered from brain damage. Only 17 patients in this group recovered without neurological deficit. Bohn [14] treated 40 children after drowning of whom 13 died and seven had permanent cerebral damage [14]. It can be concluded from these data that outcome of drowning is predominantly determined by neurological damage after circulatory arrest rather than hypothermia. At the same time, astonishing recoveries from deep hypothermia with and without circulatory arrest have been reported [48, 96]. The old adage "nobody is dead until warm and dead", should be interpreted with caution as a sensible medical statement.

9.7.1
Hypothermia Management in the Hospital

Hypothermia is a multi-system phenomenon. The treatment in the ICU focuses on many topics which are summarised in ▪ **Table 9.3.** Only the restoration of the caloric deficit is addressed in this chapter.

The main focus of the management of hypothermia in the hospital is on symptomatic treatment of vital functions and on the restoration of the caloric deficit. In severe cases this implies intensive treatment in the intensive care. Flow charts for hypothermia can be followed as a triage tool [29, 70].

9.7.2
Caloric Deficit in Hypothermia

Depending on the initial body temperature in a 70 kg water containing victim, ignoring caloric value of tissue, this deficit varies from 490 Kcal in 30°C, to 700 Kcal in 27°C and 980 Kcal in 23°C central body temperature.

To prevent a drop in central body temperature in a thermally unprotected adult, 70–80 Kcal per hour are needed. Hypothermic victims may not have sufficient thermogenesis to prevent further losses and to increase their temperature without active caloric support.

Victims of mild hypothermia to 32°C usually can be supported by insulation to normalise their body temperature if no complicating co-morbidities exist.

In moderately (28–32°C) and severely hypothermic (below 28°C) victims, exogenous caloric support is usually indicated to regain normal central body temperature.

A rewarming rate of 2°C per hour implies a caloric gain of 140–160 Kcal in addition to the Kcal provided by endogenous thermogenesis of approximately 80 Kcal per hour. Endogenous thermogenesis however may be substantially lower than 80 Kcal per hour in severe hypothermia, trauma, intoxication, in hypothyroidism and in the victim of over 60 years of age.

A caloric supply of 200–240 Kcal per hour will provide a sufficient rise in central temperature. In ◻ **Table 9.4** current therapeutic interventions used in the treatment of hypothermia are indicated. Some provide limited caloric support. Therefore, based on simple calculations, combinations of several methods can be expected to be more efficacious than single methods. It may be necessary to use a combination of methods to achieve sufficient rewarming rates if endogenous thermogenesis fails to increase temperature more than 0.5°C per hour.

9.7.3
Rewarming Strategies

Many strategies have been proposed (◻ **Table 9.4**). Most information on efficacy of these methods is derived from uncontrolled case series. A limited number of controlled clinical studies report comparisons of different methods. Rewarming strategies should fulfil the criteria listed in ◻ **Table 9.5**. Rewarming strategies include: passive external rewarming (PER), active external (AER) or active internal rewarming methods (AIR) [27, 29, 70].

9.7.3.1
Passive External Rewarming (PER)

Passive external rewarming (PER) relies for its efficacy on the minimisation of caloric loss (insulation). Rewarming is achieved by endogenous production of heat: the thermogenesis of the victims. Endogenous thermogenesis varies between 30 Kcal per hour in hypothyroidism up to 250 Kcal per hour during shivering. An active thermogenesis of over 80 Kcal per hour increases central temperature within the first hours

☐ **Table 9.4.** Theoretical rewarming rates with various rewarming strategies in a 27°C victim. (Modified from [82])

Method	Rewarming rate (Kcal/hour)	Rewarming duration (hours)
Endogenous production	30[a]	24
Shivering (above 33°C)	250	3–4
Heated aerosol	30	12
Mechanical ventilation 10 litres per minute	23	24
Blanket roll or warm water mattress	80	9
Peritoneal dialysis 4 litres per hour at 45°C	60	8
Haemodialysis 30 litres per hour at 45°C	500	1.5
Hot water bath 45°C	1000	1
Heart-lung machine	4000	0.25
Thermal ceiling; radiant heater	100	7
Veno-venous rewarming	240	3–4
Forced air rewarming	40–80	4–10
Oesophageal probe	30–60	6–12

[a]Depending on multiple factors such as age, intoxication or hypothyroidism.

☐ **Table 9.5.** Suggested criteria to be fulfilled for rewarming strategies

– Safe

– Efficacious

– Quickly and easily applicable

– Minimally invasive or non-invasive

– Low-grade technology with no specialised personnel required

– Patient access for instrumentation during rewarming

– Apparatus should be familiar to attending staff so rewarming equipment must be used in daily practise for post-surgical patients

– Cost effective

mised. Since shivering thermogenesis generates considerable heat, this condition should be used to rewarm, provided that this state does not lead to acidosis or cardiac ischaemia. However, patients are often paralysed by muscle relaxants to facilitate mechanical ventilation. This will considerably reduce endogenous thermogenesis.

In most cases of mild hypothermia (over 32°C) PER is the method of choice. Vassal also used PER in a temperature range between 22 and 32°C [124]. Mean intensive care admission temperature was 28.8±2.5°C. Seven patients were colder than 26°C. The rewarming period was 11.5±7.5 hours in the survivors. In the non-survivors (38%) rewarming period was 17.2±6.2 hours. Most patients had severe co-morbidities. Nielsen also observed good results with PER [86].

Danzl observed 1.5°C rewarming rate in the first hour with PER [27]. This rate is quite similar to the rewarming rates seen with other methods in the first hour. In the second hour of the rewarming treatment no differences between the various methods was observed (nearly 2°C per hour) apart from the rewarming rate of nearly 3°C per hour using peritoneal lavage with hot fluids [28].

If PER fails to achieve a 0.5°C temperature gain in the first hour, active methods should be employed. Especially victims over 60 years of age rewarm slowly and may need active rewarming interventions for the correction of the mild hypothermia. Hypothermic victims that need treatment in the ICU by definition will require active rewarming [72].

A review addressing the management of the hypothermia victim observed a diminishing interest for the use of space-blankets due to questionable efficacy [19].

9.7.3.2
Active External Rewarming (AER)

AER is indicated in moderate to severe hypothermic (less than 32°C) patients with stable haemodynamics if the central temperature fails to increase at least 0.5°C in the first hour with PER.

A variety of methods are available to conduct heat directly from the skin. The fear of rewarming shock withholds many clinicians from AER. Under ICU monitoring and conditioning, however, this complication should not be permitted to occur and AER can be considered as the method of choice to rewarm hypothermic victims in the ICU. Substantial volumes of intravenous infusion may be necessary to maintain adequate circulation and to prevent rewarming shock as shown in ◘ Table 9.6.

The possible explanations for the need of this substantial infusion therapy may be cardiac insufficiency due to changes in preload and afterload conditions, rheologic changes and alterations in the peripheral vascular beds [121]. Capillary leakage of plasma proteins and changes in autonomous vascular control contribute also to rewarming shock and should be counteracted by intravenous volume infusion. Moreover hypothermia leads to a systemic inflammatory response syndrome which amplifies loss of circulating volume [41, 83].

Table 9.6. Fluid infusion in 15 hypothermic victims treated in the ICU [134]

Patient	Temperatures before and after rewarming	Infusion during rewarming (litres)			Fluid balance
	°C	Total	Crystalloids	Colloids	
1	30.4–36	7	5	2	+4
2	30.6–36	6	4	2	+4
3	24.5–37	1.7	1.7	–	+1
4	31.1–37	8	6	2	+1.7
5	32.0–36	4	3.5	0.5	+1.5
6	27.1–36	8.5	7.5	1	+5.5
7	27.4–36	8.5	6	2.5	+4
8	31.5–37	3.6	2.1	1.5	+3
9	31.4–35	1.0	1.0	–	+0.5
10	25.5–36	7	3.5	3.5	+4
11	30.5–36	2.6	2.6	–	+0.8
12	29.6–36	4.3	1.0	3.3	+1
13	32.0–36	5.0	5.0	–	+2
14	32.4–36	5.7	3.7	2	+3
15	29.0–36	4.4	3.0	1.4	+1.1

Forced Air Rewarming

Forced air warming systems is an efficient and non-invasive method to transfer heat. Roggla [95] described forced air rewarming in severe hypothermia as the main part of their rewarming strategy resulting in a rewarming rate of 1°C per hour.

Steele [104] re-warmed 16 victims colder than 32°C with a forced air system or with cotton blankets. Forced warm air of 43°C induced a rewarming rate of 2.5°C per hour, 1°C more than the blanket group. Afterdrop was not observed. Koller [66] reported similar experiences, even in patients that had to be resuscitated. Rewarming rate was 1°C per hour without afterdrop.

Kornberger [67] reported forced air rewarming in nine patients with stable circulation. Observed rewarming rate was 1.9±0.8°C per hour. In six patients undergoing CPR the rewarming rate was 1.5±0.3°C per hour.

Various systems are available commercially but their heat transfer capacity varies greatly. This should be taken into account when considering efficacy and rewarming rates [47]. Systems are rapidly set up but disposables are needed. Patient instrumentation is somewhat hampered and heat transfer is impaired when instrumentation of the patient takes place. The caloric transfer varies between 40–80 Kcal per hour.

Convective warm air rewarming in combination with active vasodilatory therapy using nitro-glycerine infusion showed significantly faster rewarming than space blanket treatment, 0.75°C per hour versus 0.25°C per hour in the first 2 hours after operation [56]. In the ICU vasoactive medication is usually indicated to improve circulation.

Radiant Heating

Ledingham and Mone used torso radiant heating in 42 patients [73]. A commercial system is available [60]. The caloric gain is estimated between 50 and 80 Kcal per hour. As holds true for other AER strategies the efficacy can be improved by using vasodilators to improve peripheral circulation and thus the heat transfer via the skin. Usually these systems are operated in combination with other means of rewarming in moderate and severe hypothermia [134]. Since these systems are used in daily practise in many ICUs for postoperative rewarming they can be operational immediately. No disposables are needed and the access ability to the patient is optimal without loss of heat transfer during instrumentation of the patient.

Circulating Warm Water Mattress

These systems provide approximately 80 Kcal heat transfer per hour. Mattress water temperature can be adjusted but usually is started at 40°C. A major advantages is the possibility to cool so that the equipment can also be used to induce therapeutic hypothermia after cardiac arrest and CPR. The combination of a thermal ceiling and a circulating warm water mattress on top of the patient provides powerful rewarming rates of 2.5°C per hour [134]. No disposables are needed. In controlled clinical application in the rewarming of post cardiac surgery patients the rewarming by a circulating water blanket produced normothermia more rapidly than a warm convective air blanket [97].

Immersion in Warm Water Bath

This approach can be applied to restore caloric deficit if no other means are available. However, it is cumbersome and complicates monitoring and eventual resuscitation.

In a comparative study a warm bath of 40°C provided the fastest rewarming compared to shivering, hot air at 40 or 45°C [96]. The least afterdrop was observed with the bath method. This study, however, was performed in mild hypothermia.

The question of whether whole-body bath or just trunk immersion rewarming should be applied was studied by Hoskin [62]. Authorities in favour of trunk-only bath rewarming base their proposal on the assumption that core temperature afterdrop would be minimised by preventing peripheral vasodilation when the limbs of the subject are not immersed in the rewarming bath. In this study, trunk-only and whole-body bath rewarming are compared by rewarming eight mildly hypothermic male subjects twice, once via each technique. It was concluded that trunk-only rewarming is not superior to whole-body bath rewarming as a therapy for mild immersion hypothermia. No significant differences existed between the two techniques, either in size or duration of core temperature afterdrop or in rate of rewarming.

Heated Aerosol

Since the lungs provide a huge surface area it seems attractive to use this surface as a heat exchanging surface. Simultaneously the normal heat loss via the lungs is reduced. However, less than 10% of the metabolic heat is lost during surgery through respiration even if dry, cool gas is used for ventilation [100].

The use of heated gases as a primary rewarming strategy can therefore be challenged [127]. In clinical practice heated gases accelerated postoperative rewarming with only 0.3°C per hour [39]. This confirms that heated gases should be considered as a supplemental tool and not as a primary rewarming strategy. In patients after cardiac surgery, the use of the Thermax device, resulted in a more rapid rise in body temperature than the Humid-Vent 1, (0.3°C per hour vs 0.07°C per hour; $p=0.001$) which illustrates that the substantial caloric gain is minimal [15].

Arteriovenous Anastomosal (AVA) Rewarming

Arteriovenous anastomosal (AVA) rewarming is a non-invasive technique. Heat is applied via immersion of parts of the upper or lower extremities in hot water (44–45°C). Arteriovenous anastomoses are opened, allowing large quantities of blood to pass that can absorb the applied calories. Most authors find disappointing results when hands and feet are immersed in hot water [17, 26]. However, Vanggaard et al. [122] argue that the lower arms and legs have to be immersed as well in order to have an effective heat transfer. AVAs can be opened by high ambient temperatures, pharmacologically by vasodilators but also by the application of a negative pressure [54, 102].

The latter method is challenged recently. Core temperature increased more rapidly with forced air warming (2.6±0.6°C) than negative pressure rewarming and calories from a negative pressure rewarming device are largely constrained to the forearm. Apparently heat does not flow to the core thermal compartment [111].

9.7.3.3
Active Internal Rewarming Strategies (AIR)

Peritoneal Irrigation
This invasive method is widely used and advocated. It is performed with one or two peritoneal catheters. A flow of a simple dialysis solution from 4–12 litres per hour at a temperature of 37–43.5°C produces a rise in central temperature of about 1.5°C per hour [130]. Davis reports five patients with accidental hypothermia treated with peritoneal irrigation [30]. Admission rectal temperatures ranged from 24°C to 31.7°C and two patients had suffered circulatory arrest. Along with respiratory and circulatory management in an intensive care unit, the patients were actively rewarmed by peritoneal dialysis with fluid at 37°C. Rewarming was smooth and free of complications. All five patients made a good recovery.

Oesophageal Thermal Probes (OTP)
Thermal probes were developed from Sengstaken-Blackmore tubes and consist of an oesophageal probe wherein warm water is circulating in a closed system [74]. A system described by Kristensen operates on 42°C and circulates 3 litres per hour. Preliminary results showed a rewarming rate of 1.5°C per hour in a hypothermic victim [68]. However, less favourable results were obtained in a study in orthopaedic patients to maintain peri-operative core temperature (T_c) [69].

Fluid Warmers
The infusion of 1 litre of unwarmed fluid at 4°C causes a fall in the T_c of 0.5–1.0°C. Infusion of 8–10 litres Ringers lactate at room temperature reduces T_c about 2°C. About 16 Kcal are needed to warm 1 litre from 21 to 37°C corresponding to a decline of 0.2°C T_c per minute [68].

Usually substantial amounts of IV fluids are needed during rewarming (◘ Table 9.6). Therefore intravenous fluids should be heated before infusion. Safety and efficacy of 65°C fluids were compared with 38°C fluids in an experimental study [101]. In 18–20 kg beagles hot infusion in de vena cava superior resulted in more rapid increase in T_c. Vascular injury at the site of infusion appeared to be not significant. The rate of rewarming was 2.9°C per hour in the 65°C intravenous infusion group and 1.25°C per hour in the 38°C group. In a controlled clinical study in cardiac surgery patients a commercial available system could prevent infusion induced hypothermia [131].

Veno-Venous Systems
Extracorporeal rewarming of venous blood is an invasive option to rewarm [9, 42, 43, 55, 58]. With this technique blood is removed via a large bore lumen venous or arterial catheter heated to 40°C and returned via another venous access. Flow rates of 150–400 ml per minute can be achieved [43, 55, 58]. Acceptable rewarming rates of 1–3°C per hour can be achieved depending on flow rates and

time to get started. Problems with patency of the circuit due to clotting have been solved by heparin coated systems [99].

9.7.4
Conclusion

The treatment of accidental hypothermia in the hospital should preferably be realised via a hospital protocol. There are no randomised controlled trials, however, that definitively establish the most optimal rewarming strategy. If thermogenesis fails to increase central temperature more than 0.5°C per hour, active rewarming is indicated.

In patients with spontaneous circulation and treated by active external rewarming using forced air rewarming reproducible results have been reported. Usually the elderly patient fails adequate thermogenesis to increase sufficiently central temperature. Simultaneous use of various other rewarming strategies may be indicated to achieve and maintain normothermia. The choice for the optimal rewarming strategy depends on clinical presentation.

9.8
Hospital Treatment of Victims in Cardiorespiratory Arrest

BEAT WALPOTH and ADAM FISHER

Drowning hypothermia by submersion is associated with various levels of asphyxia is often seen in accidental hypothermia [78]. The Swiss experience with avalanche victims also suffering from asphyxia shows several similarities with drowning. Therefore, we believe that the reported clinical and laboratory data, well documented in avalanche victims, can be applied to drowning victims [98, 129].

The presence of even faint vital respiratory, cardiac or neurological signs on recovery and during rescue of a hypothermic victim is one of the most important predictors of survival [129]. This state is often called apparent death since chances of survival exist after successful rewarming. At the same time, it is well documented that such victims can go into secondary cardiac arrest during rescue survival [129]. This phenomenon is known in the literature as rescue collapse, rescue death or sheltering death (see ▶ Chapter 9.5). The pathophysiology of rescue or sheltering death is not completely understood. However, it is believed that the manipulation of the victim such as lifting in a vertical sling during a sea rescue is the main factor leading to cardiac arrest in a haemodynamically compromised and hypothermic patient [52].

All victims of drowning hypothermia in cardiorespiratory arrest should undergo immediate cardiopulmonary resuscitation (CPR) by educated public or professional rescuers [1]. Such victims must be immediately transported to a hospital with experience in rewarming and availability of cardiopulmonary bypass (CPB) rewarming [129].

The extraordinary survival cases of children reported in the literature after prolonged iced water submersion emphasises the need for maximal and continued resuscitation efforts [107]. There is no clear explanation for survival of such children compared to adults. Possibly the diving reflex in small children and their extremely fast cooling rate in cold water, favoured by the relative large body surface area of the head with maintained cerebral circulation, may delay anoxia and provide sufficient brain protection for survival [12, 13].

In hypothermic victims of drowning or avalanche admitted to the hospital in cardiorespiratory arrest with a core temperature above 30°C, asphyxia has to be considered as a main cause of death [34, 77].

Laboratory parameters may represent an aid in decision making for the hospital clinician. The main prognostic biological factor is the blood potassium level on admission [78, 81, 98]. Blood potassium level in excess of 10 mmol/l for adults and of 12 mmol/l for children have all been associated with fatal outcomes in hypothermic victims with cardiorespiratory arrest.

The main bulk of this data are from avalanche victim admissions [34, 78, 98]. Large clinical series of drowning victims do exist but very few biologic data in hypothermia from submersion have been reported. Thus, an international registry to gather more information is needed. Other prognostic factors such as asphyxia time have been reported in a retrospective analysis and in a prospective survival model by Locher [78]. Flow charts how to rescue hypothermic victims may also be of help for professional and non-professional rescuers of hypothermic drowning victims [1].

Our consensus in drowning hypothermia indicates that CPB is the state of the art method for rewarming drowning victims with core temperature below 30°C and in cardiac arrest. CPB for rewarming such hypothermic victims can be instituted in the operating room or in the emergency room depending on the available personnel and equipment. Most of the experience in CPB rewarming has been performed by open peripheral (femoral) cannulation which can now be accomplished by percutaneous cannulation of the vessels. In rewarming of children suffering from drowning hypothermia, central cannulation for CPB can be applied in order to obtain adequate blood flow during rewarming [128]. Therefore, children suffering from drowning hypothermia should be admitted to a hospital with paediatric cardiac surgical capabilities.

Improvement of CPB technology also allows its application for trauma patients using heparin coated circuits and low systemic heparinisation in order to reduce bleeding [125]. Other and new tools should be considered to prolong the resuscitative efforts, such as on-line haemofiltration during CPB or haemodialysis, cardiac-assist, or extra-corporeal membrane oxygenation (ECMO).

Recently, a debate on the speed of rewarming has emerged, since most patients rapidly rewarming on CPB (8–10°C per hour) develop severe pulmonary and probably brain oedema [129]. Hypothermic patients with a maintained circulation rewarmed non-invasively with forced warmed air (2–3°C per hour) do not show such severe pulmonary and cerebral complications [66]. Two recent reports in the *New England Journal of Medicine* of positive effects of mild hypothermia in out-of-hospital cardiac arrest patients may suggest that CPB rewarm-

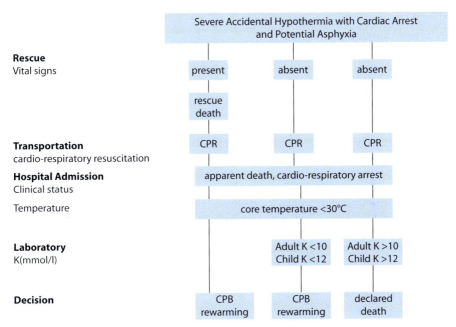

Severe Accidental Hypothermia with Cardiac Arrest
and Potential Asphyxia

Rescue
Vital signs — present / absent / absent

rescue death

Transportation
cardio-respiratory resuscitation — CPR / CPR / CPR

Hospital Admission
Clinical status — apparent death, cardio-respiratory arrest

Temperature — core temperature <30°C

Laboratory
K(mmol/l) — Adult K <10 / Adult K >10
Child K <12 / Child K >12

Decision — CPB rewarming / CPB rewarming / declared death

□ Fig. 9.5. Strategy for decision making and management of hypothermic victims suffering from potential asphyxia (submerion or avalanche) and presenting to hospital in cardiorespiratory arrest

ing of hypothermic patients in cardiac arrest should be stopped at 33–35°C [10, 57]. Further clinical experience is needed to validate this suggestion.

In the flow chart shown in □ **Fig. 9.5**, we propose a strategy for decision making and management of hypothermic victims suffering from potential asphyxia by submersion or avalanche and presenting to the hospital in cardiorespiratory arrest. For hypothermic patients with maintained circulation, active external rewarming can be considered in an intensive care unit [66].

Our clinical experience with CPB rewarming of victims from accidental hypothermia in cardiac arrest shows a good long-term recovery of the survivors [129]. In our own series, rewarming with cardiopulmonary bypass was successful in 48% of the 32 patients with prolonged deep hypothermic arrest. A total of 15 patients showed an excellent long-term outcome [129]. At follow-up, 6 years after the accident, neuropsychological examination showed normal brain function and all patients are enjoying a normal life. None of them requires any further medical treatment. Considering this excellent result, it seems reasonable to subscribe to the old saying that nobody is dead until warm and dead. These data suggest that severe hypothermia should be treated by rewarming using cardiopulmonary bypass, whereas patients with less severe hypothermia with a stable haemodynamic circulation can be treated non-invasively by forced warm air techniques.

9.9
Fluid Management
During Treatment of Immersion Hypothermia

MARIT FARSTAD and PAUL HUSBY

Hypothermia affects the microvascular fluid exchange both in accidental hypothermia as well as during controlled hypothermic cardiopulmonary bypass (CPB). CPB is the recommended first choice method for rewarming cardiac arrested victims with accidental hypothermia [35, 126, 128]. Fluid shifts in relation to CPB should therefore be considered in fluid management protocols in relation to immersion hypothermia.

CPB differs from normal circulation in several ways that may predispose to tissue oedema. Haemodilution, inflammation, perfusion techniques (flow rate, flow pattern, perfusion pressure), anaesthesia management, intraoperative fluid additions and impaired renal function may all contribute to accumulation of interstitial fluid and oedema formation. In addition, hypothermia by itself may cause an increase in microvascular fluid extravasation with an increase in total tissue water content (TTW).

Fluid exchange during accidental hypothermia, experimental hypothermia and during hypothermic CPB has been investigated in a significant number of papers. Available data may appear conflicting, but the results are principally comparable, either they are produced in non-CPB or CPB models, or obtained by clinical observation. The differences appear related to which fluid supplementation protocols are applied during the experiments and may also reflect species differences in animal studies.

Hypo-oncotic, iso-oncotic and hyperoncotic solutions have different effects on fluid accumulation in the different organs. This fact may ultimately influence clinical outcome.

9.9.1
Plasma Volume, Haematocrit,
Microvascular Fluid Exchange and Hypothermia

Studies have been undertaken for more than 50 years to clarify in more detail how lowering of body temperature affects microvascular fluid exchange [25, 63, 65, 79, 80]. Accidental hypothermia, clinical hypothermia under general anaesthesia, and experimental hypothermia have induced different and sometimes even opposite changes. The observed physiological alterations are brought about by the state of the study object prior to cooling, as well as by the depth and duration of hypothermia [90].

During hypothermia a decrease in blood volume and plasma volume in parallel with lowering of body temperature have been demonstrated in a series of studies involving different species [25, 79]. The decrease in circulating blood volume is more pronounced after a longer duration of hypothermia. The reduction may be up to 40% of normal blood volume after 6–8 hours of deep hypothermia (15°C) [90].

The decrease in blood volume is accompanied by a pronounced haemoconcentration, particularly present in deep hypothermia [63, 65, 79, 80]. Haemoconcentration has been demonstrated to occur in artificially cooled animals, in hypothermic patients [3] and even during normothermic cold exposure [5].

Species differences have been reported. In rats cooled to 15°C and maintained at this temperature level for hours, an increase in haematocrit from 42% to 70% or more has been reported [88, 89]. This finding has also been observed in artificially cooled hibernators (ground squirrels). In squirrels the increase in haematocrit did not occur after several hours as in rats, but after days [88]. Long lasting hypothermia may also represent a negative predictor for survival in man.

Hypothermia by itself contributes in addition to haemoconcentration, also to an increase in blood viscosity that may affect circulation. In fact deep hypothermia and hypothermia of longer duration has been demonstrated to cause a block of capillary flow due to formation of large blood cell aggregates. These aggregates only slowly disappear upon rewarming [80]. Profound haemoconcentration with deterioration of microcirculation may be one of the limiting factors for survival from severe and prolonged hypothermia.

The mechanism behind plasma volume reduction and haemoconcentration during hypothermia seem only partially explained. Some authors explained the reduction in plasma volume with the corresponding haemoconcentration by trapping of whole plasma in certain parts of the vascular system [25, 65], whereas another study [63] found haemoconcentration during hypothermia in dogs to be due to splenic contraction. Following splenectomy, however, there was a progressive increase in haematocrit which clearly must be explained by other mechanisms than splenic contraction.

Svanes found an increase in oncotic pressure and haematocrit during cooling of rabbits to 25°C, with no significant changes in capillary flow, capillary filtration coefficient and capillary pressure [109]. These results indicated a net transcapillary loss of fluid from circulation during hypothermia. Chen presented further support for the theory of increased microvascular fluid filtration during hypothermia [20]. Red cell volume and plasma protein concentration remained stable after cooling whereas reduction in plasma volume together with an increase in lymph flow of the thoracic duct gave support for a transcapillary fluid loss during cooling. The results further indicated a loss of plasma proteins from circulation to the interstitial space, based on a simultaneous reduction of plasma volume and a stable plasma protein concentration. Similar unpublished results were observed in ongoing studies in our laboratory.

Roberts found elevated haematocrit values in cooled dogs treated without or with saline infusion [94]. The infusion volume of 20% of plasma volume was given during stable hypothermia or just prior to rewarming. Haematocrit stayed high in all groups during the study with no between group differences even after saline was given. The results clearly illustrate how crystalloid solutions given during hypothermia are lost to the interstitial space by a cold-induced increase in fluid filtration.

Intravenous administration of warm fluids has been recommended as first aid either alone or as a contributing method, in rewarming hypothermic patients. The use of warm crystalloid solutions like Ringer solution should, according to present knowledge, be used with caution. Lauri also recommended caution with this practice as a reversal of cold-induced fluid extravasation could be present during rewarming with signs of cardiac decompensation [71].

9.9.2
Microvascular Fluid Exchange, Cardiopulmonary Bypass (CPB) and Hypothermia

CPB is associated with a 15%−30% increase in TTW, which lasts for 24−48 hours post-CPB. The increase in TTW mainly affects the interstitial space whereas the intracellular is left intact [59]. CPB may contribute to tissue oedema by factors listed above.

Recently hypothermia per se was confirmed to be one of the main contributors to an increase in TTW and generation of tissue oedema during CPB [38]. Rate of cooling did not affect fluid extravasation rate (FER) which was increased from about 0.1 ml.kg^{-1}.min^{-1} during normothermic CPB to 0.7−0.9 ml. kg^{-1}.min^{-1} during hypothermic CPB. Cooling was either within minutes or slow (about 1 hour). Tissue oedema affected principally all organs studied including skeletal muscle, skin, heart, lung, pancreas, liver and gastrointestinal tract. The extravasated fluid consisted mainly of water and small solutes. The intravascular albumin and protein masses remained unaffected [38]. The loss of fluid during CPB resembled the fluid losses seen during experimental hypothermia as reported above and is principally similar to that present in accidental hypothermia (own unpublished results). Although the mechanism responsible for an increase in FER during hypothermia is still unknown, it is apparently not related to an inflammatory reaction as methylprednisolone does not influence FER at all (◘ Fig. 9.6) [37].

Fluid extravasation during CPB depends on prime volume and quality of priming solution. Aukerman and colleagues found albumin (grams per millilitre) prime and prime volume in millilitre per kilogram were the best predictors of weight gain following extracorporeal circulation in children with prime volume being the most important [3]. Farstad found a significant reduction in need for fluid addition to the extracorporeal circuit, when the prime solution remained isooncotic (4% albumin) throughout the CPB period (◘ Fig. 9.7) [36]. This was due to a decrease in FER by albumin during hypothermic CPB. In that particular study TTW was also significantly lower and close to normal in most organs compared with results obtained when acetated Ringer solution was used for priming. Whereas hypothermic fluid extravasation could be reduced by isooncotic priming, the fluid shifts during normothermic CPB was highly unaffected [36].

Similar results have been obtained with other colloids. Yeh studied the effect of the pentafraction of hydroxyethyl starch in neonatal piglets during CPB [132]. They found significantly lower weight gain and volume requirements during

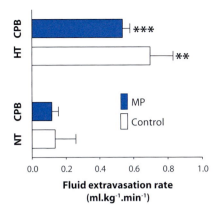

■ **Fig. 9.6.** Fluid extravasation rate (FER) during 30 min of normothermic (*NT*) cardiopulmonary bypass (*CPB*) compared with 30 min of hypothermic (*HT*) CPB in piglets. Prime was acetated Ringer solution. Induction of hypothermia resulted in an abrupt increase in the fluid extravasation rate which could not be significantly counteracted by use of methylprednisolone (*MP*)

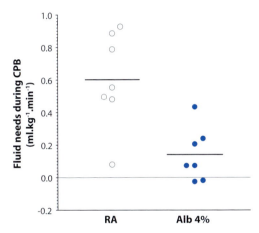

■ **Fig. 9.7.** Need for fluid addition to the machine reservoir during hypothermic cardiopulmonary bypass (*CPB*). Prime: *RA*, acetated Ringer solution. *Alb 4%*, 4% albumin in acetated Ringer solution. Values are presented as mean of each experiment (*n*=7 in each group). Mean value of the seven experiments in each group: *black line*. The fluid needs were significantly lower in the albumin group (*p*<0.01) compared with the Ringer solution group. This was also reflected by significantly lower tissue water content of most organs studied

CPB, as well as lower TTW values (kidney, pancreas, stomach, jejunum, colon and skeletal muscle) compared with a control where only crystalloids were used for priming. TTW in heart, lung, liver, spleen, skin or brain remained, however, unaffected by the addition of the pentafraction of hydroxyethyl starch.

An increase in colloid osmotic pressure of the cardiopulmonary prime was found to minimise myocardial oedema and to prevent myocardial dysfunction postoperatively in a study by Mehlhorn [84]. Similar results were recently reported by Eising, who found an increase in cardiac index by use of hyper-oncotic CPB prime [33]. Also extravascular lung water (EVLW) accumulation could be prevented, although pulmonary function was unchanged.

Töllöfsrud and Noddeland [120] mobilised fluid excess and improved cardiorespiratory function by use of hypertonic saline (75 mg·ml^{-1}) in combination with dextran (60 mg·ml^{-1}) following coronary artery surgery. Despite reduced need for fluid supplementation and decreased cumulative fluid balance following hypertonic saline/dextran infusion, their patients had increased filling pressures of the heart with improved cardiac output.

To our knowledge little information is available on cerebral fluid homeostasis in relation to hypothermia and hypothermic CPB. Hindman [61] found the mechanisms that maintain the brain fluid balance remained intact during hypo-oncotic non-pulsative CPB.

Cerebral oedema may compromise cerebral blood flow, particularly in regions of cerebral ischaemia or infarction. As accidental hypothermia may be associated with episodes of asphyxia resulting in more or less extensive ischaemic brain damage, special attention should be paid to fluid resuscitation protocols with respect to oedema formation in the brain. Prough [91] studied the effects on intracranial pressure of different fluid resuscitation protocols in dogs [91]. The intracranial pressure (ICP) was lower following resuscitation with hypertonic saline ($75 \, mg.ml^{-1}$) instead of lactated Ringer solution. They concluded that hypertonic saline fluid resuscitation could represent an alternative when aggravation of intracranial hypertension during resuscitation would place a patient at greater risk. Hypertonic saline has been proved useful in a significant number of papers in situations like head injuries and haemorrhage shock, and might even have a place in resuscitation of patients from deep hypothermia [6]. Further studies, however are needed for definite documentation.

9.9.3
Fluid Supplementation Protocols During the Treatment of Immersion Hypothermia

From available data still only a sketchy picture can be drawn about the physiological changes of fluid homeostasis induced by a decrease in body temperature. Further research is needed to round this sketch into a more complete picture permitting a better understanding of the basic physiological processes that regulate water balance during hypothermia. Despite our scanty knowledge of temperature induced fluid shifts, some guidelines on fluid management during treatment of immersion hypothermia can be drawn.

- Fluid supplementation should in general be administered rapidly enough in sufficient quantity to maintain adequate tissue perfusion without overloading the cardiovascular system. The underlying cardiac and renal functions of the patient determine how well fluid replacement will be tolerated. The rate of fluid administration must be based on the severity of hypovolaemia and the haemodynamic response to volume replacement.
- Haemodynamic parameters (central venous pressure and systemic mean arterial pressure) should be assessed regularly together with vital signs, diuresis and clinical data (breath sounds, skin colour, temperature and sensorium). Absolute values must be related to actual temperature. Definite limits are still undefined. Thermodilution catheters should be used with care as their introduction can precipitate cardiac arrhythmias. Central haemodynamics can alternatively be assessed by use of the PICCO system, a pulse contour analyser for cardiac output determination.

- Intravenous fluid can be given as crystalloid solution, or as iso-oncotic, hyperoncotic, hyperosmolar, or hyperoncotic and hyperosmolar solutions.
- Administration of isotonic crystalloid solutions (Ringer acetate/lactate) should be used with care. The main part of crystalloid solutions administered is lost from circulation to the interstitial space during hypothermia. This extravasated fluid is subsequently mobilised during rewarming and may lead to volume overload and occasionally cardiac decompensation.
- In contrast to crystalloid solutions, colloid solutions have been demonstrated to be effective in decreasing fluid extravasation and oedema formation during hypothermia. It seems therefore recommendable to use isooncotic and even hyperoncotic colloid solutions to compensate for hypovolaemia during hypothermia and rewarming.
- Hyperoncotic-hyperosmolar solutions (NaCl 7.5% with dextran 70 6%, or NaCl 7.2% with HES 6%) might be suitable for volume resuscitation during hypothermia. These solutions effectively mobilise extravascular fluid into circulation. From a theoretical viewpoint they may have a particular advantage when, for some reason, brain oedema is present simultaneously with hypothermia.

9.10
Acid-Base Management During Accidental Hypothermia

Durk Zandstra

The management of the blood pH during rewarming from hypothermia remains controversial.

Warm blooded animals, including the human, strive to maintain blood acidity (pH) at a constant value of 7.40 by means of a mechanism we call the pH-stationary, or pH-stat, regulation mechanism. Hibernators follow the same strategy [31, 92, 110].

Cold blooded animals like frogs and snakes, however, permit the blood pH to rise and the $PaCO_2$ to drop during hypothermia. This pH strategy is called alfa-stat pH regulation.

The entities pH-stat and alfa-stat have caused confusion regarding how to deal with acid-base balance in clinical and accidental hypothermia.

The pH of the blood is determined by the amount of H^+ ions dissolved in it. Since water is the most important source of H^+ ions, the dissociation constant of water (the pKw) determines predominantly the pH of the blood.

A key issue in this matter is the fact that the pKw of water lowers when cooled. This means that less H^+ ions are dissolved in the solution. The pH of cold blood will increase. The pKw of water at the iso-neutrality pH will thus also slowly increase. This iso-neutrality pH equals the intracellular pH. It is therefore claimed that intracellular processes during hypothermia are better preserved under hypothermic conditions.

Where does alfa-stat come from? The extracellular fluid from all vertebrae contain a buffer system that is composed from bicarbonates, phosphates and proteins. Histidine, in imidazole form, is the most important protein buffer. The pK from imidazole during hypothermia is almost identical to that of the pK of water. This means that the buffer capacity of the imidazole histidine is maintained over a wide range of temperature. Histidine imidazole that has lost an H^+ ion as a result of the dissociation process is called alfa imidazole. The alfa imidazole also represents the charge condition of histidine but also from the other proteins. The alfa imidazole remains constant during a fall in temperature and thereby also other proteins do not change their charge. A pH strategy allowing a constant alfa-imidazole fraction is called alfa-stat pH regulation.

The impact on clinical practice is manifold. The blood gas analyser warms the blood sample automatically to 37°C. At this temperature the acid base status of the patient is measured. In pH-stat strategy all corrections will be made solely based on results from in vitro studies. In the alfa-stat strategy a normal result at 37°C implies a good acid-base balance on all temperatures so no corrections are made for temperature of the patient

In the vision of alfa-stat strategy, pH-stat strategy results in severe acidosis inducing organ dysfunction.

For alfa-stat to be applied in clinical practice the following guidelines may be followed:

- No temperature correction for the blood gas sample. All patients are 37°C and no correction for temperature of a hypothermic patient occurs.
- Depending on the results of (1) no corrections are necessary if the acid-base results are normal.
- No additional CO_2 in the respiratory gases.
- Maintain a ventilation strategy that gives a normal pH at 37°C
- pH Adjustments should not be achieved by using bicarbonate solutions but rather by ventilation and circulation optimisation.
- A slight respiratory alkalosis seems to have a positive influence on cardiac function.

9.11
An International Data-Registration for Accidental and Immersion Hypothermia

9.11.1
Implication of Treatment and Outcome of Survivors of Accidental Deep Hypothermia: The Need for a Hypothermia Registry

BEAT WALPOTH

A transient body temperature between 35 and 32°C is common and usually without consequences for the brain or other organs. In contrast, prolonged deep hypothermia due to accidents is rare and usually associated with premature death.

However, a few people survive and can be resuscitated with appropriate means in due time. The degree of hypothermia, the exposure time and type of accident may vary but long-term survival rates without sequelae of 47% have been reported [129]. Previous reports have been based mainly on case reports with successful therapy of survival patients whereas the negative outcomes have not been reported. Larger epidemiologic studies have proposed outcome score models for facilitating triage and decision making [78].

In an effort to gain more information on the severity of sequelae and outcome of deep hypothermia victims, we propose starting an international registry. The data of this registry shall be collected world-wide using the internet as a common database for entry and retrieval of the accumulated scientific data. The registry should collect important information on body temperature, exposure time, type of accident, environmental factors and concomitant injuries. In addition, rescue modalities, prehospital treatment, hospital rewarming methods and patient outcome data should be included. This registry could be directed by an international working group which will be responsible for data safety and data analysis, as well as preparing guidelines for prevention, rescue treatment and follow-up of these patients.

9.11.2
The UK National Immersion Incident Survey (UKNIIS)

MIKE TIPTON

The UKNIIS is a survey run by the Institute of Naval Medicine, UK. It is a voluntary reporting scheme established in 1990. The aim of the survey is to validate an existing set of survival curves or propose an alternative set.

The survey does not attempt to establish a precise time of death; rather it is designed to provide an indication of the proportion of those alive at a given time. Thus it attempts to generate survival curves rather than survival times. Less precise data are accommodated by studying larger populations. Bodies recovered a considerable time after death are not included in the survey. A logistic model is used to relate probability of survival to immersion time.

The questionnaire on which the survey is based has been approved by the Defence Services Lifesaving Committee. Copies were sent to HM Coastguard, the Royal National Lifeboat Institute and other members of that committee.

The survey asks for a number of items for each incident (◘ Table 9.7).

A total of 1261 questionnaires were received between 1991–2001. The last general report was published in 1997 and was based on 900 cases [87]. It was estimated that 50% of eligible deaths were surveyed. Few incidents were reported with immersion times beyond 4 hours (14 incidents, seven deaths). Almost all the incidents occurred in salt water. The distribution of incidents by water temperature is shown in ◘ Fig. 9.8.

There were 750 reports for males, 149 for females. The death rate was 7% for males and 8% for females. Within the males, 689 of the reports involved

□ **Table 9.7.** Information required for the National Immersion Incident Survey UK

Date of rescue	Air temperature
Time of rescue	Wind speed
Duration of immersion	Location
Water temperature	Mode of rescue
Sea state	Helicopter strop used
Sex of victim	Condition on: rescue; delivery to ambulance
Age of victim	
Build of victim	Medical problems
Clothing worn	Other remarks
Lifejacket worn	

10–39 year olds: 4% died. Ninety of the reports involved 40- to 90-year-olds: 16% died. The highest death rates were in March, April and November.

Death occurred in 3% of those wearing lifejackets, 1% of those wearing buoyancy aids and 45% of those wearing neither. A substantial number of deaths occurred very early during immersion (36% of the deaths that occurred at a known time), and the period immediately following rescue was also critical (18% died shortly after rescue). This supports our current understanding of the physiological responses to immersion. Contrary to other estimations and predictions, there was no evidence of a sharp increase in survival as water temperature approached 15°C.

9.11.2.1
Conclusion

The UKNIIS survey is becoming a useful source of data. However, more reports are required to increase the database for low temperatures and long durations. Consideration should be given to making involvement in the UKNIIS a statutory requirement. Liaison is beginning with project SARRRAH in Germany (see ▶ Chapter 9.11.4).

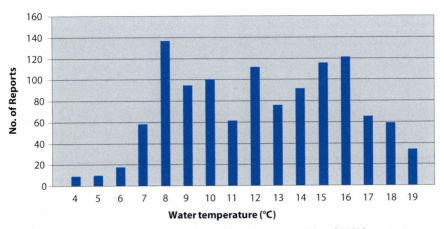

◘ Fig. 9.8. The distribution of 750 immersion incidents between 1991 and 2001 by water temperature

9.11.3
Hypothermia Research Project in The Netherlands

JOOST BIERENS

Treatment of moderate (28–32°C) and severe (below 28°C) hypothermia is complex and prolonged, because all organ systems can be seriously involved. Notably in trauma patients it has become clear that hypothermia as a complicated factor increases morbidity and mortality and prolongs hospital stay. At the same time, good outcome without side effects has been reported in patients with severe hypothermia as a single injury and in hypothermic drowning victims (submersion and immersion).

As a result of the climate in the Netherlands, hypothermia is a relatively rare event. Death rate is below 0.1 per 100.000 inhabitant per year. Yet over 150 hypothermic patients are included in the data registries of Dutch hospitals each year. The major causes are drowning (33%), accidents (17%) and violence (16%).

The low incidence of hypothermia may have consequences such as:
- The diagnosis of hypothermia is missed in a number of patients.
- Not all patients receive optimal treatment.
- The clinical experience of the individual doctor or hospital to manage the hypothermic patients is limited.

In spite of the low incidence of hypothermia, interest in the subject is high in the Netherlands. After the ferry boat disaster involving the 'Herald of Free Enterprise' in 1987, in which 194 passengers died from hypothermia and drowning, a Working Group on Hypothermia was installed by the Ministry of Health. The Working Group advised appointing a limited number of hypothermia centres in the Netherlands. These centres have never been established. An epidemiological study, performed at that time, concluded that the outcome of hypothermia victims in large or university hospitals is better than in small hospitals. This study also showed that many patients die from complications, when the body temperature is no longer hypothermic. Since 1995, ambulance nurses have a national protocol for the treatment of hypothermia. Some hospitals have developed their own in-hospital protocols for the treatment of the hypothermic patient. A multi-centred study would be a next step in improving the understanding and treatment of hypothermia patients. Preparations are currently under way.

The aims of the Dutch Hypothermia Project include:
- Inventory and standardisation of existing rewarming methods and treatment protocols which are used in hospitals
- Establishing a national network of expertise
- Advising on the best rewarming strategies and treatment, both for individual patients as well as in disasters situations

The five phases of the project are:
- Meetings between hospitals to discuss the local situation with respect to the definition of hypothermia, the several existing resuscitation, re-warming and treatment protocols and data registrations. The study group will consist of 15–25 hospitals. The aim of this phase is to acquire an overview of the current situation in the Netherlands.
- Development of national definitions, a limited number of standardised rewarming and treatment protocols and a national registration. The aim of this phase is to exchange the knowledge and clinical experiences between the participants in the study and, if possible, to standardise and limit the treatment strategies. Outcome parameters have to be defined.
- Standardisation of prehospital care and appropriate prehospital registration of data. The aim of this phase is to include prehospital data in a registry.
- Registration of the incidence, rewarming, treatment, prognostic indicators and outcome of hypothermic patients in the Netherlands. The aim of this phase is to conclude which are the best re-warming and treatment strategies in terms of re-warming speed, complications and outcome. Based on these conclusions, the existing protocols can be adapted.
- Participation in the international registration of severe (below 28°C) hypothermia. The aim of this phase is to compare the Dutch data with the data from studies in other countries.

9.11.4
The SARRRAH Project

WOLFGANG BAUMEIER

In the SARRRAH project (Search and Rescue, Resuscitation and Rewarming in Accidental Hypothermia), the progress of patients who have suffered cardiac arrest in hypothermia is extensively documented. The SARRRAH project is devised by a medical workshop of the German Maritime Rescue Service

(*Deutsche Gesellschaft zur Rettung Schiffbrüchiger,* DGzRS) and it is developed at the Department of Anaesthesiology at the University Hospital of Schleswig-Holstein, at the Lübeck campus. The project partnership includes the German Institute for Naval Medicine, the DGzRS, 11 hospitals on the North and Baltic Sea coasts, and several Institutes of Forensic Medicine. SARRRAH is supported by the Seafarers' Trust of the International Transportworkers Federation (ITF). The aim of the SARRRAH project is to improve the chance of survival in cases of severe accidental hypothermia. For that reason, algorithms for resuscitation and rewarming, which are to be used under severe conditions, have been developed. The main objective of the training program is airway management by combitube and resuscitation via active compression and decompression. The rescue crews have been provided with appropriate equipment for real emergencies. The chief objective of the training program is to initiate resuscitation early at the scene (at sea, in the SAR helicopter). All preclinical and clinical data are documented and analysed for scientific reference [7].

The second aim of the SARRRAH project is the registration of hypothermia incidents. In the case of an accident with severe accidental hypothermia, a physician of the SARRRAH project is informed by the emergency co-ordination centres or by the hospitals via telephone hotline which is available 24 hours a day. As a result, this physician contacts the rescue crew and the hospital, in order to register the data provided by the consulting physician and the emergency physician. This contact at an early stage is important because the loss of essential data is reduced and the information is close to the source of the incident. The SARRRAH protocol provides uniform documentation in its entirety and should be the basis for statistical evaluation. This entire documentation consists of eight different protocols (◘ **Fig. 9.9**): A1, sea rescue; A2, land rescue; B, primary/secondary patient transport; C, hospital admission; D, rewarming; E, discharge from hospital; F, follow up – 6 month; G, forensic medicine, patient content. The protocols, as well as information about the project, can be seen on the homepage at www.sarrrah.de. In the rescue documents, data concerning details of time, outside conditions (atmospheric conditions, sequence of accident, clothing, habitat), information with regard to vital parameters and the applied methods of resuscitation are needed. In the transport document, data concerning the progress of vital parameters due to complications are registered. The clinical document covers an extended screening with laboratory analyses and common parameters of intensive care medicine, covering the clinical process during and after rewarming. The form and duration of the rewarming therapy is of special interest. All changes of body temperature are registered. In the follow-up documentation information regarding the final diagnosis (organ failure, neurologic outcome) and possible medicolegal statements are registered. Patients who do not survive are examined by an institute of legal medicine. After analysis of the complete documentation, answers to the following questions should be sought:

— Which most common incidence of accidental hypothermia features in rescue at sea, maritime rescue and rescue on shore?
— Under which conditions can a longer period of hypoxaemia be survived in severe hypothermia?
— How often is a cardiac arrest recorded in accidental hypothermia?

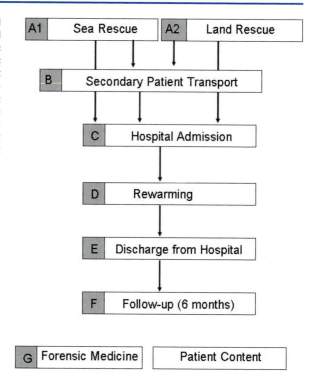

■ **Fig. 9.9.** The SARRRAH registration system is divided into eight different protocols: *A1,* sea rescue; *A2,* land rescue; *B,* primary/secondary patient transport; *C,* hospital admission; *D,* rewarming; *E,* discharge from hospital; *F,* follow up (6 months); *G,* forensic medicine, patient content

- Which techniques of preclinical therapy and rewarming are in use?
- What is the survival rate and the quality of life after cardiac arrest in accidental hypothermia?
- How often and when do hypothermia-related complications such as arrhythmias, post-immersion collapse and temperature "afterfall" occur?
- Which other complications and organ failure occur during the clinical course?

The focal point of the project at this stage is to motivate hospitals to participate and to include all areas near the German coast, perhaps even outside Germany. Recent contacts also include the Argentinian Medical Division of the Naval Hydrographic Service which is considering implementation of the same strategy to improve the treatment of hypothermic patients by using the SARRRAH databank.

References

1. AKOR SRK (1998) Richtlinien für die Behandlung der allgemeinen Unterkühlung (akzidentelle Hypothermie) und lokale Kälteschäden (Erfrierungen) (in German). AKOR SRK (Arbeitsgruppe der Aerztekommission für Rettungswesen)

2. American Heart Association in collaboration with International Liaison Committee on Resuscitation (2000) Guideline 2000 for cardiopulmonary rescuscitation and Emergency Cardiovascular Care: International Consensus on Science, Part 3: Adult basic life support. Circulation 102 (suppl I):I-22–I-59

3. Aukerman J, Voepel-Lewis T, Riegger LQ, et al. (1998) The relationship between extracorporeal circuit prime, albumin, and postoperative weight gain in children. J Cardiothorac Vasc Anesth 12:408–414

4. Axelrod DR, Bass DE (1957) Electrolytes and acid-base balance in hypothermia. Surv Anesthesiol 1:117–118

5. Baker DG (1960) Influence of cold exposure on electrolyte metabolism. Fed Proc 19 (Suppl 5):125–130

6. Battistella FD, Wisner DH (1991) Combined hemorrhagic shock and head injury: effects of hypertonic saline (7.5%) resuscitation. J Trauma 31:182–188

7. Baumeier W, Bahlmann L, Schmucker P (2004) Accidental hypothermia and the project, 'SARRRAH' – first experiences with a multicenter study. In: Oehmichen M (ed) Hypothermia. Clinical, pathomorphological and forensic features. Res Legal Med 31:129-140

8. Behn C, Gayer OH, Kirsch K, Eckert P (1969) Effects of sustained intrathoracic vascular distension on body fluid distribution and renal excretion in man. Pflugers Arch 313:123–135

9. Bergstein J, Quebbeman E, Aprahamian C, et al. (1995) Extra-corporeal rewarming, technological advances and experience in 29 patients. J Trauma 31:1297

10. Bernard SA, Gray TW, Buist MD et al. (2002) Treatment of comatose survivors of out-of hospital cardiac arrest with induced hypothermia. New Engl J Med 346:557–563

11. Bierens JJLM, Uytslager R, Swenne-van Ingen MME, et al. (1995) Accidental hypothermia: incidence, risk factors and clinical course of patients admitted to hospital. EJEM 2:38–46

12. Bigelow WG, Lindsy WK, Harrison RC, et al. (1950) Oxygen transport and utilization in dogs at low body temperatures. Am J Physiol 160:125–137

13. Biggart MJ, Bohn DJ (1990) Effect of hypothermia and cardiay arrest on outcome of near-drowning accidents in children. J Pediatr 117:179–183

14. Bohn DJ, Biggar WD, Smith CR, et al. (1986) Influence of hypothermia, barbiturate therapy and intracranial pressure monitoring on morbidity and mortality after near-drowning. Crit Care Med 14:529–534

15. Broach SD, Durbin CG Jr (2001) A randomized, controlled, clinical trial of a chemically-reactive heated humidifier. Respir Care 46:37–42

16. Brunette DD, McVaney K (2000) Hypothermia cardiac arrest: an 11 year review of ED management and outcome. Am J Emerg Med 18:418–422

17. Cahill CJ, Balmi PJ, Tipton MJ (1995) An evaluation of hand immersion for rewarming of individuals cooled by immersion in cold water. Aviat Space Environ Med 59:78–80

18. CDC news (1996) JAMA 275:510

19. Chadwick S, Gibson A (1997) Hypothermia and the use of space blankets: a literature review. Accident Emerg Nursing 5:122–125

20. Chen RY, Chin S (1977) Plasma volume, red cell volume, and thoracic duct lymph flow in hypothermia. Am J Physiol 233: H605–612

21. Cold injuries and cold water near drowning (2002) National Board of Health and Welfare, Stockholm

22. Manitoba Health Emergency Services. Emergency treatment guidelines 2003. Available at www.gov.mb.ca/health/ems/guidelines

23. Conn AW, Montes JE, Barker GA, Edmonds JF (1980) Cerebral salvage in near-drowning following neurological classification by triage. Can Anaesth Soc J 27:201–210

24. Currie J (1798) Appendix II on the treatment of shipwrecked mariners. In: The effect of water cold and warm as a remedy in fever. Cadell & Davies, London

25. D'Amoto HE, Hegnauer AH (1953) Blood volume in the hypothermic dog. Am J Physiol 173:100–102

26. Daanen HAM, Linde FJG van de (1992) Comparison of four noninvasive rewarming methods for mild hypothermia. Aviat Space Environ Med 63:1070–1076

27. Danzl DF (2002) Hypothermia. Semin Respir Crit Care Med 23:57–69

28. Danzl DF, Pozos RS (1987) Multi-centre hypothermia survey. Ann Emerg Med 16:1042–105
29. Danzl DF, Pozos RS (1994) Accidental hypothermia. New Eng J Med 331:1756–1761
30. Davis FM, Judson JA (1981) Warm peritoneal dialysis in the management of accidental hypo-thermia: report of five cases. N Z Med J 23:207–209
31. Delaney KA, Howland MA, Vassalo S, Goldfrank R (1989) Assessment of acid-base disturbances in hypothermia and their physiologic consequences. Ann Emerg Med 18:72–82
32. Dusek ER (1957) Effect of temperature on manual performance. In: Fisher FR (ed.) Protection and functioning of the hands in cold climates. Nat Acad Sci Washington, pp 63–75
33. Eising GP, Niemeyer M, Günther T, et al. (2001) Does a hyperoncotic cardiopulmonary bypass prime affect extravascular lung water and cardiopulmonary function in patients undergoing coronary artery bypass surgery? Eur J Cardiothorac Surg 20:282–289
34. Falk M, Brugger H, Adler-Kastner L (1994) Avalanche survival changes. Nature 21:368
35. Farstad M, Andersen KS, Koller ME, et al. (2001) Rewarming from accidental hypothermia by extracorporeal circulation. A retrospective study. Eur J Cardiothorac Surg 20:58–64
36. Farstad M, Husby P, Koller ME, et al. (2002) Fluid extravasation during isooncotic cardiopulmo-nasry bypass: effects of hemodilution and hypothermia. Intensive Care Med [Suppl 1]:653
37. Farstad M, Rynning SE, Heltne JK, et al. (2002) Anti-inflammatory agents do not prevent the microvascular fluid leakage induced by hypothermic CPB. Intensive Care Med [Suppl 1]:285
38. Farstad M, Heltne JK, Rynning SE, et al. (2003) Fluid extravasation during cardiopulmonary bypass in piglets – effect of hypothermia and different cooling protocols. Acta Anaesthesiol Scand 47:1–10
39. Frank SM, Hesel TW, El-Rahmany HK, et al. (2000) Warmed humidified inspired oxygen acceler-ates postoperative rewarming. J Clin Anesth 12:283–287
40. Fretchner R, Kloss T, Borowczak C, Berkel H (1993) First aid and prognosis following drowning accidents. Results of a retrospective study of 115 cases. Anasthesiol Intensivmed Notfallmed Schmerzther 28:363–368
41. Gaffin SL, Dietz FB, Brock-Utne JG, et al. (2000) Rewarming from hypothermia leads to elevated plasma lipopolysaccharide concentrations. Undersea Hyperb Med 27:1–7
42. Gentilello LM, Cobean RA, Offner PJ, et al. (1992) Continuous arteriovenous rewarming: rapid reversal of hypothermia in critically ill patients. J Trauma 32:316–27
43. Gentilello LM, Jurkovich GJ, Stark MS, et al. (1997) Is hypothermia in the victim of major trauma protective or harmful? A randomised prospective study. Ann Surg 226:439–447
44. Giesbrecht GG (2000) Cold stress, near drowning and accidental hypothermia: a review. Aviat Space Environ Med 71:733–52
45. Giesbrecht GG (2001) Emergency treatment of hypothermia. Emerg Med 13:9–16
46. Giesbrecht GG, Bristow GK (1992) A second postcooling afterdrop: more evidence for a convec-tive mechanism. J Appl Physiol 73(4):1253–1258
47. Giesbrecht GG, Ducharme MB, McGuirte JP (1994) Comparison of forced-air patiënt warming systems for perioperative use. Anesthesiology 80:671–679
48. Gilbert M, Busund R, Skaqseth A, et al. (2000) Resuscitation from accidental hypothermia of 13.7°C with circulation arrest. Lancet 355:375–376
49. Goheen MSL, Ducharme MB, Kenny GP, et al. (1997) Efficacy of forced-air and inhalation re-warming by using a human model for severe hypothermia. J Appl Physiol 83:1635–1640
50. Golden FStC, Hervey GR (1981) The „afterdrop" and death after rescue from immersion in cold water. In: Adam JA (ed.) Hypothermia ashore and afloat. Aberdeen University Press, Aberdeen
51. Golden FStC, Tipton MJ (2002) Essentials of sea survival. Human Kinetics, Champaign, IL
52. Golden FStC, Hervey GR, Tipton MJ (1991) Circum-rescue collapse: collapse, sometimes fatal, associated with rescue of immersion victims. J R Naval Med Serv 77:139–149
53. Golden FStC, Tipton MJ, Scott RC (1997) Immersion, near-drowning and drowning. Br J Anaesth 79(2):214–225
54. Grahn D, Brock-Utne JG, Watenpaugh DE, Heller HC (1998) Recovery from mild hypother-mia can be accelerated by mechanically distending blood vessels in the hand. J Appl Physiol 85(5):1643–1648
55. Gregory JS, Flancbaum L, Townsend MC, et al. (1991) Incidence and timing of hypothermia in trauma patients undergoing operations. J Trauma 31:795–798

56. Harrison SJ, Ponte J (1996) Convective warming combined with vasodilaory therapy accelerates core rearming after coronary artery bypass surgery. BJA 76:511–14

57. HCAS (Hypothermia after Cardiac Arrest Study Group) (2002) Mild therapeutic hypothermia to improve the neurologic outcome after cardiac arrest. New Engl J Med 346:549–556

58. Heise D, Rathgeber J, Burchardi H (1996) Severe accidental hypothermia: rewarming with a simple extracorporeal circuit. Anaesthesist 45:1093–1096

59. Heltne JK, Koller ME, Lund T, et al. (2001) Studies on fluid extravasation related to induced hypothermia during cardiopulmonary bypass in piglets. Acta Anaesthesiol Scand 45:720–728

60. Henneberg S, Eklund A, Joachimsson PO, et al. (1985) Effects of a thermal ceiling on postoperative hypothermia. Acta Anaesthesiol Scand 29:602–606

61. Hindeman BJ, Funatsu N, Cheng DCH, et al. (1990) Differential effect of oncotic pressure on cerebral and extracerebral water content during cardiopulmonary bypass in rabbits. Anesthesiology 73:951–957

62. Hoskin RW, Melinyshyn MJ, Romet TT, Goode RC (1986) Bath rewarming from immersion hypothermia. J Appl Physiol 61:1518–1522

63. Kanter GS (1968) Hypothermic hemoconcentration. Am J Physiol 214:856–859

64. Keatinge WR, Pry-Roberts C, Cooper KE, et al. (1969) Sudden failure of swimming in cold water. Br Med J 1:480–483

65. Klussmann FW, Lutcke A, Koenig W (1959) Über das Verhalten der Körperflüssigkeiten während künstlicher Hypothermie. Pflugers Arch 268:515–529

66. Koller R, Schnider TW, Neidhart P (1997) Deep accidental hypothermia and cardiac arrest – rewarming with forced air. Acta Anaesthesiol Scand 41:1359–1364

67. Kornberger E, Mair P (1996) Important aspects in the treatment of severe accidental hypothermia: the Innsbruck experience. J Neurosurg Anaesthesiol 8:83–87

68. Kristenson G (1988) Hypothermia Intraoperative and accidental. Principles of treatment. Intens Care World 5:13–16

69. Kulkarni P, Matson A, Bright J et al (1993) Clinical evaluation of the oesophageal heat exchanger in the prevention of preoperative hypothermia. Br J Anaesth 70:216–218

70. Larach MG (1995) Accidental hypothermia. Lancet 345:493–498

71. Lauri T (1996) Cardiovascular responses to an acute volume load in deep hypothermia. Eur Heart J 17:606–611

72. Lazar HL (1997) The treatment of hypothermia. N Eng J Med 337:1545–1547

73. Ledingham IM, Mone JG (1980) Treatment of accidental hypothermia: a prospective clinical study. Br Med J 280:1102–1105

74. Ledingham IM, Douglas IH, Routh GS, Macdonald AM (1980) Central rewarming system for treatment of hypothermia. Lancet 1(8179):1168–1169

75. Lin YC, Hong SK (1984) Physiology of water immersion. Undersea Biomed Res 11:109–111

76. Lloyd EL (1996) Accidental hypothermia. Resuscitation 32:111–124

77. Locher T, Walpoth BH (1996) Differentialdiagnose des Kreislaufstillstands hypothermer Lawinenopfer: retrospektive Analyse von 32 Lawinenunfällen. Schweizerische Rundschau für Medizin (PRAXIS) 85:1275–1282

78. Locher T, Walpoth BH, Pfluger D, Althaus U (1991) Akzidentelle Hypothermie in der Schweiz (1980–1987). Kasuistik und prognostische Faktoren. Schweiz Med Wschr 121:1020–1028

79. Löfström B (1957) Changes in blood volume in induced hypothermia. Acta Anaesthesiol Scand 1:1–13

80. Löfström B (1959) Induced hypothermia and intravascular aggregation. Acta Anaesthesiol Scand 3(Suppl III):1–19

81. Mair P, Kornberger E, Furtwaengler W, et al. (1994) Prognostic markers in patients with severe accidental hypothermia and cardiocirculatory arrest. Resuscitation 27:47–54

82. Martin (1984) Near drowning and cold water immersion. Ann Emerg Med 13:263–273

83. McInerney JJ, Breakell A, Madira W, et al. (2002) Accidental hypothermia and active rewarming; the metabolic and inflammatory changes observed above and below 32 degrees C. Emerg Med J 19:219–223

84. Mehlhorn U, Allen SJ, Davis KL, et al. (1998) Increasing the colloid osmotic pressure of cardiopulmonary bypass prime and normothermic blood cardioplegia minimizes myocardial oedema and prevents cardiac dysfunction. Cardiovasc Surg 6:274–281

85. Mills WJJ (1993) Accidental hypothermia: management approach. Alaska Med 35:54–56

86. Nielsen HK, Toft P, Koch J, Andersen PK (1992) Hypothermic patients admitted to an intensive care unit: a fifteen year survey. Dan Med Bull 39:190–193

87. Oakley EHN, Pethybridge RJ (1997) The prediction of survival during cold immersion: results from the UK national immersion incident survey. INM Report No. 97011, Alverstoke, UK

88. Popovic V (1960) Physiological characteristics of rats and ground squirrels during prolonged lethargic hypothermia. Am J Physiol 199:467–471

89. Popovic V, Kent KM (1965) Cardiovascular responses in prolonged hypothermia. Am J Physiol 209:1069–1074

90. Popovic V, Popovic P (1974) In: Hypothermia in biology and medicine. Grune & Stratton, New York San Fransisco London, pp 55–58

91. Prough DS, Carson Johnson J, Poole GV, et al. (1985) Effect on intracranial pressure of resuscitation from hemorrhagic shock with hypertonic saline versus lactated Ringer's solution. Crit Care Med 13:407–411

92. Rahn H, Reeves RB (1982) Hydrogen regulation during hypothermia: from the Amazone to the operating room. In: Applied respiratory physiology in clinical respiratory care. Martinus Nyhoff, the Hague, pp 1–15

93. Risch WD, Koubenec HJ, Beckmann U, et al. (1978) The effect of graded immersion on heart volume, central venous pressure, pulmonary blood distribution, and heart rate in man. Pflugers Arch 374:115–18

94. Roberts DE, Barr JC, Kerr D, et al. (1985) Fluid replacement during hypothermia. Aviat Space Environ Med 56:333–337

95. Roggla M, Frossard M, Wagner A, et al. (2002) Severe accidental hypothermia with or without hemodynamic instability: rewarming without the use of extracorporeal circulation. Wien Klin Wochenschr 114(8–9):315–320

96. Romet TT, Hoskin RW (1988) Temperature and metabolic responses to inhalation and bath rewarming protocols. Aviat Space Environ Med 59:630–635

97. Sanford MM (1997) Rewarming cardiac surgical patients: warm water vs warm air. Am J Crit Care 6:39–45

98. Schaller MD, Fischer AP, Perret CH (1990) Hypokalemia: a prognosis factor during acute severe hypothermia. JAMA 264: 1842–1845

99. Segers MJM, Diephuis JC, Kesteren RG van, Werken C van der (1997) Drie patienten met accidentele hypothermie; opwarmen op maat. Ned Tijdschr Geneeskd 141:1369–1373

100. Sessler DI (1997) Mild perioperative hypothermia. N Engl J Med 336:1730–1737

101. Sheaff CM, Fildes JJ, Keogh P, et al. (1996) Safety of 65 degrees C intravenous fluid for the treatment of hypothermia. Am J Surg 172:52–55

102. Soreide E, Grahn DA, Brock-Utne JG, Rosen L (1999) A non-invasive means to effectively restorenormothermia in coldstressed individuals: a preliminary report. J Emerg Med 17:725–730

103. State of Alaska cold injuries and cold water near drowning (2005) Department of Health and Social Services, Juneau, Alaska. Available at www.hypothermia.org

104. Steel MT, Nelson MJ, Sessler DI, et al. (1997) Forced air speeds rewarming in accidental hypothermia. Ann Emerg Med 27:479–484

105. Steinman A, Giesbrecht G (2001) Cold-water immersion. In: Auerbach PS (ed) Wilderness medicine, 4th edn. Mosby, St Louis, pp 197–225

106. Steinman AM (1987) Prehospital management of hypothermia. Response 6:18

107. Stotz M, Ummenhofer W (2002) Pediatric case report: near drowning in cold water. Book of abstracts, World Congress on Drowning, p 74

108. Suominen P, Baillie C, Korpela R, et al. (2002) Impact of age, submersion time and water temperature on outcome in near drowning. Resuscitation 52:247–254

109. Svanes K, Zweifach BW, Intaglietta M (1970) Effect of hypothyermia on tran scapilary fluid exchange. Am J Physiol 218:981–989

110. Swan H (1984) The importance of acid-base management for cardiac and cerebral preservation during open heart operations. Surg Gyn Obst 158:391–414
111. Taguchi A (2001) Negative pressure rewarming vs forced air rewarming in hypothermic postaneasthetic volunteers. Anaesth Analg 92:261–266
112. Tikuisis P (1995) Predicting survival time for cold exposure. Int J Biometeorol 39:94–102
113. Tikuisis P (1997) Prediction of survival time at sea based on observed body cooling rates. Aviat Space Environ Med 68:441–448
114. Tikuisis P, Belyavin AJ, Buxton AC, et al. (1997) Prediction of body cooling. DCIEM Report No. 97-TM-47
115. Tikuisis P, Eyolfson DA, Giesbrecht GG (2002) Shivering endurance and fatigue during cold water immersion. Eur J Appl Physiol 87:50–58
116. Tipton MJ (1989) The initial responses to cold-water immersion in man. Clin Sci 77:581–588
117. Tipton MJ, Golden FStC (1998) Immersion in cold water: effects on performance and safety. In: Oxford textbook of sports medicine, 2nd edn. Oxford University Press, Oxford
118. Tipton MJ, Kelleher P, Golden FStC (1994) Supraventricular arrhythmias following breath-hold submersions in cold water. Undersea Hyperb Med 21:305–313
119. Tipton MJ, Franks M, Gennser C M, Golden FStC (1999) Immersion death and deterioration in swimming performance in cold water. Lancet 354:626–629
120. Töllöfsrud S, Noddeland H (1997) Hypertonic saline and dextran after coronary artery surgery mobilizes fluid excess and improves cardiorespiratory functions. Acta Anaesthesiol Scand 42:154–161
121. Tveita T (2000) Rewarming from hypothermia. Newer aspects on the pathophysiology of rewarming shock. Int J Circumpolar Health 59:260–266
122. Vangaard L, Eyolfson D, Xu X, Giesbrecht GG (1998) Arteriovenous anastomosis (AVA) rewarming in 45°C water is effective in moderately hypothermic subjects. FASEB J 12:A90
123. Vanggaard L, Eyolfson D, Xu X, et al. (1999) Immersion of forearms and lower legs in 45°C water effectively rewarms moderately hypothermic subjects. Aviat Space Environ Med 11:1081–1088
124. Vassal T, Benoit-Gonon B, Carrat F, et al. (2001) Severe accidental hypothermia treated in an ICU: prognosis and outcome. Chest 120:1998–2003
125. Von Segesser LK, Garcia E, Turina M (1991) Perfusion without systemic heparinization for rewarming in accidental hypothermia. Ann Thorac Surg 52:560–561
126. Vretenar DF, Urchel JD, Parrot JCW, Unruh HW (1994) Cardiopulmonary bypass resuscitation for accidental hypothermia. Ann Thorac Surg 58:95–98
127. Wallace W (1997) Does it make sense to heat gases higher than body temperature for the treatment of cold water near-drowning or hypothermia? A point of view paper. Alaska Med 39:75–77
128. Walpoth BH, Locher T, Laupi F, et al. (1990) Accidental deep hypothermia with cardiopulmonary arrest: extracorporeal blood rewarming in eleven eleven patients. Eur J Cardiothorac Surg 4:390–393
129. Walpoth BH, Walpoth-Aslan BN, Mattle HP, et al. (1997) Outcome of survivors of accidental deep hypothermia and circulatory arrest treated with extracorporal blood warming. N Engl J Med 337:1500–1505
130. Wolff J, Bigler D, Drenck NE, Frosig F (1987) Chronic deep accidental hypothermia. Ugeskr Laeger 149:1177–1179
131. Yamauchi M, Nakayama Y, Yamakage M, et al. (1998) Preventive effect of fluid warmer system on hypothermia induced by rapid intravenous infusion. Masui 47:606–610
132. Yeh T, Parmar JM, Rebeyka IM,et al. (1992) Limiting edema in neonatal cardiopulmonary bypass with narrow-range molecular weight hydroxyethyl starch. J Thorac Cardiovasc Surg 104:659–665
133. Zachary L, Kucan JO, Robson MC, Frank DH (1982) Accidental hypothermia treated with rapid rewarming by immersion. Ann Plastic Surg 9:238–241
134. Zandstra DF (1997) Behandeling van accidentele en peri-operative hypothermie. In: Bakker J, de Lange B, Rommes JH (eds) Intensive care: capita selecta 1997. Stichting Venti-Care, Utrecht, 1997:247-259

Water-Related Disasters

TASK FORCE ON WATER-RELATED DISASTERS
Section editors: ROB BRONS and JOOST BIERENS

Task Force Chairs

- Rob Brons
- Rob de Bruin
- Gerard Laanen

Task Force Members

- Marileen Biekart
- Adriaan Hopperus Buma
- Menno van Duin
- Dick Fundter
- Corsmas Goemans
- Albert de Haas
- Ries Kruidenier
- Anja Nachtegaal
- Sjaak Poortvliet
- Robert Slomp
- Sip Wiebenga

Other Contributors

- Joost Bierens
- Helga Brandstrom
- Bas Jonkman
- Amanda Kost
- Martin Madern
- Jim Segerstrom
- Pieter van der Torn
- Karel Vandevelde
- Joop Wijers

10.1
Overview

ROB BRONS and JOOST BIERENS

This section gives an overview of water-related disasters. Most authors are Dutch. There are two reasons for this. During the preparation of the World Congress on Drowning, the project coordinator was unable to identify existing international experts or an expert network in the field of drowning due to large accidents at sea or floods. Only in a very late stadium, when all other task forces had kicked off, it became possible to start a task force on water-related disasters. For practical reasons, considering limitations in time and span of control, the decision was taken to make this a Dutch-only task force. The second reason is that there is a lot of expertise on these issues in the Netherlands. The expertise of the task force members is collected in this section, as well as expertise from other countries identified at a later point.

The section includes two different types of water-related disasters. In ▶ Chapter 10.3–10.6 the impact of large incidents at sea on drowning is described. In ▶ Chapter 10.7–10.12 the impact of floods on drowning is described. The content of most chapters in this section reflects aspects relevant to organisations and policymakers and relates to the national and international dimensions that most authorities in this field have to deal with. At the same time the chapters clearly indicate the important, albeit rudimentarily developed, role of rescue organisations and medical disciplines. Most of all this section should help to further stimulate international knowledge exchange in this field.

In ▶ Chapter 10.3, Helge Brandstrom overviews recent large incidents at sea. Her focus is on the impact on the human body. From her analysis it can be concluded that most people die from drowning and not from hypothermia during these mass incidents. The key issue is whether a flotation device will hold the head above water when the victim becomes unconscious. If the head is not kept above water, most victims drown when loosing consciousness. If the flotation device keeps the head above water, most victims die from hypothermia depending on temperature and condition of the sea, body size, thickness of subcutaneous fat and insulation of clothes. It is important to realise that hypothermia complicates survival already before death ensues because hypothermic victims quickly loose grip strength and the ability to coordinate swimming motions. Hypothermic victims of accidents at sea will therefore be unable to perform necessary survival actions such as hanging on to other victims, wreckage or an overturned boat. Brandstrom anticipates that the current triage criteria will be of limited value when medical personnel are confronted with large numbers of hypothermic patients and that wrong decisions will be made, leading to preventable death.

In ▶ Chapter 10.4 Dr. Karel Vandevelde, who was involved in the 'Herald of Free Enterprise' disaster in 1987, gives an explanation of this particular accident. At the same time this case report illustrates the problems mentioned in the previous chapter. There were 543 passengers and crew, 42 trucks and 84 cars on board the 'Herald of Free Enterprise'. There was no time for passengers to be evacuated to the emergency sloops: the ferry capsized in a few minutes. Within hours, two thirds of the victims were rescued by a large-scale military and civil rescue operation. At sea, emergency medical personal was unable to work effectively because they lacked experience in emergency care at sea. One third of the passengers and crew died, one third were hospitalised, while the rest were admitted to emergency shelters.

In ▶ Chapter 10.5, Sip Wiebenga, the managing director of the Royal Netherlands Sea Rescue Institute (KNRM), provides new insights into how national search and rescue (SAR) units can be prepared for large-scale incidents at sea. The KNRM is currently developing a computer model that subdivides the SAR area into a fine meshed grid. For each of the elements of the grid the annual probability of accidents and the accompanying probable number of casualties is calculated. For each sector, the estimated total number of saved casualties can be calculated based on various scenarios, such as the circumstances of the incident, the time period that the casualties are able to survive and the time for the various SAR units to reach the accident spot. In the model a drowning person becomes a saved casualty if there is enough rescue capacity within appropriate time for that person. The appropriate time is calculated with regard to the scenario of the disaster and the circumstances. The higher the number of saved casualties the better the complete SAR fleet plan is adapted to provide assistance in the given circumstances. The model also provides insight in the most effective manner to organise the national SAR organisations in case of a large scale incident at sea.

In ▶ **Chapter 10.6** Martin Madern, senior safety consultant of the Hague Fire and Rescue, and Rob Brons, Regional Chief Fire Officer in The Hague, discuss the complicated interaction of regulations between sea and land authorities when it comes to the management of large incidents that affect both land and sea. They conclude that national, as well as international, coordination between the several communication centres and dispatch centres requires further improvement. North Sea disaster planning should include clear schedules concerning warning and alarm protocols, up-grading and communication. A European or international service should be established for this purpose, but also to collect information on fighting accidents, coordination, planning, preparation and practice. Great improvement is expected from uniform phases of upgrading, an optimal network of involved organisations and better coordination of planning. As a result of combined exercises in communication, coordination and testing of each other's planning, experience is growing with these extremely complex situations.

The second part of this section is related to the drowning risks of floods. In ▶ **Chapter 10.7**, Bas Jonkman overviews the mortality statistics of worldwide fresh water floods. Death rates after floods are enormous, over 100,000 deaths per year or 30,000 deaths during one flood period. Based on a limited number of reported case studies, an initial analysis of causes of death is given in this chapter. Flood-related mortality strongly depends on the flood type. The response of people to flood exposure is a critical factor for morbidity and mortality. However, the empirical evidence for the relevance of the different causes of death is rather weak and more insight into the causes of flood mortality is needed. In addition, knowledge on the non-lethal effects of floods is limited and there is a need for more and better quantitative data on health impacts associated with all categories of flooding. This requires a centralised and systematic national reporting of deaths and injuries from floods using a standardised methodology. It is also recommended that coastal floods be included in future analyses. Such information is of practical value when preventive measures can be indicated.

Joop Weijers, Robert Slomp and Sjaak Poortvliet focus in ▶ **Chapter 10.8** on the measures taken in the Netherlands to prevent the country from flooding. Most river floods originate outside the country and the international flood warning system is based on data received from partners in Germany, Belgium and France. Expected water levels of all major waterways are communicated daily. When large quantities of water are expected, the decision to evacuate areas is taken by the provincial governor on information from water boards and the municipal governments. The population is warned by siren and informed through local television and radio stations. Another aspect of flood preparation is to know which flood defences are most likely to fail, what the consequences would probably be and what would be the best procedures to reduce casualties. In case of extreme river floods or storm surges, flood defences such as dikes, dunes and structures may wash out, collapse or fail. Infrastructural improvements can be initiated and pre-emptive evacuations or evacuations during floods can be prepared. In the Netherlands there is currently a discussion as to whether sparsely populated areas should be sacrificed to save more populated areas from flooding.

Martin Madern, Rob Brons and Amanda Kost, juridical policy maker at The Hague Fire and Rescue Service, introduce the safety chain in ▶ Chapter 10.9 as a policy concept for mass incidents. Crisis management and disaster relief in the Netherlands is based on this concept of integral safety. The safety chain contains five links: proaction, prevention, preparedness, response and recovery. The introduction of this concept has had a beneficial effect on interaction and cooperation on a national, provincial and local level. The safety chain concept can be used in all aspects of the safety and security sector such as firefighting, police force, fighting crime, health care, medical assistance and crisis and disaster management, and contributes to the coherency among their activities. It can also be considered a policy model of input, throughput and output. Output becomes input again at the beginning of the chain so that one can learn from previous mistakes. It is also important for the safety chain that every chain is as strong as the weakest link. To create a strong safety chain, all the links must be properly welded together and the policy, concerning development as well as implementation, must be as coherent as possible. The authors take the reader along the chain through mass water-related incidents.

In ▶ Chapter 10.10 Sjaak Poortvliet, policy maker for the Dutch Water Board Association focuses on risk control of flood-related drowning. He also uses the safety chain from proaction and prevention to risk control of flooding. The aim of the policy for risk control is not the limitation of flooding risks at any price but as the result of a consideration of the costs and benefits of several options. The starting point of the policy is to accept that the risks of flooding by rivers and sea cannot be entirely eliminated but can only be limited by constructing flood defences or by returning some of the space that has been reclaimed to water. The average acceptable risk determined for the upper course of the major rivers in the Netherlands is that flooding may occur every 1250 years. The acceptable risk determined for areas in the lower course, in the river delta and on the coast, is between once every 4000 and 10,000 years, depending on the population density and activities in the area concerned.

Pieter van der Torn and Bas Jonkman take you through the planning of mass emergency response to floods in the Netherlands in ▶ Chapter 10.11. The Ministry of Internal Affairs and Kingdom Relations has developed two guidelines to stimulate planning efforts for all kinds of disasters that may occur in the country. One guideline focuses on victim needs and the other guideline on the means for response to each type and severity of disaster. The input for the guidelines is based on subjective expert opinions. The guidelines were presented to the local authorities in 2000 for further study of the local consequences and have given a considerable impetus to the planning efforts of local authorities. Floods are also included as a disaster type. Using the current recommendations, the consequences of flood disaster on victim needs and means for response can be estimated by computer simulations. With these simulations an improved estimate can be made of the time factors, inundated areas, local circumstances and number of affected residents. A simulation for the Rotterdam and The Hague area shows that about one million residents will be affected in the inundated area. Such enormous scenarios emphasise the need to match the needs in various ways and to assess the trade-offs between proactive and reactive measures.

In the final chapter of this section, Jim Segerstrom confirms the enormous potential threats that can be posed by floods and states that floods may increasingly become the largest natural threat to the world. He offers some examples to support this statement: On July 12, 2003, one million civilians guarded embankments of flooded rivers in China. Millions of Chinese were displaced, at least 40 were missing and 16 perished. On August 3, 2003, large areas of New Hampshire, New Jersey, and Quebec were hit by massive flooding. Two days later the Sudan prepared for the worst flooding in the century and on August 6, 2003, floods in Pakistan affected over 1 million people and killed over 300. Motivated by his observations and practical experiences to deal with flood situations, Segerstrom proposes simple and realistic tools for policy makers about how to prepare communities for such situations.

10.2
Consensus and Recommendations

ROB BRONS and JOOST BIERENS

Although there was no consensus meeting on water-related disasters during the World Congress on Drowning, there are certainly lessons to be learned. On the basis of the contribution of the authors in this section, certain recommendations can be made:

- There is a sharp distinction between disaster handling on land and on sea, due to time and space factors. Both theoretical conclusions by Brandstrom and the case of the 'Herald of Free Enterprise' demonstrate that the logistics for emergencies on sea are quite different than on land. Wiebenga from the Royal Netherland Sea Rescue Institute shows us, that working with computer models maybe helpful in solving logistical aspects. Nevertheless, the model needs to be worked out on the basis of more scientific research.
- The prediction of flooding on the basis of computer simulation supports decision makers in their ordering of public space. Jonkman shows us that simulation is also necessary to predict certain trends in flooding. The use of such simulation will be a great help in realising the prevention of casualties in threatened areas.
- When it comes to floodings, it is useful to plan contingencies, regardless of territorial borders. International cooperation and networks of expertise are necessary for policymakers in flood prevention and response.

— Segerstrom shows us that lifesaving in flood situations is trainable, not only for lifesavers, such as policemen, firemen and lifeguards. Also, self-rescue training is possible and contributes to better awareness, especially in mass emergency response situations.

— Last but not least, people working in the field of lifeguarding need to realise that their experience in daily practice is insufficient for a mass emergency situation. There is a need to manage the expectations of the role of lifesaving organisations during water-related disasters.

10.3
Disasters at Sea

Helge Brandstrom

A large number of accidents and shipwrecks at sea have occurred over the last 20 years, some with catastrophic consequences. Some of the most well known are summarised in ◘ Table 10.1.

10.3.1
Immersion Hypothermia

Experiences from these and other accidents show that even large ships sink with astonishing rapidity and that many persons on board will abandon the ship. The

◘ **Table 10.1.** Some recent accidents at sea

Year	Name of the ship	Location of accident	Type of accident	Mortality
1987	Herald of Free Enterprise	Zeebrugge	Capsized	188
1987	Donna Paz	The Philippines	Fire onboard	2000
1990	Scandinavian Star	Swedish West Coast	Fire onboard	158
1991	Salem Express	The Red Sea	Storm, aground	480
1993	Jan Heweliusz	Baltic Sea	Capsized	55
1993	Neptune	Haiti	Storm	2000
1994	Estonia	Baltic Sea	Storm, capsized	859
1999	Sleipner	Norwegian West Coast	Storm, aground, capsized	16

low temperature of the sea leads to a rapid cooling and hypothermia ensues often in all shipwrecked victims. There has been some debate as to whether people in cold water die of hypothermia or drowning. The key question is whether the flotation device they are wearing will hold their head above water when they become unconscious. If it will not, most victims drown on losing consciousness. If it will, most victims die from hypothermia depending on temperature and condition of the water, body size, thickness of subcutaneous fat and insulation of clothes. Before death ensues, hypothermia complicates survival because the victims quickly lose the ability to coordinate swimming motions and grip strength. Victims of accidents at sea will become unable to do many of the things that are necessary for survival in cold water, including hanging on to other victims, wreckage, or an overturned boat because cooling down leads to impaired neuromuscular co-ordination and inability to grip or swim. Consciousness is in due course affected and unconsciousness ensues. Rescue equipment, including lifejackets, survival clothing and ladders to life rafts must be adapted in order to deal with these difficulties.

Rough waves are another deadly threat that affect the health and survival of victims through faster onset of hypothermia, decreased buoyancy, aspiration of water and fatigue.

10.3.2
Measures to Increase Preparedness

Measures need to be taken to prevent these accidents from happening at all, but when they occur a number of issues need to be considered.

As long as people are still on board they may be injured by trauma or burns and need attention and treatment. This is an extra problem to deal with.

If the ship has to be abandoned the organisation of the evacuation must be well known and the evacuation systems must be in good order. Evacuation routes, suited to the behaviour of people in threatening situations, must be prepared, as well as possibilities for people to get out quickly into the open.

Lifejackets must be easy to put on, have crotch straps and sufficient buoyancy to keep the head of an injured person above water and must be able to turn an unconscious person into a face upward position. Lifejackets should preferably preserve heat, including preservation of the temperature of the head. Life rafts must be constructed in a manner that they automatically turn the right way up, otherwise they can not be utilised, particularly by those in an emergency.

Instructions are of vital importance and must be brief, precise and in English as well as the local language. Information systems for passengers, intended for use in emergency situations, must have back-up systems and it must be possible for the crew to receive feed-back whether the information has been received or not.

Every minute of delay increases the risk of death in an emergency situation in a cold sea. The current call-out time for rescue boats and helicopters outside office hours of more than 1 hour is too long and people die while awaiting rescue. The time between notification of a base and start of the rescue should be less than 15 min. The rescue organisation must also have great flexibility and alternative solutions must be included in disaster plans because external circumstances, such as weather and waves, can make rapid changes in priorities necessary. Circum-rescue collapse is a threat in a patient with hypothermia or hypovolaemia from traumatic injuries. The effect of sudden loss of the hydrostatic support when taken out of the water can be fatal. Rescuers should know how to deal with the circum-rescue collapse when victims are taken out of the sea or in transition from water to air. The removal from water in a horizontal posture is preferable in all circumstances when possible.

Correct registration of passengers facilitates searches, identification and provision of information to relatives.

10.3.3
Triage Systems and Priority Guidelines

In situations like a shipwreck involving large numbers of injured people, triage is often needed. Triage is the process of sorting patients into priorities in order to establish an order for treatment and evacuation. Triage is a dynamic process and may be needed at different moments and levels of control. The overall aim however, is always the same: to provide the right patient with the right care at the right time in the right place. Triage procedures must be simple swift, reliable and reproducible.

Several triage systems exist and in ◘ **Table 10.2** an example is given of a commonly used prehospital triage system from Sweden.

The simple triage and rapid transport (START) triage system is an alternative triage system that is used in the US (◘ **Table 10.3**).

In the Triage Sieve, a system used in the UK, triage is based on the ability to move and a simple assessment of airway breathing and circulation. Another aspect of the Triage Sieve is the capillary refill time (CRT) which gives a simple and rapid to ascertain indication of peripheral perfusion. Environmental conditions, especially dark and cold, make the use of CRT however difficult. If this is the case, the pulse should be used as the indicator for perfusion (◘ **Table 10.4**).

10.3.4
Limitations of the Triage Systems

When dealing with hypothermic victims each of the triage systems has its limitations. It should be considered that clinical signs in hypothermic patients are not the same as in normothermic victims. CRT, pulse and breathing may be very difficult to assess in a hypothermic victim and these parameters are therefore not applicable as triage criteria in the hypothermic situation. Also the triage criteria for death do not apply in the hypothermic victim. A potentially deep hypothermic patient who seems to be dead and has no obvious fatal injuries, should be treated and transported with the highest priority, and not considered a hopeless and lost case. Hypothermic casualties are regarded to be alive until

□ Table 10.2. The prehospital triage system used in Sweden

Description	Colour	Priority class	
Immediate	Red	1	Immediate priority (red casualties) require immediate procedures to save life. Examples of immediate priorities are airway obstruction and tension pneumothorax
Urgent	Yellow	2	Urgent priority (yellow casualties) require medical treatment within 4–6 hours. Examples of urgent priorities are compound fractures
Delayed	Green	3	Delayed priority (green casualties) have injuries that can wait for treatment for up to 4–6 hours. This triage group also includes casualties with non-survivable injuries
Dead	Black/ white	4	Dead (black/white casualties) must be identified and clearly labelled as such to avoid re-triage

□ Table 10.3. The simple triage and rapid transport (START) triage system used in the US

Is the patient breathing?	no	=>	Open airway, breathing now?
		no	=>	*Dead*
		yes	=>	*Immediate care*
	yes	=>	Assess rate
			>30 => *Immediate care*
			<30 => check radial pulse
Radial pulse present?	no	=>	control haemorrhage
		=>	*Immediate care*
	yes	=>	assess mental state
Following commands	no	=>	*Immediate care*
	yes	=>	*Urgent care*

■ **Table 10.4.** Triage system based on the Triage Sieve

Mobility	Can the patient walk?	yes	=>	P3 Delayed
		no	=>	Assess airway and breathing
Airway and breathing	Is the patient breathing?	no	=>	Open airway, breathing now?
			no =>	Dead
			yes =>	P1 immediate
		yes	=>	Assess rate
			<10 or >29 =>	P1 immediate
			10–29 =>	Assess Circulation
Circulation	CRT	>2 Seconds or pulse >120 beats/min	=>	P1 immediate
	CRT	<2 Seconds or pulse <120 beats/min	=>	P2 urgent

CRT: capillary refill time.

rewarming and monitoring have taken place in hospital. The only exception to this advice is when a victim has been under the water for more than an hour or has obvious fatal injuries.

10.3.5
Priority Guidelines in the Hypothermic Situation

Prioritisation guidelines in case of hypothermia must be carefully prepared, as must be the handling of hypothermic patients. In a disaster with predominantly cold patients such as in situations when people are rescued from a capsized boat at sea, the temperature of the victims should be assessed. It is of great value to be able to measure body temperature in a simple and adequate manner in order to prioritise and treat patients correctly. This requires access to thermometers.

When it is impossible to measure body temperature because there is no thermometer available, high priority (very urgent) is given to suspected hypothermic patients with:
- Impaired vital functions
- Reduced consciousness or unconsciousness
- Profound hypothermia and apparently dead
- Simultaneous severe trauma

Low priority (non-urgent) is given to suspected hypothermia patients with:
- Vital functions unaffected
- No simultaneous trauma
- No signs of life, apparent mild hypothermia, reason to believe suffocation preceded cooling (submersion longer than 15 min)

If a thermometer is available and the situation permits temperature measurement, priorities are as described below.

High priority (very urgent) is given to patients:
- With vital functions impaired
- With body temperature below 28°C and/or reduced consciousness
- With significant trauma and temperature below 35°C

Medium priority (urgent) is given to patients with:
- Vital functions unaffected
- Body temperature between 28 and 32°C but no reduction of consciousness
- Body temperature between 28 and 32°C but no simultaneous trauma

Low priority (non-urgent) is given to patients with:
- Body temperature between 32 and 35°C and vital functions normal
- Body temperature between 32 and 35°C and no reduction of consciousness
- No simultaneous trauma
- No signs of life and meeting the criteria for death

10.3.6
Hospital Care or Care Onboard a Rescue Ship

In many major disasters, available resources are immediately outstripped by need. The treatment of hypothermic patients must be adapted to situations without optimal resources. This often means passive rewarming, which in itself is a good and safe therapy for many hypothermic victims. When there are sufficient resources for optimum care, such as active rewarming, the therapy can be modified accordingly. Planning of co-operation across country borders and realistic exercises with all authorities involved in rescue-operations at sea will add to the opportunity to be able to provide optimum care to a maximum group of victims.

10.3.7
Psychological Aspects

An accident at sea, a shipwreck, an onboard fire, or a drowning situation is a significant physiologic insult. It is also an emotionally charged situation during rescue, transport and in the emergency room. Those who are emotionally affected by the incident should be recognised. People who have been involved should be given the opportunity to talk about this with other involved colleagues. All personnel who has taken part in the rescue work should be given an opportunity to rest and should not immediately return to work (see also ▶ Chap. 5.20).

Further Reading

Kunskapsöversikter. Hypothermia – Cold injuries and cold water near drowning. National Board of Health and Wellfare Sweden. Modin-Tryck, Stockholm 2002

10.4
'Herald of Free Enterprise'

Karel Vandevelde

On Friday 6th March 1987, at 7.30 pm, the ferry 'Herald of Free Enterprise' accidentally capsized 1 mile out of the harbour of Zeebrugge. On board were 543 passengers and crew, 42 trucks and 84 cars. Almost immediately, and prior to the transmission of any emergency signal, a calamitous scenario arose as a result of the instantaneous loss of emergency lighting. The vessel rapidly filled with water and became a dark steel maze. There was no time for the distribution of lifejackets. The seawater temperature of nearly 0°C was too cold and it was too dark to fasten the available lifejackets. There was no time for an evacuation to the emergency sloops: the ferry capsized in a few minutes. Within hours, two thirds of the victims had been rescued by a large-scale military and civil rescue operation.

At sea, emergency medical personnel were unable to work effectively. Rescue on board the wreck was done mostly by simple means such as ropes and ladders being lowered into small openings. The complex structure of the ferry caused problems for both rescue divers and medical personnel, making the wreck and drowning victims poorly accessible. Nevertheless, seven medical teams were able to board the ship and provide medical care.

Helicopters landed at a nearby military harbour while boats with rescued victims were directed towards an empty pontoon where further transport with ambulances and busses was organised. This transportation was operational by 8.45 pm. The pontoon formed a bottleneck ensuring triage of all victims.

A total of 250 individuals were triaged within hours after the disaster by the 21 medical teams present in the harbour. Extensive available resources made it possible to start advanced life support (ALS) at the triage station. The victims who were injured were referred to the nearest hospitals according to the type and extent of their injuries. Only one patient was later referred to a higher echelon. The uninjured were transported by buses to emergency shelters managed by the Red Cross. Due to good medical triage and regulation in the harbour area, hospitals were not overcrowded. It helped that the first victims came on land 45 min after capsizing, allowing the medical coordinator to organise access and departure routes for the ambulances and to give instructions to medical personal. Visible signs of medical command and existing disaster plans were of great help. Low tide was partly the reason for opening two other triage points later on the evening.

Evaluation of the outcome showed that one third of the passengers and crew died, one third were hospitalised and the rest were sent to emergency shelters. Most of the casualties were assumed to have died due to immersion hypothermia. The majority of injuries in the hospital were orthopaedic trauma, bruises and cuts, which did not require complicated operations or investigations. Less than 7% of the victims had problems that needed intensive care treatment for drowning and pulmonary oedema. The average hospitalisation was only 5 days. A few patients in cardiac arrest and hypothermia were sent to hospital for further treatment. One young girl survived resuscitation from deep hypothermic cardiac arrest without sequelae. In addition to the provision of emergency medical care on site, normal emergency health care in the region remained undisrupted.

Disaster victim identification and post-traumatic stress disorder treatment played an important role in the post-incident management.

Disasters at sea are complex because the combination of hypothermia, drowning and trauma will always be difficult to manage.

In this disaster there were additional problems caused by the absence of a complete passenger list, the absence of a list of toxic products on board, the location of the accident, the extreme weather conditions, inadequate rescue dress and equipment for medical personnel, poor radio communication and obstruction by media and disaster tourists. Considering these circumstances and impediments this rescue operation was performed successfully.

Further Reading

Department of Transport (1987) MV Herald of Free Enterprise: Report of Court n° 8074. Formal investigation. Merchant shipping act 1894. Marine accident. Department of Transport London 09/1987. UNIPUB, London

Timperman J (1987) De medicolegale tussenkomst in het onderzoek van de slachtoffers van de veerbootramp te Zeebrugge. Belg Arch Soc Gen Hyg Arbeidsg Gerecht Gen 45:288–310

Timperman J (1991) How some medicolegal aspects of the Zeebrugge Ferry disaster apply to the investigation of mass disasters. Am J Forensic Med Pathol 12:286–290

Tischerman S, Vandevelde K, Safar P, et al. (1997) Future directions for resuscitation research. V. Ultra advanced life support. Resuscitation 34:281–293

Vandevelde K, Mullie A (1987) Over de plaats van de Medische Urgentie Groep (MUG) in de rampgeneeskunde. Het Belgisch Ziekenhuis 186:28–29

Yao Zhong Chen (2000) Sea rescue in the world. Prehosp Disaster Med 15:S75

10.5
Decision Support System for Optimising a SAR Fleet Plan to Rescue Large Numbers of Passengers

SIP WIEBENGA

The primary task of a search and rescue (SAR) organisation is to rescue persons in distress at sea. Several thousands of rescue missions are conducted annually by national SAR organisations such as the Royal Netherland Sea Rescue Institute (KNRM) of the Netherlands. A large percentage of these missions are successful in preventing further personal injury and loss of life. Rarely disasters occur with more casualties than one single SAR unit can accommodate. However, once every few decades a SAR organisation will be faced with a disaster with a passenger ship that might accommodate over 2000 persons. A SAR organisation needs to be prepared, as far as reasonably possible, for such an event. Preparing for this kind of event takes knowledge of the ferry and cruise characteristics, the casualty statistics and the SAR fleet plan.

The KNRM in combination with port and maritime consultants has developed a decision support system (DCS) that enables SAR organisations to estimate their long-term effectiveness. The model enables the SAR organisation to oversee the consequences of future changes in their fleet plan and to optimise the fleet plan with regard to seasonal changes in nature and number of distress calls per area.

The model subdivides the SAR area in a fine mashed grid. For each of the elements of the grid the annual (or in a later version the seasonal) probability of accidents and the accompanying probable number of casualties is calculated. Consequently the time that the casualties are able to survive, given the circumstances, is calculated. Finally, the time for the various SAR units, based at different locations along the coast, to reach the accident spot is calculated. This calculation will result in the estimated total number of saved casualties per year. The higher the number of saved casualties the better the SAR fleet plan is adapted to the given circumstances.

The input for these calculations is organised into three modules:

- SAR organisation information module
  In this module the available information on the SAR facilities is defined. The location of stations, their response time and the type and number of units at the stations can be changed, in order to analyse the influence of these changes on the number of saved casualties. The following parameters are used:
  - The boundaries of the SAR area
  - The SAR stations: their location, their reaction time to a call and the SAR units available at the station
  - The SAR units: their speed, capacity, radius of action and costs
- General shipping data
  In this module as much nautical data as available on the SAR area are defined. Preferably, statistical data on casualties are given, subdivided for various areas, schemes and shipping routes.
  - Approach: numbers of ship movements per area and per year, accident risk per mile, accident risk per hour
  - Separation scheme's location of numbers of ship movements per year, accident risk per mile, accident risk per hour
  - Shipping routes location of numbers of ship movements per year, accident risk per mile, accident risk per hour
  - Other area numbers of ship movements per year, accident risk per mile, accident risk per hour
  In a later version of the system, discrimination of the seasons can be made concerning the above-mentioned risks.
  Important local circumstances are water temperature, prevailing winds, general wave height, storm frequency with accompanying wave heights, shallows.
- Passenger ship module
  In this module the information on passenger shipping is defined. This information can be changed in order to estimate the influence of future changes in sailing schemes. Furthermore, the accident scenarios for various kinds of passenger ships are stored. The following parameters are used:
  - Route data: number of passengers (maximum and average), route, sailing frequency, speed
  - Accident scenario: dependent on the type of passenger ship (ferry or cruise ship), the capacity of the ship, the actual number of passengers and the sea state (wind, waves, temperature)

The model calculates the expected average number of saved casualties per year. In the model a drowning person becomes a saved casualty if there is enough rescue capacity within the appropriate time for that person. The appropriate time is calculated with regard to the scenario of the disaster and the external conditions.

The SAR fleet plan is optimised and expected to be fully operational when the average number of saved casualties is maximised, while the shipping conditions and financial consequences remain similar.

10.5.1
The Effects of Changes in Passenger Transport at Sea and SAR Operations

Passenger transport over sea has changed a lot in recent times. Modern passenger ships are larger, more luxurious and faster. The number of persons on board a ferry can exceed 2000 persons, while some cruise ships double this number. Cruise ships have become like floating cities with all conveniences available. These developments cause extra difficulties for SAR operations and evacuation of passengers from a ship in distress.

Ferries sail at speeds up to 40 knots (75 kilometres per hour). The high speeds of the modern ferries impose a series of additional risks. Navigation itself relies more strongly than before on navigational aids and sensor techniques. This greater reliance on technology imposes significant pressure on the crew to accurately interpret the data presented to them. Another risk with these high speeds is the impact of a collision. Higher speeds have a more than proportionately larger impact. This is valid for both the hull of the ship and for the individual passengers. When a collision occurs at high speed, the chance that lethal damage is caused to the hull is far greater than at lower speed. At the same time a substantially larger number of passengers will be injured during the collision and these injured persons will be less mobile in the case of an evacuation. In general, people of more advanced age and less mobility attend cruises. Therefore, the mobility of these passengers might become a problem during evacuation of a cruise ship.

During an evacuation, the large number of passengers imposes great pressure on the logistics. In the International Maritime Organisation (IMO) regulations the minimal requirements on evacuation routes are described. These are based on figures describing the evacuation of buildings. A ship in distress, however, does not resemble a building. There may be casualties because of the impact of the collision, the ship may heel and roll because of adverse sea conditions. Passengers on board a ship at sea are expected to experience greater stress during evacuation than persons in a building.

In order to minimise the risk for passengers, the IMO has tightened the safety regulations in the past few decades for passenger ships. This has resulted in increased safety. A further increase in safe passenger transport can be achieved by a stricter observation of these regulations. Both the *Estonia* and the *Herald of Free Enterprise* endangered the passengers by sailing against IMO regulations. More intense shipping, higher velocities, new highly advanced navigational aids and larger passenger numbers give all the more reason to further enhance the effectiveness of safety regulations.

Despite the reduced likelihood of a disaster with a passenger ship, the huge number of passengers on board, compel SAR organisations to anticipate sea disasters.

In order to prepare a SAR operation, scenarios of rarely occurring disasters are created, enabling SAR organisations to prepare for such large-scale accidents.

In the model now in use by the KNRM, various scenarios take into account the different properties of cruise ships and ferries, the consequences of a fire, a collision, a collision of a conventional steel ferry travelling at 20 knots and an aluminium ferry sailing at 40 knots. Becoming stranded and sinking are also taken into account. Disaster-related parameters that are described in these scenarios are:

- The time between the moment that the accident was reported and the moment that the ship became unliveable.
- The number of people hurt in the accident itself (collision, stranding or fire).
- The number of people in boats, rafts and in the water.
- The capabilities of rescue boats of the ships to rescue persons out off the water.

These parameters are, in combination with figures on sea state, water temperature and shipping activities in the vicinity, normative for the available time span for a SAR operation to take place and to produce ample rescue capacity. The scenarios are the result of analysis of disasters in the past, the probable influence of new safety regulations and the results of research on evacuation, which has recently been conducted. The scenarios can be used in the decision support system for optimising a SAR fleet plan, a statistical program predicting the occurrence of disasters and enabling one to calculate the best possible SAR fleet distribution along the SAR stations.

Current experience with the decision support system for optimising a SAR fleet plan has learned that special attention should be paid to:

- Sea-land connection in rescue: An expert meeting on this subject during the World Congress on Drowning learned that the up-scaling of the sea disaster needs appropriate action on land at the same time to be ready to handle the casualties appropriately (see ▶ Chap. 10.7). Persons who are responsible for rescue at sea and for rescue on land should communicate and carry out exercises regularly.
- Rescue capacity: Currently the biggest passenger ships can carry over 5000 passengers and crew. Considering the average number of people on board ships, one should be prepared for the rescue of 450 persons in the busiest area, within an area of 10 nautical miles along the coast within an hour, keeping hypothermia in mind.
- Fleet plan: To be able to rescue 450 people within an hour within the area of 10 nautical miles along the coast, KNRM has allocated and has future plans to develop and station different types of boats with the necessary technical specifications and survivor capacity to be able to achieve this goal. If the rescue plan in the Netherlands should only be based on the capacity of the KNRM, the lifeboat stations should on average be 8 nautical miles apart. If the plan should also be based on volunteer lifesaving stations, with boats with smaller ranges, the units should be 1.5 nautical miles apart.
- Percentage of rescued casualties: scenarios in which preparations are made to rescue 450 persons should also take into account that there will be missing persons among the passengers and crew who are likely in the sea and

swimming for their lives. These victims need to be found within as short a time possible and to this end a large number of boats need to be available. A worst-case scenario is that the accident happens between Christmas and New Years Eve; during this period there are very few lifeboats and no fishermen and yachtsmen. Only duty ships, helicopters and merchant navy ships might be at sea.

- Publicity: It seems clear that a discussion should be started about whether the percentage of rescued persons is politically and governmentally acceptable. In the case where the government were to want a higher percentage, the KNRM would require either larger or more lifeboats. But the question remains: Who pays the bill?
- Statistics: It is clear that professional shipping is becoming safer and that more accidents will happen with pleasure craft. KNRM will be ready for these accidents when the rescue capacity is 450 victims. Also based on the common incidence of these incidents, there is a clear picture of these accidents in coastal waters.
- Risk analysis for the North Sea, Dutch Continental Shelf
  - Plane: 1 accident per 10–50 years
  - Offshore platform: 1 accident per 2–10 years
  - Ferry boat: 1 accident per 2–25 years
- Shipping density: The North Sea is the busiest sea in the world. Rotterdam, the biggest port in the world, the Westerschelde, which is the entrance to the busy harbour of Antwerp, Amsterdam, as the second port in Holland, and five smaller Dutch ports all have access to the North Sea and this leads to dense traffic. Moreover, there are numerous ferry services between the Netherlands and the UK.
- Type of accident: The ideal situation for a rescue is a slow sinking ship in an upright situation. Although this is a realistic situation, experience over the last 12 years has taught that accidents can happen very fast. The Herald of Free Enterprise capsized in 3 min. The Estonia sank in 24 min. Even a helicopter could not reach the scene in time.

10.5.2
Conclusion

The issue of SAR preparedness for disaster situations needs international attention and standardisation. The availability of SAR organisations in countries is different, some have nothing while other countries have a SAR unit at 5-nautical-mile intervals along the coast.

10.6
Linking Sea and Land:
Essential Elements in Crises Decisions
for Water-Related Disasters

MARTIN MADERN and ROB BRONS

The Netherlands has traded overseas for centuries and has known periods of great prosperity. In this sense the sea has been rewarding to the inhabitants. On the other hand the Netherlands also have a history of disasters and accidents relating to its proximity to the sea. For centuries the Netherlands have fought a continuing battle against water, first by building houses on tarps, and later by building dikes and protecting the shore. Furthermore, land has been won back from the sea by mouldering. Hence the saying that the Dutch created the Netherlands in great part by themselves.

Exemplary for the Dutch battle against water has been The Great Flood in February 1953. In the night between January 31st and February 1st the southwest of Holland and a part of the island Texel, in the North of the country, were flooded. The combination of spring tide and a severe storm led to a national disaster. More than 1800 people were killed, tens of thousands of victims were evacuated. More than 200,000 animals were killed. The economic damage amounted to more than 1.3 billion Dutch guilders (0.6 billion euros). The works to restore the damaged areas took many years. To prevent any recurrence of such a disaster, the Deltaworks were initiated. The Deltaworks are a large project in which the sea-arms Westerschelde and the Nieuwe Waterweg are closed and the protection of the coast reinforced. Many laws and regulations were adapted and developed. Furthermore, many government and non-government agencies concerned with operational crisis management agreed to cooperate.

The Great Flood in 1953 is an example of a coastal flooding with disastrous consequences in the Netherlands. All coastal areas of the world, however, are threatened by disasters and accidents that take place at sea. Many of these disasters have important effects on the mainland. Examples include coastal pollution, shipping incidents, mining incidents and plane crashes in the sea.

In this chapter the administrative and operational responsibilities concerning both sea and land aspects of crisis management are described. This chapter reveals that dealing with sea and land issues implies the linking of two separate worlds which are organised in different and complex structures and disciplines. These differences require extra attention for a coordinated and synergetic effort. The approach described in this chapter can be labelled typically Dutch. The Dutch administrative culture has its premises in a *polder model*, a consultation and consensus model that integrates all different interests.

10.6.1
Territorial Jurisdiction

The complexity of the issue is demonstrated by a description of the five different jurisdictional zones which have to be taken into consideration for disaster preparedness and response (◘ **Figure 10.1**).

- Like other countries adjacent to the North Sea, the Netherlands has been appointed to manage a well-defined area of the North Sea: the Dutch Continental Shelf (DCS). The size of the DCS is based on the length of the coastal line. International agreements allow the Netherlands exclusive rights of exploration and exploitation of the DCS
- The DCS refers only to the seabed and, as a consequence, requires that other regulations are required for the water and air above the seabed. This area is called the Exclusive Economical Zone (EEZ)
- The outer-limit of the Dutch territorial waters is formed by the 12-nautical miles-line that follows the coastal line, measured from the low-tide-line along the shore
- The Dutch territorial waters are also part of municipal boundaries. The outer-limit of these boundaries is formed by the 1-kilometre line; the outer boarder of the municipalities and provinces concerned
- Within territorial waters there are territories of the ports of call. These areas do not include the 1-kilometre areas which are already municipally managed. In the Netherlands there are seven territories of ports of call, with local authorities appointed as nautical managers

Each of the aforementioned jurisdictional zones has its own legal regime. Various administrations and organisations have been assigned with different responsibilities concerning incident and disaster management.

10.6.2
Dutch Coastguard

The Dutch Coastguard is a cooperation between the Ministries of the Interior, Justice, Transport, Public Works and Water Management, Defence, Finances and Agriculture. The operational duties of the coastguard include:
- Search and rescue
- Crisis and disaster management
- Police activities
- Enforcement of environmental legislation
- Traffic control
- Emergency and safety traffic

The Director of the Coastguard heads the operational management of duties. He is also responsible for the nautical management of the territorial sea and has the authority to enforce the *Regulations for shipping on the territorial sea* and the *Shipping traffic law.*

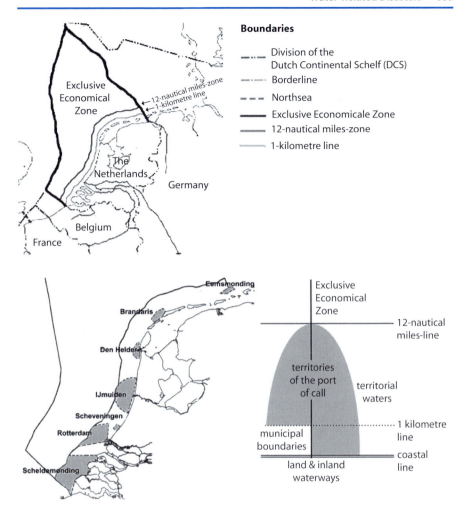

Boundaries

- – · – · Division of the Dutch Continental Schelf (DCS)
- – · – Borderline
- – – – Northsea
- ——— Exclusive Economicale Zone
- ——— 12-nautical miles-zone
- ——— 1-kilometre line

Fig. 10.1. The different areas with territorial jurisdiction: the Dutch Continental Shelf (DCS), the Exclusive Economical Zone (*EEZ*), the territorial waters (the 12-nautical-miles line), the outer limits of the municipal boundaries (the 1-kilometre line) and the territories of ports of call

   The Coastguard operates in the EEZ, the territorial waters and the aerial zone above. The Coastguard Centre is the operational command centre and the central dispatch and information centre for the Coastguard. The Coastguard Centre can activate an operational team which falls under the authority of an interdepartmental policy team during disasters at sea.

10.6.3
Crisis Management at Sea

Disaster management at sea is regulated by the Disaster Plan North Sea 2000. The aim of this plan is to coordinate crisis and disaster management on the North Sea. The procedures concern cooperation between the Coastguard Centre, all possible concerned agencies and organisations at sea, and all agencies and organisations of disaster management on land. The aim of the plan is to ensure efficient implementation of measures, resulting from international treaties concerning search and rescue, and to minimise damage to the naval environment and coastal areas.

The action of the government can be divided into search and rescue activities (SAR) and crisis and disaster management. In many accidents, SAR activities take place during the first phase of crisis and disaster management and are specifically aimed at human rescue. This task is appointed to the Coastguard and is performed according to specific legislation that regulates prevention, limitation or of harmful consequences of accidents on the North Sea. These laws enable Dutch intervention outside Dutch territorial waters in the case of consequences exceeding an explicitly defined degree of severity.

The Ministry of Transport, Public Works and Water Management governs water affairs of national interest, such as the North Sea. A special coordination centre is responsible for internal and external coordination in the case of an emergency at sea. If other Ministries are concerned, a special interdepartmental policy team takes care of interdepartmental coordination, nearby the location of the coordination centre of the Ministry of Transport, Public Works and Water Management.

10.6.4
Crisis Management on Land

In order to understand the intricate systems involving crisis management on land it is important to differentiate between the different governmental powers in the Netherlands. Different laws and regulations apply. First and foremost are the laws concerning crisis and disaster management. Legislation about crises and disaster management relate to municipalities, firefighting organisations, police and medical assistance during disasters. The combination of legislation constitutes the basis for crisis and disaster management and indicates to officials and emergency services which competences are needed. The competences are related to events that cause major disruptions to public security and situations where the lives and health of many people or great economic interests are threatened. The laws enable a coordinated effort of all involved disciplines and organisations.

The Ministry of the Interior is responsible for the system and organisation of disaster management in the regions of the Netherlands. Hereto the ministry has a round the clock staffed National Coordination Centre (NCC). The NCC facilitates interdepartmental coordination of those crises in which several ministries are involved. The role of the Ministry of Interior does not include disasters on the North Sea, for which the aforementioned interdepartmental policy team functions as coordinating authority.

Because of the importance of providing good care for inhabitants, the primary responsibility in crisis and disaster management has been placed in the hands of local officials. Therefore, the municipalities are the most important factor. The mayor carries political and governmental responsibility for the operations of municipal and emergency services during crises. This implies joint responsibility of all mayors of coastal municipalities for crises and accidents in their coastal lines, as well as for the municipally appointed 1-kilometre line of the territorial waters. In case of crises and accidents the mayor is advised by a municipal crisis team comprised of members taken from all municipal agencies and local emergency services.

Because the effects of disasters rarely respect municipal boundaries, all municipalities have made joint regional arrangements on assistance and crisis management. These arrangements apply to firefighting, the police force and medical assistance and are organised in uniform territories to improve the cooperation. Operational rescue efforts are lead by a regional operational team and a regional policy team. The regional organisation is not a separate governmental layer, but an organised inter-municipal cooperation.

There is a third governmental level between the national and municipal governments, namely, the province. Each province has a Commissioner of the Queen (a governor). The governor is appointed by law to execute coordinating activities in the case of incidents and disasters that occur on an inter-municipal level. The governor is guided by a provincial crisis team, which operates in a provincial coordination centre.

By this point of the chapter it will have become clear that, in the event of a disaster on the North Sea, with consequences for multiple coastal provinces, many authorities, coordination centres and dispatch centres, each with different appointed duties, are called into action.

10.6.5
Other Involved Parties

The palette of disciplines, governments and responsibilities concerned with North Sea incidents is still not complete. For example, port managers can be involved in the safe and swift completion of shipping traffic. District water boards, another functional governmental layer, have separate responsibilities concerning water quality, quantity and embankment. These tasks of the water boards also relate to the coastal area. Mostly this concerns the primary embankment, such as dunes and other water sources. In the case of nature and environmental protection in the coastal area there are other departments and organisations.

10.6.6
Coupling Two Systems

Situations can occur at sea which can have significant potential effects on land, and threaten the safety of many people or of the environment. The emergency evacuation of a vessel or platform can imply the need for temporary relocation of victims on a large scale. In cases like these, the system of crisis and disaster management is set into motion. This also works the other way around: a gascloud on land that drifts towards sea.

In the event of an incident on the North Sea with consequences for the land, the Coastguard Centre will inform the departmental coordination centre of the Ministry of Transport, Public Works and Water Management. Together with the NCC, the coordination with provincial and municipal government bodies is assessed. The coordinated activities can relate, for example, to landing victims on shore, receiving and registration of victims or central information for relatives.

10.6.7
Upgrading and Coordination Mechanisms

Clearly the network of disciplines, governmental layers and diverse responsibilities is rather complex. Therefore, many arrangements are made for upgrading, coordination, communication and cooperation. Exemplary are the uniform phases of coordinated upgrading that are being implemented in several regions. Regional dispatch centres and other coordination centres play a crucial role in the process of upgrading. Not all operational and governmental tasks are coherent due to distinct legal responsibilities.

10.6.8
Summary and Suggestion for Improvements

- The Netherlands has a patchwork of operational and governmental responsibilities and duties concerning crisis and disaster management on the North Sea.
- Current national coordination between the several communication centres and dispatch centres requires further investigation and improvement.
- A national consensus on *doctrine* related to coordinating mechanisms ("phases of upgrading") is needed.
- Planning related to North Sea disasters should contain clear schedules concerning warning, upgrading and lines of communication.
- A European or international service for the collection of information on fighting accidents, upgrading, coordination, planning, preparation, practice and communication is recommended.
- Intensification of functioning of the network as a whole and a joint policy on combined exercises, both on an operational and a governmental level, are necessary.

Due to Dutch legislation of the governmental organisation, some of the suggested improvements can not be implemented as yet. It is clear that great improvement is being made by uniform phases of upgrading, optimising the network and increasing coordination of planning. Furthermore, there is ever growing experience as a result of combined exercises in communication and coordination and testing each other's planning. For the Netherlands, this aspect of disaster planning remains another challenge in the coming years.

10.6.9
Website

www.noordzeeloket.nl

10.7
Drowning in Floods:
An Overview of Mortality Statistics for Worldwide Floods

Bas Jonkman

Every year floods cause enormous damage all over the world. In the last decade of the 20th century floods accounted for about 12% of all deaths from natural disasters, claiming about 93,000 lives. Furthermore, floods can have substantial impacts on public health, and indirectly lead to a decrease of socio-economic welfare. Studies carried out in the past have focused on the general documentation of various natural disasters on a worldwide scale or the analysis of flood deaths for a specific country, for example for Australia or the United States. However, a study that analyses loss of life statistics for worldwide floods in relation to their characteristics has not yet been found in the literature. This chapter provides insights into the potential magnitude of flood events and can help to develop vulnerability indicators for flood hazards. As far as we are aware, this is the first chapter that describes the loss of life statistics for different types of floods and different regions. To obtain this data, general information from the OFDA/CRED International Disaster Database on a large number of worldwide flood events which occurred between January 1975 and June 2002 has been used.

The OFDA/CRED International Disaster Database contains essential core data on the occurrence and effects of over 12,800 mass disasters in the world from 1900 to the present. The Centre for Research on the Epidemiology of Disasters in Brussels (CRED) maintains this database. Information on date and location, as well as numbers of killed and affected persons has been used. Records of 1883 flood events are analysed, although not all records have complete information.

The impact of a flood is strongly influenced by the characteristics of the inundated area and the characteristics of the flood itself. For example, rapidly rising flash floods can cause more devastation than small-scale inundations due to drainage problems, and people in developing countries might be more vulnerable to the flood hazard than the inhabitants of industrialised regions. Area characteristics such as population density and magnitude, land use, warning and emergency measures differ on a regional scale and will have a large influence on the loss of life caused by a flood. Information on the location of the flood events can be abstracted from the database. The hydraulic characteristics will depend on the type of flood. Specific problems arise with the analysis of coastal flood events. Although the majority of deaths in such events are caused by drowning, they are generally categorised in the International Disaster Database as windstorm events. Therefore the scope of this study is limited to three types of freshwater flooding: drainage problems, flash floods and river floods.

- High precipitation levels that cannot be handled by regular drainage systems cause drainage problems. This type of threat poses no, or a very limited, threat to life due to limited water levels and causes mainly economic damage
- Flash floods occur after local rainfall with a high intensity, which leads to a rapid rise in water levels causing a threat to lives of inhabitants. The time available to predict flash floods in advance is limited. Severe rainfall on the flood location may be used as an indicator for this type of flood. Flash floods generally occur in mountainous areas
- Flooding of a river outside regular boundaries causes river floods. A river flood can be accompanied by a breach of dikes or dams next to the river. The flood can be caused by various sources: high precipitation levels, not necessarily in the flooded area, melting snow and blockage of flow. In general, extreme river discharges can be predicted in advance

The flood events in the database have been classified by flood type, using information from the underlying sources of the database, such as UN and Red Cross reports and newspaper articles.

10.7.1
Analysis of Loss of Life Caused by Worldwide Floods

Worldwide flood statistics for different types of floods in different regions with respect to the numbers of persons killed or affected, as well as mortality rates can be considered as variables that indicate the magnitude of the human impact of a flood event. The relative severity of an event can be considered by analysing the mortality. Mortality is defined as the fraction of the inhabitants of the flooded area that lose their lives in the flood. Over the considered period, January 1975–June 2002, 1883 flood events in the database are reported to have killed over 175,000 persons and affected more than 2.2 billion persons.

10.7.2
Analysis by Location

It is expected that the human impact of a flood will be influenced by area characteristics, such as the available warning and emergency systems and the level of flood protection. ◘ Figure 10.2 indicates the magnitude of the floods, for events with more than 0 persons killed. The number of total affected people is shown on the x-axis and the number of killed on the y-axis. The ◘ Figure 10.2 indicates that floods with a large number of affected people are mainly Asian floods. The 45 floods with the highest number of people affected all occurred in China, India, Bangladesh or Pakistan. The event with most persons killed occurred in 1999 in Venezuela: about 30,000 people died during flash floods and extensive land and mudslides.

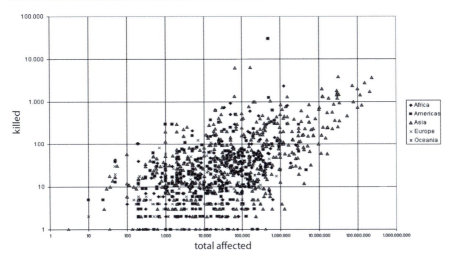

Fig. 10.2. Number of persons killed and people affected for floods with more than 0 persons killed; by continent

The average mortality per flood event is 1.14% over the whole dataset. When the mortality rate is determined for the different continents, no large differences between the continents can be observed. When Oceania is excluded due to the limited number of available data, average mortality per flood event by continent ranges between 1.1% for the Americas and 1.4% for European flood events, values for Africa and Asia are in between. When average mortality per event is considered on a more detailed level, for the 17 regions defined in the database, higher differences between regions are found. Highest mortality is found in the Southern Africa region (5.7%) and the lowest mortality is found in Western Africa (0.1%). The results do not indicate a relation between average flood mortality and the socio-economic development of a region. Mortality is for example relatively high for the European Union, while West Africa has a low average mortality.

10.7.3
Analysis by Flood Type

Three types of freshwater floods are distinguished in this study: drainage problems, flash floods and river floods. For 719 floods the type has been determined. **Figure 10.3** indicates the magnitude of the floods, for the events with more than 0 persons killed. The total number of affected people is shown on the x-axis and the number of killed on the y-axis.

Most floods with high numbers of affected persons are river floods, while a majority of the smaller floods with lower numbers of affected persons are flash floods. The average and standard deviation of mortality per flood event is shown in **Fig. 10.4.**

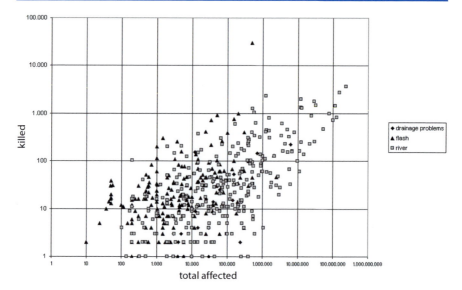

□ Fig. 10.3. Number of persons killed and people affected for floods with more than 0 persons killed; by flood type

□ Fig. 10.4. Average and standard deviation of mortality per flood event for different types of floods

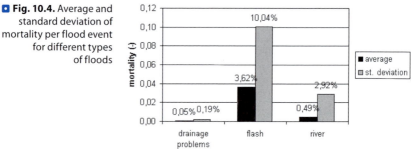

Average mortality is highest for flash floods. The other types of floods result in relatively low mortalities. As expected drainage problems have the lowest mortality.

From the results shown in **□ Figs. 10.3 and 10.4** some observations can be made. Flash floods affect relatively few people but cause relatively high mortality rates. River floods result in higher numbers of affected, but relatively lower mortality rate per event. In the case of drainage problems even more people are affected, but loss of life is low.

A combined analysis of flood type and continent shows that river floods in Asia account for 39% of the total number of persons killed and for 96% of the total persons affected. Flash floods account for 34% of the total number of persons killed. The analysis of flood mortality per event shows that average mortality

Table 10.5. Classification of flood deaths

Direct exposure	
Death	Circumstances/activity
Drowning	In water
	In vehicle
	In boat / boating
	During rescue
	In building
Deadly injury	In water
	Collapse of building
Indirect exposure	
Trauma	
Heart attack	
Electrocution	
Carbon monoxide poisoning	
Others	
Unknown	

is relatively constant between the different types of floods, while the numbers killed and affected for a certain type differs between the different continents.

10.7.4 Drowning in Floods: The Causes

While the previous analysis provides insight into the magnitude of flood mortality, it does not indicate how people drown in floods. For this reason, death statistics for some European river floods have been studied. Data were available for the 2002 Elbe river floods in Germany (27 killed), the 1997 and 2001 river floods in Poland (55 and 27 killed, respectively), the 1953 coastal floods in the Netherlands (1835 killed) and the United Kingdom (313 killed). Data from studies on Australian flood deaths and United States flash flood deaths were also included.

In **Table 10.5** a classification of flood death categories is made. A distinction is made between deaths due to direct contact with the floodwaters and indirect causes of death.

From the several sources of information on flood mortality no final conclusions with respect to the relevance of certain causes of death can be drawn. However, some patterns emerge from the limited data available. The two coastal flood events studied occurred unexpectedly without pre-warning or evacuation. Most deaths occurred amongst persons trapped in buildings and in rapidly flowing waters near the breaches in the dikes.

It appears from the studied data from the river flood cases that the main causes of death were drowning victims being swept away in water- and car-related accidents. A major percentage of deaths in European floods is believed to be caused by risk-taking behaviour. Also WHO estimates that 40% of all health problems during European floods is due to risk-taking behaviour. Several sources indicate the hazards associated with the rescue of endangered victims, especially when a voluntary would-be rescuer performs the rescue. Limited mortality occurred due to indirect causes, such as trauma, heart attack and electrocution.

The available statistics on United States flash floods show that almost half of the flash flood deaths are car-related.

For all flood types the young and elderly are more vulnerable in floods. Males are over-represented in the flood death statistics for river and flash floods, probably related to more risk-taking behaviour by males. Floods can also influence long-term mortality. More cases of diseases and illnesses may result in a rise of mortality in the months and years after the flood.

10.7.5
Conclusion

This chapter provides some insight into the loss of life in worldwide floods. The mortality rate associated with a flood event strongly depends on the flood type. Also, the way people respond to the flood exposures is a critical factor in the morbidity and mortality associated with such events. As the chapter is limited to the analysis of freshwater flood events it is recommended that coastal floods be included in future analyses.

For the prevention of flood health effects more insight into the causes of flood mortality is needed. Based on a limited number of case studies a first analysis of causes of death is given. However, the empirical evidence for the relevance of the different causes of death is rather weak. Also, knowledge on the non-lethal effects associated with floods is limited. There is a need for more and better quantitative data on health impacts associated with all categories of flooding. This includes centralised and systematic national reporting of deaths and injuries from floods using a standardised methodology.

Further Reading

Berz G, Kron W, Loster T, et al. (2001) World map of natural hazards – a global view of the distribution and intensity of significant exposures. Nat Hazards 23:443–465

Coates L (1999) Flood fatalities in Australia 1788–1996. Aust Geogr 30:391–408

French J, Ing R, Allmen S von, Wood R (1983) Mortality from flash floods: a review of the national weather service reports, 1969–1981. Public Health Rep 98:584–588

French JG, Holt KW (1989) Floods. In: Gregg MB (ed.) The public health consequences of disasters. US Department of Health and Human Services, Public Health Service. CDC, Atlanta, Georgia, pp 69–78

Mooney LE (1983) Applications and implications of fatality statistics to the flash flood problems. In: Proceedings of the 5th Conference on Hydrometeorology, Tulsa

World Health Organization, Regional Office for Europe (2002) Floods: climate change and adaptation strategies for human health. World Health Organization, Geneva

OFDA/CRED International Disaster Database: www.cred.be

10.8
Measures to Prevent the Netherlands from Flooding

Joop Weijers, Robert Slomp and Sjaak Poortvliet

Flooding can occur in the Netherlands as a result of extreme river conditions and storm surges. The low-lying areas of the Netherlands are especially vulnerable and are protected by dunes and dikes. The flood defences (dunes, sea dikes and special structures) are mainly supervised and maintained locally by water boards (*waterschappen*). The geographical boundaries of most water boards are based on secondary drainage basins, such as polders.

The Ministry of Transport, Public Works and Water Management is responsible for flood warning in the Netherlands. Flood forecasts are based on precipitation forecasts, precipitation over the last 3 days, river water levels and calibrated flow models of the rivers. Data received from partners in Germany, Belgium and France are also included. Precipitation forecasts are now available from Germany per square kilometre and are increasingly accurate and also available on-line. The perfection of the precipitation forecasts has increased the period of accurate flood forecasting.

Expected water levels for all major waterways are communicated on a daily basis to subscribers. Flood forecasts are available by fax, by a special server, on the Internet and teletext. The responsibility for flood warnings is an additional task for the office in charge of this daily information service.

Accurate flood forecasts for the Rhine are available 2–3 days in advance. Flood forecasts for the Meuse are usually available 12–24 hours before the peak water levels reach the Netherlands. The effectiveness of flood forecasts for the Vecht is currently being studied. The flood forecasts for this small river are usually available a few hours before the peak water levels reach the Netherlands.

Warnings on storm surges along the borders of the lakes (Markermeer and IJsselmeer), the seashore and in the estuaries are also given. The warning period for storm surges is several hours and is much shorter than the warning period for river floods. Also these flood forecasts are available through a central server. Storm surge forecasts are based on wind forecasts for the North Sea, tide tables, sea water levels and calibrated flow models for the North Sea and the estuaries in the Netherlands.

Water boards and provincial governments are warned in the case of expected extreme water conditions. In such circumstances, the water boards organise permanent dike inspection during the flood period and are responsible for informing the provincial government, the municipalities and the fire departments

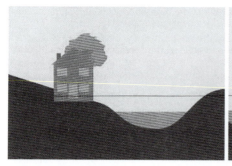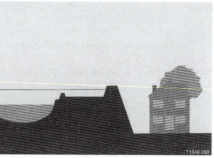

□ Fig. 10.5. Two different types of flooding and the effect of preventive measures. *Left*, the rising level of water affects larger and increasingly higher located areas. Flooding can not be prevented with dikes. Houses should not be built in potentially effected areas. *Right*, the area behind the dikes is lower than the level of the water. To anticipate an increase in water level, the height of the dikes may be increased. However, in the event of flooding over the dike, more water at a higher speed will flood the area behind the dikes, causing greater risk and damage

on the condition of the flood defences. The decision to evacuate areas is taken by the provincial Commissioner of the Queen (a governor) on information from water boards and the municipal governments. The population is warned by siren and informed through local television and radio stations.

The extreme rainfall in 1998 and subsequent flooding of parts of the Netherlands raised questions as to whether the regional and national policy towards water was the right one. Since 1998 a number of studies have been completed to evaluate whether the current national flood policy should be redefined. One of the main problems is that raising the height of dikes to compensate for rising flood levels on account of climate change causes a higher water level in the event flooding occurs in spite of the higher dikes (**□ Fig. 10.5**). When the water level in a flooded inhabited area exceeds 1 metre the risk of loss of human life increases. A current discussion is on a change of policy whereby sparsely populated areas would be sacrificed to save other more populated areas from flooding. The flooding of these areas may prevent the flooding of other areas. In this way, densely populated areas can likely be safed from flooding. This policy had been used for several centuries but the last of such areas in the Netherlands was closed off from the river in 1958. Flooding of inhabited areas was then rediscovered during three severe floods between 1994 and 1998. The government has therefore requested an independent committee of former politicians to designate the areas that are to be flooded and to set the conditions which would regulate the use of such areas. Major questions for this committee are:

- How can it be determined in advance that a dike is not high enough to prevent the low areas behind the dike from flooding. Some determining factors are: the accuracy of the flood forecast, the exact height of the dikes and the local behaviour of the river near the dikes
- How to warn the inhabitants adequately and evacuate them in the shortest time available

- Which administration (local, regional or national) will take the decision to open dikes for regulated flooding
- Which legislation has to be amended or altered to enable the sacrifice of certain inhabited areas
- How to reduce the risk of casualties due to flooding
- How will the financial and other damages be compensated
- How to gain acceptance of the population for this policy

The committee has discussed the issue with a number of parties involved, such as farmers, landowners, environmental groups, chambers of commerce, politicians and water board representatives.

10.8.1
Flood Contingency Plans

Flood defences such as dikes, dunes and other structures may wash out, collapse or fail in the event of extreme river floods or storm surges. In such situations it is important to know which flood defences are most likely to fail, what could be the consequences and what could be the best procedures to reduce casualties. Another consequence of this approach is that preemptive evacuations or evacuations during floods can be properly prepared. Modifications to strengthen planned and existing roads, dikes and other works can be considered based on these evaluations.

The water boards, the Dutch provinces, the Ministry of Transport, Public Works and Water Management and a number of Dutch research institutes and private companies collaborate to provide the different tools to answer these questions.

Both the provinces and water boards have developed tools to monitor the passage of water along river dikes and to streamline the flow of information within their own organisation and to other organisations. These tools have been designed to facilitate the permanent inspection of the dikes during a river flood period, which often lasts several days. Proper registration of the daily reports is part of this inspection. Water level forecasts can be compared to the height of dikes. Weak spots can be closely monitored and reported. For the large lakes, the deltas and the seashore, potentially threatened by the combination of storm surges and wave action, these monitoring tools are still under development.

How flooding will occur in a polder if a flood defence fails can be determined with the 1D-2D SOBEK Lowlands program developed by WL | Delft Hydraulics. Necessary data for the provincial government organisation or the regional fire brigade, such as the speed of the flooding, area covered by water at each moment of the flood, depth of the flooding, time available for evacuation and possible escape routes can be determined using this program (www.wldelft.nl). The total damage and probable number of casualties can then be calculated with the damage and casualty module. The Dutch Central Bureau of Statistics (www.cbs.nl) provide data on the value of property and the number of inhabitants per square kilometre. The ministry of Transport, Public Works and Water Management provides geographical information such as terrain heights.

The Nijmegen (Netherlands) and Kreis Kleve (Germany) regional fire departments have developed an additional tool to coordinate the evacuation of inhabitants in the common border area along the Rhine. This pilot project was partly financed by the European Community and the Dutch Ministry of Internal Affairs.

10.8.2
Websites

- www.wldelft.nl
- www.cbs.nl

10.9
Controlling the Risk of Flood-Related Drowning

SJAAK POORTVLIET

Controlling the risk of flood-related drowning involves the entire safety chain: proaction, prevention, preparation, response and recovery. This chapter describes the proaction and prevention policy, as developed in the Netherlands to control the risk of flooding, and thereby the risk of flood-related drowning. The premise of the policy is that the risk of flooding by major rivers or sea cannot be eliminated, but can be limited by constructing flood defences or by returning reclaimed space to the water.

It is also not possible to completely eliminate the risk of flood-related drowning. Complete elimination of the risk of flood-related drowning can only be achieved by evacuating areas that are susceptible to flooding. This is not a realistic option. The presence of water is a resource for food supplies (agriculture and fishing), for industry (process water and cooling water) and as a means of transport. Water is a condition for existence and the presence of water makes areas attractive as residential areas. Living in areas which are susceptible to flooding means that the risk of flooding, and thereby the risk of drowning, is accepted. In these areas proactive and preventive measures limit the risk of flooding and control the risk of flood-related drowning.

Proaction is concerned with preventing the creation of a new situation or eliminating an existing situation that could result in a disaster or accident by eliminating the risks. Proactive measures can be taken by the evacuation of areas that are susceptible to flooding. This can be done by not permitting more people to live in the stream valleys of rivers, by evacuating these areas or evacuating the areas reclaimed from rivers and sea and abandoning them to the water. The last option has the extra advantage that water can follow its natural course.

In the Netherlands, where necessary space for new developments is limited, abandoning land to make way for water is only possible to a limited extent. Moreover, as mentioned above, it is precisely the presence of water in areas that makes them attractive residential areas. It will be necessary to weigh the costs and benefits to achieve the implementation of these proactive measures.

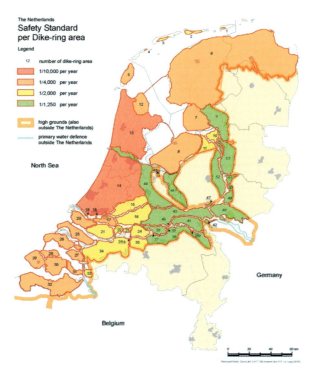

The Netherlands
Safety Standard
per Dike-ring area
Legend

12   number of dike-ring area

        1/10,000 per year
        1/4,000 per year
        1/2,000 per year
        1/1,250 per year

        high grounds (also
        outside The Netherlands)
        primary water defence
        outside The Netherlands

North Sea

Germany

Belgium

■ Fig. 10.6. Areas in the Netherlands shown according to the current standard safety levels for flood protection in the Netherlands (Meetkundige Dienst, Section CAT, Delft)

The same applies to increasing the strength of flood defences, such as dikes, dams and floodgates. No dike is strong and high enough to hold back extremely high water levels. No investment in flood defences will be capable of completely excluding the possibility of flooding. A choice has to be made. It is the task and responsibility of the national government to execute a proper cost-benefit analysis and establish which level of risk is acceptable from a political, social and economic point of view.

The Dutch government decided to establish a socially acceptable risk of flooding based on the advice of the Delta Committee and the River Dikes Committee.

The average acceptable risk determined for the upper course of the major rivers is one period of flooding every 1250 years. The acceptable risk determined for the river delta and the coastal area is between every 4000 and 10,000 years, depending on the habitation and activities that take place in the area. Risk-based and socially acceptable legislation has been proposed by the government bodies to ensure that safety standards are met and that inspections are carried out. A map that indicates the safety standard per area as the average likelihood of the highest high water level forms the basis for the design of the primary flood defences intended to protect areas from flooding (**■ Fig. 10.6**).

10.9.1
Administrative Responsibility

The government bodies that manage the primary flood defences indicated in the Flood Defences Act are responsible for establishing and maintaining the strength of the flood defences. This responsibility particularly concerns a political-social responsibility. However, citizens are entitled to call these bodies into account for their responsibility in the event of serious negligence by the managing authorities.

The plans drawn up by the managing authorities for constructing and reinforcing primary flood defences require approval of the provincial government. The purpose of submitting the dike improvement plans for approval is to ensure that the designs are sound and that other government interests are met, such as those concerning features of the landscape, natural environment and cultural heritage. The provincial government also ensures that the rights and interests of citizens are protected.

The managing authorities have to report to the provincial government every 5 years about the general hydraulic-engineering condition of the primary flood defences. If necessary, the provincial government is authorised to order the execution or cessation of reinforcement work in order to establish and maintain the strength of the primary flood defences.

The Minister of Transport, Public Works and Water Management has final responsibility for protecting the country against flooding. The minister is accountable to parliament for this responsibility. To ensure that the minister is kept properly informed about the hydraulic-engineering condition of the primary flood defences, the provincial government forwards the reports of the managing authorities, along with their comments, to the minister. In the event of the provincial government failing to submit the reports, the minister is authorised to order the execution or cessation of reinforcement work, in order to establish and maintain the strength of the primary flood defences. The minister therefore has ultimate control over the protection of the country against flooding.

10.10
The Safety Chain During Floods

Martin Madern, Rob Brons and Amanda Kost

The imbalance of the environment caused by human population pressures and economic trends, increase vulnerability to disasters. This chapter describes what can be done to prevent maritime pollution and to increase the level of preparation, coordination and communication if water-related disaster should occur.

Disasters occur when hazards meet vulnerable situations. Natural hazards, such as floods and earthquakes are part of the natural cycles of the earth. Earthquakes make buildings collapse, floods take many human and animal lives. When such hazards occur in a vulnerable society, the society will face a catastrophic situation requiring emergency relief and assistance to save lives and to protect the environment.

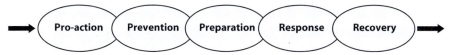

▣ Fig. 10.7. The five links of the safety chain

The distinction between natural and human-made hazards has become blurred. Hazards caused by humans, such as technological and chemical accidents, air and water pollution, have a severe effect on the environment and can lead to disaster. Hazards once considered natural and unavoidable are now thought to be partly due to human-induced environmental change. Research has shown that in many parts of the world, an increase in flooding is linked to the escalating rate of deforestation in this area. Rapid population growth increases the demand for natural resources, places pressure on the environment and raises the risk that a hazard will cause a disaster and that disasters will occur more frequently. As economies grow and technology expands, disasters caused by humans will increase. Disasters from natural hazards such as earthquakes, volcanic eruptions or flash floods may be partly attributable to humans, when unsafe settlements are built close to hazardous areas.

Assessing the vulnerability of a society to disasters by quantifying the degree to which the society is likely to be damaged by the impact of a hazard is often difficult. Measuring the financial losses of sudden disasters is easier than measuring the social losses. Furthermore, the long-term effects of disasters on the economy are difficult to assess.

This leads to the conclusion that disaster relief is not only a matter of relief when a disaster occurs. The pre-disaster and post-disaster aspects should also be taken into account. These aspects are integrated in the concept of integral safety, the safety chain. This concept has been adapted as the national concept in the Netherlands for disaster situations.

The safety chain contains five links: proaction, prevention, preparation, response and recovery (▣ Fig. 10.7). The interactions between the authorities responsible for disasters on a national, provincial and local level will benefit when all use the same concept of the safety chain. The concept is usable in all sorts of work in the safety and security sector such as firefighting, police force, fighting crime, health care and crisis and disaster management. It contributes to the coherency among the different activities.

The concept can be regarded as a policy model of input, throughput and output. Output becomes input again at the beginning of the chain so that one can learn from mistakes and can do things better in the future. To create a strong safety chain, all the links must be properly welded together. Policies concerning development and implementation must be as coherent as possible.

10.10.1
Proaction

Proaction averts structural causes of hazard by careful planning of space and environment and analysis of risk effects. It is clear that proaction cannot completely take away all risks. Floods, the topic of this chapter, cannot always be prevented. But a proactive measure is to decide not to allow houses and industries to be built in areas that may be flooded with a deluge. This decision prevents damage to houses and industries during floods. Proaction is mostly a matter of deliberation. The administration has to make choices between different interests of different stakeholders. Safety aspects may conflict with other interests. The decisions in the proactive link are often based on political issues. In recent years the Dutch government has encouraged that safety issues be taken into account, as early as possible in the national planning process. This may concern the planning of industrial areas, but also of motorways, railroads and airports. The consequence of such a proactive policy may be that an alternative location or route is chosen, which could be more expensive, but in the long run would guarantee more safety. For the next years to come, the Dutch national government also plans to stimulate the use of a proactive policy on the local and provincial governmental levels.

With regard to water disasters, the Dutch Deltaworks are a good example of such proactive and preventive measures. The Deltaworks were constructed to avoid floods such as the flood that took place in 1953 in the province of Zeeland. The flood disaster in 1953 was a rude awakening for the country. The fatal combination of a northwestern storm and spring tide resulted in the inundation of large parts of the provinces of Zeeland and South Holland. Over 1800 people died and the flood caused enormous damage to houses and property. Only one conclusion could be drawn: the country was not safe. Measures to prevent a repetition of the disaster were put forward in the form of the Deltaplan. The aim of the Deltaplan was to enhance safety by radically reducing the length of and reinforcing the safety of the coastline. The Deltaplan proposed that the dikes in Zeeland and South Holland had to be raised to delta level to be able to withstand storm surges 1.5 meters higher than those during the storm in 1953. The outlets to the sea in Southwest Netherlands had to be sealed and the water defences along the Westerschelde and the Rotterdam Waterway reinforced. These measures were laid down in 1958 in the Delta Act. The most important measures in the Delta Act were:

- The construction of 30 kilometres of primary dams in four sea inlets between the Westerschelde and the New Waterway. These dams shorten the coastline by 700 kilometres.
- No dams in the New Waterway and the Westerschelde, as the sea ports of Rotterdam and Antwerp must remain freely accessible. Reinforcement of the retaining dikes.
- Three dams inland to facilitate the construction of the primary dams. These dams also have a water management function, because they divide saltwater and freshwater delta lakes and separate waters with varying water levels.

With the completion of the Oosterschelde Barrier in 1986 (❏ **Fig. 10.8**), the province of Zeeland was safe. Following a technical and financial feasibility study, a storm surge barrier was constructed to make also South Holland safe. If a water level of 3 meters above NAP is anticipated for Rotterdam the storm surge barrier in the New Waterway is closed. This will only occur in extremely bad weather, probably once every 10 years. A test closure is conducted once a year. Because sea levels will rise in the next 50 years, the storm-surge barrier will need to be closed more frequently in the future, once every 5 years.

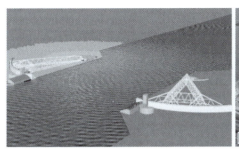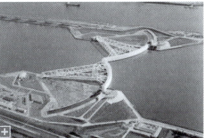

▶ Fig. 10.8. The storm-surge barrier

10.10.2
Prevention

Prevention includes two aspects. In the first place it has to ensure that existing risks will not turn into an actual disaster. The construction of dikes and storm barriers is an example of preventive measures. In the second place prevention aims to limit the consequences of a disaster as much as possible.

Examples of preventive measures are shipping-lane monitoring programs to be implemented in the most vulnerable areas that are at greatest risk for accidents involving water transportation of chemical products.

The human element is an essential factor in maritime safety and many accidents are related to human errors. This implies the necessity for preventive measures to be taken. Safe and efficient operation requires optimised man-machine interaction. Research on working conditions, on measures to improve the working environment, reduction of operator workload and increasing comfort and alertness, are good examples of a prevention policy.

10.10.3
Preparation

Preparation aims at getting ready for intervention. Preparation mainly consists of making disaster relief plans, training and exercising of relief services, and providing information to the public. Preparation of disaster plans is necessary to respond adequately to known hazards as well as to unforeseen events. It includes, for example, the arrangements for calling out key personnel and the preparation of resource registers. Clear responsibility for the disaster plans is necessary, as well as testing the effectiveness of the plans in regular exercises. More specifically, there is a need for combined international emergency planning along the coastlines.

As far as information is concerned, it is often unclear who owns a ship, with whom is the ship insured, which is the flag state, where is the ship registered and where is it coming from and where is it going. The transport sector needs more transparency as a preparation step in safety.

In June 2003 the European Committee on the Environment, Public Health and Consumer Policy made many recommendations on maritime pollution aimed at improving international cooperation, prevention and preparation. The recommendations include safety measures for the maritime transport concerning arrangements for cleaning up animals and birds, availability of specialist equipment, recovery of fuel out of sunken vessels, improved ship-monitoring programs, emergency planning, training programs for volunteers in cleaning up, effective and swift coordination of measures to remedy the situation of wild fauna when maritime disasters occur, establishing high standards and structured networks of experienced organisations, insurance, product information, polluter pays principles and developing an international compensation fund system. All these recommendations contribute to a better preparation in the case of maritime disasters.

10.10.4
Response

The aim of response is to react to and control the disaster itself. In times of flooding response would consist of rescuing the victims, evacuating the disaster area, pumping out the flooded areas, repairing dikes, guarding key facilities and providing of alternative means of transportation. In the case of maritime disasters even more aspects need to be taken into consideration.

The emergency services at sea and on land must respond in a coordinated, combined and effective fashion. Controlling the whole operational network is crucial. Taking care of the victims is essential, but dealing with the dead is also very important. Organising religious services and psychological assistance for victims and relatives must be taken care of. Reducing the environmental pollution is also a significant issue. Communication between the operational services is a vital part of the overall response to maritime disasters, also with regards to the international aspects. Furthermore, good media management is crucial. Questions such as: Why has this happened? Who is to blame? What action will be taken? What kind of insurance arrangements have been made? How do people feel about this? must all be answered quickly and accurately. If no answers can be given, the media will look elsewhere for their information. Controlling the media and distributing correct information is vital during the response phase. This can only be achieved when countries, international organisations, emergency services, ports, coastguards and other participants work closely together and are willing to exchange crucial information quickly.

There is no one-model of response and the response needs to vary with the nature and effects of the disaster. Nevertheless, any response has to be a combined and coordinated operation, and certain features will be common in the response to a variety of different forms of disaster. Some of these common key features are:

- The core of the initial response will normally be provided by the emergency services, the appropriate local authority or authorities and supported by public and private agencies and voluntary organisations. The basic objectives of the combined and coordinated response will be similar on each occasion.

- The same basic management structure will be applicable in the response to any incident. This is the fundamental, nationally agreed, basis for all emergency planning and responses.
- Accurate records will be required for debriefings, formal inquiries and disseminating of information about the lessons learned.

10.10.5
Putting the Links Together

All activities within the five links of the safety chain must be coherent. Separate or combined, they must contribute to prevent the occurrence of water-related disasters or to reduce the negative consequences of the occurring incident such as drowning. Coherent measures are only possible when actions of governments, shipping companies, emergency services, ports and other parties are embedded in an international safety policy for this kind of disaster. The concept of the safety chain can be helpful to link the diverse activities and multiple measures in a transparent way.

10.11
Planning of the Mass Emergency Response to Floods in the Netherlands

PIETER VAN DER TORN and BAS JONKMAN

The Netherlands have recently been confronted with a number of mass emergency situations, such as the explosion of a midtown firework depot (Enschede 1999) and a fire in a bar on New Year's Eve (Volendam 2001). These mass emergencies led to a state-program for mass emergency response with over 150 action points of proactive and reactive nature. The Ministry of Internal Affairs and Kingdom Relations, responsible for mass emergency response at the system level, also developed two guidelines to stimulate planning efforts of local authorities. One guideline [2] focuses on the requirements that were needed by the victims and the other guideline [3] focuses on the available means for response. An expert-based approach has been taken to draft the first edition of the guidelines.

The guidelines offer an assessment method for two questions: "Can the potential needs of the victims during a mass emergency situation match with the available means for mass emergency response?" and "What are the options in case of a discrepancy, if there are insufficient means for a timely response?" These questions were put to the regional authorities who were asked to identify the most severe scenario of a mass emergency situation in their region, to investigate the available means of response in the region and to strike a balance between the regional victim needs and the available means for response.

Fig. 10.9. The scheme of the planning process of needs and demands for mass emergency response

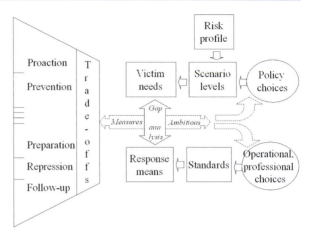

To answer the questions, a gap analysis had to be made comparing the victim requirements with the available means for response (**Fig. 10.9**).

Options to strike a balance are: increasing the response capacity, invest in prevention, prepare the public for self-rescue and bystander assistance or, inform the public that the gap between risk and response can only be bridged against unwarranted high costs. In addition, politicians and policymakers might have to decide to settle for less ambitious scenarios and operation managers and professionals might have to lower their working standards.

10.11.1
Scenarios

Overall 18 types of mass emergencies were considered relevant for the Netherlands. Among these, two types of water-related mass emergency situations were distinguished: traffic accidents on water (ferry, cruise ship, recreational area, plane crash) and floods. Each type of mass emergency was scaled by level of severity on an ordinal five-point scale based on the expected number of victims. In this chapter, these guidelines are described with special emphasis on their application in floods.

10.11.2
Victim Requirements

Victim needs were parameterised and quantified for fire services, health care, police, local authorities and multidisciplinary needs. The quantification was based on expert opinion (best guess).

Victim needs obviously vary depending on the type of mass emergency. Floods were thought to score high on mechanical trauma and psychosocial needs, material and financial damage, as well as a need to evacuate and secure the area. The number of inhabitants living within the area at risk for flooding was thought to be the major determinant within a range of less than 5000 inhabitants (level 1) up to over 75,000 inhabitants (level 5).

10.11.3
Means for Response

An inventory was made of all response processes and teams and their potential capacity to meet the needs of the victims. The quality level of the regular daily care was taken as a point of reference for the capacity estimates. The most important response measures consist of rescue operations and medical assistance. Other relevant parameters for floods were thought to be: registration and operating evacuation centres. The engagement of shallow water rafts by volunteer or military organisations was seen as a local responsibility and was not quantified. The estimated capacity for evacuation is presented in ◘ **Table 10.6**. The estimates for operating an evacuation centre are presented in ◘ **Table 10.7**.

10.11.4
Definition of Flood Risks and Hazards

A broad definition of floods was adopted, including both seaside and inland water floods, as well as flooding of polders. Only serious floods were considered and defined as an inundation depth of more than 1 meter above surface level. Floods were scaled by level of severity with the use of the historical record. The following historical floods were selected:

- The inland drainage problems in the Southeast part of the Netherlands (Limburg 1993 and 1995) were scaled level 1–2. Problems during these floods led to extensive measures on the local and supra-regional level but did not result in casualties.
- The inland floods in the Central East part of the Netherlands (Rivierenland 1995) resulted in the preventive evacuation of 250,000 inhabitants and of all cattle and was scaled level 4–5.
- The seaside flood in the South West part of the Netherlands (Zeeland 1953) resulted in 67 dike failures, a death toll of 1835 persons and the reactive evacuation of 72,000 persons. This was thought to be an unrealistic event in the present day situation and was scaled above level 5.

To determine what level of severity of flooding might occur in a specific area already existing maps for flood-risks were used. The current safety standards for dike heights was used as a measure for the level of severity. Currently, the standards of accepted safety is based on water levels that occur once every 1250 to 10,000 years (◘ **Fig. 10.6**), depending on the costs for realising a certain level of protection.

▶ Table 10.6. Estimated emergency response needs in the area to be evacuated

Start of the evacuation of people from the area: within 1,5 hours

Start of planning of the evacuation of cattle: within 2 hours

Security established in the evacuated area: within 2 hours

Estimated capacity of emergency respone personnel during evacuation:

  per 50 persons in the area: 1 emergency relief worker

  per 1000 persons in the area: 1 medical assistant

Estimated capacity of public transport:

  per 800 persons in the area: 1 bus with the capacity for 65 persons*

  per 200 persons in the area: 1 special transport vehicle with the capacity for 1 disabled person

  per 100 persons in the area: 1 ambulance with the capacity for 1 sick person

* the other persons in the area will have their own means of transportation

▶ Table 10.7. Estimated response needs at the evacuation reception center with a capacity of 2500 persons

Start opening evacuation reception center within 1 hour

Estimated capacity of emergency response personnel:

  150 emergency assistance workers per 2500 persons in the evacuation reception center

  100 first aid workers per 2500 persons in the evacuation reception center

  100 psychosocial support workers per 2500 persons in the evacuation reception center

10.11.5
Current Status of the Guidelines

The two guidelines were presented to the local authorities in 2000 and 2001, respectively. Most local authorities chose an ambition level for the response that should become available in their region in 2002 and drafted inventories of the available means for response in 2003. Also the means for interregional assistance were explored in many regions.

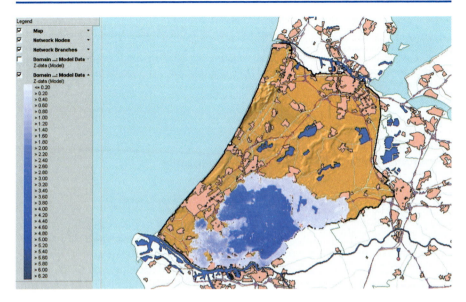

◘ Fig. 10.10. Simulation of a dike failure in the Rotterdam area. This model indicates the water depth in the different parts of the region. (From [1], Asselman and Jonkman 2003)

The guidelines gave a considerable impetus to the planning efforts of the local authorities. With the attention however also came critique. If the available means proved to be insufficient to meet the needs of the estimated number of victims, the underpinning of the estimates for the potential number of victims was questioned The weight of evidence proved to be too small to enforce decisions. A more evidence-based approach with computer simulations is needed to substantiate the estimates for the different types of mass emergencies.

Computer simulation programs are available for floods. Time sequences, locations, inundated areas, local circumstances and number of affected residents may be defined this way. In ◘ **Fig. 10.10** a computer simulation for the Rotterdam area is presented that demonstrates that about one million residents in the inundated area may be affected by floods [1]. Based on the data from the computer simulation, it can also be estimated that thousands of drowned victims are to be expected. Such a scenario indicates how important it is to match the needs in various ways, to assess the trade-offs between proactive and reactive measures and to prepare rescue organisations and medical organisations for their roles in case of floods.

References

1. Asselman N, Jonkman SN (2003) Consequences of floods: the development of a method to estimate the loss of life. Delft Cluster Research paper

2. Ministry of Internal Affairs and Kingdom Relations (2000) Guideline Disaster Measures (only available in Dutch: Leidraad Maatramp, Min. van BZK, Directie Brandweer en Rampenbestrijding, 2000)
3. Ministry of Internal Affairs and Kingdom Relations (2000) Guideline Operational Performances (only available in Dutch: Leidraad Maatramp, Min. van BZK, Directie Brandweer en Rampenbestrijding, 2000)

10.12
Current Trends in Swift Water, Moving Water and Flood Rescue Response

JIM SEGERSTROM

Floods remain the principal weather-related killer and may increasingly become the largest natural threat to the world. Some very recent examples: On July 12, 2003, one million civilians guarded embankments of flooded rivers in China. Millions of Chinese were displaced, at least 40 were missing and 16 dead. On August 3, 2003, large areas of New Hampshire, New Jersey, and Quebec were hit by massive flooding. Two days later the Sudan prepared for the worst flooding of the century and on August 6, 2003, floods in Pakistan affected over 1 million persons and killed over 300. Floods are becoming progressively more severe, particularly in developing countries (◘ **Figs. 10.11–10.12**).

At the same time, the international community remains focused on responding to other threats such as terrorism. Yet while terrorist attacks directly lead to 11,000 fatalities in 2000–2002, nearly 300,000 drowned in weather-related disasters, primarily flooding, during the same time period.

The title of this chapter ("Current trends...") gives the impression of a positive move towards dealing with this potential global pandemic. Such is not the case.

In 1999 there were 96 catastrophic floods in 55 countries and in 2002 there were 134 in 67 countries. In the near future these figures are likely to increase. The world is gradually warming, exacerbating the drought-flood cycle. As a result, glaciers are disappearing. Oceans will rise an average of 0.5 metre in the next 50 years, creating coastal flooding, particularly in northern Europe. Some expect that a large portion of the Ross Ice Shelf in Antarctica will soon calve, creating an iceberg the size of Australia. The rise of the water level in the seas and oceans will heavily affect occupied coastal zones and there will be massive population displacements. It is expected that 94 million people each year will be affected significantly by flood events by 2030.

If the increasingly severe drought-flood cycle leads to an increase in unstable totalitarian governments in the third world, the international response system will be even less able to cope with the problems than it is today. Currently the global insurance industry can only replace a small portion of the losses in property and infrastructure. The World Bank spends tens of billions of dollars in response to such disasters, but little of that money benefits the large proportion of third world populations. This money is spent on sophisticated equipment, such as a few helicopters, that will have little impact in large-scale floods.

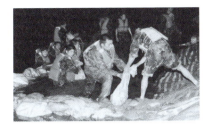

▪ Fig. 10.11. Flood guarding levees in China, July 2003

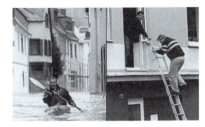

▪ Fig. 10.12. Flooding in Germany, June 2003

Most national governments perceive floods as unique events. This perception is leading to a fragmented response, with little exchange of information, knowledge and experiences. Instead of mitigation through relocations and building flood resistant structures, governments persist in directing efforts towards flood control, but with little success.

Since 2002, both national and international governments appear unable to cope with the increasing scale of the flooding in Europe. Homeowners in Germany have re-built their houses in the same spots as the 2002 floods and are warned by their government that they are likely to be destroyed again in the next flood. Most responsible officials of the world's governments have little idea of current technologies, training and equipment with which to deal with these events.

Standardised training information is rarely distributed. As a result, public safety and military personnel are losing their lives during flood fighting operations. Basic water rescue equipment, such as buoyancy aids, is generally unavailable, even in first world countries. At the same time a substantial number of first responders around the world, in the United States as high as 26%, do not know how to swim (**▪ Figs. 10.13–10.15**).

These trends will continue until a flood event occurs that causes fatalities on a scale where several thousand people are killed by a flood-related dam collapse in a few minutes, for instance, in either Europe or North America. Drowning will be the leading cause of death in such events due to moving water, mudslides and debris flows.

Fortunately there are solutions at hand. Educational information about flooding is readily available. Information from the Federal Emergency Management Agency (FEMA) in the United States and the Emergency Agency (EA) in the United Kingdom are both good examples. Simple standard flood rescue training can be delivered worldwide and international standards of these trainings have

◻ **Fig. 10.13.** Flooding in Germany 2002

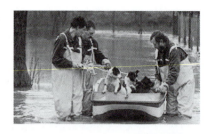

◻ **Fig. 10.14.** Flooding in Slovakia June 2002

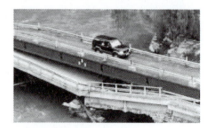

◻ **Fig. 10.15.** Flooding in Mozambique 2002

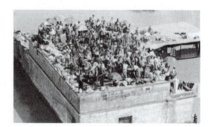

been developed. This is extremely important because education and training always saves more lives than responses and are inexpensive to disseminate. Local responders will always save most lives, while international rescue teams are just receiving word of the flooding while they are still in their home countries. At the same time, increasing efforts are being made to coordinate effective international flood assistance in the third and fourth stages of the flood, particularly by non-governmental organisations.

The impact of flooding in third world countries can be mitigated and reduced primarily by modern engineering practices on hillsides, and attention to agriculture and building out of flood plains, domestic typing and listing of available resources. Along with modern incident command systems, this can provide an organisation to flood responses that will save even more lives.

◘ Table 10.5. Practical Tips for Flood Rescue Personnel

- Do not let urgency and emotion effect rescue decisions. Both are killers
- All rescue personnel within 4 meters of the edge of any water should be wearing personal flotation devices
- The power of moving water is deceptive without training. Water moving at only 20 kilometres per hour will exert nearly 220 kilos of pressure on the average person
- Common causes of flood deaths are failure to evacuate houses that are going to be submerged, and driving cars through floods. Therefore, civilians should evacuate when ordered, and should not drive cars across flooded roadways, under any circumstances. Public safety authorities should advertise the slogan: "Turn around! Don't drown!"
- Do not tie ropes to rescuers in moving water. Rescuers die tied to the end of ropes, when pushed downstream and trapped under cars every year
- A rope thrown from shore is effective in 90% of all flood rescues
- Conduct a thorough hazard assessment of the flood area. Consider such problems as floating debris, hazardous materials and contaminated water, deteriorated roadways, poles and fences, night, bad weather, inadequately trained rescue team members, poor communications, levee failures, poor evacuation plans, poor coordination with air rescue resources, poor flood plain maps, increasingly bad weather, poor crowd control, storm drains and dam failures. Most of these hazards can be mitigated before the flood
- There are four distinct phases to major flood events and critical issues for which emergency managers must be prepared in each phase. If you are an emergency management official responsible for flood response, and do not know what those four phases are, or the issues within each phase, you are not ready for the flood
- There is no such thing as 'flood control'. Floods go wherever they want
- There is no such thing as 'flood disaster management'. There is such a thing as 'flood disaster response'. A disaster is an event in which many lose their lives and local resources are overwhelmed. Management implies that officials were ready for the scale of the event. In which case, it would not be a disaster, since few would lose their lives. Floods are best managed before they occur, through education and mitigation
- Do not consider using boats for flood rescue, unless the boat crew members feel confident they can survive without the boat. Boats sinking during flood operations are a growing trend
- Always make sure that the rescuers are deployed upstream of any rescue sites to warn of debris coming down. And that other rescuers are deployed downstream, as additional safety

10.12.1
Rescue Programs

There are many river rescue programs, including those taught by boating safety organisation in several states in the US, provinces in Canada, and by the National Association for Search and Rescue. All of these courses deliver generally recognised competency standard training for emergency responders. Flood rescue trainings should provide information on three levels of response: awareness, operations and technicians.

Awareness training can be provided to all public safety personnel and private individuals who may be involved in flood rescue operations. Awareness concentrates on personnel safety, necessary equipment, scene and accident assessment, hazards, and rescue alternatives. Awareness training is not rescuing training, and can be conducted entirely in the classroom, or over the Internet.

Operation training includes personal self-rescue skills in moving water. Swift water and flood operations training is ideal for the isolated villages and rescue workers in developing countries, since it requires simple technology, techniques and equipment, and will effectively save many lives. Operation trainings take 2–3 days.

Technician training is comprehensive and is equipment and time intensive. Such training is limited by the swimming skills of responders, the need for constant practice of those skills, and the necessary equipment to perform them. Swift water Flood Technician training takes 6–10 days. Recertification, at least every 2 years, is required in order to keep up to date with new equipment and technologies.

Flood events will become more severe in the coming decades but public safety agencies around the world are not keeping pace. The pneumonic PREP nicely summarised the efforts that governmental and private organisations can focus their efforts in order to save lives:

- P for 'prevention' of flood deaths, by
- R for 'recognition' of local flood problems, both historic and potential, and
- E for 'education' so that civilians will respond correctly in the event, and finally,
- P for 'preparation' of rescue resources, the most expensive part of the solution.

Decreasing the global pandemic of drowning in flood events will take a major focus, but not necessarily an expensive one. The warning signs are there; now is the time to act.

10.12.2
Websites

- www.t-rescue.com/articles/Swiftwater/Swiftwater.htm
- www.alertnet.org
- www.dw-world.de

- www.english.eastday.com
- www.montreal.cbc.ca
- www.specialrescue.com
- www.theage.com
- Flood videos: www.noaa.gov
- No Way Out: njrigg@comcast.net
- Low water crossings: www.noaa.gov/oh/tt2/xwater/index.shtml
- Swiftwater Newsgroup: SwiftH2O-News-subscribe@yahoogroups.com
- FEMA: www.fema.gov/home/nwz96/autofld.shtm
- Flood Hazard Maps: www.fema.gov/mit/floodp.shtm
  or www.fema.gov/MSC/femahome.shtm
- Dam Failures through the years: www.fema.gov/mit/damprgm.shtm
- Pictures and graphs of floods:
  www.cgrer.uiowa.edu/research/exhibit_gallery/Great_floods.html
- Floods: http://www.eastnc.coastalnet.com/weather/nwsmhx/flds.html
- Northwest floods of 1996: http://www.teleport.com/~samc/flood1.html
- National Weather Service: http://www.nws.noaa.gov/

Further Reading

BBC News (2003) Fifty years on, UK flood risk remains. BBC News, 29 January 2003
New York Times (2003) The Antarctic is melting. New York Times, 6 February 2003
Ray F (1998) Swiftwater rescue. CFS Press
Segerstrom J (1999) THE ,Weapon of Mass Destruction. Fire International, June 1999
Segerstrom J (2001) Safe management of moving water and flood rescue responses. Special Rescue
    Services
Segerstrom J (2001) Current trends in training and equipment for flood disaster response. In: Pro-
    ceedings of the 22nd Annual International Disaster Management Conference, Florida. Emer-
    gency Medical Foundation, Tampa, Florida, 31 March 2001
Segerstrom J (2001) Emergency management aspects of flood response. In: Proceedings of the
    22nd Annual International Disaster Management Conference, Florida Emergency Medical
    Foundation, Tampa, Florida, 31 March 2001
Segerstrom J (2003) Flood rescue: an oxymoron. A review of the European floods of 2002. Technical
    Rescue, April
The Economist (2003) The impact of disaster. The Economist, 19 July 2003
The Washington Post (2003) , 3 January 2003

Breath-Hold, SCUBA and Hose Diving

Task Force on Breath-Hold, SCUBA and Hose Diving
Section editors: David Elliott and Rob van Hulst

"Water is a hazardous and unforgiving environment
but if the hazards are controlled, the risks of diving are low"

Task Force Chairs

- David Elliott
- Rob van Hulst

Task Force Members

- Alfred Bove
- Glen Egstrom
- Des Gorman
- Maida Taylor
- Jürg Wendling

Other Contributor

- Jim Caruso

11.1
Overview and Recommendations

Diving is defined as an underwater activity during which a person breathes from a source of compressed gas. For the purposes of this chapter it also includes breath-hold diving in which the participant extends his underwater excursion for the duration of breath-hold time and then returns to the surface for a further breath. The definition does not include diving by head-first entry by a swimmer into the water (board diving).

Water is a hazardous and unforgiving environment but if the hazards are controlled, the risks of diving are low. The objective of this chapter is to outline ways in which the risk of drowning among divers may be reduced and also to focus on those additional features of management that do not feature routinely in the treatment of a non-diver. Although there is no difference in physiology or physics between recreational and working divers, there are sufficient differences in motivation and procedures for them to be considered in separate categories. The boundaries between them are not always clear but, for the prevention and management of drowning, diving can be put into at least three very different categories.

Working divers represent a wide range of activity from offshore saturation diving and military diving to inland rescues and construction work. For many there are accepted training and diving procedures. Diving by the navies of the world and commercial diving companies, includes the use of oxy-helium at deeper depths, and rarely leads to death by drowning, probably because it is well regulated and well supervised. This population is not excluded from this review but they are not a major consideration when compared with other divers. Reliable data on fatalities among working divers is not available except in a very few sectors but it is widely agreed that self-regulation and the enforcement of national regulations have been effective in many countries and their seas. Improvements in diving health and safety for some nations would come from a broader definition of the types of professional diver to be included within their existing standards and more rigorous enforcement. An observation by many is that safety begins with a competent risk assessment of each dive when it is planned and that this is more effective than the traditional application of a prescriptive rule book. In the UK, at least, failure to comply with health and safety regulations is dealt with under criminal law. In some other nations improvements could start from the introduction of the simplest standards.

At the World Congress on Drowning it was agreed that:
- Well-constructed national regulations have been effective where enforced and that any significant improvements in health and safety would arise only from a more inclusive definition of working divers and a wider application of existing procedures.

Recreational divers are a large and independent group ranging from SCUBA tourists to deep mixed-gas wreck divers. They dive for pleasure and not for reward, and not for other people. They can choose when, where and how to dive. Many get suitable training from a recognised training agency. Recreational divers are not required to follow detailed regulations and so, within the worldwide recreational diving industry, self-regulation is dominant. The expense of diving has kept it in a minority role as a relatively elite sport although it is practised around the world and in many places far from the sea. Diving is a safe recreational activity when performed sensibly even though, due to the nature of the environment, the few underwater accidents that do occur have a high risk of a fatal outcome and drowning is the mode of death in around half the fatalities. The cause of drowning is usually due to some underlying medical or procedural error.

At the World Congress on Drowning it was agreed that:
- Self-regulation within the worldwide recreational diving industry continues to be the practical route for further improvement but that there is a need to counter a perception that there is a conflict between commercial interests and safety.
- The training agencies comply with international quality assurance and control procedures (QA/QC) such as the International Standard ISO 9000 and also encourage independent monitoring to assure the effective and safe use of existing and new procedures.

Subsistence fishermen are found predominantly in the poor countries around the world. It is common to find that untrained persons using minimal and possibly inappropriate equipment use diving to catch fish to feed themselves and their families or to collect shellfish. Some may be provided with self-contained breathing apparatus (SCUBA) by fishing boat owners, while others just use a compressor in their boat and hold the compressed-air hose between their teeth. For them training, regulations and medical support appear to be zero. It is known that their morbidity is high but there is no hard data on drowning and fatalities.

At the World Congress on Drowning it was agreed that:

- Subsistence fishermen who are predominantly found in the poor countries around the world, use diving equipment that is minimal and that their training, regulations and medical support appear to be zero.
- To improve diving-fishermen safety and reduce drowning there is a need to collect data on accidents and drowning among representative populations of diving fishermen around the world. This should be followed up with international non-governmental organisations (NGO), other charities and appropriate UN development initiatives so that existing academic societies, training organisations and others could deliver suitable medical and diving advice and training for fishermen compatible with the limits of available local resources.

11.2
The Underlying Physics and Applied Physiology

A detailed knowledge of the physics and physiology of diving is not needed by those concerned with the prevention and management of drowning but it is necessary to know that increased environmental pressure is a unique physiological variable that affects all those who descend below the surface of the sea. By definition man is exposed to one atmosphere of pressure (1 bar) at sea level and to increasing pressure while descending through the water, such that each additional 10 m (33 feet) of sea water or so increases the environmental pressure by one additional atmosphere. Some knowledge of the natural laws that relate to the hyperbaric environment is needed in order to understand the hazards to which divers are uniquely exposed. A full account of the relevant aspects of environmental physiology is available elsewhere and so a summary can suffice.

Barometric pressure is transmitted throughout the body just as it is through a fluid and so the diver should not usually sense its direct effects. Pressure:

- Acts at the molecular and cellular level in a complex manner
- Acts directly on the gas-containing spaces of the body (ears, sinuses, lungs) in accordance with Boyle's Law
- Causes the pulmonary gases at increased pressure to be dissolved into the body's tissues until equilibrium (saturation) is achieved. Beyond a brief threshold duration, the diver needs to surface by following a predetermined slow ascent in order to assist their safe elimination
- Causes an increase in the partial pressure of the respiratory gases to the extent that some significant effects, such as seizures due to toxicity, can occur that endanger the individual

11.2.1
Gas Pressure and Volume

The ideal gas law is $PV=nRT$ where P is the absolute pressure, V is the volume of gas, n is the number of moles of gas, R is the universal gas constant and T is the absolute temperature. In other words, Boyle's Law states that the volume of a given mass of gas is inversely proportional to the pressure. Thus 1 litre of gas at sea level (100 kPa) decreases to 0.25 litres at 30 m (400 kPa; 100 feet). Of equal importance to the pathogenesis of dysbaric illnesses is the converse of this, that 1 litre of compressed gas at 30 meters (400 kPa; 100 feet) will expand on ascent to 4 litres at the surface.

11.2.2
Compression Barotrauma

During descent, the reduction in volume of gas contained in the body needs to be compensated by the addition of an appropriate supplementary volume of compressed gas. Thus the respiratory gases must have easy access to compensate the gas-filled spaces of the sinuses and middle ear, otherwise the diminishing volumes of their gas may cause pain and possibly vertigo. This can be the start of a cascade of events that may lead to death by drowning but is not a primary concern during treatment if that happens.

11.2.3
Partial Pressures

The application of Dalton's law, that the partial pressure of a gas in a mixture is equal to the product of its fractional concentration and the absolute pressure, has a special importance in the hyperbaric environment. Thus at 50 meters (600 kPa; 165 feet) the partial pressure of oxygen in compressed air is 126 kPa which is equivalent to breathing a hypothetical 126% oxygen at the surface.

11.2.4
Gas Solubility and Uptake

Henry's law determines how much gas dissolves in a particular liquid with which it is in contact. In accordance with Henry's Law, the quantity of gas dissolved in a liquid is proportional at constant temperature to the partial pressure of that gas. Some gases are more soluble than others and their solubility in the watery and the fatty tissues of the body are not the same. Also, the uptake of the inert components of the respiratory gases into solution in the body depends upon the characteristics of the circulation during the transient dynamic phase until the steady state of tissue gas equilibrium (saturation) has been achieved.

11.2.5
Lack of Oxygen

Hypoxia is a particular hazard of some types of diving in which errors can be made in the content of the respiratory gas supplied to the diver or when there is a failure of complex breathing apparatus. With persons breathing compressed air, hypoxia should not be a hazard. A hazard arises when divers are required to breathe a gas mixture which is meant to be in the partial pressure range of 20–150 kPa and either the wrong oxygen percentage is provided, or the oxygen make-up system of a closed-circuit or semi-closed-circuit breathing apparatus fails. With a scrubber in the circuit, there is no concurrent accumulation of carbon dioxide then, unlike hypoxia from most other causes, its onset may not be noticed by the subject who gently passes through unconsciousness towards an anoxic death.

11.2.6
Oxygen Toxicity

The toxic effects of oxygen on the lungs and the central nervous system are especially important in diving where not only is partial pressure of oxygen in the air increased by descent, but also because pure oxygen and oxygen-enriched mixtures are used as respiratory gases. Pulmonary oxygen toxicity is not likely to arise in diving of the type associated with the commoner causes of drowning. Most compressed-air divers are exposed only briefly to such moderate pressures that oxygen neurotoxicity does not usually occur in that category of diving. However, it does occur among working divers and more advanced types of recreational diving and so, for practical purposes, the important aspects are those of recognition.

Neurotoxicity, however, is important. The partial pressure threshold for the neurological effects of oxygen is in excess of 150 kPa and can easily be exceeded by divers. This form of oxygen toxicity is relatively quick in onset. Nitrogen narcosis, heavy exercise and carbon dioxide build-up are considered to be synergistic with oxygen in causing this toxicity. The classic presentation is that of a sudden seizure. If this occurs in the water, it may have a fatal outcome.

11.2.7
Carbon Dioxide Effects

To prolong breath-hold duration hyperventilation may be intentional for the purposes of reducing CO_2 levels. It may be unintentional, in association with near panic. The latter is likely to be concurrent with other factors contributing towards a perceived in-water emergency and may contribute to an unfavourable outcome.

Excess CO_2 may be due to extrinsic causes such as the failure of carbon dioxide scrubbing in closed-circuit breathing apparatus or intrinsic, such as voluntary hypoventilation to conserve breathing gas. This hypercapnia alone can account for dyspnea and headaches, even seizures and unconsciousness, but it is perhaps more significant as just one of several synergistic factors in cases of unexpected loss of consciousness underwater.

11.2.8
Nitrogen Narcosis

At increased partial pressures nitrogen behaves as a narcotic agent, the mechanism of its action being analogous to that of alcohol and volatile anaesthetics. Euphoric irresponsibility is not compatible with the safe use of complex procedures and equipment and for this reason commercial compressed-air diving is limited, in the North Sea, to 50 meters (165 feet). In other places slightly deeper limits may be in force but, in general, at deeper depths than this nitrogen is replaced by helium as the necessary oxygen diluent. Compressed air in the past has been used successfully by experienced divers to 90 meters but, much beyond that, there is the probability of narcosis leading to unconsciousness. Helium has no significant narcotic properties at depths down to around 700 meters (2300 feet).

11.2.9
Decompression Illnesses

A few diving deaths are precipitated by decompression illness but drowning is rare in these circumstances.

The pathology of burst lung during ascent (pulmonary barotrauma) may lead to the passage of air bubbles in the blood to the brain (arterial gas embolism). Characteristically this can lead to unconsciousness on arriving at the surface and the victim may sink. If then found and recovered, the diagnosis of drowning may hide the need to treat underlying cerebral arterial gas embolism.

The pathology of decompression sickness arising from bubbles formed from dissolved gases means that its onset is usually after the dive. Thus it is a concern only when a drowning diver with an inert gas load is recovered to the surface with no opportunity to off-gas by completing the appropriate decompression protocol. There is then a risk of the onset of neurological deficits during the next 24 hours.

11.3
Diving Techniques

11.3.1
Breath-Hold Diving

The first divers, historically, were the breath-hold divers who, through the centuries, have dived for sponges, shellfish and salvage. This type of diving is still a practical activity in many parts of the world.

The duration underwater for a diver with no breathing apparatus is limited by the individual's breath hold endurance (apneic diving). No equipment is needed for this type of diving but many use a snorkel. A half-mask or, in poorer places, goggles made from sea-shells assist viewing underwater. Fins may be used.

11.3.2
Compressed-Air Diving

The majority of divers use compressed air for breathing. This may be from bottles of compressed air which the diver carries (self-contained breathing apparatus: SCUBA). The gas must be made available for breathing, breath-by-breath (on demand), at the same pressure as that exerted by the depth of water around them. This is done by a demand valve opened by inspiration after which the exhaled gas is discharged into the sea (open circuit). The term *SCUBA* is generally reserved to mean that the diver is carrying compressed gas that is delivered to the diver as needed, at a pressure to match that of the surrounding water.

The compressed gas may also be supplied by a hose from the surface to a demand valve from which the diver breathes as needed. Because this provides a facility for a communication link to the surface plus a potentially unlimited supply of air, it is a common technique for working divers but is not used by recreational divers because it limits mobility and freedom. Some fishermen divers use a simpler but more hazardous technique in which the hose is no more than a pipe held between the teeth of the diver with compressed air free-flowing into the mouth.

The use of compressed-air diving should be limited in depth because of the narcotic consequences of raised partial pressures of nitrogen. Beyond around 50 meters (165 feet) divers breathe a mixed gas, usually containing helium which has no significant narcotic effect but which is expensive.

To reduce nitrogen uptake and to prolong bottom time, oxygen-rich nitrogen mixtures, also known as nitrox and EAN, are used by some recreational and working divers at depth, but these dives are limited by the hazard of oxygen neurotoxicity.

11.3.3
Deep Mixed-Gas Diving

To dive deeper some recreational divers use sequences of various mixed gases, usually including helium. The hazards of this type of diving, especially when performed solo, are significant. For teams of working divers, who use diving bells and saturation techniques, the controls mean that this type of diving is relatively safe. Saturation divers are those who live for some days at raised environmental pressure in a deck chamber and make excursions to work at depth being supplied by a hose from the diving bell. These working procedures are generally safer than shallower bounce-diving and a description of their techniques is not needed in this review.

11.3.4
Rebreathers

Some divers may use a semi-closed circuit or closed-circuit breathing apparatus but because this equipment is more complex, there is a greater risk of failure. Examples include the use of closed-circuit oxygen apparatus in waters less than 8 meters (25 feet) particularly for military purposes. An oxygen-nitrogen mixture in semi-closed breathing apparatus of various types, originally for the military, is now used by recreational divers. With CO_2 being continuously produced by the diver and scrubbed from the breathing circuit, such apparatus can present special hazards such as an insidious hypoxia if the flow rate becomes too low. This type of equipment requires greater technical support, different diving procedures and additional training.

11.4
Epidemiology of Drowning While Diving

Drowning is the mode of death in 40%–60% of recreational diving fatalities. This observation comes from several national sources where some form of accident reporting is available, but the data are not collected universally and the results are not comprehensive. The data from divers at work are also largely unknown. Divers working in an industrial or military environment are usually well monitored and drowning appears to be rare. In contrast, accidents around the world among those who dive to catch fish go almost totally unreported. The focus of this task force is upon the causes of the accidents that may lead to drowning and the possibilities for their prevention.

All attempts at analysing the demographics of recreational divers involved in drowning are limited by the lack of complete information on deaths and probably some underestimate of the numerator in assessing risk. More importantly, even where there are some data for recreational diving, there are no denominators since there is no idea of the active diving population, defined as those persons making one or more dives in the past calendar year. For example, the number of certified divers far exceeds that of active divers, since re-certification is not required and the apparent population may be inflated by including those who have ceased diving. Nonetheless, working with the limited information available, some characteristics of diving deaths from drowning in recreational diving can be projected for some geographical areas.

Some data are available for commercial divers in a few geographical areas but drowning is a rare industrial accident among working divers. At the other extreme, numerous diving fishermen work largely untrained and unregulated around the world and appropriate data are simply not available.

At the World Congress on Drowning it was agreed that:
- The collection of diver morbidity and mortality data and the associated contributory factors for each incident is a necessary first step in reducing drowning incidents among divers. Also needed are the denominator data that will allow the calculation of risk.

11.5
Physical, Mental and Medical Fitness

The prevention of drowning among divers depends upon their physical and mental fitness because an underwater emergency may occur at any time and the lives of the diver and others may depend on their ability to respond fully.

Drowning during or after a dive may also be a consequence of a number of factors related to medical and mental fitness. Examples include:
- Loss of consciousness in the water
- Extreme breathlessness
- Panic or other inappropriate behaviour
- Disorientation or vertigo
- Cardiac disease

Screening of divers for fitness to dive is designed to identify those at risk but the extent to which such screening is implemented is very varied. In recreational diving the unfit participant puts his diving partner (buddy) at increased risk of an accident. In well-regulated military, commercial and some recreational activities there is likely to be a structured program for health monitoring. In some groups of divers, such as student scientists and emergency rescue divers the requirements differ between nations, but for many divers, medical review never happens.

Components of an ideal screening procedure include:
- Accepted standards of physical, mental and medical fitness for each specific type of diving
- A method of screening that usually includes some degree of self-assessment
- An evaluation of that initial assessment that in many cases leads to a medical examination

■ A medical practitioner who has a relevant understanding of the unique physiology of increased environmental pressure and the hazards of the underwater environment

After some form of self-assessment, some recreational diving agencies refer the candidate diver for a review by a doctor identified as having appropriate competencies. In some countries, when completion of a self-assessment form has revealed a medical query, the diver can be referred to any medical practitioner. This system, though not perfect, can be effective in places where no alternative is available. The self-assessment form may be a once-in-a-diving-lifetime event for most recreational divers but it needs to be repeated as the diver gets older. The diving fisherman in poorer communities is among the group that probably is unaware of many of the hazards and is never assessed.

Fitness to make the next dive is also a responsibility of the individual diver to confirm that there is no potential limit to his or her underwater performance that might shortly be needed.

At the World Congress on Drowning it was agreed that:
■ Recreational divers are free to dive when, where and how they like but the diver also has an obligation to the public. Any underwater accident to a diver can put buddy divers and rescuers at considerable risk.
■ Greater stringency is needed in the assessment of the physical, mental and medical fitness of all who choose to dive. A single assessment of fitness for diving at the beginning of diver training should not be considered valid throughout the rest of the diver's life. Re-assessments are recommended at intervals that may diminish with advancing years and re-assessment may also be needed after illness or injury.
■ To give a medical opinion on a diver's fitness, the doctor should have prior knowledge of the unique hazards faced by a diver. Whenever possible, the medical assessment should be conducted by a doctor acknowledged as competent in this special subject. It is recommended that the training of diving doctors, both for the medical examination of divers and also for the treatment of medical emergencies in diving, complies with guidance such as that published by the European Diving Technology Committee (EDTC) and the European Committee for Hyperbaric Medicine (ECHM). Periodical revision training is also important.
■ The mental, physical and medical standards of fitness in each category of diving should be harmonised internationally.

11.6
Causation of Drowning Accidents in Relation to Training

The prevention of drowning among divers depends largely upon their training because a large proportion of those who drown have been found to be diving beyond their competency.

Thus the major contributors to recreational fatalities are poor dive planning and preparation, inexperience, exhaustion of gas supplies, problems with buoyancy and unfamiliarity with the equipment or the environment. A feature of too many recreational diving deaths is the finding that the dead diver had no relevant training. Between one-third and half of all diving deaths by drowning involve young, inexperienced male divers. A significant number of diving deaths by drowning involve students participating in instructional classes. Standards that provide a clearer picture of the nature of a calculated risk, preferably for each diver on each dive, need to be established.

Through legislation there are high standards for most commercial and naval divers, but little safety guidance is available for the subsistence fisherman in poorer regions. Most intending divers undergo some training when attention can be directed at identified causes of accidents that suggest human error and/or violations of procedure.

Most underwater accidents occur as a direct result of a loss of control on the part of the diver. This may be mitigated by the actions of the diver or buddy in an effort to regain control, or it may result in drowning, injury or death. The causes of the loss of control, which are most often traced back to diver error, may be catastrophic or they may be cumulative resulting in panic in the face of minor emergencies.

One example is called avalanching in which stressors from relatively benign problems become additive until the diver cannot tolerate the ultimate stress load and a loss of control ensues. Another example is the case in which buddy separation may increase stress as well as breathing rate with a resultant diminution of air supply and increased breathing resistance leading to panic and a loss of control. These are only two of the many scenarios that may lead to panic in a loss of control. When control is lost an emergency is born. To regain control quickly the emergency procedure must be appropriate, reliable, over-learned and practised regularly. For the individuals to learn it, it must also be tolerable.

At the World Congress on Drowning it was agreed that:
- Greater emphasis should be placed at all levels of training on the causation and prevention of in-water fatalities.
- After some 3–5 years without regular diving, the individual should be subject to a formal re-assessment of competence before re-entering the water.

11.7
Introducing Children to Diving

At the World Congress on Drowning it was agreed that:
- The policy of training children as young as 8 year olds to dive should emphasise the immaturity of mental outlook that many young persons may have when an emergency occurs.

11.8
Underwater Self-Rescue and Assisted Rescue: Training to Cope With Emergencies

Man makes highly specific adaptations to the demands associated with the surrounding environment and thus training programs must be focussed upon similar psychomotor elements present in the desired end behaviour. This requires that an analysis of the skill components of critical diving procedures must be undertaken *before* an effective training program is developed for any specific procedure.

The large scale proliferation of non-standardised diving equipment has led to a wide variety of configurations that require large and small changes in the execution of effective emergency procedures. The effectiveness of emergency air sharing is one example as its procedure is complicated by the large number of currently available solutions to the problem. As examples:

- Buddy breathing from a donor's regulator
- Sharing air through an octopus (an optional second regulator attached to SCUBA)
- Sharing air with a variety of dual purpose auto-inflation devices with breathing capability
- The use of an independent air source such as a pony bottle or spare air device

Each option can be expected to be effective only if the donor and receiver are comfortable with it. Effective changes in procedure are best developed by retraining while using the new configuration.

Training programs should progress from the simple to the complex elements of the emergency procedure. Achieving proficiency with the emergency procedures under ideal conditions before training for proficiency under simulated emergency conditions is fundamental to effective progression. Critical skills must become over-learned if they are expected to operate successfully in an emergency. Over-learning implies the skill can be readily accomplished without a great deal of conscious thought. Once over-learned, periodic practice of the emergency procedures is necessary to retain an effective level of proficiency: "use it or lose it".

Crisis management during underwater emergencies requires that the individual diver must ultimately be responsible for his or her own safety. In order to accomplish this goal the diver must have a reasonably complete knowledge and understanding of the nature of the calculated risk to which they are exposing themselves. They must also develop an appropriate level of awareness of the risks involved and their ability to be able to accept those risks. The analysis of hundreds of diving accidents in the USA has resulted in a national Responsible Diver Program for several years. The individual diver must be prepared to accept the responsibility for his or her own welfare on every dive and the skills that are critical to safety must be identified and proficiency in each developed.

While there is no guarantee that training programs can prepare the diver for all emergency situations, it is clear that training for coping with emergencies will result in the development of divers with an increased ability to utilise rational problem solving capability in underwater emergency circumstances.

Diving has a number of inherent risks that, by and large, are acceptable to the diving population. The steps needed for the assessment of risk are the relationship between a dose and the response to that dose, identification of the hazards, the analysis of exposure and describing the risk. Risk–benefit analysis would be a more effective solution for enhancing safety than prescriptive regulations and standard procedures imposed by government or training agencies.

A significant part of the current dilemma is associated with the proliferation of recreational diving equipment with limited regard for impact of equipment changes on diver training. Emergency procedures in particular have become significantly more difficult to teach because of the variation and increased complexity of current equipment configurations such as the Buoyancy Compensation Device (BCD). We are faced with the need for a re-examination of the effectiveness of the methodology that we use to teach self-rescue and emergency procedures. The communication of the best information available to the widest membership in the diving community is clearly in the best interest of the safety of all divers. This information must be accompanied by the recognition that there can be no guarantee of safety and that all risks are relative to the specific conditions of each dive. Diving does and always has involved a calculated risk that the diver needs to assess for every dive that is made.

Risk assessment procedures are already in place for naval, commercial and other working divers but, for example, are probably non-existent among diving fishermen of the poorer countries.

At the World Congress on Drowning it was agreed that:
- Emergency procedures should be consistent with a variety of equipment in a variety of configurations
- Programs of refresher training should be established to maximise practical re-learning and updating of basic emergency skills. This is needed particularly after an individual's equipment has been modified
- Self-rescue and buddy rescue procedures should be compatible with the equipment used and the environmental conditions
- Training of rescuers should include the procedures for recovery of the victim from the water into a boat and transfer of the patient from the deck of a boat to a helicopter or some other emergency transport vehicle
- Hand signals and basic procedures used in diving emergencies, whether at depth or on the surface, should be standardised and promoted through rescue and diving agencies throughout the world

11.9
Immediate Treatment of the Diver Who Almost Drowned

In the United States alone, some 90 recreational SCUBA fatalities occur each year, and drowning is reported as the leading cause of death. In diving-related drowning incidents, entanglement, out-of-air emergencies at depth and overhead environment (cave diving and wreck diving) are common circumstances. In cold water, the maximum breath-hold time drops dramatically, further compromising ability to survive. In divers who sustain pulmonary barotrauma and cerebral arterial gas embolism, unconsciousness will lead to water aspiration and drowning.

Treatment can be divided into the immediate phase that is part of the rescue and resuscitation effort, and a later in-hospital phase. The training of those who will respond immediately to an incident is based on procedures that are generally available in numerous publications. A limiting factor may be the dissemination of that knowledge to the appropriate individual.

After water aspiration, victims may present with minimal respiratory complaints or with severe pulmonary oedema due to direct lung injury from the aspirated water. Patients who have aspirated a significant quantity of water will frequently have a widened alveolar-arterial oxygen gradient and mild to severe hypoxaemia. P_aCO_2 can be low or elevated depending upon alveolar ventilation.

The drowning victim who presents in cardiac arrest should be treated vigorously, since salvage with normal neurological function has been described even after prolonged cardiac arrest. Cardiac arrest in this setting is due to hypoxaemia and acidosis, and a reliable airway must be established to supply a high inspired oxygen concentration; 100% oxygen through a high flow system should be used. Aspiration of stomach contents is a constant threat in the comatose drowning victim, so the preferred method of establishing an airway is endotracheal intubation. There is also the possibility of a concomitant unstable neck injury and the risk of aspiration. At present there is insufficient data on the efficacy of the Heimlich manoeuvre in non-fatal drowning victims. Patients with cardiac arrest secondary to non-fatal drowning can have a severe metabolic acidosis and may require large doses of bicarbonate to reverse the acidosis. Concurrent with the above resuscitative measures, a nasogastric tube should be inserted to decompress the stomach, and measurement of body temperature should be obtained to evaluate hypothermia. In the presence of a significantly lowered body temperature, a patient should not be declared dead and appropriate rewarming measures should be instituted while resuscitation proceeds.

Immediate therapy should consist of establishing a functional airway, providing 100% oxygen concentrations in inspired breathing gas, nasogastric intubation, rewarming, and cardiopulmonary resuscitation if cardiac arrest has occurred. Use of positive pressure ventilation with a mechanical or manual resuscitator may provoke aspiration, and should be delayed until gastric contents are removed. However, if the patient is apneic, assisted ventilation is necessary and should be provided with the knowledge that vomiting and aspiration are likely. A portable, battery-operated device for measuring arterial oxygen saturation (pulse oximetry) is a useful guide for therapy prior to reaching a hospital.

Non-fatal drowning when SCUBA diving may be associated with problems of toxic gas mixtures, decompression related disorders, and venomous marine animals. In cases of non-fatal drowning associated with any of these other disorders, treatment strategy should include therapy for each of the disorders.

At the World Congress on Drowning it was agreed that:
- Rescuers must be made aware that the treatment of drowning in a diver might be complicated by other medical conditions such as carbon monoxide poisoning, envenomation and omitted decompression arising from that same dive.
- National and international standards of medical care should be written for all medical emergencies in diving by suitable academic bodies.

11.10
Accident Investigation and Autopsy

At the World Congress on Drowning it was agreed by the task-force Breath-Held, SCUBA and Hose Diving that:
- Drowning is mostly a diagnosis of exclusion and often is a presumptive diagnosis based on purely circumstantial evidence. All diving related deaths should be thoroughly investigated, including a complete autopsy, evaluation of the equipment and a review of the circumstances surrounding the fatality by knowledgeable investigators with appropriate training and experience.
- The post-mortem examination of a drowned diver should be conducted by a pathologist who is knowledgeable about diving (or who is advised by a doctor who is knowledgeable about diving).

Further Reading

Bennett PB, Elliott DE (2003) The physiology and medicine of diving, 5th edn. Brubank AO, Neuman TS (editors). Saunders, Edinburgh, ISBN 0-7020-2571-2

Bove AA, Davis JC (2004) Bove and Davis' diving medicine, 4th edn. Bove AA (editor). Saunders, Philadelphia, ISBN 0-7216-9424-1

Divers Alert Network (2002) Report on decompression illness, diving fatalities and project dive exploration. DAN America

Edmonds C, Lowry C, Pennefather J, Walker R (2002) Diving and subaquatic medicine, 4th edn. ISBN 0-340-80630-3

European Journal of Underwater and Hyperbaric Medicine (ISSN 1605-9204), published quarterly by the European Underwater and Baromedical Society, Speyerer Strasse 91–93, 68163 Mannheim, Germany

Undersea and Hyperbaric Medicine (ISSN 1066-2936), published quarterly by Undersea and hyperbaric Medical Society, 10531 Metropolitan Avenue, Kensington, MD 20895, USA

Walker D (1998) Report on Australian diving deaths 1972–1993. JL Publications, Australia

11.11
Diving Accident Investigations

Des Gorman

The risk of injury and death from diving varies with the nature of the diving. The mortality rate for offshore occupational divers approaches zero. By contrast, diving fishermen have a considerable mortality and morbidity rate. For example, prior to the introduction of a relevant code of practice, abalone divers in South Australia had an annual decompression illness (DCI) risk of almost 1% and a prevalence of radiologically apparent dysbaric osteonecrosis of about 50% [1]. By contrast, in Australasian recreational divers, for whom reasonable anecdotal exposure data exist, the incidence of DCI is approximately 1 for every 10,000 hours of exposure and the mortality rate is less than 1.5 deaths for every 100,000 hours of exposure. Although these risks compare favourably with other adventure sports [2], they are nevertheless excessive and associated with considerable personal and social cost. Careful investigation of accidents is required to identify causative factors so that corrective strategies can be identified and implemented.

As is the case for almost all human endeavour [3], human error rather than equipment malfunction, is responsible for most diving deaths [4–9]. Investigation of fatal diving accidents is often relatively unrewarding because of the multiple interactive factors that characterise such events.

Issues of culpability often predominate in analyses; these comments are also true for non-fatal accidents, although to a less extent. Many models have been proposed to explain accidental events in terms of system flexibility and responsivity. These models have applicability to diving, but the key outcome of the modern discipline of human factor analysis is the central role of incident monitoring [3]. Such incident monitoring has been put in place in diving [4–6] and has already been productive in terms of identifying latent and active errors, violations and some key ergonomic issues which are involved in diving accidents. Consequently, a system of diving accident prevention should be based on the following active hierarchy.

First, ongoing anonymous critical incident monitoring is needed [4–6]. This is the only vehicle by which some appreciation of diving exposure can be obtained, which is essential for meaningful accident statistics. It is also the only way in which the incidence of factors that could contribute to an accident can be determined relatively free of confounders and bias.

Second, systematic diving accident investigation is necessary. In fatalities, this requires careful autopsy (see also ► **Chapters 12.5 and 12.7**).

Third, there is a need for a forum of diving physicians, medical examiners (pathologists), diving instruction agencies, diving instruction companies and divers. Data derived from incident and accident analyses can be analysed and corrective strategies determined. Errors in technique would be addressed by educational programs and adoption of appropriate procedures.

Fourth, the efficacy of the corrective measures has to be monitored by ongoing incident and accident analyses.

Clearly, this sequence is a conventional risk management hierarchy of hazard identification, risk assessment, corrective measures, and finally, ongoing monitoring. The corrective measures exist in a sub-hierarchy of elimination, substitution, isolation, and protection. In this context, improving the safety of diving is no different from that of any occupation.

References

1. Edmonds C, Walker D (1989) Scuba diving fatalities in Australia and New Zealand. The human factor. SPUMS J 19:94–104
2. Anonymous (2001) ACC Injury Statistics, 2nd edn. www.acc.org.nz
3. Reason JT (1990) Human error. Cambridge University Press, New York
4. Acott CJ (1992) Scuba diving incident reporting, the first 125 reports. SPUMS J 22:218–221
5. Acott CJ (1994) Diving incident monitoring, an update. SPUMS J 24:42–49
6. Acott CJ (2001) 457 Equipment incident reports. SPUMS J 31:182–195
7. Divers Alert Network (2002) Report on decompression illness and diving fatalities. DAN, Durham, NC, USA
8. Edmonds CW (1986) The abalone diver. NSCA, Sale, Victoria, Australia
9. McAniff JJ (1988) United States underwater diving fatality statistics 1986–1987. Report number URI-SSR-89-20. University of Rhode Island, National Underwater Accident data Centre

11.12
The Investigation of SCUBA Diving Fatalities

JIM CARUSO

Diving using compressed air, or a similar breathing gas, and SCUBA (self-contained underwater breathing apparatus) equipment is a popular pastime throughout the world. Recreational diving fatalities include most types of diving for personal pleasure and without remuneration. This also includes diving for personal game collection (for example spear-fishing, abalone and lobster collecting). Fortunately, fatalities related to recreational diving are infrequent. In the United States there are an average of 90 recreational diving fatalities each year. These deaths, however, are often catastrophic events that involve young individuals (many lost years of productive life) and in the majority of cases they are totally preventable. They are also frequently litigated. It is extremely important to thoroughly investigate recreational diving fatalities and use the case reports as a lessons learned with the hope of reducing the number of diving-related deaths in the future. That is exactly the role played by the Divers Alert Network (DAN).

11.12.1
Military and Commercial Diving Fatalities

These were once dangerous environments with frequent accidents, many of them fatal. However, fatal accidents have become a very rare occurrence in both the military and commercial diving setting. The rare accidents that do occur are often due to equipment malfunctions or unsafe work practices. This is very different from what is seen in recreational diving deaths.

11.12.2
Basic Diving Physiology

In order to be able to interpret the circumstances surrounding a fatal diving incident, a basic understanding of diving physiology is required. The vast majority of diving-related injuries are due to effects of pressure, effects of inert gas, mechanical trauma, or insufficient breathing gas. Occasional injuries and fatalities are due to hazardous marine life and problems such as oxygen toxicity. Of course, natural disease plays a role in many diving fatalities, especially as the diving population ages and older adults take up diving.

Pressure

Boyle's Law describes the relationship between pressure and volume. As pressure decreases, volume increases and the converse is true. SCUBA equipment delivers compressed gas (usually air) to the diver at depth (increased pressure). So if the diver inhales and then ascends without exhaling, the result will be over-expansion of the lungs. Pulmonary over-expansion can lead to any or all of the following: mediastinal emphysema, subcutaneous emphysema, pneumothorax, arterial gas embolism. Usually less catastrophic but more common injuries due to the effects of pressure include barotrauma to the middle ear, inner ear, sinuses, and teeth.

Inert Gas

In diving terminology an inert gas is defined as basically any gas except oxygen. In diving it is often the nitrogen contained in air but divers can use mixtures containing helium and oxygen, enriched air with higher than 21% oxygen content, or pure oxygen. Nitrogen has an intoxicating effect at high partial pressures which most divers can feel when they descend below 100–130 feet (30–40 metres) breathing air. Divers going too deep will become progressively disoriented with increasing depth. Substituting helium for nitrogen can prevent nitrogen narcosis. Both nitrogen and helium progressively dissolve in tissues when breathed at hyperbaric partial pressures. This is also depth-dependent and a diver must limit the exposure at deeper depths as well as ascend slowly, often stopping at shallower depths in order to off-gas. If the tissues of the diver become supersaturated with inert gas the gas may bubble out of solution as he or she ascends, which can lead to venous bubbles causing decreased tissue perfusion. This can potentially lead to decompression sickness (caisson disease) with classic symptoms of joint pain, neurological deficits and various atypical presentations. The venous bubbles can arterialise in divers with a patent foramen ovale who shunt the bubbles to the left side. This is called a paradoxical embolism.

Mechanical Trauma

There are always a few deaths every year due to a diver being hit by a boat propeller or other forms of mechanical trauma. In many cases, the source of the injury is the boat that the diver is using as a platform. Sometimes the accident is due to reckless boaters who speed through the dive site without regard for the welfare of those who are in the water. In other instances, the diver failed to use a marker buoy or dive flag to warn boaters of his or her location.

Insufficient Breathing Gas

It may seem unconscionable for a diver to run out of air, but it unfortunately is an all too common occurrence. The result can include drowning or a rapid ascent, which can cause pulmonary barotrauma or air embolism. Entrapment or entanglement in a cave, wreck, or kelp can result in a diver running out of air and subsequently drowning.

Hazardous Marine Life

This is rarely a cause of mortality but more commonly causes morbidity. Envenomation, bites, stings, and simple wounds can result from contact with various sea creatures. Sharks rarely attack divers while on the bottom. More likely shark targets include free divers and surfers who spend considerable time on the surface or moving up and down in the water column.

Oxygen Toxicity

This is rarely a problem if the diver breathes air since the diver would have to go to extreme depths to reach the point where CNS oxygen toxicity would occur. High partial pressures of oxygen can cause seizures, which would be catastrophic at depth. Using breathing mixes that contain a high percentage of oxygen is increasing in popularity and several recent fatalities related to seizures at depth have occurred.

Disease

As you might expect, cardiovascular disease is the most common natural cause implicated in a fatal diving incident. Some divers have undiagnosed health problems while others dive with known health problems that may put them at increased risk for morbidity and mortality. Diving often takes place in remote areas or at least far from advanced emergency medical care. Suffering a seizure at depth or having myocardial ischaemia or infarction while diving off a remote island would have increased morbidity compared to the same events taking place on land in a large metropolitan area.

What Kills SCUBA Divers?

A thorough investigation usually reveals a critical error in judgement, the diver going beyond his or her level of training and experience, or a violation of generally accepted safe diving procedures. In other words, the cause is diver error.

Cardiovascular disease is the most common natural disease process associated with a recreational diving fatality.

Drowning is the most common cause of death with various events leading up to the drowning including running out of air at depth, entrapment, air embolism, cardiac dysrhythmia, and trauma. However, to simply sign a case out as a death due to drowning may not be accurate and certainly does very little to prevent future similar incidents. It also offers little closure for the family. It is absolutely essential to determine, to the extent possible, the events leading up to the drowning and any significant contributing factors.

Important observations on recreation diving fatalities from the DAN database include the following:

- Nearly half of all fatalities involved a diver who had made 20 or fewer lifetime dives.
- Buddy separation occurred in 40% of diving-related deaths and solo divers made up at least 14% of the fatalities.
- Barely a third of divers who died while engaged in more challenging types of diving (cave, wreck penetration, deep) documented training specific to that type of diving.

11.12.3
Autopsy Protocol for Recreational SCUBA Diving Fatalities

Since most pathologists and autopsy technicians rarely perform an autopsy on someone who died while SCUBA diving, few offices of medical examiners' offices will have significant experience in performing appropriate post-mortem examinations. The following is a guideline that can be followed with the understanding that some of the recommended procedures will be impractical and may only take place in a facility with significant laboratory resources available (see also ◘ Table 11.1). In all cases, expert consultation should be obtained if there are any questions regarding diving procedure, autopsy findings, or equipment.

A thorough investigation of the events surrounding the fatality, including witness accounts, the scene investigation, and a professional evaluation of the equipment is essential.

A complete autopsy with standard toxicology for drugs of abuse and therapeutic medications, as well as a carboxyhaemoglobin level should be performed in every diving related fatality. A short post-mortem interval is desirable to minimise artefacts.

11.12.4
History

The medical history is without doubt the most important part of the evaluation of a recreational diving fatality. Ideally, one should obtain significant past medical history with a focus especially on cardiovascular disease, seizure disorder, diabetes, asthma, and chronic obstructive pulmonary disease. Medications

□ Table 11.1. Basic investigation

Review past history, clinical history and resuscitation efforts

Scene investigation and circumstances of the death, evidence

External exam and evidence of injury, X-rays, pay special attention to head and neck

Autopsy to include thorough cardiovascular, respiratory, musculoskeletal and brain exam

Sinuses and middle ear exam may be useful

Toxicology

taken on a regular basis as well as on the day of the dive should be recorded and information regarding how the diver felt prior to the dive should be obtained. Any history of drug or alcohol use must also be noted.

Also, the dive history is extremely important. If possible, the investigator should find out the experience and certification level of the diver. The most important part of the history will be the specific events related to the dive itself. The dive profile (depth, bottom time) is an essential piece of information and if the diver was not diving alone (they are taught never to do so), eyewitness accounts will be invaluable. Questions to be asked include:

- When did the diver begin to have a problem (pre-dive, descent, bottom, ascent, post-dive)?
- Did the diver ascend rapidly, which may be a factor leading to air embolism and pulmonary barotrauma?
- Did the diver panic?
- Was there a history of entrapment, entanglement or trauma?
- If resuscitation was attempted, what was done and how did the diver respond?
- What were the weather and water conditions at the time of the mishap?

11.12.5
External Examination and Preparation

A thorough external examination including signs of trauma, animal bites or envenomation should be carried out. Palpate the area between the clavicles and the angles of the jaw for evidence of subcutaneous emphysema. X-rays of the head, neck, thorax and abdomen should be taken to look for free air.

Modify the initial incision over the chest to make a tent out of the soft tissue with a T-shaped incision and fill this area with water. A large bore needle can be inserted into the second intercostal spaces bilaterally. If desired, any escaping air can be captured in an inverted, water filled, graduated cylinder for measurement and analysis. This is a very difficult procedure and unlikely to be undertaken in most medical examiner offices. The oxygen content of the captured gas may give some clues to its origin. As the breastplate is removed, note any gas escaping from vessels.

Open the pericardial sac under water and note if pneumopericardium is present. Repeat the needle insertion manoeuvre, this time into the right and left ventricles with capture of any escaping gas if practical. After the mediastinum, heart, and great vessels have been examined under water for the presence of air, the water may be evacuated and a standard autopsy may be performed.

Carefully examine the lungs for bullae, emphysematous blebs and haemorrhage.

Note any inter-atrial or inter-ventricular septal defects, particularly note if there is a patent foramen ovale. Carefully check for evidence of cardiovascular disease and any changes that would compromise cardiac function.

Obtain blood, urine, vitreous, bile, liver, kidney and stomach contents for toxicological analysis. Not all specimens need to be run, but at least look for drugs of abuse. If an electrolyte abnormality is suspected or if the decedent is a diabetic, the analysis of the vitreous may prove useful.

Prior to opening the skull, tie off all of the vessels in the neck to prevent artefact air from entering the intracranial vessels. The skull may be opened prior to the examination of the chest. Tie the vessels at the base of the brain once the skull is opened. Disregard bubbles in the superficial veins or venous sinuses. Examine the meningeal vessels and the superficial cortical vessels for the presence of gas.

Carefully examine the circle of Willis and middle cerebral arteries for bubbles.

Have an expert evaluate the dive gear. Are the tanks empty? If not, the gas should be analysed for purity because little carbon monoxide goes a long way at depth. All gear should be in good working order with accurate functioning gauges.

11.12.6
Possible Findings

- Air embolism
Intra-arterial and intra-arteriolar air bubbles in the brain and meningeal vessels, petechial haemorrhages in grey and white matter, evidence of COPD or pulmonary barotrauma (pneumothorax, pneumomediastinum, subcutaneous emphysema), signs of acute right heart failure, pneumopericardium, air in coronary and retinal arteries.
- Decompression sickness
Lesions in the white matter in the middle third of the spinal cord including stasis infarction, if there is a patent foramen ovale (or other potential right to left heart shunt) a paradoxical air embolism can occur due to significant venous bubbles entering the arterial circulation.
- Venomous stings or bites

A bite or sting on any part of the body, unexplained oedema on any part of the body, evidence of anaphylaxis or other severe allergic reaction. A serum tryptase level may prove useful in these cases.

11.12.7
Interpretation

The presence of gas in any organ or vessel after a SCUBA diving death is not the conclusive evidence of decompression sickness or air embolism. During a long dive inert gas dissolves in the tissues and the gas will come out of solution when the body returns to atmospheric pressure. This, combined with post-mortem gas production, will produce bubbles in tissue and vessels. This has caused many experienced pathologists to erroneously conclude that a death occurred due to decompression sickness or air embolism.

Intravascular bubbles, especially if present predominantly in arteries, found during an autopsy performed soon after death occurred is highly suspicious for air embolism. The dive history will help support or refute this theory.

Gas present only in the left ventricle, or if analysis shows that the gas in the left ventricle has a higher oxygen content than that present on the right side, would lead the pathologist to correctly conclude that an air embolism probably has occurred.

Intravascular gas from decomposition or off-gassing from the dive would have little oxygen and be made up of mostly nitrogen and carbon dioxide.

Deeper longer dives can cause decompression sickness and significant intravascular, mostly venous, gas. Rapid ascents and pulmonary barotrauma are associated with air embolism.

11.12.8
Selected Diving Fatality Cases
Where the Investigation and Autopsy Made a Difference

Case 1. A 52-year-old male was in good health except for hypertension that was controlled with a single medication. After an uneventful dive, the man returned to the boat but collapsed on the deck within minutes of completing the dive. The autopsy showed a massive cerebrovascular accident. The history would make an air embolism a likely diagnosis and the autopsy was the key part of the investigation to distinguish between an accidental and a natural manner of death. The fact that he was diving prior to the CVA was pure coincidence.

Case 2. A 38-year-old male made a short dive to a fairly shallow depth and collapsed shortly after returning to the boat. The story is similar to case 1, except a key piece of evidence was the dive computer (very commonly used and very handy for the investigation). The computer showed a bottom time of 7 min and a maximum depth of 34 feet (11 metres). It also had an ascent rate display that was 'pegged' to the red 'dangerously rapid ascent' area. The autopsy showed intravascular bubbles in the cerebral arteries. The case was correctly interpreted as an air embolism.

Case 3. A very experienced technical diver was using multiple breathing gas mixes during a long and deep dive profile. After ascending from 160 feet (48 metres) to 120 feet (36 metres) the diver suffered a witnessed seizure and drowned. The autopsy disclosed abundant intravascular gas and the medical examiner incorrectly determined the cause of death to be an air embolism. Further investigation into the dive profile and an examination of the equipment revealed that the diver had mistakenly used a high oxygen containing decompression mix instead of the bottom and travel mixes he should have been breathing at 120 feet (36 metres). The correct interpretation of the circumstances is that the diver drowned due to a seizure (central nervous system oxygen toxicity) while breathing from the wrong regulator at depth.

Case 4. A 45-year-old man became separated from his dive buddy and was found unconscious on the bottom. The cause of death was presumed to be a cardiac event, but a complete autopsy with appropriate toxicology was performed. Coincidentally, another diver on the boat became ill during the dive and aborted the dive due to an equipment problem. The dead diver had an extremely high carboxyhaemoglobin level and a full investigation disclosed several contaminated tanks, all from the same dive shop.

Case 5. A 52-year-old man was a novice diver who had been having chest pains for a few days prior to his dive. He made the dive anyway and became separated from his dive buddy. The diver was found on the bottom unconscious and could not be resuscitated. The autopsy disclosed severe coronary atherosclerosis and a ruptured plaque in the left anterior descending coronary artery.

Case 6. A 19-year-old man was diving off a party boat in a large group but without a designated dive buddy. One of the boat crew remembers giving the diver a small bag prior to his departure from the surface. All of the other divers returned to the boat but the missing diver was not found despite an extensive search. Days later the body of the diver was recovered by fishermen. X-rays and a complete autopsy revealed the cause of death, which was a single gunshot wound to the head. This case represents a rare suicide while diving. Additional investigation revealed that the diver had recently dropped out of school, had a dispute with his parents, and purchased a handgun at a pawnshop.

11.12.9
Drowning

To many in the healthcare field, particularly in forensic medicine, the term drowning is applied to any individual who was known to enter the water alive and subsequently was found dead and still in the water. The reason for this is that some believe that drowning is a diagnosis of exclusion and certainly anyone who is immersed in a liquid is at risk for drowning. A thorough medicolegal investigation is required in each case of drowning. Nowhere is this truer than in recreational diving deaths. Some divers die of other conditions while in the water.

11.12.10
Key Points

Prior to arriving at the conclusion that one has drowned, other causes of death must be ruled out, such as trauma, natural disease processes, drug overdose or disposal of a homicide victim in water. Therefore, a complete autopsy including toxicology is always indicated.

A drowning death is death by asphyxiation with subsequent hypoxaemia and cerebral anoxia. The amount of water inhaled is variable and some believe that in 10%–15% of cases, laryngeal spasm can result in a drowning without aspiration.

Absorption of significant amounts of water, which can especially occur in cases of freshwater drowning, was once thought to cause serious electrolyte abnormalities and potential fatal dysrhythmias. This is no longer felt to be the case as the amount of water aspirated varies from case to case and is often small. Also, it is likely that a healthy heart and kidneys would compensate for the increase in volume and electrolyte abnormalities do not seem to play a large role.

The break point is defined as the time when a person can no longer voluntarily breath-hold. This occurs in response to blood levels of CO_2 and O_2. The person will breathe regardless of his or her immersion status and if submerged, continued inhalation of water will occur.

The type of water inhaled, fresh or saltwater, usually has little bearing on survival. Freshwater drowning results in larger amounts of fluid absorbed and damage to pulmonary surfactant. This may become clinically important if the victim survives. Saltwater drowning usually results in greater pulmonary oedema, pleural effusions, and haemoconcentration.

In the past, near drowning was defined as resuscitation of a submersion victim with subsequent survival for at least 24 hours regardless of whether or not death occurs after this period. Discussions before and at the World Congress on Drowning questioned whether this is an appropriate terminology and recommended it be abandoned (see ▶ Chapter 2.3).

No definitive diagnosis of drowning can be made based on autopsy findings alone. The circumstances, autopsy findings, and toxicology results are combined to arrive at the cause of death. Autopsy findings in drowning deaths may include oedema fluid in the airways, large and bulky lungs filled with froth, foam or fluid, water in the stomach, right ventricular dilatation, cerebral oedema, and haemorrhage in the petrous or mastoid bones.

External findings that may occur prior to or after death include washerwoman palms (wrinkled skin), gooseflesh, and bites from animals living in the water.

Because the drowning victim usually struggles, rigour mortis sets in earlier and rapid cooling slows the decomposition process. Immersion leaches blood from wounds so distinguishing between an ante-mortem or a post-mortem wound may be difficult. Animal bites may have occurred prior to or after death.

Various chemical tests, especially electrolyte studies, have been proposed to aid in the diagnosis of drowning or in determining freshwater versus saltwater drowning. None has proved consistently useful and most are of no value.

Diatom analysis has long been a favourite and controversial topic when discussing drowning deaths. Diatoms are ubiquitous, microscopic, unicellular algae with a silica skeleton in the shape of two valves. Because these organisms are found everywhere, their presence in the body could be due to inhalation, ingestion or aspiration. Laboratory glassware and water may contain diatoms. Various techniques for evaluation include ultrasonic or acid digestion of the tissue and often a part of the body less likely to be exposed to post-mortem diatoms, such as bone marrow and solid organs, is examined. One attempts to find diatoms in the deceased that are specific to the body of water from which the body was recovered. Of course there has been drowning in water where the victim regularly swam eliminating the usefulness of this technique.

Further Reading

Calder IM (1985) Autopsy and experimental observations on factors leading to barotrauma in man. Undersea Biomed Res 12:165–182

Caruso JL (1996) Recreational diving fatalities in the United States, 1990–1994: patterns and trends. Undersea Hyperb Med 23(Suppl):60–61

Caruso JL (1997) Fatalities related to cardiovascular disease in the recreational diving population. Undersea Hyperb Med 24(Suppl):26

Caruso JL (1998) Carbon monoxide poisoning in recreational diving: an uncommon but potentially fatal problem. Undersea Hyperb Med 25(Suppl):52

Caruso JL (1998) Inexperience kills: the relationship between lack of diving experience and fatal diving mishaps. Undersea Hyperb Med 25(Suppl):32

Caruso JL (1999) 1997 fatality case reports with autopsy findings, 1999 report on diving accidents and fatalities. Divers Alert Network, Durham, NC

Caruso JL (1999) Fatalities involving divers making technical dives. Undersea Hyperb Med 26(Suppl):28

Caruso JL (2000) Ten years of diving fatality epidemiology: the DAN database, 1989–1998. Undersea Hyperb Med 27(Suppl):32

Caruso JL, Mebane GY (1996) 1994 fatality case reports with autopsy findings, 1996 report on diving accidents and fatalities. Divers Alert Network, Durham, NC

Di Maio DJ, Di Maio VJ (2001) Forensic pathology, 2nd edn. CRC Press, Boca Raton

Kindwall EP, Pellegrini JP (1993) Autopsy protocol for victims of scuba diving accidents. 1991 report on diving accidents and fatalities. Divers Alert Network, Durham, NC

Levin DL (1993) Drowning and near-drowning. Pediatr Clin North Am 40:321–336

Matsumoto H, Fukui Y (1963) A simple method for diatom detection in drowning. Forensic Sci Int 60:91–95

Modell JH (1968) Blood gas and electrolyte changes in human near-drowning victims. JAMA 203:99–105

Modell JH (1999) Drowning without aspiration: is this an appropriate diagnosis? J Forensic Sci 44:1119–1123

Pachar JV, Cameron JM (1993) The diagnosis of drowning by quantitative and qualitative diatom analysis. Med Sci Law 33:291–299

U.S. Navy (1993) U.S. Navy Diving Manual, vol 1, Revision 3

Investigation of Drowning Accidents

Section editor: JEROME MODELL

Editor

- Jerome Modell

Authors

- Roger Bibbings
- Eke Boesten
- Ian Calder
- Peter Cornall
- Walt Hendrick
- James Howe
- Peter MacGregor
- Germ Martini
- Jerome Modell
- Rutger Schimmelpenninck
- Adee Schoon
- John Stoop
- Robert Williamson
- Andrea Zaferes

Editing Assistant to Jerome Modell

- Anita Yeager

12.1
Introduction and Overview

JEROME MODELL

This section contains several chapters dealing with state-of-the-art techniques for identification and retrieval of drowning victims, accident investigation and legal recourse when injury is sustained either by the victim or the rescuer. These issues initially had not been considered as a potential topic for the project and for this reason no task force was established and no recommendations were made during the World Congress on Drowning. However, in the final program a large body of knowledge and several discussions on the investigation of drownings and retrieval of drowning victims were included. Therefore, it was felt important to the coordinating editor to include a section in this *Handbook on Drowning*.

Inherent in the discussion of these items is that social expectations and culture play a large role in determining the importance and finances allocated to investigate these accidents and to recover the deceased. It is, perhaps, ironic that, in many locales, it appears that society is willing to invest larger sums of money to retrieve dead victims than it is to ensure the proper elements are in place prospectively to promote water safety and effective rescue.

My intent is not to belittle the importance placed on retrieval of drowning victims but, rather, to point out that while society seems to be willing to retrieve a dead body at any price, it is not always willing to provide adequate finances and personnel necessary to avoid such catastrophes. I would advocate that prevention of fatal and near-fatal aquatic accidents is far more cost effective than retrieval efforts after the fact.

Furthermore, emphasis should be on learning from each drowning episode as to what could have been done proactively to prevent it. To experience a drowning in an environment that is unsafe or takes unnecessary chances, is tragic. But, to permit such conditions to persist, thereby inviting further drownings, to me, is incomprehensible.

Several of the chapters in this section deal with the methodology of finding dead bodies. I certainly hope that this methodology will also be expanded to identify the hazards that may have contributed to the drowning episode in order that they can be modified or eliminated completely. Investigations of accidents in maritime events should not be focused merely to assign blame for the disaster at hand but, rather, to recommend improvements in safety so as to avoid such disasters in the future.

▶ Chapter 12.9 on legal claims in drowning cases is particularly fascinating to me because it almost assumes that in any drowning episode, someone should be compensated financially for injury or loss. This merely is a testimony to our litigious society whereby one person's unfortunate disaster results in another person's financial gain. I have a difficult time dealing with that concept and believe that one should attempt to rescue a drowning victim because it is the right thing to do, not because one may be sued if they do not act as a lifesaver, or they may sue the drowning victim himself/herself if they, as the voluntary rescuer, suffer any injury.

Obviously, a great deal still needs to be done in regard to investigation of aquatic accidents in order to determine their cause and to institute preventive measures to decrease their incidence. It is only through such investigations that we will continue to make the water a safer environment for recreation and business.

12.2
Behaviour of Dead Bodies in Water

JAAP MOLENAAR

Knowing the behaviour of dead bodies in water is very important for rescue services. This knowledge facilitates completion of the search operation. Effective procedures may result in a timely, successful rescue within a time frame that resuscitation can potentially still be useful. In other situations the recovery of a body can be done quickly and the operation can be limited in size and duration. A limited period also minimises the length of the emotional and uncertain period of the family and beloved ones of the missing person.

Worldwide there is very little adequate research data or knowledge available in this field that allow a systematic, fast and effective search procedure. Data usually reflect gathered incident information, which is often incomplete and has not been subjected to scientific analysis.

The behaviour of dead bodies in water depends largely on the type of water in which the incident has taken place. If we focus on the types of water, the following two categories emerge:

- Still water, such as canals and lakes
- Current water (or flowing water)
  - Slow current water
  - Medium current water
  - Fast current water
  - Seasonal current water, which can change in appearance. Medium speed current water becomes fast current due to water from melting ice in the spring or heavy rainfall, or into slow current in the summer due to a dry period.

12.2.1
Still Water

Frequently the location where the body has submerged is the location where it will be found afterwards. A possible influence on the behaviour is the system of refreshing or flushing of a canal or lake. If the body enters the water close to an entry point of fresh water, the movement of the water at the intake can influence the behaviour of the body by the turbulence in the water. Similar results can be found for exit points by the use of locks.

If sufficient vessels sail through still water and the body is in balance with the water, the power of propellers can move the body to another location. This only happens, however, when the bottom of the canal or lake is flat, hard, without obstacles and the water is relatively shallow. Another potential influence is the difference in the temperature of the water layers. It has been postulated that the body hovers through the water on these layers as the water increases in mass when it is colder. However, this concept remains to be proven.

12.2.2
Current Water

There is a diversity in current water caused by:

- The difference in height between two points
- The amount of water that is transported per unit of time

The velocity and intensity of the current is of great influence on the possible behaviour of dead bodies in water. Other aspects that can be important are the bottom contour and the bottom type. The bottom contour depends on the presence of obstacles on the water bed, such as large stones or rocks, steel cables and other objects. The bottom type is what the water bed is made up of, such as mud, sand or solid.

The most common cases reported in current water are:

- The dead body was found where the submersion occurred
- The dead body was found 300–500 meters downstream
- After several months the dead body was found at a long distance (as far as 160 kilometres) from the location of submersion
- The dead body was found across a river or between two breakwaters in a river.

Variation in the velocity of the current has an influence on behaviour. For example, a river that normally has a velocity between 0.5 and 1 metre per second can at some times have a velocity of 4 or 5 metres per second. Such a difference can have a substantial influence on the behaviour of a dead body in this water.

In 1999 the Council of Regional Chief Fire Officers in the Netherlands launched a research program to gain more knowledge about the behaviour of dead bodies in different types of water. The first step of this research program was to gather information. All fire brigades with a rescue diving team were asked to complete a questionnaire after the recovery of every dead body. In the past few years, questionnaires have been received but often the information was not complete. Often the location or time of submersion was unknown. Thus it is not possible to draw scientifically valid conclusions based on the information received. The research program will continue until at least 100 cases with complete and useable questionnaires are received. Those cases will then be analysed according to scientific methods. The hypothesis of the research program is that there is a relationship between the location of submersion, the velocity of the water and the expected location where the body is found. Based on this study, search attempts may become faster and more effective. However, the results could also show that there is no relation at all and every prediction is based purely on speculation. Material from other research programs from around the world will be used for reference and comparison in the analysis phase of the report.

12.3
Search and Recovery in Near-Shore Waters

JAMES HOWE

Search and recovery efforts for missing persons conducted in near-shore waters are those conducted in waters no more than 1 mile from a shoreline. Near-shore waters might also be accurately called the recreation zone because most ocean recreation activities are undertaken in this area. Nearly all recreational surf areas are found here.

The environment of near-shore water is very hydrodynamic. This is where streams, rivers, and storm water drainage channels run-off into the ocean. It is typical to find permanent, recurrent, and temporary water currents (rip currents, long shore currents) in these areas. The presence of currents generated by either wave action or run-off causes bottom scouring. Bottom scouring in turn affects the intensity, location, and direction of the water currents and negatively affects water clarity.

Near-shore waters are the home to a thriving eco-system. This well-developed eco-system includes a wide array of marine organisms. As in any fully developed eco-system, there are multiple levels of predation and many of the organisms have developed powerful defense mechanisms.

Shoreline topography and geology have both direct and indirect effects on the near-shore waters they abut. Ease of access to the shoreline is a major determining factor in the level of water use for recreational activity. Shoreline composition (sand, pebbles, boulders, coral) is a factor in the ocean skill level of persons accessing the waters. The more foot friendly the beach, the lower the ocean skill level of persons going into the water.

Near-shore waters are where the vast majority of ocean sport participants are found. Activities include swimming, snorkelling, diving (into the water), surf sports (body surfing, surfing, body boarding), wind sports (wind surfing, kite surfing, small sailboats), and small scale harvesting of shells, seaweed, fish, and other animate and inanimate objects. Near-shore waters are, in effect, a highly dynamic wilderness area where the vast majority of ocean recreation activity happens. The implications for search and recovery professionals are evident.

Successful search and recovery efforts in all wilderness environments have common elements. The first is a strong base of local knowledge of the area. This includes the terrain, common hazards, unusual hazards, weather impacts, animal life and behaviours, common entry and exit points, shelter areas, common activities and, recollection of past search efforts and the results. It is not always the rescue professional who will have the most extensive local knowledge of the search area. In most cases, local fishermen, surfers, divers, and community residents should be included in the pre-planning, execution and de-briefing phases of search and recovery efforts.

Initial information regarding a missing person, or persons, is often not complete or totally factual. It is important to qualify witnesses as to their level of local knowledge to determine the type and extent of search effort to undertake. It is common that visitors to near-shore water areas may confuse the behaviour of some marine life with that of a person in distress. There are also many other circumstances in which the initial report may need to be qualified prior to a search effort being undertaken, especially when children or young adults are reported missing. Information regarding the location, activity, experience level, and emotional and physical health of the missing person should continue even after a search is initiated to help define the search area.

A second common element required for all effective searches is a coordinated communications system. Near-shore searches present special challenges. In designing a communications plan for water searches the first priority is to establish a link from the water search site to shoreline assets. Sea-to-shore communications can be established by either visual signal or radio communication. The use of radio communications normally requires the use of a boat, personal watercraft, or aircraft. In-water communications are essential to ensure rescuer safety and to coordinate the search effort. In-water communications are best accomplished by use of the buddy system. In this system, teams of two or more searchers are designated and assigned search areas. Each team member is required to keep visual contact with all other team members at all times. Each team must check in with the surface search coordinator to report findings and receive new search assignments. This system allows for specialised search teams (surface swimmers, craft assisted snorkel divers, SCUBA equipped bottom searchers) to be used in a coordinated effort.

A third common element is command and control protocols for the search effort. A basic incident command model is recommended to effectively manage this aspect of the effort. This emergency management system, widely used in the US, designates roles and responsibilities for everyone involved in the search and recovery effort.

An often overlooked aspect of search and recovery efforts are the needs of family members or associates of the missing person. It is important to address their needs during the search effort. This could include access to information and personal communications; counselling or faith-based services; and basics such as food, shelter, clothing and transportation. Media inquiries and access to the search area must also be managed. The incident command model designates a role for media management and public information dissemination.

The specialised work of near-shore search and body recovery begins with training the rescuer. All rescuers who work in this highly dynamic environment need extensive hands-on training, on a continuing basis, to be effective. It is the basic ocean skills of swimming, surfing, and diving underwater that form the basis of competence for these men and women. Mechanical devices or technological solutions are not a substitute for these skills.

Specialised mechanical devices can, however, greatly enhance the abilities of near-shore rescuers. SCUBA apparatus allows rescuers to access deep-water areas with greater speed and efficiency, and for longer periods. Rescue craft give rescuers speed and area coverage advantages. They also provide rest and recovery platforms. Aircraft and helicopters provide excellent area coverage. They also allow searchers excellent water and bottom surveillance if water clarity is good.

Technology also provides professional rescuers with additional tools to assist in the search. Depth finders and fish finders can assist in locating specific bottom structures. Global positioning systems (GPS) help in determining and maintaining search grid areas. Infrared light may be of assistance in certain low-light situations. There are some indications that thermal imaging technology will prove to be beneficial in locating bodies underwater.

The search for missing persons in near shore waters continues to be a skill-intensive and dangerous activity. The most prudent investment professional rescue organisations can make is in the training of their personnel in basic ocean skills, physical fitness, and local knowledge of their near-shore areas. Risks to rescue personnel can be minimised and mission success maximised by using the aforementioned systems, equipment, and technologies.

12.3.1
Website

■ http://training.fema.gov/EMIWeb/IS/is195.asp

12.4
Search Techniques

12.4.1
Search Techniques for Dead Bodies:
Searching with Dogs

ADEE SCHOON

In general, police dogs are associated with well-trained attack dogs. These dogs are trained to obey their handlers under all circumstances and are faithful partners during patrol duty. However, there is also a less well-known type of police dog, the search and detection dogs. These dogs are trained to detect certain odours, and to respond to them in such a way that their handlers realise it has discovered an odour source. This is done through what is known in animal learning behaviour as instrumental learning: specific odours lead to a response, which in turn leads to a play reward. To the dog it is a game, to the police it is a useful detection tool.

Search and detection dogs have been in use by the police for almost a century, and have been used to detect many substances. Today, they are trained to detect narcotics, explosives, tobacco, accelerants, human scent, and dead bodies. There are two important aspects to their training. The first relates to the odours the dogs are trained on. This needs to be varied: the full range of products that the dog needs to respond to, as well as significant differences in concentration. The second aspect concerns the searching itself. The dog must learn to locate the odour source precisely and to search under all circumstances, ignoring distractions. Two different kinds of search and detection dogs can be used when searching for victims of drowning: human scent tracking dogs and dead body detection dogs. In the Netherlands, the National Police Agency coordinates the deployment of these dogs.

12.4.1.1
Training Search Dogs

The human scent tracking dog is trained to follow human scent on a trail, to find human scent on small and large objects that have been touched, and to find people themselves. They are taught to do so in- and outside of buildings, in urban and industrial areas, in rural areas, woods, heath, and in and on water. Dead body detection dogs are taught to detect human blood remains and corpse odour in different stages of decomposition. They are taught to search in the same areas as the human scent-tracking dog.

For the water training, some special techniques are used. The odour sources used to train the human scent tracking dogs are worn clothes and hair. Dead body detection dogs are trained on last-worn clothes from the deceased people. The dogs are taught to search from the waterside and from a boat. The handler and the dog start downwind, and work their way towards the source. From the banks, this is relatively straightforward. In a boat, the dog sits on an elevation in the bow, allowing it to hang over the side and smell the water surface. The handler watches his dog and directs the helmsman. The boat is steered in a zig-zag pattern, starting downwind and gradually moving upwind. To pinpoint the odour source more precisely, the dog is then worked in the reverse direction. The handler has to learn to 'read' his dog, especially when in the boat, where the dog catches a whiff but cannot move independently towards the odour source, the handler has to watch his dog closely and instruct the helmsman towards the source.

12.4.1.2
Deploying Search Dogs

Whether to use a human scent tracking dog or a dead body detection dog depends on the duration that a person has been missing. Depending on a number of factors, amongst others the temperature, it takes some time before the typical corpse odour is emitted. So, human scent tracking dogs need to be called in after a recent disappearance, and dead body detection dogs if a person has been missing a long time.

It is relatively easy to get the dogs to make a reliable response. It is much more difficult to then locate the body. The volatile molecules move away from an odour source in a plume: narrow at the source, and widening as the molecules float away in the air current. Independently moving dogs will zoom in on such an odour plume, detecting its boundaries and keeping within the plume moving towards higher concentrations until they reach the source. However, when such an odour source is located under water, the movement of the volatile molecules is influenced by both water and wind movements. If the direction of the current is in line with the wind direction, the dog can alert to the odour hundreds of meters away from the source depending on the strength of the wind and water currents. However, if the direction of the current is opposite to the wind direction, the dog will alert much closer to the source, or even upwind depending on the relative forces of water and wind movement. Add to this the circular water movements caused by cribs in rivers, undercurrents and other curious water and wind movements, and the complicated relationship between the place where the dogs alert and the position of the dead body becomes clear. On top of this, divers who have to go under water for the actual search have very poor vision in murky waters and often have difficulty in finding the body, even in stagnant water, sometimes even when at less than arm's-reach distance.

In spite of these difficulties search and detection dogs prove to be valuable in searching for dead people. In a case where the victim was in relatively stagnant water, the dead body dogs indicated a spot near a bridge after a one-hour search. The day before, several policemen had searched the area from a boat, and on the day the dogs were deployed 20 people and a helicopter were also searching. Following the indication from the dogs, four diving teams searched the area and located the body after 3.5 hours at the spot the dogs had indicated. In a second case in a canal, a person had gone missing one night. Human scent tracking dogs were called in the next day and indicated a spot after searching the area for 1 hour. The area was searched by divers for 5 hours and by using a tow net for an additional 8 hours without result. Almost a month later, dead body detection dogs searched the area and located a spot some 50 meters south of the initial area after a 3-hour search. Again, divers searched the area for 4 hours without result. Two weeks later, the dead body dogs were called in again. While coasting the canal north of the area indicated before, the handlers saw the dead body floating in the water. This was some 500–600 metres north of the earlier indication areas, and the body was still floating with the current further north quite rapidly. This was remarkable, because the general water movement in the canal is south, and the earlier searches had been conducted on these premises.

12.4.2
Search Techniques for Drowning Victims: Recovery Using Side Scan Sonars

ROBERT WILLIAMSON

Recent technology improvements in side scan sonar have provided the search and rescue community with a relativity new search tool for identifying the location of drowning victims and thereby facilitating their recovery. When deployed and used properly, the side scan sonar allows a systematic and thorough search of an area by creating real time sonar images of the water bottom and a drowning victim. Only when the victim has been located or a suspect target identified is it necessary to deploy divers. Side scan sonar is the tool for conducting the search while divers are used for the recovery. The information contained in this chapter is provided to assist teams, which have already been trained on their specific equipment.

12.4.2.1
Establishing a Search Area

The establishment of a drowning victim side scan sonar search area is based on information gained from talking to eyewitnesses or locals familiar with the body of water to be searched. Information regarding the water entry of the victim and area where last seen can establish a starting point for the search. If no entry point can be established but an empty boat was located, then the wind and water current effects on the boat would be critical in establishing a search area. Once this basic information is known the four corners of the search area should be marked on the navigation plotter of the system. Navigation waypoints should then be entered to delineate the track lines that will be used to conduct the search. These track lines should be established to allow for a minimum of 10% overlap of the swath lines, which will be created by the sonar scanning range selected. The search swath, if using both sides of the towfish, will be double the scanning range selected. For example, if a range of 40 meters is selected for the search then the swath coverage will be a total of 80 meters. By overlapping the swath lines by 10%, 100% bottom coverage is guaranteed.

When conducting sonar operations, information regarding water depth, bottom contour and type should be taken into account in establishing track lines. Track lines should be established to run parallel contours of equal depth to allow the towfish to be run at a consistent depth. If the track lines are perpendicular to contour lines then additional work will be required to constantly adjust the altitude of the towfish so it remains the correct distance off the bottom. If during the search the victim is not located and bottom conditions created extensive shadows that would hide a victim, then it will be necessary to establish track lines that run 90° to the original track lines. This provides visibility to areas that were hidden by shadows during the initial search.

12.4.2.2
Determining Scanning Ranges

Victim searches are best conducted on a 50-meter or less scanning range scale. The bottom conditions will in part dictate the maximum range on which a successful search can be conducted. If the bottom is flat and featureless, then a maximum scanning range of 50 meters can be used. The victim will appear small on the screen using this range but with the shadow cast by the body, it should still be recognisable. The 50-meter scanning range is normally the longest range that can be used to allow for recognition of a human body.

If the bottom is littered with rocks and debris then the scanning range should be reduced to a range that will allow the operator to distinguish between bottom objects and the victim. In some situations, especially with trees either still standing or lying on the bottom, locating and identifying a victim can be difficult. When searching in debris littered waters it may be necessary to mark suspect targets and then have a diver ground truth the target to either verify or discount that the target is the drowning victim.

There are trade-offs when selecting a scanning range. Longer scanning ranges (40–50 meters) allow for a shorter search period but a drowning victim will present as a smaller target on the screen and will possibly be missed. Searches using a smaller scanning range (10–20 meters) will present the victim as larger on the screen making it easier to identify but requires a longer search time. If the area to be searched is large and the bottom conditions will allow, it is advised to search on a scanning range of 40–50 meters and mark all suspect targets so that if the victim is not positively identified, then the marked suspect targets can be re-scanned at a shorter range.

12.4.2.3
Setting Towfish Scanning Altitudes

A proper towfish scanning altitude is based on the sonar scanning range select-ed for the search. A minimum altitude is necessary to allow the sound to reach out to the scanning range selected. A maximum altitude is one that will allow imaging of the bottom while at the same time providing clearance for the tow-fish from obstacles. Normally, the towfish is flown above the bottom 10%–20% of the scanning range. If the scanning range selected is 50 meters, then the tow-fish should be flown 5–10 meters off the bottom. When the bottom conditions are unknown, the initial search should be flown at 20% or 30% of the scanning range in an effort to avoid the towfish striking or snagging debris. Once the bottom conditions become known, the towfish should be flown at 10% of the scanning range for the best possible images. When scanning at higher towfish altitudes the range delay feature of the system can be employed to reduce the amount of water column displayed on the screen and increase the amount of bottom displayed. The higher the towfish is flown off the bottom, the smaller the shadow cast by the victim. Conversely, the closer to the bottom the towfish is flown the larger the shadow cast by the victim.

12.4.2.4
Drowning Victim Recovery

Once the image of a drowning victim is identified it should be marked on the plotter so that a recovery can be made. Several techniques can be used to re-duce a divers exposure to depths and challenging water conditions. With most side scan sonar systems the global positioning system (GPS) is used to provide the system with speed and location information. With some systems the image is geo-referenced allowing the operator to select the victim in the image and to know the latitude and longitude position. If proper system layback has been entered and if differential GPS positioning is available, the latitude and longi-tude location of the victim could be within a 3 to 5-meter radius of accuracy. In shallow water a weighted marker could be placed over the victims latitude and longitude position and a diver could conduct a circle search of the area using the marker as a reference point.

Another method that can be used for shallow water dives, but is more useful for deeper dives where diver bottom time is limited, is a marker target. Con-structing a 3'×3'×3' cage using copper tubing for the frame, covered with chick-en wire, and with no plastic covering on the wire, and lined with thin sheets of Styrofoam, makes an easily identifiable marker target. This target would be weighted and attached to a polypropylene line. The line would run to a buoy and sheave at the surface. The line would pass through the sheave and be terminated with a small weight. This will allow the buoy to be positioned directly over the target at all times. The target would be placed in the water based on the lati-tude and longitude position of the victim. Both the target and victim would be scanned and then the target would be moved closer to the victim. This scanning and moving would be conducted until the target was relatively close to the victim. A distance and heading from the target to the victim could be provided to the diver after marking both the target and victim on the plotter. Upon descent of the diver he would use this information to establish a limited search pattern to recover the victim. On one documented recovery the marker cage was positioned directly over the victim allowing the diver to make his descent, remove the cage and complete the recovery.

12.4.3
Infrared Detection Systems for Maritime Search and Rescue Units

GERM MARTINI

In the night of 27 July 1999 a fatal accident occurred when a small boat in the shallow waters of the Waddenzee, the Netherlands, could not be found in time in spite of extensive search and rescue (SAR) operations by lifeboats and helicopters. In their conclusions of the investigation of the tragedy, the Shipping Chamber of the Dutch Council for the Transportation Safety, recommended the introduction of thermal imagers as a resource for maritime and air-borne units engaged in SAR operations. This chapter overviews the operational aspects of infrared detection systems in SAR operations.

12.4.3.1
Infrared Detection Systems

An infrared detection system is a thermal imaging system integrated in an infrared video camera. The system measures the thermal energy of an object in relation to background energy of the environment. The camera generates a real-time video signal that allows an operator to view all movements of a thermal picture on the scene. Infrared cameras can provide continuous day and night visual surveillance.

All natural and manmade objects emit infrared energy. The ability to distinguish and to register on-line subtle temperature differences adds a whole new dimension to sight and reveals what was once thought to be invisible.

12.4.3.2
Practical Use of Infrared Detection Systems

The development of infrared cameras was initiated in response to the military demand for night vision systems based on infrared thermal imaging. Since then, thermal imagers have become accepted internationally as a vital piece of equipment for the army, firefighters and police. Thermal imaging devices decrease search and rescue times in buildings filled with smoke. Infrared detection systems have proven their effectiveness in the war on drugs and crime, in traffic investigations and surveillance.

Infrared detection systems are also employed to check clothes, boots and tents for heat loss in below zero temperatures. Other infrared detection systems

□ Table 12.1. Requirements for use of infrared detection systems for maritime SAR operations

- Simple and fully automatic to operate, leaving the crew free to concentrate on SAR activities

- Resistant to spray, water, short-term immersion in water, cold, heat, shocks and vibrations produced by lifeboats

- Short warm-up time to thermal image

- Long battery life and rechargeable battery packs

- A video signal for connection to a compatible monitor

- A full colour camera and monitor

- The choice between a black or a white background, if the monitor is displaying in black-and-white

- Unaffected by rapidly changing light levels or by the level of ambient light

- Camera with folding-screen

- If mounted, a camera with pan/tilt can achieve 360° continuous pan

- Anti-ice feature and wiper to avoid freezing at low outdoor temperatures

- Training

- Technical support and repair service

are used by companies engaged in process control, predictive maintenance and automotive, electrical and mechanical applications.

The past 4 years have seen an explosion in activity in companies manufacturing thermal imagers to the point where the choice is now both extensive and confusing.

12.4.3.3
Marine Applications of Infrared Detection Systems

There are marine applications using infrared detector systems for SAR operations to detect unlit buoys, small vessels, and other hazards to navigation. Often the systems are used to complement radar by viewing selected objects in real-time video. Infrared detection systems are used for marine law enforcement such as to detect if a vessel has been operated recently and if asylum seekers are thought to be in hiding.

Based on available information on infrared cameras, requirements for the use of infrared detection systems by the Royal Netherland Sea Rescue Institute for maritime SAR operations have been identified (□ **Table 12.1**).

◘ Fig. 12.1. Handheld camera

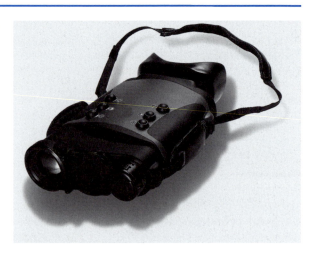

Current experiences on board KNRM lifeboats show a large detection range of humans between 50 and 1800 meters in an open and calm sea. A limitation with infrared detection systems, however, is that they are not always water or spray proof and not weather proof in adverse weather conditions. Also, the infrared detection systems do not detect persons drifting in open seas as easily as radar systems.

Based on the current set of experiences, the KNRM is considering a number of options for the future use of infrared detection systems:

- To equip all 30 larger lifeboats with a mounted infrared camera allowing the operator to view a thermal picture of the scene on a monitor in the wheelhouse
- To equip all 30 smaller lifeboats with a handheld infrared camera
- To equip all 20 KNRM trucks with a mounted or a handheld infrared camera

It has already been decided that it would be extremely expensive to provide infrared detection systems on board all KNRM lifeboats and trucks. Therefore, locating infrared handheld cameras at centrally chosen places in the Netherlands is being considered. When the need for an infrared system arises, the camera would be supplied on location to be used by a lifeboat or a helicopter. Another option is to provide only some lifeboat stations permanently with infrared handheld cameras.

To identify the best solution, two lifeboat stations will be equipped with a handheld infrared camera (◘ **Fig. 12.1**). This will allow the acquisition of first-hand experience, practice and the collection of data and information from the crew members for review later. One element of the evaluation will be to observe whether the essential basic skills of the crew members of lifeboats are not compromised by the use of modern technology. Also, the effect of the introduction of infrared systems on the use of 'bridge resource management' principles during both exercises and SAR operations (◘ **Fig. 12.2**) will be observed.

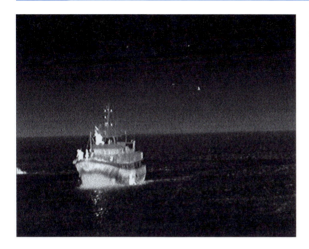

◘ Fig. 12.2. Infrared picture of a ship

12.5
Homicidal Drowning

Andrea Zaferes and Walt Hendrick

- An adolescent drowns in a lake where he frequently swam, and it is ruled accidental. Twenty years later his brother confesses that he and his friends watched a man drown the teenager.
- A woman is found drowned in a bathtub. The ruling is accidental drowning. When the husband of the woman drowns his second wife, the truth is discovered. Both were murders.
- An investigation for possible foul play ensues when a non-swimmer, college student is reported missing. When he is found submerged off a friend's dock, the investigation immediately ceases. Accidental drowning is ruled. Later foul play was detected.

The initial determinations of these actual drowning incidents as accidents are not uncommon. What is uncommon is the discovery of their red flags and the ensuing investigations. This chapter intends to contribute to a general awareness that many homicidal drowning cases are being missed.

12.5.1
Drowning Investigations

As many as 20% of child drowning incidents may be homicides. Notably, drowning in females may be a red flag for foul play in illogical child and adult drowning. A large percentage of these homicidal drowning incidents are either not sufficiently investigated or are not investigated at all. There are several reasons for this. "Tragic accident" is often a mindset that causes tunnel vision. The red flags normally found on homicide victims or at the scenes are rarely present, and law enforcement and medical personnel are not trained to recognise the red flags specific to homicidal drowning. The body may not have been recovered. Rescue personnel may inadvertently destroy evidence. Because drowning evidence is usually circumstantial rather than hard, cases are difficult to investigate and prosecute. Hence drowning cases may be pushed back when case loads are heavy. The drowning determination by process of exclusion can make it difficult to prove whether a victim drowned or was disposed of in the water. Witnesses are often grieving family members, which adds to the 'tragic accident' mindset. And very importantly, if a drowning is investigated, it is usually motivated by hindsight, after valuable scene evidence has been lost. Therefore a standard information gathering incident form to use on every drowning incident would be very helpful.

12.5.2
Land and Water Deaths Are Treated Differently

A hunter finds the body of a young man in the woods. A detective, crime scene technician, and coroner arrive to search for signs of foul play. The site is taped off and an officer is stationed to prevent scene contamination. The exact position and condition of the body is documented. Potential evidence is collected.

What if a fisherman discovers this body underwater, and similarly, neither the cause nor manner of death is obvious? Our experience shows that accidental drowning is the most likely mindset for arriving personnel. The dive team is called in to recover the body, which may or may not be bagged as it is dragged to shore. Is the exact condition and location of the body documented, along with wind, current, and depth? Are water samples taken? Are detectives and a medical examiner called in? Are the underwater and shore areas taped off and searched for possible evidence? Many departments have to answer "no" to most or all of these questions.

Compare a dispatch for a toddler found dead at the bottom of the basement steps in her home with a call for a toddler found drowned in a bathtub. The crying mother states that she went to answer the phone, was gone for less than 2 min, and, when she returned, found Sally not moving. How are these incidents managed? Are crime scene technicians called in? Is the house well photographed? Are scene temperatures taken? Are family members, neighbours, and babysitters interviewed? Is the family checked for any previous child or spouse deaths? The answers are likely to be "yes" for the basement incident and "no" for the drowning. Without obvious evidence to the contrary, the occurrence of drowning is typically treated as a tragic accident.

The tendency to see drowning incidents as accidents may cause red flags and evidence to be missed at every level from first responders to medical examiners. Compounding this is that drowning scenes present little or no typical signs of foul play. Victim trauma, signs of struggle at the scene, and signs of previous abuse, are not typically visible at pure-drowning homicide incidents where there has been no other violence or cause of death other than drowning.

Foul play is easily perceived when victims have a bullet in their head or bricks tied to their body, or when the available information is illogical. The vast majority of drowning homicides that do get reported in research papers and coroner reports involve additional forms of violence, such as strangulation, stabbing, or beating [1–8]. There is no evidence that the majority of drowning homicides include other forms of violence. Rather, it more likely demonstrates that police and medical personnel more frequently recognise such aggravated drowning homicide incidents, and miss, or fail to gain convictions on, pure drowning homicides.

Holding the head of a child underwater in a tub takes little effort. The little water splashed from the tub is easily wiped away. A non-swimmer pushed into deep water may not even have subcutaneous bruising. Pure drowning homicides can be medically undetectable, are effortless to perform, require no perpetrator skill, require little or no clean up, the body does not need to be disposed of, and the perpetrator often receives much sympathetic attention and possibly accidental death life insurance money.

- A father calls for help when his 4-year-old son drowns in a bathtub. Deputies find the father performing CPR. The investigators, who had initially accepted accidental drowning, later obtain a confession of premeditated murder.
- An infant death is ruled as SIDS by an experienced medical examiner. A later tip sparks an investigation. The boyfriend of the mother drowned the infant in a sink because it cried.
- While on a boat with her family, a young girl falls out and drowns. Accidental drowning is ruled. Two years later the mother admits that the father hit the girl out of the boat.

The investigative mind should be kept alert when responding to drowning incidents. Hospital physicians should consider notifying police in each drowned patient. Pathologists should routinely check the full torso for subcutaneous bruising and other signs of foul play on drowning victims. This is especially important when there are no witnesses, the witnesses knew the victim prior to death, or when the drowning incident seems illogical. If examination of the lungs of the victim does not show evidence of water aspiration, other causes of death must be considered [9]. Departments should consider homicidal drowning investigation training.

It could prove helpful to use a standard incident form on all drowning incidents to better collect and recognise potentially valuable evidence of foul play. This record would also provide research data.

12.5.3
Website

- www.rip-tide.org

References

1. Copeland A (1986) Homicidal drowning. Forensic Sci Int 31:247–252
2. Fanton L, Miras A, Tilhet-Coartet S, et al. (1998) The perfect crime: myth or reality? Am J Forensic Med Pathol 19:290–293
3. Lucas J, Goldfeder LB, Gill JR (2002) Bodies found in the waterways of New York City. J Forensic Sci 47:137–141
4. Missliwetz J, Stellwag-Carion C (1995) Six cases of premediated murder of adults by drowning. Arch Kriminol 195:75–84
5. Oishi F (1970) A typical case of homicide and head injuries. Tokyo ika daigaku Zasshi 28:541–548
6. Pollanen MS (1998) Diatoms and homicide. Forensic Sci Int 91:29–34
7. Trubner K, Puschel K (1991) Todesfalle in der Badewanne. Arch Kriminol 188:35–46
8. Heinemann A, Puschel K (1996) Discrepancies in homicide statistics by suffocation. Arch Kriminol 197:129–141
9. Modell JH, Bellefleur M, Davis JH (1999) Drowning without aspiration: is this an appropriate diagnosis? J Forensic Sci 44:1119–1123

12.6
The Approach of the Pathologist to the Diagnosis of Drowning

Ian Calder

Drowning is defined by the 1978 Oxford Dictionary as "to perish by suffocation under water (or other liquid)" [1]. This encompasses a wide spectrum of environments in which death can occur. In 2002, a group of international experts was convened at the World Congress on Drowning to update the definition of drowning. Their consensus was "Drowning is a process of experiencing primary respiratory impairment from submersion/immersion in a liquid medium. Implicit in this definition is that a liquid-air interface is present at the entrance of the airway of the victim, preventing the victim from breathing air. The victim may live or die after this process, but whatever the outcome, he or she has been involved in a drowning incident" [2]. Water obviously is the most common medium for drowning. Nevertheless, drowning can result in a wide variety of pathological appearances due to the physical, chemical and biological nature of the immersion fluid.

Survival following immersion in contaminated water may subsequently result in complications and death. The features of this may be bacterial pneumonia with lung abscesses, but also atypical pneumonia with features of viral infection with inclusion bodies. In the industrial scenario there may be immersion or submersion in fluids other than water, for example oil or solvents. The immediate physiological effect of aspiration of liquid is to reduce the oxygen exchange in the lungs. The confounding factors of the toxic effects of the chemical substances must also be considered in these circumstances.

The scientific and reasoned diagnosis is one of the most difficult problems with which a pathologist has to deal, especially if there is a period of delay in the recovery of the body. Thus the only certainty is that there is a history of immersion. It is important that all immersion deaths are approached objectively with the assimilation of facts and observations, thus facilitating a logical and defensible conclusion (personal communication, GA Gresham, 1971). There may be no true stigmata of drowning and a clinical-pathological diagnosis may have to be made based on circumstantial evidence.

The following differential diagnosis should be considered in approaching the investigation of bodies recovered from water:

- Death due to drowning
- Death due to injury or other factors before entering the water
- Death due to natural causes during immersion such as sudden fatal arrhythmia or cardiac arrest
- Death due to injury during immersion
- Death due to other factors, such as hypothermia, during the time of immersion

External evidence of immersion discussed below should be taken into consideration:

- Skin slippage may commence within a matter of minutes following immersion in warm water, but this may extend to many hours, or days in cold water. The early changes occur in areas where there is thickened keratin on hands, fingers and the soles of feet. The result is the development of wrinkling of the skin referred to as washer-woman skin. Such changes do not so readily affect skin protected by clothes.
- Immersion in cold water can result in the development of cutis anserina (goose flesh). The cause is contraction of the erector pilae, which are attached to the hair follicles. This causes dimpling of the skin. As there are other causes such as rigour mortis, the finding has to be regarded with some circumspection.
- The distribution of post-mortem hypostasis has little or no value in the diagnosis of drowning, as there may be much variation of posture during the period of immersion or submersion.
- External contamination may give some indication as to the environment in which the body was submerged. Examination of fluid in the lungs is considered later in the text.

12.6.1
Estimation of Time of Death

Estimation of time of death is an enigma of pathology and an aspect for which there is rather imprecise science. However, there are certain signs following immersion in temperate climates that may be helpful:

- Absence of wrinkling of the skin of hands: less than a few hours
- Wrinkling of the skin of hands and feet: 1–3 days
- Early putrefaction of exposed skin: 4–12 days
- Marbling of the skin with gaseous distortion of the face and abdomen: 14–28 days
- Liquefaction and early skeletonising: 2 months

These observations are extremely variable and may be modified by environmental factors such as water contamination, water flow, temperature and animal interference.

12.6.2
Death Before Entering Water

Death before immersion has to be considered in the differential diagnosis of all cases of bodies recovered from water. At one end of the spectrum is the use of immersion to dispose of a body as the result of a crime. At the other end are natural causes causing involuntary fall into water. The diagnosis of ante-mortem injuries, such as from road accidents with vehicles becoming immersed, is an important factor in such investigations. In cases where the victim was dead before becoming immersed, there will not be signs of water aspiration in the lungs.

12.6.3
Immersion Other Than Drowning

Sudden immersion in cold water of persons who are intoxicated with alcohol is recognised as a cause of sudden death, with the mechanism possibly related to vaso-vagal inhibition or other fatal cardiac arrhythmias.

12.6.4
Autopsy Technique

It is not possible to be prescriptive on autopsy techniques, as pathologists have developed or been taught a fundamental technique, which is flexible and modified for individual circumstances.

There are special findings, which have to be considered in immersion deaths in relation to diving. The ultimate diagnosis may be drowning, but the reason for such has to be carefully considered, as to why an individual well experienced in the aquatic environment dies. Factors such as equipment failure need to be considered, and the all-important effects of pressure physiology resulting in barotrauma. Simple palpation of tissues of the mediastinum or chest wall may give the characteristic crepitant feeling of surgical emphysema, reflecting the presence of gas in tissues.

Photographic or diagrammatic recording of external lesions is vital. Pneumothorax has to be included or excluded by appropriate technique. Diving is not necessarily a cause of pneumothorax as uncontrolled pressure changes of half a metre can provoke alveolar rupture [3, 4]. In 1921, Gettler suggested blood samples be taken from left and right ventricles for electrolyte measurement to aid the differential diagnosis of fresh and salt water immersion [5]. Subsequent studies demonstrated this to be unreliable [6].

12.6.5
Autopsy Observations

There may be no abnormal findings in bodies found in the water. This leads to an unexplained sudden death. This happens, for example, in circumstances of sudden immersion in cold water, and the cause has been proposed to be vaso-vagal inhibition, producing cardiac arrest. There are no pathological findings in these cases. Although in these cases death occurs in water, it is not appropriate to classify such victims as having drowned. If these victims were alive when they entered the water, their death is likely due to a primary cardiac event, not as the result of submersion precluding respiration. Thus, dry drowning is not an appropriate label because these victims die of a fatal cardiac arrhythmia, not of respiratory impairment secondary to immersion/submersion [2, 7].

It has to be recognised that there are no specific features or markers of drowning. However, the finding of froth in the air passages lends support to the inhalation of water. The froth is formed by the mixture of water and air with proteinaceous exudate and surfactant. It is usually white when submersion occurs in sea water; however, it may be pink or red-tinged due to rupture of red blood cells by the absorption of hypotonic liquid in the presence of hypoxia when fresh water is aspirated. This releases free haemoglobin into the plasma, which colours the pulmonary oedema fluid. The physical distribution of pulmonary oedema from drowning is somewhat different from that of cardiac failure as it may form a continuous column from trachea, bronchi, and bronchioli. The lungs in such circumstances show oedema, with characteristic fluid exuding from cut surfaces. External examination of the lungs frequently show hyperinflation with anterior fringes of the lungs overlapping. Petechial haemorrhages in the interlobular fissures of the lungs, face or eyelids are not a constant feature, but such findings must be taken into the appropriate clinical-pathological context.

The lungs of victims of immersion/submersion who have aspirated water may vary in weight from one victim to the next. However, as a rule, they are heavier than normal. In the experience of the author, lungs that weigh more than a kilogram usually do not reflect drowning, but some other cause of the oedema due to heart failure, especially in the case of post immersion shock due to hypothermia. Histology is non-specific, but the detail of the oedema is important to differentiate from inhaled or endogenous fluid. There may however be dilatation and rupture of alveoli. Amorphous and bi-refringent material due to inhalation of water may be present in the alveoli, and food particles secondary to aspiration of regurgitated stomach contents.

The appearances of the lung may be altered as a result of resuscitation. In view of the fact that dissection can confound the appearances, especially when it is necessary to identify the presence of gas, standard radiography is a useful diagnostic tool [8].

The following experiences are of proven value in the forensic laboratory experience of the author:

- A definitive diagnosis of immersion and submersion can be helped by the identification of diatoms. These are organisms with a silica shell, which is resistant to both decomposition and concentrated acids. The principle of the technique is digestion of lung and/or bone marrow, and then microscopic examination of the precipitate of the fluid. It is of paramount importance that a control sample is obtained from the environment in which the immersion incident occurred.

- Centrifuged lung oedema fluid can be subjected to toxicological analysis. In a series of six cases it was possible to identify contaminants of the immersion fluid in the lungs. This technique can be of value where there is a presence of significant amounts of chromium or ferrous salts, pesticides or industrial waste.
- Fatal immersion in swimming pools presents diagnostic problems to interpretation of fluid in the lung. A lung placed in a sealed non-permeable plastic container can be subjected to headspace analysis for the bactericidal agent, usually chlorine. Two cases have proved positive.

References

1. Anonymous (1978) The Oxford English Dictionary, 3rd edn, p 684
2. Idris AH, Berg R, Bierens J, et al. (2003) Recommended guidelines for uniform reporting of data from drowning: the "Utstein Style." Resuscitation 59:45–57
3. Kidd DJ (1973) Small pressure differentials causing barotraumas. Defence and Civil Institute of Environmental Medicine, 73-CP960:232
4. Calder IM (1985) Autopsy and experimental observations on factors leading to barotraumas in man. Undersea Biomed Res 12:165–182
5. Gettler AO (1921) A method for determination of death by drowning. JAMA 77:1650–1652
6. Modell JH, Davis JH (1969) Electrolyte changes in human drowning victims. Anesthesiology 30:414–420
7. Modell JH, Bellefleur M, Davis JH (1999) Drowning without aspiration: is this an appropriate diagnosis? J Forensic Sci 44:1119–1123
8. Calder IM (1987) Use of post-mortem radiographs for the investigation of underwater and hyperbaric deaths. Undersea Biomed Res 14:113–132

12.7
Accident Investigations in Drowning

Peter Cornall, Roger Bibbings and Peter MacGregor

Although most organisations have made progress with risk assessment, many are still failing to adopt a professional approach to the investigation of accidents and incidents. Consequently, they are failing to learn vital lessons to improve their overall management of health and safety and reduce the incidence of drowning. Water-based accidents can sometimes cause professional accident investigators to be unsure of their findings. This can be due to the powerful and frequently misunderstood environment in which the accident has occurred.

This chapter reviews important elements of proper investigations of drowning incidents and the lessons that can be learned from these investigations. It seeks to demystify the misgivings and to provide investigators with the confidence and a framework to follow, to successfully investigate water-based accidents. The chapter also discusses other essential aspects of investigation and concludes with a ten point prompt list designed to help organisations identify ways to improve their ability to learn from their safety failures.

12.7.1
Some General Points

Drownings are extremely costly in both human and financial terms but, if investigated correctly, can represent valuable learning opportunities to help future prevention methods and strategies. However, drowning accidents can occur at individual sites or within single organisations and are quite rare. It is, therefore, important that we learn collectively from the experience of others. Individual findings need to be pooled and systems need to be in place for rapid sharing of information. For this reason, all involved organisations should develop a strong capability to dig deep following accidents and to develop a clear understanding of their immediate and underlying causes.

Good investigations can provide unique opportunities for learning and change in organisations. Also, investigation can be a powerful educational experience for those directly involved, by improving understanding of health and safety management principles and embedding the resulting lessons in the memory of the organisation.

12.7.2
Essential Steps

The essential steps involved in investigation are described in ◘ **Table 12.2**.

12.7.3
Barriers to Learning from Failure

Accidents and incidents often arouse powerful emotions, particularly where they have resulted in death or serious injury. On the positive side, this means that the attention of everyone can be focused on improving prevention. On the negative side, however, the same emotions can also cause organisations and individuals to become defensive. This is natural and understandable but needs to be addressed positively. Only if a culture of openness and confidence is engendered, a mature approach to learning from these events can be supported.

All too often, in the wake of an accident, the tendency is to seek to attribute blame rather than to search for causes. Yet, the most important thing to establish about accidents is not just how they happened but why they were not prevented. Some of the major pitfalls in drowning and incident investigation are included in ◘ **Table 12.3**.

◼ **Table 12.2.** The essential ten steps involved in investigation of drowning incidents

1. Taking prompt emergency action: provide first aid, make things safe

2. Prompt reporting within the organisation and to other agencies where necessary

3. Securing the scene

4. Deciding on the level of investigation required and establishing terms of reference and allocating responsibilities in the investigation process

5. Gathering the evidence

6. Analysing and integrating the evidence

7. Identifying gaps in the evidence and seeking further evidence and clarification by studying previous events that may be relevant

8. Developing and testing hypotheses: what happened, how, why

9. Generating conclusions and recommendations

10. Communicating recommendations and tracking closure with stakeholders

12.7.4
Team-Based Investigation

Research carried out for the UK-based Royal Society for the Prevention of Accidents (RoSPA) has confirmed that a team approach to learning from accidents, involving employees and including safety representatives, can be extremely powerful. This is particularly true if it is led by senior managers and supported by health and safety professionals acting as facilitators.

Team-based investigation can provide access to local, expert knowledge, particularly about local conditions, tides, weather, water flow rates, and operational issues. Team-based investigations can also support the building of trust and the development of open and fair cultures, develop an understanding of risk management in practice among participants and promote learning about how to investigate in general. While performing team based investigations, workforce experts for drowning prevention are created, which are particularly useful for informal support for closure on recommendations. Finally, the team will provide a check and audit of safety management standards. Team-based investigation works best where organisations have clear and well-used near miss procedures. Although water incidents in many situations have only two outcomes, drowning or drying off, daily informal investigation of lower risk safety issues and problems is important in creating a positive climate for more structured investigation when major safety failures occur.

◘ Table 12.3. Pitfalls in drowning and incident investigation

- No reporting of accidents and near misses due to employee fear of consequences

- No investigation at all and under-reporting to enforcing authorities

- No clear procedures for investigation

- No workforce involvement even though trade union safety representatives have a legal right to investigate accidents

- No matching between investigation effort, safety significance and learning potential

- Failure to gather all the relevant facts

- No use of structured methods to integrate evidence

- Distortions in evidence gathering and analysis due to uncritical biases

- Concluding the investigation too early

- Simply focusing on the errors of individuals

- No search for root causes

- No examination of safety management system failures

- Failure to think outside conventional rules and operating systems

- Poor communication of lessons learned

- Failure to secure closure on resulting recommendations

12.7.5
Learning from Drowning Incidents: Ten Point Prompt List

The following prompt list has been developed by RoSPA to help competent persons in organisations carry out effective self-assessments of the current situation:

— Commitment to learning
Does everyone understand and accept that the organisation is fully committed to learn from its health and safety failures and that it is more interested in learning lessons that can help improve its performance than in merely allocating blame?

— Reporting
Does everyone involved feel obliged and empowered to report promptly and accurately all accidents, incidents and safety significant issues that come to their attention?

Are they actively encouraged to report errors and safety failures? Can they be confident that they will be valued for doing so? Do health and safety performance targets tend to act as a disincentive to reporting accidents and incidents?

- Scaling and terms of reference
  Are there adequate and suitable processes and criteria (for example, risk/consequence or learning potential) in place to enable the organisation to decide on the scale and depth of investigation and to draw up initial terms of reference? Does the organisation simply scale its investigation response according to the severity of injury or does it consider the safety significance of each accident or incident and its potential for improving safety in the future?
- Team-based approaches
  To what extent does the organisation adopt an open, team-based approach to investigation, with effective involvement of operative level employees, safety representatives, and supervisors, drawing on their practical knowledge and providing opportunities for them to learn more about safety and become champions for necessary safety change?
- Training, guidance and support
  Have all team members received necessary training and guidance to enable them to play their part effectively in the investigation process; such as training in interview techniques? Is practical guidance and technical support available to the team from qualified professionals?
- Information gathering
  How adequate are existing procedures in enabling investigators to gather necessary data following accidents and incidents – including among others: securing the scene, gathering essential physical and documentary evidence, taking photographs, interviewing witnesses?
- Use of structured methods
  Does the organisation make use of structured methods to identify the circumstances of which the accident or incident is the outcome? Does it use such methods to integrate evidence, generate and test hypotheses and reach conclusions so it can make recommendations?
- Immediate and underlying causes
  Do investigations seek to identify and discriminate between immediate and underlying causes? Is there a clear link between the outcome of investigations and revision of risk assessments, for example to establish if and why risk assessments for the activities concerned were inadequate, had not been properly implemented or had been allowed to degrade.
- Communication and closure
  Are there effective means in place to communicate conclusions back to stakeholders and to track closure? Is the implementation of recommendations managed to an agreed timetable with reporting back to the investigation team?
- Reviewing investigation capability
  Does the organisation undertake a periodic review of the adequacy of its approach to investigation with a view to improving its capability to learn lessons from incidents and to embed these lessons in the corporate memory?

12.8
Legal Aspects and Litigation in Aquatic Lifesaving

JEROME MODELL

The material in this chapter is from insight gained from reviewing over 200 legal cases in the United States. Whenever someone experiences a drowning episode at a public or private facility at which the public believes lifesavers should be present and have an obligation to ensure safety, the potential for a lawsuit exists. In the US, lifesavers and the owners of facilities frequently have lawsuits brought against them when a patron drowns, or survives after a drowning episode but with permanent disability. Much of the problem results from unrealistic expectations on the part of the plaintiff. In other cases, the facility and lifesavers, clearly, are not providing the optimum environment to ensure safety.

The expectations of the plaintiffs are that no one should drown while at a pool or beach staffed by lifesavers. It is also believed that their loved ones could not possibly have died from anything but drowning, even when the victims either have a medical disease or exhibited behaviour that contributes to the fatal event. Plaintiffs believe that the lifesaver should be able to stop any inappropriate behaviour on the part of the patrons of the facility without injury to anyone. This is despite the fact that the victim or the acquaintances or friends of the victim may engage in dangerous activities. The plaintiff also expects that lifesavers should be skilled in prompt rescue and resuscitation and should not be distracted from their primary function. This is important because some lifesavers have never been taught prompt rescue techniques nor the basics of basic life support (BLS). Other lifesavers are required to attend to other responsibilities such as selling tickets, beach chairs and towels or cleaning locker rooms and toilets while they are on lifeguard duty.

The plaintiff also expects that lifesavers should always be in attendance and attentive to those in the water, and they should be properly trained and certified in basic (BLS) and advanced cardiac life support (ALS). However, while BLS training should be routine for lifesavers, ALS expectations are not realistic except in large facilities that have multiple lifesavers in attendance who make this their profession. The plaintiff also expects that extensive emergency rescue and resuscitation equipment should always be available and working. Here again, the facility might be of such size that, economically, this is not feasible. But if the equipment is available, it should be tested periodically to ensure that it is in working order. The plaintiff also expects that lifesavers should always be able to rescue and resuscitate victims if they are performing their duties properly. This may not always be a reasonable expectation.

There are many conditions that compromise the ability of a defence attorney to defend the lifesavers. If less than optimum conditions are present at the pool, such as murky water that precludes unrestricted visual access of the entire pool this is an obvious problem. If standard equipment is absent or if it is present but malfunctioning, has not been tested frequently or if the lifesavers have never been trained in its use, this will not play well to a lay jury.

In other situations, there is delayed recognition that the victim is in trouble. For example, some lifesavers may tell other patrons that the submerged individual is 'just playing or horsing around' or that this particular individual always holds his breath underwater. That is not an excuse for proper retrieval of the victim. Poor maintenance at the pool, such as covers off of suction drains, have been the source of persons literally being held by suction at the bottom of the pool and causing their drowning. Distraction of lifesavers by other patrons, their friends, spouses or others should never be permitted. Not infrequently, lifesavers will go on break without proper relief or another properly trained person being present to assume their duties. The patrons are then at risk for getting into difficulty and drowning during that period of time. The same is true if there are too few lifesavers for the number of bathers. If the lifesaver does not know proper rescue and resuscitation procedures, that is totally unacceptable. Furthermore, there are liability cases where the lifesavers were not physically able to enter the water and perform their duties. Some lifesavers are reluctant to enter the water, so they send other bathers to do their job. Poor construction of the pool, which prevents prompt access by emergency medical service (EMS) teams, can be problematic, and an EMS team that is not properly trained to recognise cardiopulmonary collapse or to perform endotracheal intubation, makes it difficult to defend such cases.

There are a number of things that lifesavers should do in order to decrease the risk of their successfully being sued. Lifesavers should become certified in rescue techniques and become certified in BLS. In some cases, at larger beaches where full-time professionals are present, being certified in ALS is certainly desirable. They should never be distracted by pool or beach patrons and should always be attentive to monitoring potential victims. They should never be engrossed in other activities such as selling tickets, towels or beach chairs while they are on duty at the water site. They should position themselves so they can easily visualise every part of the water to depth for which they are responsible. There is no substitute for continuously scanning the water. They should enter the water immediately for any suspicious situation or for any submerged victim who is not actively moving at the time. They should never assume that the victim was 'playing or horsing around'. Also, they should never send a patron into the water to rescue a victim, that is their job. Lifesavers should ensure that all appropriate rescue and resuscitation equipment is present and functioning. Routine drills should be held at frequent intervals to ensure that not only the equipment is functioning, but that the lifesaver personnel are capable of using such equipment for the intended use. They should be sure that water conditions are kept optimal, particularly, as it applies to the quality of the water and the ability to visualise the entire pool to depth. They should disallow dangerous behaviour on the part of the patrons and immediately eject persons whose behaviour puts them or others at risk. They should have an action plan for rescue and resuscitation and practice this at frequent intervals.

It is important to point out that, not infrequently, it is the facility or the owner of the facility that is the primary target of lawsuits in the event that someone has drowned or has been rescued from drowning, only to have residual complications. Many courts will view the lifesaver as an agent of the owner of the facility.

The attorneys for many plaintiffs will look to the facility itself as a 'deep pocket' because lifesavers, as a rule, are not financially affluent nor do they have large insurance policies to protect themselves.

In any case, lifesavers are at the water site to protect the patrons as much as possible and to rescue and resuscitate them when an adverse event occurs. Neither their behaviour nor the acts of the facility owner should compromise their ability to perform their job. If lifesavers are cognisant of the reasons they get into trouble legally and fulfil their responsibilities in optimum fashion, they should have little fear of a litigant being successful against them. On the other hand, compromise in safety, regulations and techniques only invites catastrophic verdicts in lawsuits.

12.9
Legal Claims in Drowning Cases

RUTGER SCHIMMELPENNINCK

■ A stewardess on her way to work in uniform sees a tractor overturn while cutting grass along a canal in a residential area. The driver is caught under the tractor half under the water. While shouting "help" he slowly submerges. Passers-by do nothing, but the stewardess takes off her shoes, walks into the water and with all her strength, lifts part of the tractor and frees the driver. She feels a sharp pain in her back and goes to the doctor who tells her that she has lifted too much and will be unable to work for the rest of her life. Can she recover damages from the driver of the tractor even if it is alleged that she should have waited for passers-by or the fire brigade to help?

This chapter considers the legal claims which can arise from rescue operations in the event of drowning in unsupervised situations. The case described above is just one of the many examples of a drowning in the abundant waterways of the Netherlands that raise the question of who is responsible for the damages. In this example, the rescuer, the stewardess, sustained damages. In addition, the rescued person could also have sustained damages as a result of a badly performed rescue. Rescuers fear that they will suffer physical or other material damages from which they cannot recoup, or that they will be held liable for a poorly performed rescue attempt. This could keep potential rescuers from helping people in need.

Drownings can be divided into supervised and unsupervised situations. In a supervised situation, an agreement frequently exists or at least an owner or manager of the property can be sued for failing to perform his/her duty by preventing the drowning or for failing to make a timely rescue attempt. The owner of a swimming pool or the swimming teacher can be sued. Jerome H. Modell writes in the previous chapter of this handbook on the legal aspects of drowning accidents in private or public supervised situations.

In the abundant waterways of the Netherlands, many drownings occur annually. Hundreds of accidents occur every year to people swimming or sailing in open water, or who end up in the water as a result of car accidents. The current legal situation in the Netherlands is described below.

12.9.1
When the Rescuer Sustains Damages

Can a rescuer claim damages sustained by him from the person rescued? This question depends to some extent on the professional or non-professional capacity of the rescuer. When a professional rescuer sustains damages as a result of his activities, he will probably be able to hold his/her employer liable, who is frequently insured for these sorts of claims. This makes holding the rescued person liable a less obvious course of action. More interesting is the question of whether an amateur rescuer, such as the stewardess in the above example, who sustained damages as a result of the performance of the rescue, can hold the victim liable. Amateurs who act altruistically in emergencies and sometimes risk their own lives should not have to sustain damages. However, the question arises as to where they can claim compensation for damages and on what grounds.

Consider the scenario in which the hazardous situation resulted from dangerous behaviour of the person who was drowning: a suicide attempt, sailing, swimming, water skiing, skating or diving in dangerous circumstances, or when intoxicated. The dangerous situation could have been caused by someone pushing the victim into the water. In such cases, it is possible for the rescued person or the third party to be held liable for compensation for the damages arising from his/her unlawful behaviour.

Whom can the rescuer hold liable if no parties cause a dangerous situation? The rescuer has a legal duty to do so under the Netherlands Penal Code. Those who do not rescue when they could do so can be held liable. Should rescuers have no right to compensation if no one can be held responsible?

The theory of caretaking offers a solution. Caretaking means that someone looks after the interests of another without being obliged to do so on the grounds of any agreement. In this way, a non-professional rescuer (in this example the stewardess) can be considered a caretaker. A caretaker has a right to compensation for all reasonable expenses incurred. Therefore, in principle, the stewardess can recoup the damages she sustained from the tractor driver. Neither any culpability on the part of the drowning victim nor the success of the rescue are important to the right to compensation for damages sustained. This only differs if the caretaking was performed improperly. Considering the fact that non-professional rescuers have no experience in rescuing drowning victims and that an emergency situation is stressful, the courts rarely consider caretaking to have been performed improperly.

12.9.2
When the Rescued Person Sustains Damages

The rescued person can suffer significant physical damages if the rescue is not carried out properly. If the rescuer fails to act in a timely manner, the rescuer violates his legal duty to provide help and can be held liable on the grounds of an unlawful act. If the rescuer does act as reasonably expected of him but later it appears that he/she could have acted better, the question as to the liability of the rescuer depends on the professionalism of the rescuer. Rescuers can usually be divided into three categories:

- Professional rescuers such as firemen
- Trained rescuers with a first aid certificate
- Amateurs without rescue experience

Higher demands are made of the rescuer according to his/her degree of professionalism.

It would be a violation of the principle of reasonableness and fairness if amateurs who act in emergency situations and sometimes risk their own lives were held liable for damages sustained by the victim as a result of an unsuccessful or incorrectly performed rescue operation. Liability for an unsuccessful or incorrectly performed rescue operation by amateurs or professionals cannot be based on an agreement, since none exists, but only on the grounds of an unlawful action. The obligation vested in the rescuer to perform to the best of one's ability cannot guarantee a certain result. Only when it is shown that obvious errors were made during the performance of a rescue operation could a claim be awarded against professional rescuers.

12.9.3
Conclusion

Non-professional rescuers should not have to fear that they will be unable to claim compensation for damages sustained by them, nor should they have to fear that they can be held liable for damages sustained by the rescued person if they perform in a prudent manner. Claims against professional rescuers on the grounds of unsuccessful or incorrectly performed rescue operations have more chance of success. As a rule, professional rescuers or their employers are insured for this eventuality.

12.10
The M/S Estonia Disaster
and the Treatment of Human Remains

Eke Boesten

On 27 September 1994, the M/S Estonia, a Roll-on Roll-off (Ro-Ro) ferry vessel flying the Estonian flag, departed from Tallinn at about 7:17 p.m. for a scheduled voyage to Stockholm. She was carrying 989 people, of which 803 were passengers and 186 crew members. The ferry was also carrying 40 trucks and trailers, 25 passenger cars, 9 vans and 2 buses. The conditions were stormy, with a strong south-westerly wind. Waves 6–8 meters high were striking the bow of the ship.

As the ferry ploughed through the waves, continual loud noises were heard. Investigation by those in charge showed nothing. However, shortly after 1:00 a.m., the ferry began to react to what may have been the accumulation of water inside. In a sudden movement, the ferry listed approximately 30° to one side. After initially righting herself, the ferry took a final and fatal lunge to the side and started to fill with water. The few passengers who could get out of their cabins, fought to make their way up the stairs, which were tilted sideways. They tried to escape through the doors, but it seems that the doors could not be opened. The alarm was given to the crew at 1:20 a.m.; but it was too late to be of much help. The Estonia put out a distress call, which was picked up by the M/S Silja Europa and the Turku Sea Rescue Centre in Finland and by several others. The radio of the Estonia went silent just after 1:30 a.m.. The vessel sank in less than 30 min from the time anyone had sensed that there was a problem.

Approximately 200 persons on board managed to get out of the ferry. An organised evacuation with the launching of lifeboats and life rafts was not possible because of the extreme conditions. The first vessels to approach the scene of the accident had to decide, independently, how they could best help rescue people. The heavy weather, however, prevented the lowering of lifeboats and rescue boats. Most vessels, therefore, lowered rope ladders down the sides into the sea.

The vast majority of persons on board the Estonia did not survive the disaster. "We found mayhem on the ship", said Johan Fransson, head of Sweden's Maritime Administration. He had supervised dives to the wrecks in 1994. "A lot of bodies were found in the stairwells. This was chaos". [1]. In fact, 852 people died. One of the aftermaths of this tragedy is that a substantial number of bodies remained in the sea after the rescue operations were terminated.

This disaster of massive proportions had considerable legal consequences. Legal proceedings were commenced in all the countries involved, and in others too. The country most involved was Sweden as 500 Swedish nationals died in the disaster. The final resting place of the Estonia is close to Swedish waters, although on the Finnish part of the continental shelf. The ferry itself, although Estonian, was operated in conjunction with Swedish interests. The press repeatedly referred to the Swedish co-operator as the party responsible for the wreck. The Swedish government took immediate control of the inquiries after the accident and made a remarkable proposal about what to do with the wreck and the bodies that were entombed within it.

Soon after the disaster, both the Swedish Prime Minister and the opposition leader stated that the wreck must be salvaged and the bodies retrieved at any price. After an investigation by the Swedish Maritime Administration, however, it was found that salvaging the wreck, at a depth of 75–80 meters, was not practicable and the cost of such an operation would be enormous. The Swedish government then appointed an ethics council to look into the matter. It recommended that the vessel not be salvaged and that the bodies be left entombed in the ship. The Swedish, Finnish and Estonian governments thereupon decided that a special agreement would be enacted to protect the wreck and the surrounding area as a graveyard. This resulted in the Estonia Agreement (*"The Agreement, done at Tallinn on 23rd February 1995 and at Stockholm on 23rd April 1996, between the Republic of Estonia, the Republic of Finland and the Kingdom of Sweden regarding the M/S Estonia with Additional Protocol"*). The Agreement expressed the intention of the contracting parties "to undertake or institute legislation aiming at the criminalisation of any activities disturbing the peace of the final place of rest, in particular any diving or other activities with the purpose of recovering victims or property from the seabed".

However, the M/S Estonia had sunk in international waters. Thus, measures taken pursuant to the Agreement would only be applicable to persons subject to Swedish, Finnish or Estonian law. The Swedish survivors themselves hired divers of other nationalities to dive on the wreck to recover bodies. In addition, the concern was expressed that divers without any connection to the tragedy might dive at the wreck and steal property from it. To solve the problem of the limited application of the Agreement, Sweden decided, with the approval of the other two countries and in conjunction with the wreck owners, that 25 million US dollars would be spent on constructing a concrete shield that would cover the entire wreck. This would make the Estonia accessible only with great difficulty. However, this decision was made without consulting any of the survivors or the organisations representing them.

The organisations of survivors protested and commenced legal proceedings. It is not within the scope of this manuscript to describe the legal aspects in detail, but it is worth noting that one of the arguments made was that a state has a duty to retrieve as many corpses as possible after a decision is made that salvage of a wreck is unrealistic. This argument, however, has no foundation in international law.

The events that followed this tragedy raise the issue of whether diving on a wreck that is considered to be a grave site is permitted in international law. Because there have been deaths in almost every shipping disaster of any magnitude, every shipwreck site could be considered a grave site. International legal documents do not often mention this issue. National laws on shipwrecks all too often lack any provision on this subject as do bilateral or regional agreements between states.

In February 2001 a panel of experts convened in New Orleans, USA, to discuss the legal aspects of human remains and grave sites under water, specifically the legal issues surrounding the protection of human remains at shipwrecks, the absence of clear legal documentation and the discussions on the Estonia, Titanic and war wrecks (Panel at Underwater Intervention 2002, New Orleans, Chairman: Gregg Bemis, gbemis@swcp.com). First, the panel identified the various interest groups involved: survivors, relatives of the deceased, owners, explorers, researchers, developers, divers, the general public, governments, flag states and coastal states. Second, it was noted that although there is a variety of national laws dealing with these issues, these laws only apply to wrecks within a particular jurisdiction. Although these laws generally require that the sites be treated with respect and that unnecessary disturbance of human remains should be avoided, they do not provide any guidance on specific activities such as forensic research or recovery. Third, the group looked at the international rules that currently exist. The *UNESCO Convention for the Protection of the Underwater Cultural Heritage* addresses this issue, but only partly. The convention is applicable to underwater cultural heritage that is more than 100 years old (adopted on 2 November 2001 by the plenary session of the 31st General Conference. For the full text, see www.unesco.org). The broad definition of underwater cultural heritage of the convention does include human remains. Article 2 specifies that parties to the convention are to ensure that proper respect is given to all human remains located in maritime waters. An annex to the convention provides rules concerning activities directed at underwater cultural heritage. Rule 5 also provides that "Activities directed at underwater cultural heritage shall avoid the unnecessary disturbance of human remains or venerated sites".

The panel concluded that, although some guidance can be found in international and national legal documents, there is little law directly pertaining to undersea human remains, even though the issue generates attention from political, archaeological, historical, forensic, scientific and cultural perspectives. The outrage of the public and media after the Swedish government decided not to recover the bodies on the Estonia demonstrates the strong public interest as well. The public nature of this issue is further supported by discussions about diving at the wreck of the Titanic and by cultural differences concerning the treatment of human remains. In some countries a seaman's grave is a valid burial place; in other cultures the dead should be buried in the ground. People everywhere are generally guided, both in law and practice, by the ideals of paying the proper respect and respectful treatment.

Where has the controversy over the Estonia led? The process of protecting the human remains on the Estonia has resulted in an agreement that forbids the nationals of the signing states from diving on the wreck. This eliminates the option of a new investigation into the cause of the disaster. Additionally, the construction of a concrete shield over the wreck was stopped after the first few loads of sand were deposited in response to the relatives of the victims making their strong objections known.

It may be asked whether proper respect and respectful treatment guided the decisions that were taken regarding the treatment of these human remains. Survivors and relatives of the victims were never consulted and remain dissatisfied with the way this disaster has been dealt with. Will the aftermath of the Estonia disaster serve as an example of how these matters should not be conducted? One can hope that further discussions will contribute to an awareness that the issue of human remains in the sea is in need of thoughtful attention.

12.10.6
Website

▬ www.unesco.org

Reference

1. Wilson D (2003) Suspicions surround sunken ferry. Washington Times, 12 January

12.11
Maritime Accident Investigations

JOHN STOOP

Investigations of accidents in the maritime sector may serve as performance indicators for policy making, data for scientific research, information for courts to allocate blame, liability, to take disciplinary actions against the officers of sea-going vessels, and to incite the prevention of reoccurrence of similar accidents. Consequently, accident investigations are focused at various levels of the maritime system and different causal factors. The degree of sophistication and analytical tools may vary with the nature of the incident. Three major categories of investigations are minor accidents, major accidents, and disasters. This chapter focuses on accident investigation conducted by transportation safety boards, advocating their potential for a wider and more generic application. It elaborates on their present and possible new missions, working processes, and primary investigative questions.

In analysing major accidents in aviation, shipping or railways, the instrument of single-event, in-depth investigation is frequently applied. Such accident analysis focuses on technical investigations, human factors and operational practices. Their purpose is mainly to learn, irrespective of blame, and to prevent similar accidents in their sector. Finally, inquiries do not specifically focus on an industrial sector, but emphasise governance, responsibilities and systematic changes, which are required to restore public faith in society. Although infrequently applied, they have had major impacts on safety. National authorities have responsibility to investigate major accidents. Accidents that include fatalities and hull losses are referred to as naval disasters and are subjected to the responsibility of accident investigation committees or maritime courts. If disruption of public faith is involved in accidents with high numbers of casualties and media attention, a parliamentary inquiry may be conducted.

12.11.1
Accident Investigation: A Concept

The principal goal of a transport safety board is to provide knowledge that can be used to prevent accidents or to mitigate the resulting harm. To achieve that goal, the mission of a safety board covers four principal purposes:
- Determine preventable or mitigable causes of major accidents, disasters and catastrophes
- Identify precursors to potential major events
- Increase safety by making and implementing recommendations
- Assure public confidence in safety on a national or sectorial basis

The first purpose of a safety investigation board is to uncover evidence that can be used to prevent the next accident. Fixing blame for the accident is the responsibility of the justice system. The second component is recognition that accidents are the tip of a causal iceberg, and, therefore, identifying precursors to potential events is as important as identifying direct causes of events. The third component takes the investigation board into the real world of change; by deriving recommendations that actually enhance safety and are feasible. The final component acknowledges that the board will act as a spokesman for safety, crossing governmental, sectorial and public communities.

To guarantee a successful mission, five primary working processes have been identified in an international survey of best practices of multi-modal boards in the USA, Canada, Sweden and Finland and a number of single mode boards in the Netherlands. These five processes move the board from the decision to undertake an investigation through the analysis of the events into formulations of recommendations to prevent or mitigate future accidents and to assessing the effects of those recommendations. These five processes are:
- An initiation process to decide whether to take action. A board obtains information about specific transportation incidents, statistical information on transportation conditions and events, and the results of research relevant to transportation safety. The board has a mechanism that helps it decide which events merit an intensive investigation.
- A fact-finding process to assemble all relevant data bearing on an event and to determine findings about the main factors contributing to the event. There are three forms that the fact-finding may take: a reactive event investigation of an incident, a retrospective safety study to determine the factors associated with and preceding events or a pro-active safety study in which the board plans a research study that includes primary data collection of events as they occur.
- A safety deficiency identification process that takes the facts at hand and determines systematic threats to transport safety. The safety deficiency identification process can use pattern recognition, multivariate regression, modelling, operational experience, or a combination of these.
- A recommendation process that formulates effective steps to prevent or mitigate the harm of incidents. These steps should be economically and politi-

cally acceptable. The recommendation process may include consideration of how proposed actions might be implemented.

- A feedback process that maintains contact between the work of the board and the external public world. A central feature of this feedback process is a systematic monitoring of the recommendations of the board, in terms of the actions taken in response to the recommendations and the effects of these actions on transportation safety.

12.11.2
Five Primary Questions

To be independent, credible and influential, investigations should be of indisputable quality and have access to all relevant information and knowledge. Essentially, five questions are to be answered during the investigations [3]:

- What happened
- How did it happen
- Why did it occur
- What can be done to prevent a reoccurrence
- What can be done to minimise consequences

These questions can be categorised and allocated to various phases of the investigation process, fact-finding, analysis and recommendations [6]:

- Fact-finding focuses on collection of facts and other volatile information. This phase provides information about 'what' and 'how'. It concentrates on the sequence of events and provides information on the accident by collecting incontestable facts. A wide variety of forensic and classic scientific techniques are available during on-scene and post-scene investigations [2]. This phase takes advantage of inductive as well as deductive methods and provides information on a case study basis [8].
- The analysis phase is focused on 'why' the accident could occur and supplies additional post-scene information. Collection of background information takes place and in-depth specific analyses are performed. This phase focuses on arriving at a satisfactory explanation of the occurrence and identification of systemic deficiencies. The analysis applies scientific and operational expertise.
- Recommendations focus on lessons to be learned and what can be done by whom to prevent repetition of similar occurrences. This phase leads to a final report and recommendations. Recommendations are based on the products of the previous phases; the sequence of the event and accident scenarios, explanatory factors of technical, organisational, managerial or institutional nature, system deficiencies on various system levels to incorporate the multicausal and systemic nature of the event. All three phases are closely connected and require cooperation between all actors involved in the investigation process.

The investigation process is essentially iterative, and requires a team effort and the management of expertise and resources. During the fact-finding phase, a basic operational background knowledge is required to assess the need for specialist expertise for the investigations and to assess which information might be relevant to proceed with the investigations. It is crucial to be aware of methodological pitfalls and shortcomings in accident investigation methods.

During analysis, data collected in the fact-finding phase are analysed. Additional information is collected by specific investigations and through research in various disciplines. The investigator controls and manages the overall investigation process and assesses the methodological aspects.

12.11.3
The Public Safety Assessor: A New Mission

A possible next step in the evolution of safety boards will be defining the role of public safety assessor [5]. Present safety boards already function to gather information across stakeholders and actors. It is a small step to an information dissemination role. During the TWA 800 and Swissair 111 disasters, the National Transport Safety Board (NTSB) and the Canadian Transport Safety Board acted as a clearinghouse for informing the public and relatives of victims after the disasters. In the future, safety boards may be seen as safety ombudsmen, the principal advocate for safety and appropriate care of accident victims [1, 4].

Expansion of independent investigations is considered a duty of society [7]. It is considered the only way to establish what has happened and put an end to public concern. It can help victims and their families come to terms with their suffering.

12.11.4
Conclusions

Evaluating accident investigation methodology, questions can be raised about a more general applicability of the instrument outside its conventional scope in the maritime world. Questions from an injury control and safety promotion view include:
- Are the available principles and techniques more generally applicable
- Is there proof for safety deficiency identification
- Is it possible to structurally change the system

These questions are especially important for minor cases where no hull losses or multiple fatalities are involved, and where single casualties like drowning may occur. Also wider applicability may be possible in inland shipping, leisure craft sailing, surfing and other water-related activities where drowning is involved.

References

1. Bosterud H. (2001) Emergency management in a changing world. International Conference on Emergency Management TIEMS 2001, 19–22 June 2001, Oslo
2. Carper K (2001) Forensic engineering, 2nd edn. CRC Press LLC
3. ETSC (2001) Transport accident and incident investigation in the European Union. European Transport Safety Council, Brussels
4. Hovden J (2001) Regulations and risk control in a vulnerable society: points at issue. International Conference on Emergency Management TIEMS 2001, 19–22 June 2001, Oslo
5. Kahan J, Frinking E, de Vries R (2001) Structure of a board to independent investigate real and possible threats to safety. RAND Europe, May 2001
6. Stoop JA (2002) Harmony in diversity. Methodological issues in independent accident investigation. The International Emergency Management Society. 9th Annual Conference proceedings, 14–17 May 2002, Waterloo, Ontario, Canada
7. Van Vollenhoven P (2002) Independent accident investigation: every citizen's right, society's duty. Chairman Dutch Transport Safety Board, The Hague, October 2002
8. Yin RK (1994) Case study research. Design and methods. Applied social research methods series, vol 5. Sage Publications, Newbury Park

Important Websites

www.aetsas.com
www.alsg.org
www.apola.asn.au/
www.blueflag.org
www.cc.uoa.gr/health/socmed/hygien
www.cdc.gov/injury
www.childsafetyeurope.org/watersafety
www.dlrg.de
www.dnr.state.ak.us/parks/boating
www.drenkeling.nl
www.drowning.nl
www.drowning-prevention.org
www.ehbo.nl
www.epsa.org.ar
www.hss.state.ak.us/dph/chems/injury-prevention/kids_don'tfloat.htm
www.hvrb.org
www.ilsf.org
www.imo.org
www.intensive.org
www.intensiv-innsbruck.at/education/ertrinken_hasibeder.htm
www.iria.org
www.itsasafety.org
www.iws.ie
www.keepwatch.com.au
www.kidsalive.com.au
www.kindveilig.nl
www.knrm.nl
www.marine-medic.com.au
www.minvenw.nl
www.nationalwatersafety.org.uk
www.polmil.sp.gov.br/salvamarpaulista/
www.rcc-net.org
www.reddingsbrigade.pagina.nl
www.redcross.ca
www.redned.nl
www.resuscitationcouncil.nl
www.rlss.org.au
www.rnli.uk
www.rospa.com

www.royallifesaving.com.au
www.safewaters.nsw.gov.au
www.slsa.asn.au
www.sobrasa.org
www.socorrismo.com
www.sossegovia.com
www.sshk.nl
www.surflifesaving.com.au
www.swimandsurvive.com.au
www.szpilman.com
www.thelifeguardstore.com
www.uscg.mil
www.uscg.mil/d17/d17rbs/d17rbs.htm
www.usla.org
www.vaic.org.au
www.watersafe.org.nz
www.watersafety.com.au
www.watersafety.gr
www.watersafety.vic.gov.au
www.who/int
www.who.int/violence_injury_prevention/
www.who.int/violence_injury_prevention/publications/other_injury/en/
drowning_factsheet.pdf

Final Recommendations of the World Congress on Drowning
Amsterdam 26 – 28 June 2002

The World Congress on Drowning is an initiative of
de Maatschappij tot Redding van Drenkelingen
Established in Amsterdam in 1767

As a result of an interactive process that was initiated in 1998 by nine task forces, including some 80 experts, and finalized during plenary sessions, expert meetings and research meetings in 2002 at the World Congress on Drowning, recommendations were made in the field of drowning prevention, rescue and treatment. This was the first time that many of these subjects were addressed in a global forum.

The congress was attended by more than 500 persons. Although not every participant was directly involved in the development of each recommendation, these recommendations can be considered to be the most authoritative recommendations on the issue of drowning prevention, rescue and treatment at this moment.

Many of the foremost authorities have been involved in the preparations during the four years prior to the congress and have been actively involved during the congress. The draft version of the 13 final recommendations was presented at the plenary closing ceremony of the congress. That preliminary version of the recommendations was distributed by e-mail and adapted as a result of the comments received. An additional series of detailed recommendations in the areas of rescue and diving (breath hold, scuba and hose diving) were agreed upon within the nominated task forces.

This final version of the recommendations was then agreed upon by the members of the scientific steering group and the chairs of the nine task forces (epidemiology, prevention, rescue, resuscitation, hospital treatment, brain and spinal protection, immersion hypothermia, diving and drowning and water-related disasters).

All recommendations, together with the preparatory documents as consensus papers, reports of expert and research meetings, will be published in 2005 in the Handbook on Drowning.

A list of names of the members of the scientific steering group, task forces and attendees of the World Congress on Drowning is included.

1. A new, more appropriate, world-wide uniform definition of drowning must be adopted

A uniform definition of drowning is important for purposes of registration, diagnosis and research.

The following definition was accepted: "Drowning is the process of experiencing respiratory impairment from submersion/immersion in liquid."

All organisations involved in epidemiological research and vital statistical data collection as well as rescue organisations and the medical community should consider and preferably accept this new definition as a basis for useful communication and include it in their glossary. Further consultation of drowning experts is needed to uniformly classify morbidity and mortality due to drowning.

2. There is a great need of adequate and reliable international registrations of drowning incidents

International and national registration procedures of the number of drowning victims, immersion hypothermia victims, rescues, and hospital data are needed to better appreciate the world-wide burden of drowning. Also clinical data, for example on resuscitations and rewarming techniques, are needed to improve treatment.

International organisations, such as The World Health Organisation (WHO), the International Red Cross and Red Crescent organisations (IRCRC), the International Life Saving Federation (ILS), the International Life Boat Institute (ILF) and Diver's Alert Network (DAN), as well as national organisations, institutions and medical research consortiums are advised to set up and coordinate data-collection.

3. More data must be collected and knowledge gained about drowning in low-income countries and societies

According to repeated WHO reports, over 80% of all drownings occur in low-income countries or in low-income groups in high income countries. Nevertheless only few epidemiological data about these risk groups are available. The WHO, IRCRC, ILS, ILF and the European Consumer Safety Institute (ECOSA) are encouraged to expand the research on drowning risk factors in these low-income groups because this is expected to have a major impact in reducing the risk of drowning.

4. Preventive strategies and collaboration are needed

The vast majority of drownings can be prevented and prevention (rather than rescue or resuscitation) is the most important method by which to reduce the number of drownings. The circumstances and events in drowning differ across many different situations and in different countries world wide. Considerable differences exist in the locations of drowning and among different cultures.

Therefore, all agencies concerned with drowning prevention – legislative bodies, consumer groups, research institutions, local authorities and designers, manufacturers and retailers - must collaborate to set up national and local prevention initiatives. These will depend on good intelligence and insightful research, and must include environmental design and equipment designs as a first route, in conjunction with education, training programs and policies which address specific groups at risk, such as children. The programs must be evaluated and the results of the evaluations must be published.

5. All individuals, and particularly police officers and fire fighters, must learn to swim

Knowing how to swim is a major skill to prevent drowning for individuals at risk. International organisations such as WHO, IRCF and ILS, and their national branches must emphasize the importance of swimming lessons and drowning survival skills at all levels for as many persons as possible. The relationships between swimming lessons, swimming ability and drowning in children needs to be studied. In addition, certain public officials who frequently come in close contact with persons at risk for drowning, such as police officers and fire fighters, must be able to swim for their own safety and for the safety of the public.

6. Rescue techniques must be investigated

Most of the current rescue techniques have evolved by trial and error, with little scientific investigation. Rescue organisations such as the ILS, ILF, IRCRC but also the International Maritime Organization (IMO) must be encouraged to evaluate the self-rescue and rescue techniques in their training programs in accordance with current scientific data on the effectiveness and efficiency. Based on the data, the best rescue techniques must be selected for education and training programs.

7. Basic resuscitation skills must be learned by all volunteer and professional rescuers as well as lay persons who frequent aquatic areas or supervise others in water environment

The instant institution of optimal first aid and resuscitation techniques is the most important factor to survive after drowning has occurred. Resuscitation organisations, such as organisations, in particular those related to International Liaison Committee on Resuscitation (ILCOR), as well as professional rescue organisations and other groups who frequent aquatic areas, must promote training programs in first aid and Basic Life Support for anyone who frequently visits or is assigned to work in the aquatic or other water environment.

8. Uniform glossary of definitions and a uniform reporting of drowning resuscitation must be developed and used

To increase the understanding of the dying process and the resuscitation potential in drowning, a uniform reporting system must be developed and used for the registration of resuscitation of drowning.

International resuscitation organisations, such as ILCOR-related organisations and medical groups, must establish a uniform reporting system, facilitate its use, be involved in the analysis of the data and support of recommendations based on the studies.

9. Hospital treatment of the severe drowning victim must be concentrated

The optimal treatment of drowning victims includes dealing with specific severe complications such as the Acute Respiratory Distress Syndrome, pneumonia, hypoxic brain damage, hypothermia and cervical spine injuries. Due to the limited exposure and experience of most physicians with drowning victims, these victims should ideally be treated in specialised intensive care centres for optimal treatment and promotion of clinical research.

10. Treatment of the patient with brain injury resulting from cardiopulmonary arrest attributable to drowning must be based on scientific evidence. Due to the absence of interventional outcome studies in human drowning victims, current therapeutic strategies must be extrapolated from studies of humans or animals having similar forms of acute brain injury

The following recommendations for care of drowning victims who remain unresponsive due to anoxic encephalopathy are made on the basis of best available scientific evidence. The highest priority is restoration of spontaneous circulation. Subsequent to this, continuous monitoring of core and/or brain (tympanic) temperature is mandatory in the emergency department and intensive care unit (and in the prehospital setting to the extent possible). Drowning victims with restoration of adequate spontaneous circulation who remain comatose should not be actively rewarmed to temperature values >32-34°C. If core temperature exceeds 34 °C, hypothermia (32-34°C) should be achieved as soon as possible and sustained for 12-24 hours. Hyperthermia should be prevented at all times in the acute recovery period. There is insufficient evidence to support the use of any neuro-resuscitative pharmacologic therapy. Seizures should be appropriately treated. Blood glucose concentration should be frequently monitored and normoglycemic values maintained. Although there is insufficient evidence to support a specific target $PaCO_2$ or oxygen saturation during and after resuscitation, hypoxemia should be avoided. Hypotension should also be avoided. Research is needed to evaluate specific efficacy of neuroresuscitative therapies in drowning victims.

11. Wearing of appropriate and insulating life jackets must be promoted

Without floating aids, a subject generally drowns within minutes due to swimming failure in cold water. Therefore, the development of insulating and safe garments for aquatic activities is needed. Life jackets should always be worn when immersion can occur to prevent submersion in an early stage. When only non-insulating floating aids can be used, the victim should consider whether swimming ashore is achievable.

12. The balance between safety and profitability of recreational diving must remain critically observed

It was agreed that self-regulation within the world-wide recreational diving industry continues to be the practical route for further improvement but that there is a need to counter the perception that there is a conflict between commercial interest and safety.

13. Safety of diving fishermen needs more attention

Subsistence fishermen, who are predominantly found in the poor countries around the world, use equipment that is minimal and their training, regulations and medical support appear to be zero.

To improve diving-fishermen safety and reduce drowning there is a need to collect data on accidents and drowning among representative samples of diving fishermen around the world.

This should be followed up with international non-governmental organisations, other charities and appropriate UN development initiatives so that existing academic societies, training organisations and others could deliver suitable medical and diving advice and training for fishermen compatible with the limits of available local resources.

Several more specific recommendations have been proposed and need the full support of related organisations
These recommendations refer to the further development of existing research projects such as:
- Global uniformity of beach signs and safety flags
- Risk assessment of beach hazards
- Determination of optimal visual scanning techniques
- Construction of the most adequate rescue boats, including alternatives such as jet boats, hovercrafts, with minimum risk of injuries for the drivers

Other recommendations were made to improve practical aspects related to:
- Legal aspects of drowning incidents
- Evacuation planning of large passenger ships
- Uniformity in training programs for lifeguards
- Fund raising for aquatic safety activities

All recommendations, together with the preparatory documents as consensus papers, reports of expert and research meetings, will be published in the Handbook on Drowning. The Handbook will be available in 2005.

A large number of additional recommendations were elaborated before and during the World Congress on Drowning by the members of the task forces rescue and diving (breath hold, scuba and hose diving). These detailed recommendations are included in the appendices.

All recommendations need full support from governments, organisations, institutions and individuals to enable reduction of the last remaining field of neglected injuries. Each year some 500,000 persons world-wide are still dying from drowning. This is too much.

Overview Recommendations Task Force Rescue

During the preparation of the World Congress on Drowning, experts have prepared documents on a wide variety of topics. These topics have been further elaborated at the congress by the members of the task force recsue. Because of practical limitations in time, and the wide variety of subjects to be covered, there were no opportunities to include these recommendations in the final procedures.

Recommendations aimed at all national and international governmental bodies, including IMO, Search and Rescue organisations, the International Lifeboat Institution and prevention institutions

1. The existing standard for the evaluation of hazard presented at beaches should be implemented as the world-wide standard to enable the development of appropriate drowning prevention strategies at beaches.
2. Communities throughout the world which can expect to face flooding, must prepare themselves and the emergency workers they designate, to effectively respond to flood rescue.
3. Search and rescue response must be ensured in areas around the world where there is significant maritime traffic, whether it be cruise liners, cargo ships, fishing boats or leisure craft.
4. The International Aeronautical and Maritime Search and Rescue Manual should be reviewed and incorporated by the sea rescue organisations of all of the nations of the world to ensure a coordinated and effective approach to maritime emergencies.
5. The Incident Command System, which has been developed to allow for effective oversight and organisation of emergency responses, should be adopted by all aquatic rescue organisations worldwide.

Recommendations aimed at all national and international bodies in the area of rescue, including the International Red Cross and Red Crescent organisations, the International Lifeboat Institutions and the International Life Saving Federation

1. Scientific study should be undertaken to form a basis for determining the skills and minimum competencies required to rescue another human in an aquatic emergency.
2. Further research is needed in the area of surveillance, scanning and vigilance by lifeguards from a physiological and psychological perspective to determine the best methods of instruction and practice.
3. Further research should be undertaken to identify appropriate use and training of the personal watercraft (PWC) in aquatic rescue.

4. Rescue communications must provide dependable, robust, integrated, and effective command and control for all involved segments of the response system, not simply point to point communications.

5. Sea rescue providers should ensure that their rescue craft keep pace with available technology, evaluating and embracing effective new types of surface rescue craft and air rescue craft.

6. It is recommended that common terms for spinal injury immobilization techniques be adopted by all lifesaving organisations and that the terms should be vice grip, body hug, and the extended arm grip. Studies should be conducted on each of these methods to establish the best possible methods of extrication.

7. All lifesavers should be taught the standing backboard technique, to allow for immediate stabilization of the spine of a person who walks up to the lifeguard complaining of spinal pain post trauma.

8. An international study of fund-raising activities by aquatic lifesaving organisations should be commenced to identify the most effective methods.

Overview Recommendations Task Force Diving (breath hold, scuba and hose diving)

During the World Congress on Drowning, experts of the task force Breath hold, scuba and hose diving have finalised a consensus document on a variety of topics.

It was agreed that
1. Well-constructed national regulations have been effective where enforced and that any significant improvements in health and safety would arise only from a more inclusive definition of working divers and a wider application of existing procedures.
2. Self-regulation within the world-wide recreational diving industry continues to be the practical route for further improvement but that there is a need to counter a perception that there is a conflict between commercial interests and safety.
3. The training agencies comply with international quality assurance and control procedures (QA/QC) such as the International Standard ISO 9000 series and also encourage independent monitoring to assure the effective and safe use of existing and new procedures.
4. Subsistence fishermen who are predominantly found in the poor countries around the world, use equipment that is minimal and that their training, regulations and medical support appear to be zero.
   To improve diving-fishermen safety and reduce drowning there is a need to collect data on accidents and drowning among representative samples of diving fishermen around the world.
   This should be followed up with international non-governmental organisations (NGOs), other charities and appropriate UN development initiatives so that existing academic societies, training organisations and others could deliver suitable medical and diving advice and training for fishermen compatible with the limits of available local resources.
5. The collection of diver morbidity and mortality data and the associated contributory factors for each incident is a necessary first step in reducing drowning incidents among divers. Also needed are the denominator data that will allow the calculation of risk.
6. Recreational divers are free to dive when, where and how they like but the diver also has an obligation to the public. Any underwater accident to a diver can put buddy divers and rescuers at considerable risk.
7. Greater stringency is needed in the assessment of the physical, mental and medical fitness of all who choose to dive. A single assessment of fitness for diving at the beginning of diver training should not be considered valid throughout the rest of the diver's life. Re-assessments are recommended at

intervals that may diminish with advancing years and re-assessment may also be needed after illness or injury.

8. To give a medical opinion on a diver's fitness, the doctor should have prior knowledge of the unique hazards faced by a diver. Whenever possible, the medical assessment should be conducted by a doctor acknowledged as competent in this special subject. It is recommended the training of diving doctors, both for the medical examination of divers and also for the treatment of medical emergencies in diving, complies with guidance such as that published by the European Diving Technology Committee (ECHM) and the European Committee for Hyperbaric Medicine (EDTC). Periodical revision training is also important.

9. The mental, physical and medical standards of fitness in each category of diving should be harmonised internationally.

10. Greater emphasis should be placed at all levels of training on the causation and prevention of in-water fatalities.

11. After some 3 to 5 years without regular diving, the individual should be subject to a formal re-assessment of competence before re-entering the water.

12. The policy of training children as young as 8 years old to dive should emphasise the immaturity of mental outlook that many young persons may have when an emergency occurs.

13. Emergency procedures should be consistent with a variety of equipment in a variety of configurations.

14. Programs of refresher training should be established to maximise practical re-learning and updating of basic emergency skills. This is needed particularly after an individual's equipment has been modified.

15. Self-rescue and buddy-rescue procedures should be compatible with the equipment used and the environmental conditions.

16. Training of rescuers should include the procedures for recovery of the victim from the water into a boat and transfer of the patient from the deck of a boat to a helicopter or some other emergency transport vehicle.

17. Hand signals and basic procedures used in diving emergencies, whether at depth or on the surface, should be standardised and promoted through rescue and diving agencies throughout the world.

18. Rescuers must be made aware that the treatment of drowning in a diver might be complicated by other medical conditions such as carbon monoxide poisoning, envenomation and omitted decompression arising from that same dive.

19. National and international standards of medical care should be written for all medical emergencies in diving by suitable academic bodies.

20. Drowning is mostly a diagnosis of exclusion and often is a presumptive diagnosis based on purely circumstantial evidence. All diving-related deaths should be thoroughly investigated, including a complete autopsy, evaluation of the equipment and a review of the circumstances surrounding the fatality by knowledgeable investigators with appropriate training and experience.

The post-mortem examination of a drowned diver should be conducted by a pathologist who is knowledgeable about diving (or who is advised by a doctor who is knowledgeable about diving).

Acknowledgements

Foundation Drowning 2002
Hans Knape
Rutger Schimmelpenninck
Herpert van Foreest

National Steering Group
Ed van Beeck
Henk Beerstecher
Joost Bierens
Jan-Ewout Bourdrez
Rob Brons
Rob de Bruin
Hein Daanen
Jan Carel van Dorp
Rob van Hulst
Hans Knape
Wim Rogmans
Rutger Schimmelpennick
Lambert Thijs
Paul Touw

Task-force chairpersons
Christine Branche
Chris Brewster
David Elliott
Paul Pepe
Jean-Louis Vincent
Beat Walpoth
David Warner
John Wilson

Task-force members
Peter Barss
Elizabeth Bennett
Robert Berg
Marileen Biekart
Leo Bossaert
Alfred Bove
Ruth Brenner
Jean Carlet
Daniel Danzl
Michel Ducharme
Menno van Duin
Glen Egstrom
Anton Fischer
Dick Fundter
Luciano Gattinoni
Gordon Giesbrecht
Corsmas Goemans
Des Gorman
Tom Griffiths
Albert de Haas
Anthony Handley
Moniek Hoofwijk
Adriaan Hopperus Buma
Jim Howe
Paul Husby
Ahamed Idris
Udo Illievich
Cor Kalkman
Laurence Katz
Gabriel Kinney
Olive Kobusingye
Patrick Kochanek
Ries Kruidenier
John Langley
Gerard Laanen
Ian Mackie (†)
Peter Mair
Jordi Mancebo
Andrej Michalson
Peter Morley
Anja Nachtegaal
Bengt Nellgård
Martin Nemiroff
Beverly Norris
John Pearn
Eleni Petridou

SJAAK POORTVLIET
LINDA QUAN
SLIM RAY
PETER SAFAR (†)
TAKEFUMI SAKABE
IAN SCOTT
ANDREW SHORT
ANTONY SIMCOCK
ROB SLOMP
GORDON SMITH
DAVID SZPILMAN
MAIDA TAYLOR
PETER TIKUISIS

MICHAEL TIPTON
HANS VAN VUGHT
MAX HARRY WEIL
JÜRG WENDLING
VOLKER WENZEL
PETER WERNICKI
SIP WIEBENGA
JANE WIGGINTON
KLAUS WILKENS
MIKE WOODROFFE
RICK WRIGHT
DURK ZANDSTRA

Contact Data and Affiliations

Stathis Avramidis, MSc
European Lifeguard Academy Greece,
El. Venizelou 12A,
18533 Kastella-Pireas, Greece
S.Avramidis@leedsmet.ac.uk;
elagr@hotmail.com
www.ela.pre.gr
PhD student, Part Time Lecturer
of Aquatics, Leeds Metropolitan
University (UK) // Director,
European Lifeguard Academy Greece

Wolfgang Baumeier, Dipl. Ing, MD
Department of Anaesthesiology,
University Hospital Schleswig-
Holstein, Campus Lübeck,
Ratzeburger Allee 160, 23538 Lübeck,
Germany
baumeier@uni-luebeck.de
www.sarrrah.de
Consultant
Coordinating Physician in Maritime
Disaster Management

**Peter Barss, MD, ScD, MPH, DTMH,
FACPM, FRCPC**
United Arab Emirates University,
Faculty of Medicine and Health
Sciences
PO Box 17666, Al Aïn,
United Arab Emirates
peter.barss@uaeu.ac.ae
www.fmhs.uaeu.ac.ae
Associate Professor

**Steve Beerman, MD, BSc, BSR,
CCFP, FCFP**
Lifesaving Society Canada,
287 McArthur Avenue,
Ottawa Ontario, K1L 6P3, Canada
sbeerman@shaw.ca
www.lifesavingsociety.com
Family Physician, Clincial Instructor,
Department of Family Practice,
Faculty of Medicine,
University of British Columbia
Chair, Medical Committee,
International Life Saving Federation //
Medical Advisor, Lifesaving Society –
Canada

Elizabeth Bennett, MPH, CHES
Children's Hospital and Regional
Medical Center, Health Eduction,
PO Box 50020/S-217, Seattle,
WA 98145-5020, USA
elizabeth.bennett@seattlechildrens.
org
www.drowning-prevention.org
Health Education Manager
Clinical Instructor,
University of Washington

Robert A. Berg, Professor, MD
The University of Arizona College of
Medicine,
1501 N Campbell Avenue, Tucson,
AZ 85724-5073, USA
rberg@peds.arizona.edu
Professor of Pediatrics (Critical Care
Medicine) // Associate Dean for
Clinical Affairs, The University of
Arizona College of Medicine //
Member, Emergency
Cardiovascular Care Committee,
Amercian Heart Association //
Member, Pediatric Resuscitation
Committee, American Heart
Association

**Roger E.Bibbings, MBE, BA, FIOSH,
RSP**
Royal Society for the Prevention of
Accidents, RoSPA House,
Edgbaston Park, 353, Bristol Road,
Birmingham B5 7ST, UK
rbibbings@rospa.com
www.rospa.com
Occupational Safety Adviser

**Joost J. L.M. Bierens, Professor,
MD, PhD, MCDM**
Department of Anesthesiology,
VU University Medical Center,
De Boelelaan 1117,
1081 HV Amsterdam,
The Netherlands
jbierens@vumc.nl
www.vumc.nl
Professor in Emergency Medicine
Member, medical committee,
International Life Saving Federation //
Advisory board, Maatschappij tot
Redding van Drenkelingen //
Member, Medical Commission Royal
Netherlands Sea Rescue Institution

Jenny Blitvich, PhD
School of Human Movement
and Sport Sciences,
University of Ballarat, Victoria 3353,
Australia
j.blitvich@ballarat.edu.au
Senior Lecturer, School of Human
Movement and Sport Sciences,
University of Ballarat
Member, Consultative Committee for
Water Safety Research

Eke Boesten, LLM, PhD
Celebesstraat 86, 2585 TP The Hague,
The Netherlands
Lawyer

Leo L. Bossaert, Professor, MD, PhD
University Hospital Antwerp,
Department of Intensive Care,
Wilrijkstraat 10, 2610 Antwerp,
Belgium
leo.bossaert@ua.ac.be
Director, Department of Intensive
Care // Professor of Medicine,
University of Antwerp, Belgium
Executive Director,
European Resuscitation Council

Alfred A. Bove, Professor, MD
Cardiology Section,
Temple University Medical School,
3401 N. Broad Street, Philadelphia,
PA 19140, USA
fred@scubamed.com
www.scubamed.com

Christine M. Branche, PhD
National Center for Injury
Prevention and Control,
Centers for Disease Control
and Prevention,
4770 Buford Highway NE,
Mailstop K-63,
Atlanta GA 30431-3724, USA
cbranche@cdc.gov
Director, Division of Unintentional
Injury Prevention

Helge Brandstrom, MD
University Hospital, Department of
Anaesthesiology and Intensive Care,
Umea, Sweden
helge.brandstrom@vll.se
Senior Consultant Anaesthesiology
and Intensive Care
Scientific Secretary, KAMEDO,
Swedish National Board of Health
and Welfare

Ruth A. Brenner, MD, MPH
National Institute of Child Health
and Human Development,
National Institutes of Health,
Department of Health and Human
Services, Room 7B03-7510,
6100 Executive Blvd, Bethesda,
MD 20892-7510, USA
brennerr@mail.nih.gov
Medical Officer

B. Chris Brewster
3850 Sequoia Street, San Diego, CA
92109, USA
brewster@lifesaver1.com
www.lifesaver1.com
Lifeguard Chief (ret.), San Diego
Lifeguard Service
President, United States Lifesaving
Association // President,
Americas Region, International Life
Saving Federation

Rob K. Brons, LLM
Fire and Rescue The Hague Region,
PO Box 52158, 2505 CD The Hague,
The Netherlands
commandant@brw.denhaag.nl
www.denhaag.nl/brandweer;
www.usar.nl
Chief Fire Officer
National Commander, Urban Search
and Rescue Team, The Netherlands //
Chairman, Examination Committee,
Dutch Life Saving Association

**Christopher J. Brooks, OMM, CD,
MBChB, DAvMed, FFOM**
Research & Development,
Survival Systems Limited,
Dartmouth, Nova Scotia, Canada
chrisb@sstl.com
www.survivalsystemsgroup.com
Director, Research & Development

David Calabria
D&D Technologies (USA), Inc.,
7731 Woodwind Drive,
Huntington Beach, CA 92647, USA
dcalabria@ddgroup.com.au
www.ddtechglobal.com
Chief Executive Officer,
D&D Group of Companies
(Australia) // President,
D&D Technologies (USA), Inc.
Founding board member, National
Drowning Prevention Alliance, USA

Ian M. Calder, MD
University of Cambridge, Thorpe,
Huntingdon Road,
Cambridge CB3 0LG, UK
calderpath@hotmail.com
Pathophysiologist

Jim Caruso, MD
1413 Research Blvd, Rockville,
MD 20850, USA
James.caruso@afip.osd.mil
Commander, US Navy // Chief Deputy
Medical Examiner, Diving Medical
Officer and Flight Surgeon // Office
of the Armed Forces Medical
Examiner, Rockville, MD, USA //
Consulting Physician, Divers Alert
Network // Associate Consulting
Professor, Department of
Anesthesiology, Duke University
Medical Center

Davide Chiumello, MD
Istituto di Anestesia e Rianimazione,
Universita' degli Studi di Milano,
Ospedale Maggiore Policlinico-
IRCCS, Via Francesco Sforza 35,
20122 Milano, Italy
chiumello@libero.it

**Veronique G.J.M. Colman,
Professor, PhD**
Faculty of Movement and
Rehabilitation Sciences,
Catholic University Leuven,
Tervuursevest 101, 3001 Leuven,
Belgium
Veronique.colman@faber.kuleuven.
be
www.faber.kuleuven.be
Assistant Professor, Faculty of
Movement and Rehabilitation
Sciences of the Katholieke
Universiteit Leuven // Responsible in
the Faculty for courses on didactics
of swimming, life saving, didactical
software, multimedia // Educating
toplevel coaches and lifesavers
Member, Education Commission of
the Flemisch Life Saving Federation

Peter N. Cornall
Water and Leisure Safety,
Royal Society for the Prevention of
Accidents, ROSPA house,
Edgbaston Park, 353 Bristol Road,
Birmingham B5 7ST, UK
pcornall@rospa.com
www.rospa.com
Head of Water and Leisure Safety
Secretary, UK National Water Safety
Forum // UK Safety Expert on ISO
Water Safety Information
Standardization Committee //
Chair, UK's BSI Water Safety
Information Standardization
Committee PH/8/2/1

**Günter Cornelissen, Dipl.Pol,
Dipl.Ing**
DIN Deutsches Institut für Normung
eV, Verbraucherrat,
Postfach 301107, 10772 Berlin,
Germany
guenter.cornelissen@din.de
www.verbraucherrat.din.de
Head of Consumer Council's offices
Safety Standardisation

Hein A. M. Daanen, Professor, PhD
Department of Performance &
Comfort,
TNO Human Factors, PO Box 23,
3769 ZG Soesterberg, The Netherlands
daanen@tm.tno.nl
www.tno.nl
Head, Department of Performance &
Comfort, TNO Human Factors //
Professor in Thermal Physiology,
Faculty of Human Movement
Sciences, Free University of
Amsterdam

Peter Dawes
Surf Life Saving Queensland,
PO Box 3747,
South Brisbane QLD 4101, Australia
pdawes@lifesaving.com.au
www.lifesaving.com.au
Operations Manager,
Surf Life Saving Queensland

Michel B. Ducharme, PhD
Human Protection and Performance
Group, Operational Medicine Section,
Defence Research and Development,
1133 Sheppard Avenue West, Toronto,
Ontario, M3M 3B9, Canada
Michel.ducharme@drdc-rddc.gc.ca
Defence Scientist, Head of Human
Protection and Performance Group at
DRDC Toronto
Adjunct Professor, Faculty of Physical
Education and Health, University of
Toronto // Adjunct Professor, School
of Human Kinetics, University of
Ottawa

Glen Egstrom, PhD
University of California Los Angeles,
Department of Physiological Sciences,
3440 Centinela Avenue, Box 951606,
Los Angeles, CA 90095-1606, USA
gegstrom@ucla.edu
Professor (Emeritus)
President, Glen H. Egstrom Inc.

**David H. Elliott OBE, Professor, MD,
DPhil, FRCP, FFOM**
40, Petworth Road, Rockdale,
Haslemere, Surrey GU27 2HX, UK
Davidelliott001@aol.com
Specialist in diving physiology
and medicine

Mike Espino
American Red Cross National Headquarters,
8111 Gatehouse Road, 6th floor,
Falls Church, Virginia 22042, USA
espinom@usa.redcross.org
www.redcross.org
Manager Aquatics Technical
Development

Marit Farstad, MD
Department of Anesthesia
and Intensive Care,
Institute for Surgical Sciences,
Haukeland University Hospital,
5021 Bergen, Norway
fars@helse-bergen.no

**Peter J Fenner AM, MD, DRCOG,
FACTM, FRCGP**
School of Medicine, James Cook
University, Townsville, Queensland,
PO Box 3080, North Mackay,
Qld 4740, Australia
pjf@occupationalhealthmackay.com.
au
Associate Professor

Adam P. Fischer, MD
Department of Cardiovascular
Surgery, Centre Hospitalier
Universitaire Vaudois,
Rue du Bugnon 46, 1011 Lausanne,
Switzerland
Associated medical doctor in
Cardiovascular Surgery

Andrea Gabrielli, MD
Division of Critical Care Medicine
University of Florida, 1600 Sw Archer
Road, Gainesville, FL 32610-0254,
USA
AGabrielli@anest.ufl.edu
Associate Professor of Anesthesiology
and Surgery // Medical Director,
Hyperbaric Medicine // Medical
Director, Cardiopulmonary Services

Luciano Gattinoni, Professor, MD, PhD
Maggiore Hospital, Department of
Anesthesia and Intensive Care,
Via F. Sforza 35, 20122 Milan, Italia
gattinon@policlinico.mi.it

Harry P.M.M. Gelissen, MD
Radboud University Medical Centre,
Department of Intensive Care,
PO Box 9101, 6500 HB Nijmegen,
The Netherlands
H.Gelissen@ic.umcn.nl

Gordon G. Giesbrecht, Professor, MD, PhD
211 Max Bell Centre,
University of Manitoba, Winnipeg,
MB, R3T 2N2, Canada
giesbrec@ms.umanitoba.ca
www.umanitoba.ca/physed/
giesbrecht
Professor, Department of Anesthesia
and Faculty of Physical Education
and Recreation Studies,
University of Manitoba
Board Member, Wilderness Medical
Society // Revision Committee
Member for State of Alaska Cold
Injuries Guidelines

Julie Gilchrist, MD
National Center for Injury
Prevention and Control, Centers for
Disease Control and Prevention,
Division of Unintentional Injury
Prevention, 4770 Buford Highway NE,
Mailstop K-63, Atlanta, GA 30341,
USA
jrg7@cdc.gov
www.cdc.gov/injury
Medical epidemiologist
LCDR, US Public Health Service

Frank St. C. Golden, MB, MD, BCh, PhD
15 Beech Grove, Gosport,
Hants PO12 2EJ, UK
golden_biomed@ntlworld.com
University of Portsmouth, UK,
Consultant in Environmental
Medicine and Applied Human
Physiology

Des Gorman, Professor, MD
Occupational Medicine Unit,
University of Auckland,
Private Bag 92019, Auckland,
New Zealand
d.gorman@auckland.ac.nz
Professor of Medicine

Ralph S. Goto
Ocean Safety and Lifeguard Services
Division, City and County of
Honolulu, 3823 Leahi Avenue,
Honolulu, HI 96815, Hawaii
rgoto@honolulu.gov
www.aloha.com/~lifeguards;
www.co.honolulu.hi.us/esd/
oceansafety/index.htm
Administrator, Ocean Safety and
Lifeguard Services Division,
Honolulu // Emergency Services
Department, City and County of
Honolulu
Chair, Signage Committee,
United States Lifesaving Association //
Certification Officer, Southwest Re-
gion, United States Lifesaving
Association

Shirley A. Graves, MD
University of Florida,
College of Medicine, PO Box 100254,
Gainesville, FL 32610, USA
sgraves@anest.ufl.edu
Emeritus Professor,
Anesthesiology and Pediatrics

Tom Griffiths, EdD
Aquatics and Safety Office,
Penn State University, Department
of Intercollegiate Athletics,
University Park, PA 16802, USA
Tjg4@psu.edu
www.aquaticsafetygroup.com
Director,
President,
Aquatic Safety Research Group, LLC

Ivar Grøneng
Norwegian Maritime Directorate,
PO Box 8123, 0032 Oslo, Norway
ivar.groneng@hellyhansen.no
www.sjofartdir.no; www.hhsp.no
Project Coordinator //
Master Mariner

Ton Haasnoot
KNRM, (Royal Netherlands Sea
Rescue Institution), PO Box 434,
1970 AK IJmuiden, The Netherlands
t.haasnoot@knrm.nl
www.knrm.nl
Head Training Department
2nd Coxswain of IJmuiden Lifeboat

Katrina Haddrill
New South Wales Department of
Tourism, Sport and Recreaction,
PO Box 1422, Silverwater NWS 2128,
Australia
khaddrill@dsr.nsw.gov.au
www.safewaters.nsw.gov.au
Senior Project Officer
Executive Officer, New South Wales
Water Safety Taskforce

Jack J. Haitsma, MD, PhD
Department of Anesthesiology,
Erasmus University Medical Centre,
PO Box 1738, 3000 DR Rotterdam,
The Netherlands
J.Haitsma@erasmusmc.nl
Staff Member, Department of
Anesthesiology // Secretary,
Acute Respiratory Failure,
Diagnosis and Treatment of the
Respiratory Intensive Care Assembly,
European Respiratory Society

Anthony J. Handley, MD, FRCP
40 Queens Road, Colchester,
Essex CO3 3PB, UK
tony.handley@btinternet.com
Honorary Consultant Physician,
Essex Rivers Health Authority,
Colchester, UK
Consultant Physician, Cardiologist
Chief Medical Adviser,
Royal Life Saving Society UK //
Honorary Medical Officer,
Irish Water Safety // Honorary
Medical Adviser, International Life
Saving Federation of Europe //
Secretary, Medical Committee,
International Life Saving
Federation // Chairman, AED
Subcommittee Resuscitation Council
(UK) // Chairman, European
Resuscitation Council International
BLS Course Committee // Chairman,
BLS Task Force International Liaison
Committee on Resuscitation

W. Andrew Harrell, Professor, PhD
Centre for Experimental Sociology,
University of Alberta, 5-21 Tory,
Edmonton, Alberta T6G 2H4, Canada
harandrw@aol.com
Director, Population Research
Laboratory, University of Alberta

Walter Hasibeder, MD
Department of Anesthesiology
and Intensive Care Medicine,
Krankenhaus der Barmherzigen
Schwestern, Schlossberg 1,
4910 Ried im Innkreis, Österreich
Walter.Hasibeder@bhs.at
www.bhs.ried.at
Head, Department of Anesthesiology
and Intensive Care Medicine

Balt Heldring, LLM
PC Hooftstraat 204,
1071 CH Amsterdam,
The Netherlands
mrbheldring@xs4all.nl
www.itlawyers.nl
Lawyer, Member of the Amsterdam
Bar Association

Walter Hendrick
PO Box 548, Hurley, NY 12443,
USA
butch@teamlgs.com
www.teamlgs.com;
www.rip-tide.org
President, Lifeguard Systems //
President, RIPTIDE // Ulster County
Sheriff's Office Special Consultant

Robyn M. Hoelle, MD
Emergency Medicine, University of
Florida, PO Box 14347, Gainesville,
FL 32604, USA

James D. Howe Jr
Honolulu Emergency Services
Department, Ocean Safety and
Lifeguard Services Division,
3823 Leahi Avenue,
Honolulu Hawaii 96815
jhowe@honolulu.gov
www.co.honolulu.hi.us/esd/
oceansafety/index.htm
Chief of Lifeguard Operations,
Island of Oahu
Lecturer, University of Hawaii, Maui,
Kauai, and Windward Community
Colleges, Ocean Safety Education
Course (Personal Water Craft and
Tow-in Surfing Certification) and
Ocean Safety Management, Principals
and Practices // Expert/Consultant,
Ocean Safety International, Inc.,
Hawaii

Paul Husby, Professor, MD, PhD
Department of Anesthesia
and Intensive Care, Institute for
Surgical Sciences,
University of Bergen,
Haukeland University Hospital,
5021 Bergen, Norway
paul.husby@kir.uib.no

Ahamed H. Idris, Professor, MD
Surgery and Emergency Medicine,
University of Texas Southwestern
Medical Center,
5323 Harry Hines Blvd, Dallas,
TX 75390-8579, USA
Ahamed.idris@utsouthwestern.edu
Professor of Surgery and Emergency
Medicine, University of Texas, Dallas //
Director, Dallas Center for Resuscita-
tion Research // Medical Consultant,
NASA

Udo M. Illievich, Professor, MD
Neuroanesthesiology and Critical
Care, Clinic of Anesthesia and
General Intensive Care,
Medical University of Vienna,
1090 Vienna, Austria
udo.illievich@meduniwien.ac.at
www.anaesthesiology.at
Supervising Anaesthesiologist
Critical Care Physician, Head of the
Task Force Neuroanesthesiology
and Critical Care

Nicolaas J.G. Jansen, MD, PhD
Pediatric Intensive Care Unit,
Wilhelmina Children's Hospital,
University Medical Center Utrecht,
PO Box 85090, 3508 AB Utrecht,
The Netherlands
N.J.G.Jansen@wkz.azu.nl
Senior staff Member,
Pediatric Intensive Care,
Department of Pediatrics

Bas N. Jonkman, MsC
Road and Hydraulic Engineering
Institute, Ministry of Transport,
Public Works and Water Management
and Delft University of Technology,
Faculty of Civil Engineering,
PO Box 5044, 2628 CS Delft,
The Netherlands
s.n.jonkman@dww.rws.minvenw.nl
Engineer working for the Ministry of
Transport, Public Works and Water
Management, Road and Hydraulic
Institute, the Netherlands //Research-
er at Delft University, Faculty of Civil
Engineering // involved in the
research and policy on flood
protection in the Netherlands

Cor J. Kalkman, Professor, MD, PhD
Division of Perioperative Care,
Anesthesia, Emergency Medicine
and Pain Management,
University Medical Center Utrecht,
PO Box 85500, 3508 GA Utrecht,
The Netherlands
c.j.kalkman@azu.nl
Professor of Anesthesiology

Laurence M. Katz, MD
University of North Carolina
at Chapel Hill,
Department of Emergency Medicine,
Neurosciences,
101 Manning Dr,
Chapel Hill, NC 27599, USA
lkatz@med.unc.edu
Associate Professor, co-Director,
Carolina Resuscitation Research
Group

Gabriel Kinney
Business Development,
Martime Systems and Sensors,
Lockheed Martin, Syracuse,
New York NY 13221 4840, USA
gabesnewfsar@yahoo.com
Director, Association for Rescue at
Sea (AFRAS) // Council Member,
International Lifeboat Federation
Captain, USCG (Ret), Former Chief,
US Coast Guard Office of Search
and Rescue

Alexandra Klimentopoulou, MD
1st Department of Pediatrics,
Athens University Medical School,
Aghia Sophia Children's Hospital,
Thivon & Levadias str,
11527 Athens, Greece
alkliment@hotmail.com
Paediatrician, Senior house Officer 3
Research Assistant,
Department of Hygiene
and Epidemiology,
Athens University Medical School

Johannes T.A. Knape, Professor, MD, PhD
Division of Perioperative Care, Anesthesiology, Emergency Medicine and Pain Management, University Medical Center Utrecht, PO Box 85500, 3508 GA Utrecht, The Netherlands
J.knape@azu.nl
Chairman, Department of Anaesthesiology
Honorary Secretary, Section and Board of Anaesthesiology, Union Europeènne des Médècins Specialistes.

Olive C. Kobusingye, MD, MBChB, MMed (Surg), MPH
WHO Regional Office for Africa, PO Box 6, Brazzaville, Republic of Congo
kobusingyeo@afro.who.int
Regional Advisor on Disability / Injury Prevention and Rehabilitation // WHO Regional Office for Africa Accident and Emergency Surgeon

Patrick M. Kochanek, MD
Safar Center for Resuscitation Research, Department of Critical Care Medicine, University of Pittsburgh School of Medicine, 3434 Fifth Ave, Pittsburgh, PA 15260, USA
Kochanekpm@ccm.upmc.edu
www.safar.pitt.edu
Director, Safar Center for Resuscitation Research // Professor and Vice Chairman

Amanda Kost, LLD
Fire Department of The Hague, PO Box 52155, 2505 CD The Hague, The Netherlands
a.kost@brw.denhaag.nl
Legal Policy Advisor

Gerard D. Laanen, MSc
Ministry of Transport, Public Work and Water Management, PO Box 20906, 2500 EX Den Haag, The Netherlands
g.d.laanen@hkw.rws.minvenw.nl
www.dccvenw.nl
Director, Ministerial Coordination Centre for Crisismanagement

Burhard Lachmann, MD, PhD
Department of Anaesthesiology, Erasmus Medical Center, PO Box 1738, 3000 DR Rotterdam, The Netherlands
b.lachmann@erasmusmc.nl
Research Director

John Langley, PhD
Injury Prevention Research Unit, Department of Preventive and Social Medicine, Dunedin School of Medicine, University of Otago, PO Box 913, Dunedin, New Zealand
john.langley@ipru.otago.ac.nz
www.otago.ac.nz/ipru
Director, Injury Prevention Research Unit

Laurie J. Lawrence, Dip. Phys Ed, Dip. Ed, BA
D&D Technologies Inc, PO Box 379, Sydney, Brookvale, NSW 2100, Australia
laurie@kidsalive.com.au
www.kidsalive.com.au;
www.laurielawrence.com.au
Company Director // Motivational Speaker Safety Institute of Australia Fellow // Patron AUSTSWIM Queensland // Founder of Kids Alive Water Safety Program
Master Coach Australian Swimming, International Hall of Fame

John Leech, Lt Cdr, MNI, MIIMS
Irish Water Safety Association, The Long Walk, Galway, Ireland
johnleech@iws.ie
www.iws.ie
Chief Executive,
Irish Water Safety Association
Commander, Irish Navy // Officer i/c Naval Diving Section in Ireland // Lecturer, Naval College

Jennifer M. Lincoln, MS
4230 University Drive, Suite 310, Anchorage Alaska 99508, USA
jlincoln@cdc.gov
www.cdc.gov/niosh/injury/traumafish.html
PhD canididate, Occupational Safety and Health Specialist, NIOSH Project Officer for the Injury Prevention Project in the Commercial Fishing Industry

Bo Løfgren, MD
Department of Cardiology, Research Unit, Aarhus University Hospital, Skejby Sygehus, Brendstrupgaardsvej 100, 8200 Aarhus N, Denmark
bo.loefgren@ki.au.dk

John B. Long
Royal Life Saving Society, Commonwealth Headquarters, River House, High Street, Broom, Warks, England B50 4HN, UK
commonwealth@rlss.org.uk
Royal Life Saving Society, Commonwealth Secretary
Secretary, ILS Development Committee // Chairman, WHO/ILS Liaison Committee // Commonwealth Vice-President, Royal Life Saving Society

Marilyn Lyford, BHsc
The Royal Life Saving Society Australia (NSW Branch), PO Box 753, Gladesville NSW 1675, Australia
mlyford@rlssa.org.au
www.nsw.royalifesaving.com.au
Health Promotion Manager

Peter MacGregor, RSP MIFire DMS, FIM MIOSH
Royal Society for the Prevention of Accidents, RoSPA House, Edgbaston Park, 353 Bristol Road, Birmingham B5 7ST, UK
pmacgregor@rospa.com;
www.rospa.com
Water Leisure Safety Consultant

Ian Mackie, AM, FRACP †

Martin H.E. Madern
Fire Department of The Hague,
PO Box 52155,
2505 CD The Hague,
The Netherlands
m.madern@brw.denhaag.nl
www.denhaag.nl/brandweer
Bachelor of public administration,
Senior Safety Consultant (Senior Policy Adviser) // Substitute local coordinator emergency planning & crisis management, City of The Hague

Denise M. Mann, BS, EMT-P
12006 Glenway, Houston,
TX 77070, USA
denisemann@sbcglobal.net
Patient Outcome Manager/
EMS Community Relations &
Research, City of Houston EMS,
Houston, TX, USA
Harris County Child Fatality Review
Board, Save a Life – Prevent a Drowning, Houston CPR Task Force,
National CPR Task Force,
Greater Houston EMS Council

Ruy Marra
Superfly, Estrada das Canoas,
1476 casa 2 Sao Conrado,
22610-210 Rio de Janeiro, Brasilia
superfly@visualnet.com.br
www.paralife.com.br
Creator and Pilot

Fernando Neves Rodrigues Martinho, PhD
Casa Patrão de Salva Vidas Ezequiel
Seabra, Praia de Angeiras 4455,
204, Lavra, Matosinhos, Portugal
fmartinho@epesajms.coop,
www.epesajms.coop
Pedagogic Director, Social Economy
Professional School, that promotes
the Professional Course in Aquatic
Safety and Rescue // President of
Portuguese Life Saving Association
(AsNaSA), delegate to the International Life Saving Federation
Trainer in Life Saving Techniques –
First Aid for Water Life Saving //
Animator for Life Saving Associations
in Portuguese Spoken Countries

Germ Martini
KNRM (Royal Netherlands Sea
Rescue Institution), PO Box 434,
1970 AK IJmuiden, The Netherlands
g.martini@knrm.nl
www.knrm.nl
Operational Lifeboat Inspector
Honorary Secretary,
KNRM Lifeboat Station

John T. McVan, MEd
United States Military Academy,
Aquatic Instruction,
735 Brewerton Road, West Point,
NY 10966, USA
John.Mcvan@usma.edu
Assistant Professor,
Director of Aquatic Instruction

Bart-Jan T.J. Meursing, MD
Canisius-Wilhelmina Hospital,
Weg door Jonkerbos 100,
6532 SZ Nijmegen, The Netherlands
b.meursing@chello.nl
Cardiologist // Interventional
Cardiologist

Robyn J. Meyer, MD, MS
Department of Pediatrics,
The University of Arizona College
of Medicine,
1501 N Campbell Avenue, Tucson,
AZ 85724-5073, USA
rjmeyer@peds.arizona.edu
Assistant Professor, Pediatric Critical
Care, University of Arizona
Medical Director, Pediatric ECMO,
University of Arizona

Andrej Michalsen, MD, MPH
University Medical Center Utrecht,
Division of Perioperative Care,
Anesthesia, Emergency Medicine
and Pain Management,
PO Box 85500, 3508 GA Utrecht,
The Netherlands
a.michalsen@azu.nl

Rebecca Mitchell, MA, MOHS
Injury Prevention and Policy Branch,
New South Wales Health,
North Sydney, Australia
RMITC@doh.health.nsw.gov.au
PhD student

Jerome H. Modell, MD, DSc (Hon)
Department of Anesthesiology,
University of Florida,
College of Medicine,
PO Box 100254,
Gainesville, FL 32610, USA
modeljh@shands.ufl.edu
Professor Emeritus of Anesthesiology
Courtesy Professor of Large Animal
Clinical Science

Jaap Molenaar
NIBRA (Netherland Institute for Fire
Service and Disaster Management),
PO Box 7010, 6801 HA Arnhem,
The Netherlands
j.molenaar@nibra.nl
www.nibra.nl
Project Manager // Senior Trainer //
Consultant and Dean Operational
Branch
Developer of the courseware for
rescue divers and instructors in the
Netherlands Fire Service

Kevin Moran, MEd
Centre for Health and Physical
Education,
Symonds Street, 74 Epsom Av.,
Private Bag 92601, Epsom, Auckland,
New Zealand
k.moran@auckland.ac.nz
Principal Lecturer in Physical
Education
Chairman, Watersafe Auckland
Incorporated (WAI), Auckland,
New Zealand // Senior Advisor,
Surf Life Saving Northern, Auckland,
New Zealand

Luiz Morizot-Leite, MS
Beach and Marine Safety,
Miami Dade County Fire Rescue,
10800 Collings Avenue,
North Miami Beach, FL 33154, USA
lmorizo@miamidade.gov
American Red Cross Lifeguard
Instructor Trainer
Ocean Rescue Lifeguard-Paramedic
Lieutenant

Peter Morley, MD
Intensive Care Unit,
Royal Melbourne Hospital,
Parkville, Grattan Street,
Melbourne Victoria 3050, Australia
peter.morley@mh.org.au
Senior Specialist Intensive Care,
Royal Melbourne Hospital
Chairman, Advanced Life Support
Committee, Australian Resuscitation
Council

Bengt Nellgård MD, PhD
Neuro Intensive Care Unit,
Sahlgrenska University Hospital,
413 45 Gothenburg, Sweden
bengt.nellgard@vgregion.se
Director, Neuro Intensive Care Unit
Associate Professor, Department of
Anesthesiology and Intensive Care
Medicine, Gothenburg University,
Sweden

Martin J. Nemiroff, MD
US Public Health Service/
US Coast Guard,
20829 Via Colombard,
Sonoma California CA 95476 – 8059,
USA
martinsgate6@sbcglobal.net
Captain, USCG (ret)

Michael A. Oostman
1912 Dimmitt Court,
Bloomington, IL 61704, USA
Michael@thelifeguardstore.com
www.thelifeguardstore.com
Vice President, Jeff Ellis & Associates,
Inc.

**Linda Papa, MD, CM, MSc, CCFP,
FRCP(C), FACEP**
Department of Emergency Medicine,
University of Florida College of
Medicine, PO Box 100186,
Gainesville FL 32610-0186, USA
lpstat@aol.com
Assistant Professor and Director of
Clinical Research, Department of
Emergency Medicine //
Director of Clinical Studies in Mild
Traumatic Brain Injury, McKnight
Brain Institute

Luis-Miguel Pascual-Gómez
Buena Vista 4, Esc-3, 2-b,
40006 Segovia, Spain
dtecnica@sosseggovia.com
www.sossegovia.com
Professor, Technical and Educational
Director-E.S.S. (Segovia Lifesaving
School) // Lifesaving Instructor //
Co-Founder and former President
of ESS

**John Pearn, Professor, MD, AM,
RFD**
Department of Paediatrics and Child
Health, University of Queensland,
Royal Children's Hospital, Herston,
Brisbane, Queensland 4029, Australia
j.pearn@uq.edu.au
Senior Paediatrician, Royal Children's
Hospital Brisbane
Former Surgeon General, Australian
Defence Force // Leader, Major
Research Team in Immersion Studies

Margie M. Peden, PhD
Department of Injuries and Violence
Prevention, World Health
Organization, Appia Avenue 20,
1211 Geneva 27, Switzerland
pedenm@who.int
www.who.int/violence_injury_pre-
vention/
Coordinator, Unintentional Injury
Prevention, Department of Injuries
and Violence Prevention,
WHO Geneva

Tommaso Pellis, MD
Cardiac Mechano-Electric Feedback
Lab, The University Laboratory of
Physiology, Oxford, OX1 3PT, UK
thomas.pellis@physiol.ox.ac.uk
Senior Research Scientist,
University Laboratory of Physiology,
Cardiac Mechano-Electric Feedback
Lab // Consultant in Anaesthesia
and Intensive Care

**Paul E. Pepe, MD, MPH, FACP,
FCCM, FACEP, FCCP**
Emergency Medicine Administration,
5323 Harry Hines Blvd, MC 8579,
Dallas, TX 75390-8579, USA
Paul.Pepe@UTSouthwestern.edu
Professor of Surgery, Medicine,
Public Health and Riggs Family Chair
in Emergency Medicine, University of
Texas Southwestern Medical Center
and the Parkland Health and Hospital
System, Dallas, USA
Director, City of Dallas Medical
Emergency Services (EMS, Fire,
Police, Health) // Medical Director,
Dallas Metropolitan Medical
Response System (for Anti-Terrorism) //
Medical Director for the Dallas Met-
ropolitan BioTel (EMS) System

David E. Persse, MD
The City of Houston Emergency
Medical Services, USA
david.persse@cityofhouston.net
Director, Emergency Medical
Services, Public Health Authority,
City of Houston // Associate Professor
of Emergency Medicine, University of
Texas Medical School at Houston //
Associate Professor of Surgery,
Baylor College of Medicine

Ulrik Persyn, Professor, PhD
Faculty of Movement and
Rehabilitation Sciences,
Catholic University Leuven,
Tervuursevest 101, 3001 Leuven,
België
Ulrik.Persyn@faber.kuleuven.be
www.faber.kuleuven.be
Responsible in the Faculty for courses
on movement and training science of
swimming

Eleni Petridou, MD, MPH
Department of Hygiene and
Epidemiology, Athens University
Medical School,
75 Mikras Asias Street, Goudi,
115 27 Athens, Greece
epetrid@med.uoa.gr
www.cc.uoa.gr/socmed/hygien/
cerepri
Associate Professor of Preventive
Medicine and Epidemiology
Director, Center for Research and
Prevention of Injuries among the
Young (CEREPRI) // Director,
Hellenic Society for Social Pediatrics
and Health Promotion

Francesco A. Pia, PhD
Pia Consulting Services,
3 Boulder Brae Lane, Larchmont,
NY 10538-1105, USA
frankpia@optonline.net
www.Pia-Enterprises.com
President, Independent Researcher //
Member, American Red Cross
Advisory
Council on First Aid and Safety //
National Technical Advisor,
American Red Cross' Lifeguard
Training Program

Sjaak Poortvliet
Association of Water Boards,
PO Box 80200, 2508 GE The Hague,
The Netherlands
spoortvliet@uvw.nl
www.uvw.nl
Policyworker, Association of Dutch
Water Boards

Rolf Popp, Dipl.-Ing
Binnenschiffahrts-Berufsgenossen-
schaft, Präventionsbezirk West D IV-1,
Frankenweg 2, 56337 Eitelborn,
Germany
BSBG-Eitelborn-Popp@t-online.de
www.bsbg.de
Senior Surveyor // Health and Safety
Inspector
Convenor CEN TC 162 WG 6, ISO TC
188 WG 14, FA PSA SG 13, scope of all:
PPE against drowning

Linda Quan, Professor, MD, MPH
Department of Pediatrics,
Children's Hospital and Regional
Medical Center,
4800 Sand Point Way NE cm-09,
Seattle, WA 98105, USA
Linda.quan@seattlechildrens.org
Professor in Pediatrics,
University of Washington School of
Medicine, Seattle, Washington, USA
Pediatric Emergency Medicine
Attending, Children's Hospital and
Regional Medical Center, Seattle,
Washington, USA

Slim Ray, PhD
CFS Press, 68 Finalee Avenue,
Asheville NC 28803, USA
slimray@cfspress.com
www.cfspress.com
International Rescue Instructor-
Trainer

Monique Ridder, MSc, PhD
Christelijke Hogeschool Windesheim,
PO Box 10090, 8000 GB Zwolle,
The Netherlands
mam.ridder@windesheim.nl
www.windesheim.nl
Professor in health science
and nutrition

Rienk Rienks, MD, PhD
Heart Lung Center Central Military
Hospital,
Heidelberglaan 100, 3584 CX Utrecht,
The Netherlands
r.rienks@chello.nl
Cardiologist
Chairman of the Task Force on
Cardiology and Diving // Chairman,
Committee on Cardiology and Sports,
Netherlands Society of Cardiology

Wim H.J. Rogmans, PhD
Consumer Safety Institute,
PO Box 75169, 1070 AD Amsterdam,
The Netherlands
w.rogmans@consafe.nl
www.veiligheid.nl
Director, Consumer Safety Institute

Marcia L. Rom, JD
Alaska Injury Prevention Center,
3701 East Tudor, Suite 105,
Anchorage, AK 99508, USA
Marcia_rom@hotmail.com
www.alaska-ipc.org
Projects Director

**Peter Safar, Professor, MD,
DSc (Hon) †**

Takefumi Sakabe, professor, MD
Department of Anesthesiology and
Resuscitology, Yamaguchi University
School of Medicine,
1-1-1 Minami-Kogushi, Ube,
Yamaguchi, 755-8505, Japan
takefumi@po.cc.Yamaguchi-u.ac.jp
Professor and Chairman,
Department of Anesthesiology-
Resuscitology, Yamaguchi University
School of Medicine // Director,
Intensive Care Unit, Yamaguchi
University Hospital // Secretary-
General, The Japanese Society of
Reanimatology // Secretary-General,
Japanese Society of Neurosanesthesia
and Critical Care // Deputy Secretary-
General, Western Pacific Association
of Critical Care Medicine

Paloma Sanz
Morillo n° 11, 1° D, 40002 Segovia,
Spain
sanzvel@usuarios.retecal.es
Doctor Specialist of Physical
Education and Sport
President, Cultural Association ESS
(Segovial Lifesaving School)

Justin P. Scarr, BEd, MBA (MGSM)
Royal Life Saving Society Australia,
Suite 201, 3 Smail Street,
Broadway, NSW 2007, Australia
jscarr@rlssa.org.au
www.royallifesaving.com.au
National Operation Manager

**Gert-Jan Scheffer, Professor, MD,
PhD**
Radboud University Medical Center,
Department of Anesthesiology,
PO Box 9101, 6500 HB Nijmegen,
The Netherlands
g.scheffer@anes.umcn.nl
Professor and Chairman

Rutger J. Schimmelpenninck, LLM
Keizersgracht 814,
1017 EE Amsterdam, The Netherlands
r.schimmelpenninck@houthoff.nl
Lawyer

Adee Schoon, PhD
Leiden University,
Institute of Biology,
Animal Behaviour Group,
PO Box 9516, 2300 RA Leiden,
The Netherlands
adee.schoon@klpd.politie.nl
Researcher

**Michael Schwindt, Professor,
Dipl.-Pädagoge**
Rolandstraße 35, 31137 Hildesheim,
Germany
www.sarrrah.de
Research and Development
of Life-Saving Systems

Ian Scott, PhD
PO Box 302, Abbotsford,
Victoria 3067, Australia
ianscott@virtual.net.au
Department of Injury and Violence
Prevention, World Health
Organisation, Geneva

Jim Segerstrom, MICP
Special Rescue Services Group,
World Rescue Service, PO Box 4686,
Sonora CA 95370, USA
jim@specialrescue.com
www.specialrescue.com
President, Special Rescue Services
Group
Executive Director, International
Rescue Instructors Association //
Technical Specialist to Special
Operations, Fire and Rescue Branch,
California Office of Emergency
Services // Founder, Swiftwater/Flood
Rescue Technician Program, US //
International Legal Consultant,
Investigater and Expert Witness on
Life Safety

Andrew D. Short, Professor, PhD
Coastal Studies Unit,
School of Geosciences,
University of Sydney,
Sydney, NSW 2006, Australia
a.short@geosci.usyd.edu.au
www.geosci.usyd.edu.au/about/
people/staff/short.html
Professor of Marine Science,
University of Sydney
National Coordinator, Australian
Beach Safety and Management
Program

Antony Simcock, MD, MB BS, FRCA
Royal Cornwall Hospital, Truro,
Cornwall TR1 3LJ, UK
tonyds@onetel.com
Honorary Consultant Anaesthesist

Brian V. Sims
Royal Life Saving Society – United
Kingdom, River House, High Street,
Broom, Warwickshire B50 4HN, UK
rlssbs@globalnet.co.uk
Member, ILS Rescue and Education
Commission // Secretary,
ILSE Rescue Commission //
Member, International Standards
Organisation: Water Safety Signs
and Beach Safety Flags Committee //
Member, British Standards
Institution

Paul E. Sirbaugh, DO, FAAP, FACEP
Texas Children's Hospital,
6621 Fannin Ste A210,
MC 1-1481, Houston, TX 77030, USA
sirbaugh@bcm.tmc.edu
Director of EMS, Assistant Professor
of Pediatrics // Assistant Medical Director, Section on Emergency Medicine, TCH // Director of Prehospital
Medicine, TCH // Assistant Physician
Director, City of Houston, EMS

Robert M. Slomp, Msc
Works and Water Management
Department Water Systems,
Safety Against Flooding,
Ministry of Transport,
PO Box 17, 8200 AA Lelystad,
The Netherlands
R.slomp@riza.rws.minvenw.nl
www.rijnenmaas.nl
Team Leader, RIZA (Disaster
management flood risk Rhine and
Meuse) // Advisor Risk Analysis

Gordon S. Smith, MD, MPH
Liberty Mutual Research Institute
for Safety, 71 Frankland Road,
Hopkinton, Massachusetts 01748,
USA
gordon.smith@libertymutual.com
www.libertymutual.com/research/
Epidemiologist // Associate Professor,
Center for Injury Research and Policy,
Johns Hopkins Bloomberg School of
Hygiene and Public Health, Baltimore

Luiz Smoris
jlesmoris@112.gsc.rcanaria.es

Robert K. Stallman, PhD
Sandvollvn. 80, 1400 Ski, Norway
robert.stallman@nih.no
Associate Professor, Norwegian
University of Sport & Physical
Education
Member, Board of Directors,
Norwegian Life Saving Association

Alan M. Steinman, MD, MPH
1135 Harrington Place,
DuPont, WA 98327, USA
asteinman@aol.com
Rear Admiral, US Public Health
Service / US Coast Guard (Retired) //
Advisor to the US Coast Guard in
the areas of drowning, sea-survival,
hypothermia, flotation devices and
protective clothing // Professional
Affiliate, Health Leisure and Human
Performance Research Institute,
Univ. of Manitoba, Winnipeg,
Manitoba, Canada

Carla St-Germain, BA, BEd
Lifesaving Society,
287 McArthur Avenue,
Ottawa, Ontario K1L 6P3, Canada
experts@lifesaving.ca
www.lifesaving.ca
Project Manager Education

John A. Stoop, PhD
Faculteit TBM, Technical University
Delft, PO Box 5015, 2600 GA Delft,
The Netherlands
stoop@kindunos.nl
www.kindunos.nl
Associate Professor, Safety Science,
Delft University of Technology //
Managing Director, Kindunos Safety
Consultancy Ltd
Accredited Aviation Accident
Investigator // Board Member,
Dutch Road Victim Organisation

Martin Stotz, MD
Bloomsbury Institute of Intensive
Care, The Middlesex Hospital,
Mortimer Street, London, W1T 3AA,
UK
stotzm@hotmail.com
Anaesthesiologist

David Szpilman, MD
Socieda Brasiliera de Salvamento
Aquatico, Av. das Américas 3555,
bloco 2, sala 302, Barra da Tijuca,
Rio de Janeiro, Brasil 22631-004
david@szpilman.com;
szpilman@globo.com
www.szpilman.com;
www.sobrasa.org
Medical & Rescue Helicopter
Service – GSE – CBMERJ // Head,
Adult Intensive Care Unit,
Hospital Municipal Miguel Couto
Founder, Ex-President and Former
Medical Director of SOBROSA
(Brazilian Life Saving Society)
Medical Commission and Board
Member of International Life
Saving Federation // Member
of CLAR (Comitê Latino-Americano
de Ressuscitação)

Richard Ming Kirk Tan
73 Farrer Drive,
#02-01 Sommerville Park,
Singapore 259280, Singapore
mingkirk@yahoo.com
www.slss.org.sg
Consultant, Shook Lin & Bok //
Adjunct Associate Professor,
National University of Singapore
Honorary Secretary-General,
Singapore Life Saving Society

Greg Tate
Royal Life Saving Society Australia,
Floreat Forum, Perth WA 6014,
Australia
gtate@rlsswa.com.au
www.lifesavingwa.com.au
Manager Community Health

Maida Taylor, MD
785 Foerster Street,
San Francisco, CA 94127, USA
mermaida@pol.net
Clinical Professor, University of
California San Francisco,
Department of Obstetrics Gyneology
and Reproductive Sciences // Clinical
Director for Women's Health, Medical
Affairs, Novo Nordisk
Pharmaceutical, Princeton, NJ, USA

Andreas Theodorou, MD
Pediatric Critical Care Medicine,
Department of Pediatrics,
The University of Arizona Health
Sciences Center, PO Box 245073,
Tucson, AZ 85724-5073, USA
aat@peds.arizona.edu
Professor of Clinical Pediatrics //
Associate Head, Department of
Pediatrics

Lambert Thijs, Professor, MD, PhD
Department of Intensive Care,
VU University Medical Centre,
PO Box 7057, 1007 MB Amsterdam,
The Netherlands
lg.thijs@vumc.nl
Emeritus Professor of Intensive Care

Peter Tikuisis, PhD
Human Modelling Group,
Simulation, Modelling,
Acquisition, Rehersal,
and Training Section, Defence
Research and Development Canada,
1133 Sheppard Avenue West, Toronto,
Ontario, M3M 3B9, Canada
peter.tikuisis@drdc-rddc.gc.ca
Defence Scientist
Adjunct Professor, Faculty of Physical
Education and Health, University of
Toronto

Michael Tipton, Professor, MD
Institute of Biomedical &
Biomolecular Sciences,
Department of Sport & Exercise
Science, University of Portsmouth,
Portsmouth PO1 2DT, UK
michael.tipton@port.ac.uk

**Nigel M. Turner, MB ChB, FRCA,
EDICM**
Pediatric Intensive Care Unit ,
Wilhelmina Children's Hospital,
University Medical Center Utrecht,
PO Box 85090, 3508 AB Utrecht,
The Netherlands
Nigel.turner@zonnet.nl
Paediatric Anaesthesiologist
Director, Dutch Advanced Paediatric
Life Support (APLS) Course //
Secretary, Dutch Foundation for the
Emergency Care of Children

Wolfgang Ummenhofer, MD, PhD
Department of Anesthesia,
University Hospital, Basel,
Switzerland
wummenhofer@uhbs.ch
Associate Professor

Ed van Beeck, MD, PhD
Institute Public Health Care,
Erasmus University Rotterdam,
PO Box 1738, 3000 DR Rotterdam,
The Netherlands
e.vanbeeck@erasmusmc.nl
www.erasmusmc.nl/mgz
Associate Professor of Public Health

Giel van Berkel, MD
Beatrixziekenhuis, PO Box 90,
4200 AB Gorinchem, The Netherlands
g.van.berkel@rivas.nl
Internist-Intensivist

Pieter van der Torn, MD, DEnv
Foundation for Cooperation of
Technique & Care,
Blankenburgerpark 154,
3042 HA Rotterdam, The Netherlands
vandertorn@wttz.info
Consultant for risks assessment
and disaster response

Josephus P.J. van Gestel, MD, PhD
Pediatric Intensive Care Unit,
Wilhelmina Children's Hospital,
University Medical Center Utrecht,
PO Box 85090, 3508 AB Utrecht,
The Netherlands
J.vanGestel@wkz.azu.nl
Staff Member,
Pediatric Intensive Care Unit

Robert A. van Hulst, MD, PhD
Diving Medical Center,
Royal Netherlands Navy,
PO Box 10.000, 1780 CA Den Helder,
The Netherlands
ravhulst@planet.nl
http://www.marine.nl/schepen/
mijnendienst/duiken/
duikmedischcentrum/
Senior Medical Officer,
Diving and Submarine Medicine
Director, Diving Medical Center,
Royal Netherlands Navy
Consultant, National Sportdiving
Association // National Representa-
tive, European Diving Technology
Committee (EDTC)

Joost van Nueten
Belgium Medical Crash Team
Sea Eagles vzw,
Vloeiende 26, 2950 Kapellen, Belgium
bmct@pandora.be
www.powerboat-rescue.com
Chief Nurse, Emergency Care
Department, Jan Palfijn Hospital
Antwerpen, Belgium
Rescue diver and helicopter
jumper // Chairman BMCT – Sea
Eagles Rescue Team

**Adrianus J. van Vught, Professor,
MD, PhD**
Pediatric Intensive Care Unit,
Wilhelmina Children's Hospital,
University Medical Center Utrecht,
PO Box 85090, 3508 AB Utrecht,
The Netherlands
a.vanvught@wkz.azu.nl
Director, Pediatric Intensive Care
Unit

Hans Vandersmissen
KNRM (Royal Netherlands Sea
Rescue Institution), PO Box 434,
1970 AK IJmuiden, The Netherlands
info@knrm.nl
www.knrm.nl
Free-lance maritime journalist

Karel R.R. Vandevelde, MD
Emergency Department,
AZ Sint-Jan,
Ruddershove 10, 8000 Brugge,
Belgium
Karel.Vandevelde@azbrugge.be
Consultant Anaesthesiologist,
Critical Care Medicine

Harald Vervaecke, PhD
International Life Saving Federation,
Gemeenteplein 26, 3010 Leuven,
Belgium
ils.hq@pandora.be;
haraldvervaecke@hotmail.com
http://www.ilsf.org
Senior Advisor, Qatar National
Olympic Committee // Senior
Advisor, Doha 2006 Asian Games
Secretary General, International Life
Saving Federation // President,
Belgian Life Saving Federation //
President, Flemish Life Saving
Federation

**Jean-Louis Vincent, Professor, MD,
PhD**
Department of Intensive Care,
Erasme University Hospital,
Route de Lennik 808, 1070 Brussels,
Belgium
jlvincent@ulb.ac.be
www.intensive.org
Head, Department of Intensive Care
President, International Sepsis Forum //
Past President, European Society of
Intensive Care Medicine // Past
President, European Shock Society

Michael Vlasto, FRIN, FNI
The Royal National Lifeboat
Institution (RNLI), West Quay Road,
Poole, Dorset BH15 1HZ, UK
mvlasto@rnli.org.uk
Operations Director, RNLI
Chairman, National Water Safety
Forum // Chairman, UKSAR
Organisation Maritime and Aviation
Consultative Committee

Wiebe de Vries, MSc
Royal Foundation of National
Organisation Providing Accident
Rescue Services and First Aid
"The Orange Cross",
Scheveningseweg 44,
2517 KV Den Haag, The Netherlands
vriesw@xs4all.nl; devries@ehbo.nl
Head, Research and Development
Professional Secretary,
Dutch Resuscitation Council

Beat H. Walpoth, MD, FAHA
Cardiovascular Research,
Service for Cardiovascular Surgery,
Department of Surgery, HUG,
University Hospital, 1211 Geneva 14,
Switzerland
beat.walpoth@hcuge.ch
Director of Cardiovascular Research //
President-Elect, European Society of
Artificial Organs

David S. Warner, Professor, MD
Department of Anesthesiology,
Box 3094, Duke University Medical
Center, Durham, NC 27710, USA
warne002@mc.duke.edu
Professor, Departments of
Anesthesiology, Neurobiology,
and Surgery, Duke University
Medical Center

Max Harry Weil, MD, PhD, ScD (Hon), Distinguished University Professor
35100 Bob Hope Drive,
Rancho Mirage, CA 92270, USA //
The Keck School of Medicine,
University of Southern California,
Los Angeles, CA, USA
weilm@911research.org
www.911research.org
President, The Institute of
Critical Care Medicine

Jürg Wendling, MD
Fbg du Lac 67, 2505 Biel-Bienne,
Switzerland
mail@wendling.ch
EDTC, Vice Chairman,
Surgery, Hand Surgery,
Diving Medicine SUHMS
National Director, Divers Alert
Network Hotline in Switzerland

Volker Wenzel, Professor, MD, PhD
Department of Anesthesiology and
Critical Care Medicine, Innsbruck
Medical University, Anichstrasse 35,
6020 Innsbruck, Austria
volker.wenzel@uibk.ac.at
www.anaesthesie.uibk.ac.at
Associate Professor of Anesthesiology
and Critical Care Medicine//Respon-
sible Coordinator, Experimental
Anesthesiology

Peter G. Wernicki, MD
Pro sports, 1355 37th Street,
Vero Beach, FL 32960, USA
wernicki@hotmail.com
Vice Chair Medical Commission,
International Lifesaving Federation
Medical Advisor, United States
Lifesaving Association – Board of
Directors // Past Chief of
Orthopaedics, Indian River
Memorial Hospital

Andrew G. Whittaker, BHMS
Victorian Aquatic Industry
Council, 44–46 Birdwood Street,
Box Hill South, Victoria 3128,
Australia
executive@vaic.org.au
www.vaic.org.au
Chief Executive Officer

Sip E. Wiebenga
KNRM (Royal Netherlands Sea
Rescue Institution), PO Box 434,
1970 AK IJmuiden, The Netherlands
se.wiebenga@knrm.nl
www.knrm.nl
Director, Royal Netherlands Sea
Rescue Organisation

Jane Wigginton, Professor, MD
University of Texas Southwestern
Medical Center,
5323 Harry Hines Blvd,
Dallas, TX 75390-8579, USA
Jane.Wigginton@UTSouthwestern.
edu
Assistant Professor, Emergency
medicine // Assistant Medical
Director, EMS // Resuscitation
Research Coordinator

Klaus Wilkens, PhD
Holunderweg 5, 21365 Adendorf,
Germany
president@ilseurope.org
www.ilseurope.org
Lecturer for Management,
University of Hamburg
President DLRG, (German Life
Saving Society) // President,
International Life Saving Federation
of Europe (ILSE)

Ann M. Williamson
NSW Injury Risk Management
Research Centre,
University of New South Wales,
Sydney NSW 2052, Australia
a.williamson@unsw.edu.au
www.irmrc.edu.au
Associate Professor, Deputy Director

Robert L. Williamson, BS, MS
Marine Sonic Technology, Ltd.,
5508 George Washington Memorial
Highway, PO Box 730,
White Marsh, VA 23183-0730, USA
rwmson@marinesonic.com
www.marinesonic.com
Marketing Director Side Scan Sonar
Trainer

John R. Wilson, Professor, MSc, PhD
Institute for Occupational
Ergonomics, University of
Nottingham,
Nottingham NG7 2RD, UK
John.Wilson@nottingham.ac.uk
Professor of Human Factors

Michael Woodroffe
International Lifeboat Federation c/o
The Royal National Lifeboat
Institution, West Quay Road,
Poole, Dorset, BH15 1HZ, UK
thewoodies@hotmail.com
Commander// Overseas Training and
Development Advisor // Deputy Chief
of Operations, RNLI // Master
Mariner // Commander RNR
Director, Seahorse Marine
Consultancy

Rick Wright
Rescue and Education Commission,
International Life Saving Federation,
PO Box 451, Swansea NSW 2281,
Australia
rickwright50@hotmailcom
Past Chairman, ILSF Rescue and
Education Commission

Andrea Zaferes
Lifeguard Systems/RIPTIDE,
PO Box 548, Hurley, NY 12443, USA
az@teamlgs.com
www.teamlgs.com, www.rip-tide.org
Vice President // Dive Team Trainer //
Death Investigator //
Medicolegal Death Investigator
Water and ice rescue Instructor

Durk F. Zandstra, MD, PhD
Intensive Care,
Onze Lieve Vrouwe Gasthuis,
PO Box 95500, 1090 HM Amsterdam,
The Netherlands
d.f.zandstra@olvg.nl
www.olvg.ziekenhuis.nl
Medical Director ICU // Director,
Postgraduate Intensive Care Training
Program

Edward Zwitser
KNRM (Royal Netherlands Sea
Rescue Institution), PO Box 434,
1970 AK IJmuiden, The Netherlands
et.zwitser@knrm.nl
www.knrm.nl

Subject Index